Revision Shoulder Arthroplasty

Francesco Franceschi
George S. Athwal
Alexandre Lädermann
Edoardo Giovannetti de Sanctis
Editors

Revision Shoulder Arthroplasty

Springer

Editors
Francesco Franceschi
Orthopaedics and Trauma Surgery
UniCamillus-Saint Camillus
International University
of Health Sciences
Rome, Italy

Alexandre Lädermann
Div. of Orthopaedics
and Trauma Surgery
Hôpital de la Tour
Meyrin, Switzerland

George S. Athwal
Upper Limb Centre
Roth McFarlane Hand
London, ON, Canada

Edoardo Giovannetti de Sanctis
IULS-Institut Universitaire
Locomoteur et Sports
Pasteur 2 Hospital
CHU, Nice, France

ISBN 978-3-031-45943-6 ISBN 978-3-031-45944-3 (eBook)
https://doi.org/10.1007/978-3-031-45944-3

This Springer imprint is published by the registered company Springer Nature Switzerland AG
The registered company address is: Gewerbestrasse 11, 6330 Cham, Switzerland

Paper in this product is recyclable

Preface

Dear readers,

The editors are proud to offer you this book regarding revision shoulder arthroplasty, which remains a major debated topic.

In the last two decades, better understanding of shoulder replacement has allowed the shoulder community to develop much more of a consensus in the treatment of failed shoulder arthroplasty and with this book we want to give you the keys for a successful approach to this surgery.

The *Revision Shoulder Arthroplasty* contains 7 parts and 35 chapters written by more than 100 authors.

In Part I, the background includes the explanation of hemiarthroplasty, anatomic and reverse total shoulder failure. Part II includes updates on preoperative evaluation and planning of a failed shoulder replacement. Parts III and IV pertain to most updated surgical techniques for revising, respectively, the glenoid and humeral components. Parts V, VI, and VII presents the most current ways of managing shoulder arthroplasty complications.

To our knowledge, this is the most comprehensive compendium of an exhaustive discussion on revision shoulder arthroplasty in one textbook.

These parts represent an international approach to revision shoulder arthroplasty and all the authors comprising the majority of worldwide shoulder arthroplasty innovators, surgeons, and academicians, are pioneers and active clinicians in this discipline.

This book we believe will be a must read for any serious student in the field of shoulder arthroplasty.

We would like to thank personally all the contributors, residents, fellows, and attendings that had worked in this project.

Rome, Italy — Francesco Franceschi
London, Canada — George S. Athwal
Meyrin, Switzerland — Alexandre Lädermann
Nice, France — Edoardo Giovannetti de Sanctis

Contents

Part I Background

1 **Why Do Total Shoulder Replacements Fail?** 3
Jonathan Peter Evans and Gregory Bain

2 **Why Reverse Shoulder Arthroplasties Fail** 19
Robert Z. Tashjian and Christopher D. Joyce

3 **Shoulder Hemiarthroplasties: How Do They Fail** 27
Juan David Lacouture, Aníbal Debandi, and Pascal Boileau

Part II Planning and Operative Technique

4 **Management of a Painful Shoulder Arthroplasty** 43
Sumit Raniga and Antonio Arenas-Miquelez

5 **Preoperative Planning for Revision Arthroplasty: Imaging, Instruments, and Implants**. 59
Giuseppe Porcellini, Matilde Delvecchio, Andrea Giorgini, Gian Mario Micheloni, and Luigi Tarallo

6 **PSI, Navigation, AR, and MR in Revision Shoulder Arthroplasty** 69
Jessica L. Churchill, Conner Paez, Jason C. Ho, Vahid Entezari, Joseph P. Iannotti, and Eric T. Ricchetti

7 **Surgical Approach in Shoulder Arthroplasty Revision**. 83
Arnaud Godenèche, Joris Tiercelin, Jérôme Garret, and Thais Dutra Vieira

8 **Custom Glenoid Implants for Revision Shoulder Arthroplasty** 89
Jay D. Keener, Ben Zmistowski, and Anand Murthi

Part III Glenoid

9 **Classifying Bone Loss in Revision Arthroplasty** 107
Khai Cheong Wong, Bryan H. G. Loh, and Denny T. T. Lie

10 **The Convertible Glenoid in Revision Shoulder Arthroplasty** ... 121
Riccardo Ranieri, Mario Borroni, Giacomo Delle Rose, Marco Maria Minelli, and Alessandro Castagna

11 **How to Remove a Well-Fixed Glenoid Component in a Failed Anatomic Total Shoulder Arthroplasty** ... 127
Kristian Efremov and Andrew Jawa

12 **Revising the Glenoid in Hemiarthroplasty** ... 135
Giuseppe Sircana, Giovanni Merolla, and Paolo Paladini

13 **Revising the Failed Glenoid in TSA** ... 145
Gianluca Ciolli, Edoardo Giovannetti de Sanctis, and Lionel Neyton

14 **Revising a Failed Glenoid in Reverse Total Shoulder Arthroplasty** ... 157
Akshay V. Daji and Howard Routman

15 **Options for Glenoid Reconstruction: Graft vs. Metal vs. Combined** ... 169
Marko Nabergoj, Patrick J. Denard, Philippe Collin, Tiago Martinho, Arash Amiri, Jeanni Zbinden, and Alexandre Lädermann

16 **Single-stage vs. Two-stage Reconstruction of Glenoid Defects in Revision Shoulder Arthroplasty** ... 187
Ashish Gupta, Kristine Italia, Roberto Pareyon, Mohammad Jomaa, Marine Launay, Jashint Maharaj, Luke Gilliland, James Nielsen, and Ludwig Seebauer

17 **Surgical Management of Periprosthetic Scapular Spine and Acromion Fractures** ... 209
Ludwig Seebauer, Kristine Italia, Roberto Pareyon, Mohammad Jomaa, and Ashish Gupta

Part IV Humerus

18 **Humeral Stress Shielding and Bony Adaptations in Shoulder Arthroplasty** ... 227
E. Fumina Kobayashi and William R. Aibinder

19 **Classifying Humeral Bone Loss in Revision Shoulder Arthroplasty** ... 239
Chad W. Parkes and Peter N. Chalmers

20 **Convertible Humeral Component in Revision Shoulder Arthroplasty** ... 245
Su Cheol Kim and Jae Chul Yoo

21 **How to Remove a Well Implanted Humeral Component and Complications Associated** ... 255
Amir Abdelmalek, Robert Hurley, Andrew McBride, Phillip Duke, and Mark Ross

22 Revision of a Failed Humeral Stem with Sufficient Bone Stock . . . 263
Edoardo Giovannetti de Sanctis, Alessio Palumbo, Angelo Baldari, Gian Mauro De Angelis D'Ossat, Luca Saccone, Luca La Verde, and Francesco Franceschi

23 Revision of the Failed Stem Without Sufficient Bone Stock . . . 269
Yousif Atwan, Joseph T. Labrum IV, and Joaquin Sanchez-Sotelo

24 Periprosthetic Humeral Fracture: Management and Outcomes . . . 277
Fabrizio Mocini, Lorenzo Proietti, Dario Candura, Gianluca Ciolli, Katia Corona, and Simone Cerciello

Part V Infection

25 Diagnosing Shoulder Prosthetic Joint Infections . . . 289
Corey J. Schiffman and Surena Namdari

26 Managing the Infected Arthroplasty: Antibiotic Suppression, Debridement, One- Versus Two-Stage Revision . . . 295
Franziska Eckers, Bettina Hochreiter, Gregory A. Hoy, and Eugene T. Ek

27 Preventing Infection in Revision Shoulder Arthroplasty . . . 307
Adam Z. Khan, Mohamad Y. Fares, and Joseph A. Abboud

Part VI Instability and Soft Tissue Management

28 Defining Risk Factors for TSA and RSA Instability . . . 321
Emma Lewis, James Conville, Andrew McBride, Phil Duke, and Mark Ross

29 Management of Shoulder Arthroplasty Instability . . . 329
Jimmy J. Chan, Niraj V. Lawande, and Gregory P. Nicholson

30 Pectoralis Transfer for Deltoid Deficiency After Reverse Shoulder Arthroplasty . . . 337
Ryan Lohre, Abdulaziz F. Ahmed, Karan Dua, and Bassem Elhassan

31 Tendon Transfers in Shoulder Arthroplasty . . . 349
Arno A. Macken, Eric R. Wagner, Wouter J. van der Poel, Geert Alexander Buijze, and Thibault Lafosse

Part VII Others

32 The Role of Arthroscopy After Shoulder Replacement . . . 369
Javier Ardebol, Simon Hwang, Theresa Pak, Mariano E. Menendez, and Patrick J. Denard

33 The Role of Resection and Hemiarthroplasty After RSA 379
Michael Warnock and Ruth A. Delaney

34 The Role of Hemireverse in Revision Shoulder Arthroplasty. . . 385
Arnaud Walch and Gilles Walch

35 What Is the Value of Revision Shoulder Arthroplasty?. 395
Evan K. Stieler, Evan A. O'Donnell, and Jon J. P. Warner

About the Editors

Francesco Franceschi completed his residency training at the *Catholic University of Sacred Heart*, Rome, Italy. His clinical interests include shoulder arthroscopy and arthroplasty. He is on the staff at *Villa San Pietro, Fatebenefratelli*, Rome, Italy. He is Professor of Orthopedic Surgery at *Unicamillus Medical School*, Rome, Italy, and Consultant for the *Vatican State Health Care (FAS)*. He has published scientific articles and book chapters on various topics related to shoulder surgery and has presented his scientific research at several academic meetings.

George S. Athwal is originally from Vancouver and completed his M.D. at the *University of British Columbia*. Following completion of his orthopedic surgery residency at *Queen's University*, he spent 2 years sub-specializing in upper extremity reconstruction and trauma. He completed a 1-year fellowship at the Hospital for Special Surgery, *Cornell University*, New York, NY. Following this, he completed 1 year at the *Mayo Clinic* in Rochester, MN, specializing in shoulder and elbow surgery. In 2005, he joined the *Roth-McFarlane Hand and Upper Limb Centre at the University of Western Ontario*. He is actively involved in biomechanical and clinical research pertaining to the shoulder and elbow. He is the author of more than 400 publications, chapters, and books pertaining to the shoulder and elbow.

Alexandre Lädermann is Privat Docent at the *University of Geneva*, founder of *BeeMed* and *Med4Cast*, and president of the *Foundation for Research and Teaching in Orthopedics, Sports Medicine, Trauma, and Imaging (FORE)*. He is a leading specialist in the field of shoulder and elbow surgery. Dr. Alexandre Lädermann is placed in the top 0.1% of scholars writing about Shoulder Surgery over the past 10 years by *Expertscape's PubMed*-based algorithms, a level labeled as "*World Expert*." He is the author of more than 200 publications in journals and books concerning the shoulder joint.He is also a member of the *Central Committee of the French Arthroscopic Society (SFA)*, past president of *Swiss Shoulder Society (Expertengruppe Schulter und Ellbogen (Swiss Orthopaedics))*, and past president of the Membership Committee and Member of the *Central Committee of the European Society for Surgery of the Shoulder and the Elbow (SECEC/ESSSE)*. Moreover, he is chairman of the *12th Val d'Isère Advanced Shoulder Course* and has been president of congress of the *European Society for Shoulder and Elbow Surgery (SECEC/ESSSE)* in Geneva and of the *International Congress on Adipose Stem cell Treatment (iCAST)* in Zurich.

Edoardo Giovannetti de Sanctis is a shoulder specialist orthopedic surgeon at the *Institut Universitaire Locomoteur et du Sport (IULS), Hôpital Pasteur 2* (Nice, France). He attended medical school in *Campus Bio-Medico University* (Rome, Italy) and underwent orthopedic training at the *Catholic University of the Sacred Heart* (Rome, Italy). He completed fellowships in San Antonio, Texas (Dr SS. Burkhart), and Lyon, France (Dr Lionel Neyton). He is a member of the *European Society for Surgery of the Shoulder and Elbow (ESSSE/SECEC).*

Part I

Background

1 Why Do Total Shoulder Replacements Fail?

Jonathan Peter Evans and Gregory Bain

1.1 Background

A total shoulder replacement (TSR) is an intervention employed for end-stage degenerative shoulder pathology in the context of adequate rotator cuff function. Critically, the success of this intervention is dependent upon careful patient selection and a thorough understanding of the anatomical considerations, indications, and limitations of the procedure.

The procedural volume and incidence of total shoulder replacement (TSR) have increased dramatically over the last 40 years. The modern era of shoulder arthroplasty began with the first generation of anatomical total shoulder replacements reported by Charles Neer in 1974 [1]. The contemporary reports of TSRs show an exponential rise in use, with a 250% increase between 2000 and 2008 [2] and 367% increase between 1993 and 2007 [3].

National joint registries have provided a wealth of data for the short- to mid-term survival of total shoulder replacements. The Australian Orthopaedic Association National Joint Replacement Registry (AOANJRR) currently provides the best 10-year estimates at the implant level, with pooled all-cause survival at 92% (95% confidence interval (95% CI) 91–93) [4, 5] (Table 1.1) (Fig. 1.1).

Beyond 10 years, evidence is limited to case series analysis. Pooled case series survival at 15 years has been reported to be 88% (95% CI 84–93) [5]. At the 20-year mark, only two series have been reported at the single implant level: Schoch et al. reported the Neer total shoulder arthroplasty (TSA) ($n = 19$) [6] and Evans et al. reported the Aequalis ($n = 40$) [7], the all-cause revision was reported to be 83% and 84%, respectively.

Evans et al. also reported that within their series, no implant survived to 20 years without showing evidence of radiographic lucency of the glenoid. Radiographic evidence of humeral head migration was 83% at 20 years, and, temporally, the mean onset of humeral head superior migration occurred at 9 years and preceded radiographic glenoid failure by 3 years. Clearly, the second decade of implant survival is a crucial time point, which is not currently served with adequate data (Fig. 1.2).

The concept of "implant failure" can be dependent upon the clinician and patient's viewpoint. Typical end points include the dichotomies of revision, radiographic features, or functional milestones. Increasingly, we are

J. P. Evans (✉)
Department of Orthopaedic Surgery, Flinders Medical Centre, Adelaide, Australia

University of Exeter, Exeter, UK
e-mail: j.p.evans2@exeter.ac.uk

G. Bain
Department of Orthopaedic Surgery, Flinders Medical Centre, Adelaide, Australia

Flinders University, Adelaide, Australia
e-mail: greg@gregbain.com.au

F. Franceschi et al. (eds.), *Revision Shoulder Arthroplasty*,
https://doi.org/10.1007/978-3-031-45944-3_1

Table 1.1 Total shoulder replacement survival from single implant case series and registry reports with more than 10 years of follow-up. *AOANJR* Australian Orthopaedic Association National Joint Replacement Registry

Author	Country	Implant	Number of implants	Follow-up duration	All-cause survival (%)	Lower 95% confidence limit (%)	Upper 95% confidence limit (%)
Case-series							
Khan et al. [75]	United Kingdom	Aequalis with cemented, keeled, all-polyethylene flat-back glenoid	39	10	92	85.7	100
Khan et al. [75]	United Kingdom	Aequalis with cemented, keeled all-polyethylene flat-back glenoid	39	12	86.2	72	99
Levy et al. [76]	United Kingdom	Copeland TSR	17	11	71	68	75
Levy et al. [76]	United Kingdom	Copeland TSR	17	14	71	68	75
Levy et al. [76]	United Kingdom	Copeland TSR	17	22	61	58	64
Raiss et al. [32]	Germany	Aequalis	46	13	98	83.7	98.9
Schoch et al. [77]	United States	Neer TSR	19	20	83.2	70.5	97.8
Sperling et al. [78]	United States	Neer TSR	19	10	97	91	100
Sperling et al. [78]	United States	Neer TSR	19	15	84	70	100
Tammachote et al. [79]	United States	Neer TSR with cemented metal-backed glenoid	100	10	97	93	100
Tammachote et al. [79]	United States	Neer TSR with cemented metal-backed glenoid	100	15	93	87	99
Young et al. [33]	European	Aequalis with cemented, keeled, all-polyethylene flat-back glenoid	308	10	94.5	91.4	97.7
Young et al. [33]	European	Aequalis with cemented, keeled, all-polyethylene flat-back glenoid	308	15	79.4	70.3	88.5

Table 1.1 (continued)

Author	Country	Implant	Number of implants	Follow-up duration	All-cause survival (%)	Lower 95% confidence limit (%)	Upper 95% confidence limit (%)
Evans et al. [7]	United Kingdom	Aequalis with cemented, keeled, all-polyethylene flat-back glenoid	44	20	83·2	70·5	97·8
National Joint Registry							
AOANJRR [4]	Australia	Aequalis	1564	10	93.8	91.8	95.3
	Australia	Bigliani/Flatow	142	10	91.2	83.9	95.2
	Australia	Global AP	2716	10	93.5	90.7	95.5
	Australia	Global advantage	694	10	93.3	90.3	95.3
	Australia	SMR (Systema Multiplana Randelli)	436	10	94.3	91.1	96.4
	Australia	SMR	1930	10	80.4	77.6	82.8
	Australia	Solar	169	10	96.1	91.5	98.3

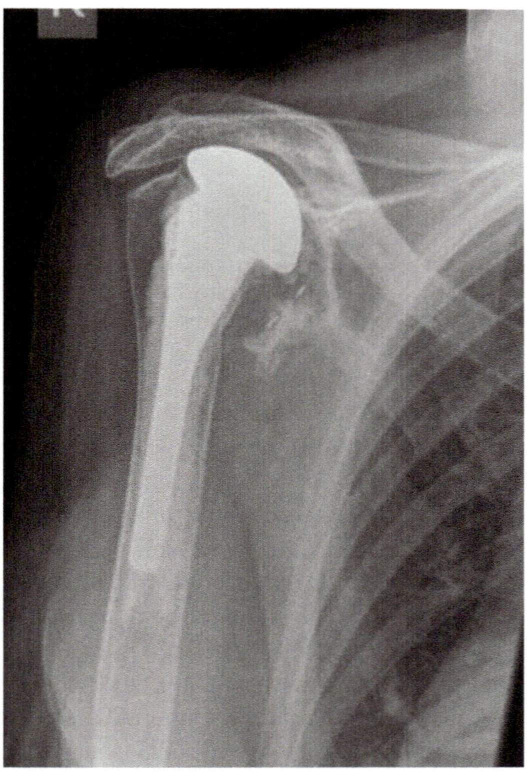

Fig. 1.1 Failure of the glenoid component at more than 15 years follow-up. The humeral head position suggests complete rotator cuff failure, and the cemented glenoid component has become completely loose. The significant glenoid erosion should also be noted

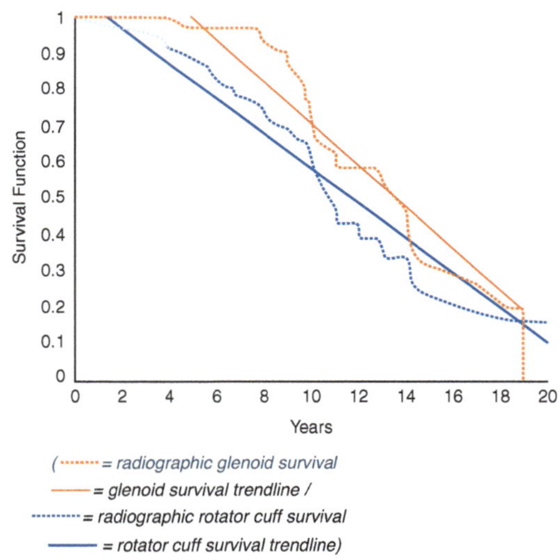

Fig. 1.2 Radiographic survival function of the glenoid and rotator cuff up to 20 years follow-up. It should be noted that the rotator cuff function precedes glenoid loosening. Primary data from Evans et al. [7]. (= radiographic glenoid survival; = glenoid survival trendline; = radiographic rotator cuff survival; = rotator cuff survival trendline)

combining these metrics with the patient-focused assessment of how the surgery has impacted their life. Patient-reported outcome measures (PROMs) are validated questionnaires that aim to quantify the patient's perception of latent variables such as pain and physical function. Long-term data suggest that the improvement in pain and function afforded by a TSR is sustained from the baseline to a 10-year follow-up, with the most recent meta-analysis estimates showing an effect size of 2.13, where a value greater than one suggests significant improvement [5].

1.2 Failure Mechanisms

The failure of total shoulder replacements can be subclassified in numerous ways. As an overview in this introductory chapter, we present the failed outcome in three broad subcategories: implant-, surgery-, and patient-related.

1.3 Implant-Related Outcome

1.3.1 Design Evolution

Total shoulder implants aim to recreate normal kinematics at the glenohumeral articulation. This can only be achieved when normal articular anatomy is reestablished and passive and active stabilizers of the shoulder are balanced. Therein, in concordance with Neer's principles, anatomical considerations are bound to the tolerance of a TSR, and consistently regarding these factors in a consistent manner is directly related to the outcome.

There has been considerable evolution in the design of total shoulder replacements, born through the desire to reduce failure rates. From the initial implantation of the early Neer prostheses, where a choice of two sizes limited the attainment of normal kinematics and conferred a high rate of resultant loosening, the pursuit of an implant that recreated "normal anatomy" was then applied to the first modular designs in the early 1990s (Biomet, Cofield, and Global models), which attempted to match the wide variations in the dimensions of the humeral head and the diameter of the medullary canal. Although an improvement, these second-generation prostheses did not truly mimic the complex three-dimensional anatomy of the proximal humerus.

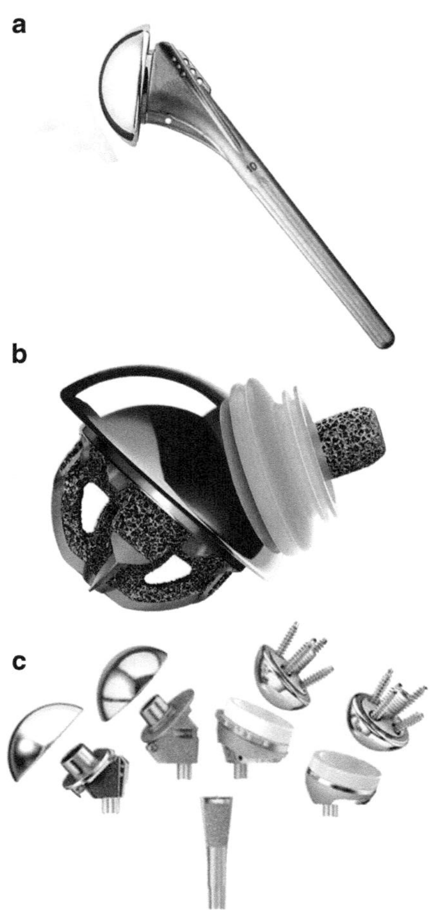

Fig. 1.3 Examples of modern total shoulder prosthesis designs: (**a**) a stemmed total shoulder with a pegged all-polyethylene glenoid; (**b**) a metaphyseal fit humeral component with a hybrid glenoid; and (**c**) a modular system

The work of Boileau and Walch revealed that the shape of the proximal humerus was much more complicated than previously described [8]. This then led to the development of third-generation prostheses where additional variable neck angles and eccentric heads recreated the tridimensional bony anatomy. The current fourth-generation humeral implants follow these design principles and further improve the flexibility of the construct by applying interchangeable platform-based systems. Further contemporary modifications have focused on the fixation of the humeral implant, and the modern portfolio of humeral implants includes stemmed, stemless, metaphyseal fit or resurfacing designs (Fig. 1.3).

The glenoid has been deemed the "weak link" in the total shoulder replacement construct. Like the humeral component, there have been consistent efforts to improve its design. The evolution in its design was influenced by an improved understanding of glenohumeral kinematics, which includes both rotation and translation. A commonality of the design is the use of polyethylene as the glenoid-sided articular bearing; however, the fixation to the native glenoid has utilized cemented and uncemented approached, keeled, or pegged designs, screw fixation, metal back, and all-polyethylene designs. With a 10-year survival of 83–100%, the cemented all-polyethylene glenoid remains the gold-standard prosthesis [9].

1.3.2 Preimplantation Native Anatomy and Rotator Cuff Integrity

Careful appreciation of the status of the rotator cuff and the level of glenoid deformity are the primary anatomical considerations that predict the failure of a TSR.

The principal role of the rotator cuff is to maintain the glenohumeral center of rotation. This is achieved through the triad of providing a platform for rotation about the scapula, compression of the humeral head into the glenoid, and providing muscle balance to the glenohumeral joint [10] (Fig. 1.4). Tears of the rotator cuff are common and increase with age [11]. Coexistent preoperative tears of the rotator cuff have been shown to prejudice the outcome of a total shoulder replacement by reducing strength and range, having a predisposition to subluxation, and loosening of the glenoid component [12–15]. Careful preoperative evaluation of the rotator cuff is vital and should be conducted clinically and radiographically. Instability after a TSA is one of the most frequent causes of reoperation. In a meta-analysis of instability patterns reported in 33 studies, Bohsali et al. highlighted the importance of rotator cuff integrity and tension and attributed anterior instability to a combination of soft tissue tensioning, subscapularis integrity, and component position, superior instability due to a deficiency of the rotator cuff, posterior instability due to excessive component retroversion, and inferior instability due to a failure to restore humeral length [16]. Godenèche et al. and Edwards et al. postulated that preoperative fatty degeneration, particularly of the infraspinatus and subscapularis, leads to poorer results and early postoperative rotator cuff failure, superior migration, and subluxation, findings that are also highlighted in the long-term follow-up of Young et al. [17–19] (Fig. 1.5).

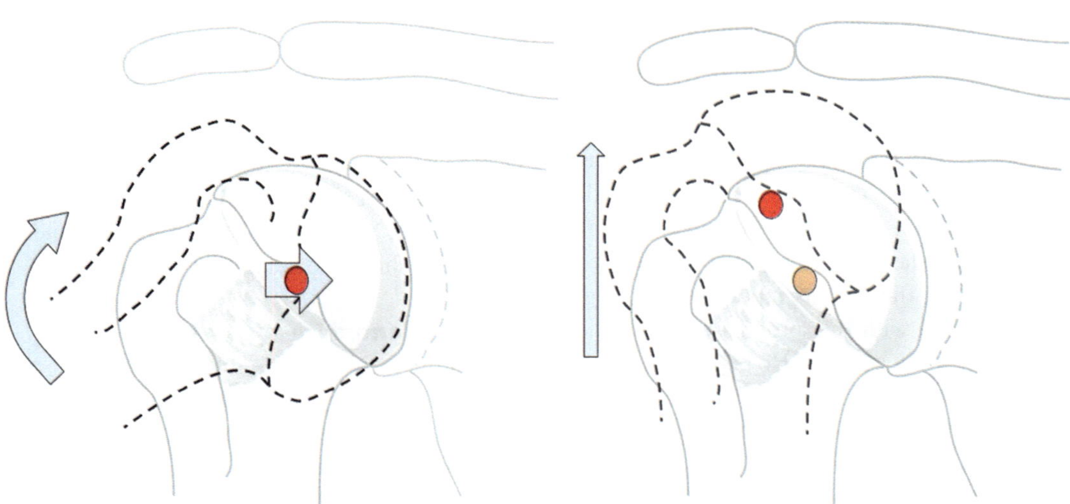

Fig. 1.4 Humeral head movement with deltoid contraction with an intact rotator cuff (left) where the center of rotation is maintained. In a deficient rotator cuff (right), the humeral head elevates, leading to poor function, instability risk, and early glenoid wear through eccentric loading

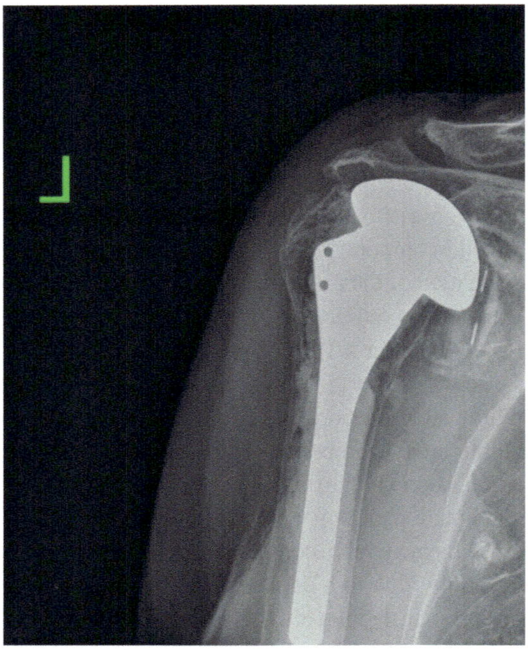

Fig. 1.5 A total shoulder replacement at 10 years follow-up demonstrating superior migration of the humeral head indicative of rotator cuff failure

A preoperative glenoid assessment is essential and requires an analysis of bone loss and alignment. The glenoid regularly endures contact forces of >50% body weight in activities of daily living [20]. Standard radiographs provide an assessment of wear patterns but can overestimate retroversion by 86% [21]. Computed tomography provides a much greater level of detail for bone loss, version, and vault anatomy. The vault itself must adequately receive the glenoid component dependent upon fixation design (pegged, keeled). Walch et al. noted that retroversion greater than 27° resulted in a 44% rate of implant loosening [22]. In the instance of 92 retroverted and biconcave glenoids, the authors reported loosening in 21% at 6 years, with 16% progressing to revision. In a review of 66 patients, Ho et al. reported glenoid osteolysis with more than 15° of retroversion [23]. In a synthesis of the available evidence, Malhas et al. suggested that in cases where retroversion is greater than 15°, consideration should be given to patient-specific instrumentation or bone graft [24]. Walch et al. also reported that preoperative humeral posterior subluxation of 80% or greater is associated with an 11% risk of postoperative posterior instability [22].

Although the emphasis is often placed on the glenoid morphology and rotator cuff, a preoperative assessment of the humerus also plays a pivotal role in reducing failure risk. An assessment of the true size of the humeral head is vital in the selection of an appropriately sized humeral component. An appreciation of the osteophyte morphology and position using three-dimensional imaging assists in their operative removal. Failure to achieve this can compromise the impingement-free range of motion and appropriate head sizing, both with consequent effects on implant success.

The humeral head is elliptical, with a ratio of frontal to sagittal size demonstrating a consistent 10% mismatch [25]. Therefore, matching a circular prosthetic head can be a challenge, and, although the true clinical effect remains unknown, a lateral overlap should be avoided as this could confer an impingement risk with the rotator cuff.

Lastly, the shaft of the humerus should be assessed. Variability in this zone can result in patients for whom standard straight stems may not be viable. Furthermore, in a small proportion (less than 10%), a straight stem will disrupt the cuff insertion.

1.3.3 Glenoid Failure

Glenoid fixation has remained the most important factor in the survival of a total shoulder replacement. Although considerable effort has been put into evolving the design of the glenoid prosthesis from Neer's original cemented, keeled polyethylene concept, substantial improvements in survivorship have not been realized.

1.3.3.1 Glenoid Design

Recreating the complex biomechanics of the shoulder is a challenge; it is neither a ball and socket nor a hinge but is rather a joint that demonstrates translation and rotation [26].

The level conformity of the articular geometry has been shown to have a significant impact on survival. The native shoulder demonstrates a mismatch between the articular surfaces to allow the rotation and translation interface. Smaller mismatches between joint surfaces, although imparting improved joint stability, increase shear stresses and edge loading, which leads to glenoid loosening [27–29]. Nho et al. performed a retrieval study and demonstrated greater abrasion and delamination in more conforming implants [30]. The optimal mismatch remains unknown, but less evidence of radiographic loosening has been shown with implants of a radial mismatch of between 6 and 10 mm [31] (Fig. 1.6).

A further consequence of the lack of constraint within the articular surface is the impact that the rotator cuff can have on loading symmetry. Franklin et al. proposed the "rocking horse phenomenon" that postulates that eccentric loading of the glenoid component, resulting in an asymmetric compression and distraction force, can lead to early failure [14]. The resultant micromotion leads to eventual cement–implant interface failure. Although proper implant positioning and posterior humeral head subluxation are important factors in this phenomenon, as previously emphasized, the rotator cuff's integrity has a significant role to play in influencing asymmetrical motion, and, therein both the preoperative integrity of the cuff and the strength of the subscapularis repair are reasons for secondary glenoid component loosening.

The cemented all-polyethylene glenoid component remains the gold-standard glenoid prosthesis. In studies with more than 10 years of follow-up, glenoid implant survival with revision as an end point has been reported to be 100% [32] and 94.1% [7, 33]. In the large series reported by Young et al. of Aequalis TSRs, radiographic loosening was reported to be 19.7% at 10 years and as high as 66.5% at 15 years [33].

The back of the glenoid component can be either flat or curved (convex), matching the native curve of the glenoid. Anglin et al. reported the tensile displacement of the glenoid component as almost double in flat-back vs. curved-back components [34]. In the short-term postoperative period, the radiolucency behind the component is higher in flat-back components, but a comparison of longer-term revision-free survival characteristics is not known.

The cement–implant interface and fixation device in all-polyethylene components has been broadly divided into keeled and pegged designs. A meta-analysis of eight studies found similar rates of radiolucencies but higher revision rates in keeled designs [35]. A radiostereographic analysis has revealed that both designs migrate in an anteroposterior direction but that the keeled designs show significantly greater rotation and maximum total point movement [36]. However, Kilian et al. randomized 59 patients to receive keeled or pegged designs, and, at a mean follow-up of 7.9 years, the implants radiolucency and revision rates were equivalent [37].

The glenoid component material utilized has been developed in line with hip and knee arthro-

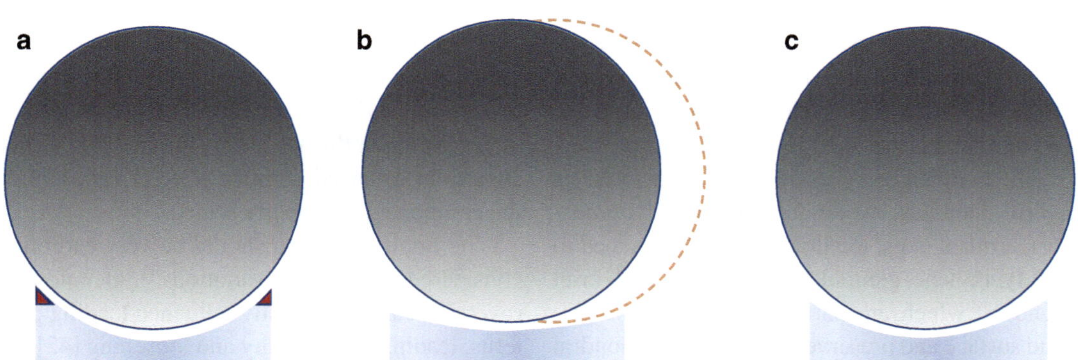

Fig. 1.6 The radius of curvature mismatch. (**a**) A conforming glenoid with minimal mismatch that does not allow translation and would be prone to edge loading. (**b**) Too great a mismatch leads to increasing contact stress over a reduced area. (**c**) The current consensus in radii mismatch is between 6 and 10 mm

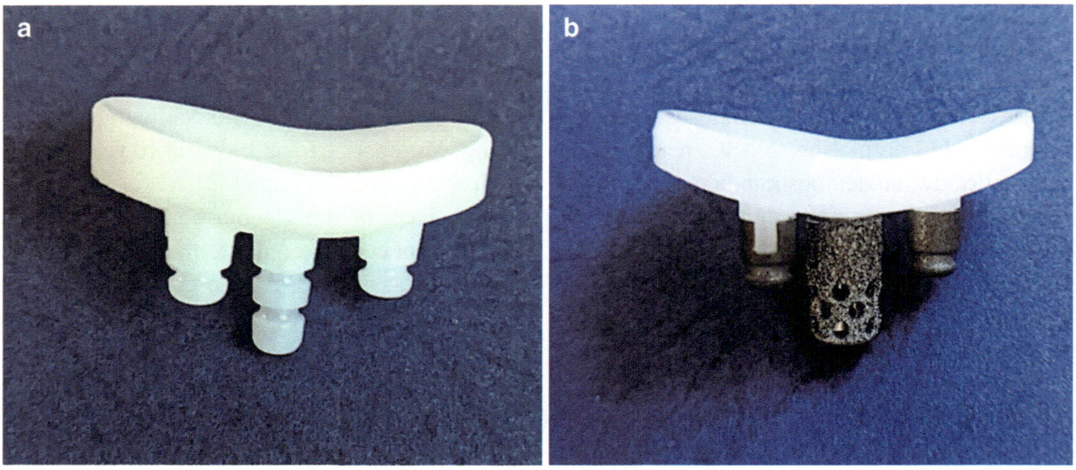

Fig. 1.7 Examples of modern glenoid components: (**a**) a pegged, all-polyethylene curved-back glenoid and (**b**) a hybrid, pegged curved-back glenoid

plasty. The Australian registry (AOANJRR) reports a lower revision rate with cross-linked polyethylene than with conventional polyethylene components at 5 years (2.7% vs. 6.7%) [38].

Metal-backed glenoids have been developed in an attempt to improve the fixation. The first point to note is that the additional layer creates an extra interface and reduces the potential thickness of the polyethylene. Dissociations at the metal polyethylene interface have been reported, and lateralization is increased due to the size of the component, both of which contribute to higher failure rates. AOANJRR analysis has demonstrated significantly lower revision rates with all-polyethylene glenoids versus metal-backed designs at 5 years (3.7% vs. 17.9%) [39]. This area continues to evolve with the use of screw augmentation and hydroxyapatite coatings, particularly in the revision scenario. However, long-term data on these implants, which remain novel devices, are required.

The contemporary design evolution includes hybrid glenoids, which utilize longer porous-coated metal pegs, to allow ingrowth, attached to a polyethylene glenoid back surface, and inset glenoids, which are partially rooted to the glenoid surface and preserve the natural subchondral bone. Although laboratory-based loading analysis shows promise, longer-term clinical data remain sparse and these should be cautiously considered, with studies needed to delineate the potential adverse effects and survival (Fig. 1.7).

1.3.3.2 The Glenoid Surgical Technique

Regardless of the component design used, surgical technique has a significant role to play in the causality of TSR failure [40]. This extends to the surgical approach, adequacy of the exposure, glenoid preparation and implantation technique, and soft tissue management.

The use of modern cannulated reaming systems and cement pressurization techniques has been shown to decrease the incidence of radiographic lucency around the glenoid component. The glenoid should be carefully reamed to the denuded bone but to preserve the subchondral plate [24]. Removal of the subchondral plate makes the implant fixation reliant on the inferior and significantly weaker cancellous bone, which is known to influence early failure [41]. This should be balanced with the need to ensure that the component is properly seated.

The implant version should be very carefully considered. Even small variations in glenoid retroversion can significantly influence loading patterns, leading to instability and loosening [42]. In a study of 122 failed TSRs, the glenoid component was implanted in excessive retroversion in up to 46% [43]. Finite element analysis has demonstrated that retroversion beyond 10° significantly reduces contact area, increases contact pressures, and increases micromotion more than sevenfold, thus promoting early loosening [44].

An adequate cementing technique is required, as failure most commonly occurs at the implant–cement interface. There is debate over the application of cement to the backside of the implant, which is discouraged in most current designs [9]; however, cadaveric studies have shown that the loading characteristics are more favorable when the cement is along the entire surface of the implant contacting the subchondral bone [45]. Other authors have shown that in experimental models, loosening takes place in traction if there was cement at the back of the polyethylene [46], but in cyclic loading, loosening with an associated cement fracture occurs only when the interface is 2–3-mm thick. The cement mantel should therefore be as thin as possible at the back of the implant but should be optimized around the keel or pegs.

1.3.4 Humeral Failure

The humeral component design seeks to conform to the native anatomy to optimize function and reduce the risks of failure. The important geometric parameters include the humeral head diameter and thickness, neck inclination, humeral head height, humeral head retroversion, acromiohumeral distance, and medial and posterior head offset [47]. Although the failure of the TSR construct has predominantly been on the glenoid side, the area that has seen the biggest design evolution is the humerus. Currently, there are large offerings in modularity, stem length, fixation choice, and platform systems; however, there is a relative paucity of long-term evidence on the survival and failure mechanisms of these design developments.

1.3.4.1 Humeral Design

Since the development of the third-generation prosthesis in the 1990s, there has been an ever-increasing emphasis on modularity. Modularity greatly assists in the matching of natural anatomical variability, and, although this has not been translated into definitively improved outcomes, there is evidence that there is a beneficial effect on the adjacent glenoid replacement [48].

Clinically significant loosening of the humeral component is much less common than on the glenoid side. The overall prevalence of loosening is believed to be 1.1% [49], and some case series in cemented humeral components have reported no humeral loosening at more than 20 years of follow-up [7]. Radiological rates of aseptic loosening occur most frequently in uncemented stems (49–55% of patients at 4.2–12 years) [50, 51]. Osteolysis secondary to polyethylene wear debris has been described; however, the clinical significance has not manifested in higher revision rates [52].

Cementation of the humeral component was the standard of treatment for a considerable period. Good results have been reported in long-term outcome studies; however, newer uncemented designs have been developed under the rationale that they decrease operative time, simplify revision, and avoid proximal stress shielding. The meta-analysis performed by Uy et al. on the humeral component fixation technique for osteoarthritis identified similar revision rates and therefore promotes press fit due to the potential gains in patients with sufficient bone stock [53]. There is consensus that in the scenario of trauma, the humeral component should be cemented.

Stem length has also evolved, with an emphasis on shortening the stem to reduce stress shielding. Evidence of the impact of this on failure rates is emerging. Godenèche et al., in their evidence synthesis, identified that the incidence of revision and adverse radiographic observations were lower in coated short stems, compared with short and long uncoated stems, but caution that longer follow-up is required [54]. Indeed, the need for a stem at all is being questioned. Although the registries have reported reduced rates of bone-preserving total shoulder resurfacings, the use of metaphyseal fixation is rapidly rising. Equally good outcomes in the short to medium term, with lower intraoperative fracture rates, have been reported [55]. Dillon et al. reported a failure rate of 2.1% at 3.3 years in 3026 metaphyseal TSRs [56]. The overall failure rate of these prostheses needs to be evaluated in longer-term studies (Fig. 1.3b).

1.3.4.2 The Humeral Surgical Technique

The humeral head size should be matched to optimize the rotator cuff function. Increasing the thickness of the humeral head by 5 mm has been shown to reduce the range of motion by between 20° and 30° and stress the rotator cuff, and, for every 1 mm of oversizing, there is a loss of 3–4° [57]. Overstuffing the joint can also cause obligate translation on the glenoid component [58]. It is also vital that the humeral head does not overlap laterally, as to avoid impingement on the rotator cuff that, over time, would precipitate early failure (Fig. 1.8).

Careful soft tissue handling and repair of the subscapularis is required to avoid intraoperative tears and postoperative failure. Diligent and cautious mobilization of the tendon should be conducted with the release of subcoracoid adhesion as well as the middle and inferior glenoid ligaments [59]. The release of the subscapularis is the workhorse approach to a TSR and, as such, a secure repair of the subscapularis is essential. Failure of this repair has the potential for poor outcomes and early TSR failure. In general, three techniques are used: a tenotomy, a peel, and a lesser tuberosity osteotomy. Multiple cadaveric, biomechanical, and clinical trials comparing these techniques have been undertaken. Overall, while tenotomy and peel preserve bone stock, osteotomy benefits from bone-on-bone healing and is biomechanically superior [60]. In clinical studies, there is a broad equivalence between all three techniques.

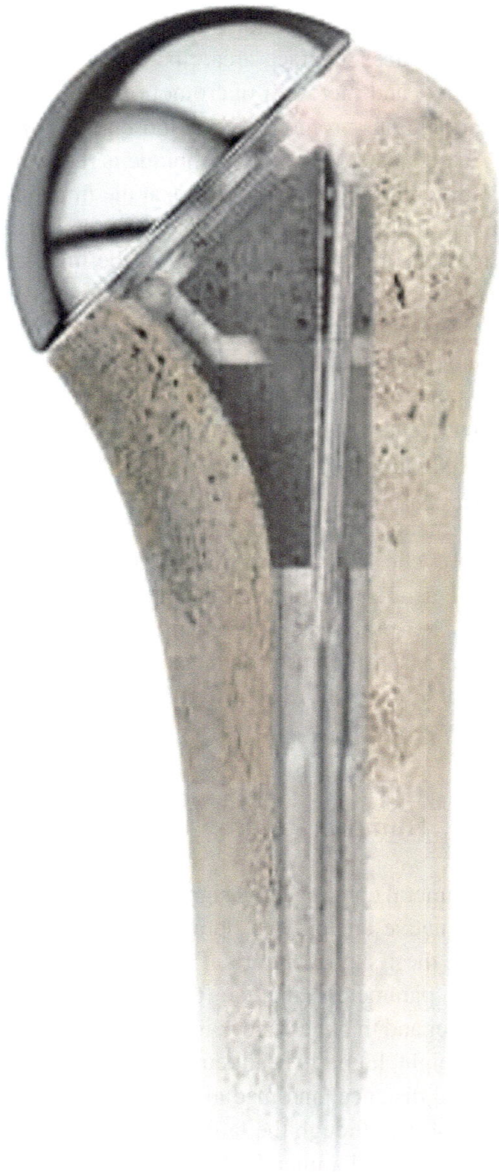

Fig. 1.8 Matching the humeral head size to the native anatomy is vital for correct rotator cuff tension. Over- or undersizing can lead to early failure

1.4 Surgery-Related Outcome

The overall complication rate in shoulder arthroplasty is 11% [61], with the previously discussed complications of component loosening, glenoid wear, instability, and rotator cuff failure being the most common. However, there are important surgical factors that influence the patient outcome and failure rate of a TSR. Fractures, neural injury, and infection, although less common, all contribute to the potential failure of the surgery and should be carefully considered.

As with all surgeries, there is an important learning curve and surgical volume effect associated with TSR. Beazley et al. reported the early career learning curve of a single surgeon and found a trend for consistent performance in TSRs after 16 cases and a complication rate under 10% with statistical significance seen in 40 cases [62]. Hammond et al. assessed the effect of surgeon volume, finding that high-volume surgeons had half the risk of complications [63].

Periprosthetic fracture is an extremely rare occurrence in anatomical TSR. There is a reported prevalence of 0.69%, with the majority occurring intraoperatively. Implant selection, an understanding of the implantation technique, and surgical diligence are all vital, but the patient's comorbidity profile also plays a significant role, including osteopenia and cortical thinning by osteolysis.

Nerve injury has been reported to occur in 0.63% of 3360 TSR cases [61]. The most common injuries are to the axillary nerve. Many of these injuries are traction relates, rather than iatrogenic lacerations or incorporation in suture repair, as most such cases recover over time. Neurological damage to the brachial plexus is exceedingly rare but carries a grave prognosis, and, therefore, the appreciation of relevant anatomy is vital.

The choice of surgical approach may have a bearing on the failure rate of a TSR. The traditional deltopectoral approach, with subscapularis management, has been previously discussed. More recently, subscapularis sparing approaches through either the anterolateral approach or deltopectoral interval have been described. The proposed benefit is avoidance of violating the subscapularis attachment. Development in the TSR approach is warranted, but caution should be advised as the evidence remains at the case series level and most authors comment that the approaches are technically demanding. The consequent trade-off in visualization and implant positioning may have a bearing on the ultimate failure rate, and a future medium- to long-term follow-up is required.

An infection represents a truly devastating complication. An infection following a TSR has been reported to occur in 0.51% of cases [61]. A stiff and painful shoulder should always alert the surgeon to the possibility of an infection, even if the serological markers are normal [64]. A reduction in risk is in the surgeon's realm as inoculation of microorganisms often occurs at the time of surgery and includes antibiotic prophylaxis, operating room management, surgical site preparation, and meticulous implant and tissue handling.

1.5 Patient-Related Outcome

The success and failure of a total shoulder replacement surgery can be significantly influenced by preexisting patient factors. These aspects should be carefully regarded by the treating team and should be discussed as part of the decision-making process. Knowledge of certain indicators of poor post-op prognosis, and their consequent integration into the patient discussion, may alter the course of treatment. As the number of TSRs has been increasing over the last two decades, so has the proportion of patients with significant comorbidities, with a particular emphasis on obesity, diabetes, and chronic obstructive pulmonary disease [65].

Patient factors have been found to be equally associated with the outcome as technical aspects. Matsen et al. found that an American Society of Anesthesiologists (ASA) Class I categorization, shoulder problems not related to work, lower baseline simple shoulder test, and no history of prior surgery had similar odds ratios associated with better outcome in their prediction model to the absence of humeral head superior displacement and glenoid erosion type other than A1 [66]. Leschinger et al. found that ASA 3 and smokers had a higher chance of complications [67]. Fu et al. reported that insulin-dependent diabetes conferred a significant increase on the risk of complications, whereas non-insulin-dependent diabetes did not [68].

The relevance of psychosocial aspects has been highlighted by Vajapey et al., who postulated that depression and anxiety were associated with an increased risk of perioperative complications and lower functional scores; they commented that psychosocial factors may play as just an important role as technical factors [69].

Younger age at surgery is strongly associated with a lifetime risk of revision. This is related to higher physical demands and is likely to be related to relative mortality rates and revision thresholds. The Australian registry demonstrates higher revision rates in patients under the age of 65 [4]. Craig et al., using a large national dataset, found the lifetime risk of revision to be 1 in 37 in women aged 85 years and older down to 1 in 4 in men aged 55–59 years [70]. The influence of male gender on revision risk has also been highlighted by Singh et al. and Bekerom et al., who found that it conferred a 1.7- and twofold increase on revision, respectively [71, 72].

A diagnosis of osteoarthritis as the index pathology is predictive of superior outcomes compared to other pathologies [66]. Although a TSR in inflammatory arthritis is associated with a predictable improvement in pain, it carries a higher risk of secondary rotator cuff insufficiency compared to osteoarthritis [73]. Boileau et al., in a large Aequalis multicenter trial, demonstrated that patients with an index diagnosis of rheumatoid arthritis (RA) had a greater complication (10%) and revision rate (7.5%) at 2 years [33]; interestingly, the Australian registry (AOANJRR) found that RA has the lowest revision rate [4]. Burrus et al. found that patients with an index diagnosis of avascular necrosis (AVN) were at a higher risk of a wide spectrum of complications, including revision surgery [74]. Those with post-traumatic AVN and steroid-induced AVN were at a significantly higher revision risk.

1.6 Summary

Total shoulder replacements confer excellent pain relief and function in the treatment of end-stage degenerative shoulder pathology with an intact rotator cuff. All-cause survival estimates are approximately 90% at 10 years. Robust long-term evidence is lacking, which may be of concern, with case series demonstrating substantial failure of the glenoid component in the second decade after implantation.

The failure of total shoulder replacements is dependent on multiple aspects, including implant-, surgery-, and patient-related factors. Although significant emphasis has been placed on evolving the implant design and developing surgical techniques, patient-related factors are likely to play an equal role in the success of the surgery.

The survivorship of the glenoid remains the most significant implant-related failure point. Meticulous attention to the preoperative anatomy, implantation position, and implantation technique are all vital. However, changes in the implant design and technique have failed to significantly improve the failure rate. This remains the most important area of future research.

Humeral components are increasingly uncemented and use shorter bone-preserving designs. Currently, short- to medium-term revision rates are favorable for this design change.

Reducing the risk of failure of total shoulder replacements is contingent on the surgeon working within the constraints of the native anatomy, the application of the anatomical principles in the arthroplasty implantation, evidence-based component selection, and a focus on safe surgical practice and the influence of patient factors.

References

1. Neer CS II. Replacement arthroplasty for glenohumeral osteoarthritis. JBJS. 1974;56(1):1–13.
2. Kim SH, Wise BL, Zhang Y, Szabo RM. Increasing incidence of shoulder arthroplasty in the United States. J Bone Joint Surg. 2011;93(24):2249–54.
3. Day JS, Lau E, Ong KL, Williams GR, Ramsey ML, Kurtz SM. Prevalence and projections of total shoul-

der and elbow arthroplasty in the United States to 2015. J Shoulder Elb Surg. 2010;19(8):1115–20.
4. Australian Orthopaedic Association National Joint Replacement Registry. Hip, Knee & Shoulder Arthroplasty Annual Report 2019. 2019. https://aoanjrr.sahmri.com/annual-reports-2019.
5. Evans JP, Evans JT, Craig RS, Mohammad HR, Sayers A, Blom AW, et al. How long does a shoulder replacement last? A systematic review and meta-analysis of case series and national registry reports with more than 10 years of follow-up. Lancet Rheumatol. 2020;2(9):e539–48.
6. Schoch B, Schleck C, Cofield RH, Sperling JW. Shoulder arthroplasty in patients younger than 50years: minimum 20-year follow-up. J Shoulder Elb Surg. 2015;24(5):705–10.
7. Evans JP, Batten T, Bird J, Thomas WJ, Kitson JB, Smith CD. Survival of the Aequalis total shoulder replacement at a minimum 20-year follow-up: a clinical and radiographic study. J Shoulder Elb Surg. 2021;30(10):2355–60.
8. Boileau P, Walch G. The three-dimensional geometry of the proximal humerus. Bone Joint J. 1997;79-B(5):857–65.
9. Trivedi NN, Shimberg JL, Sivasundaram L, Mengers S, Salata MJ, Voos JE, et al. Advances in glenoid design in anatomic total shoulder arthroplasty. J Bone Joint Surg Am. 2020;102(20):1825–35.
10. Provencher MT, Parada SA, Gross DJ, Golijanin P. Kinematics of the rotator cuff. In: Normal and pathological anatomy of the shoulder. Springer; 2015. p. 221–32.
11. Minagawa H, Yamamoto N, Abe H, Fukuda M, Seki N, Kikuchi K, et al. Prevalence of symptomatic and asymptomatic rotator cuff tears in the general population: from mass-screening in one village. J Orthop. 2013;10(1):8–12.
12. Sperling JW, Galatz LM, Higgins LD, Levine WN, Ramsey ML, Dunn J. Avoidance and treatment of complications in shoulder arthroplasty. Instr Course Lect. 2009;58:459–72.
13. Favard L, Katz D, Colmar M, Benkalfate T, Thomazeau H, Emily S. Total shoulder arthroplasty–arthroplasty for glenohumeral arthropathies: results and complications after a minimum follow-up of 8 years according to the type of arthroplasty and etiology. Orthop Traumatol Surg Res. 2012;98(4):S41–7.
14. Franklin JL, Barrett WP, Jackins SE, Matsen FA. Glenoid loosening in total shoulder arthroplasty. Association with rotator cuff deficiency. J Arthroplast. 1988;3:3.
15. Foruria AM, Sperling JW, Ankem HK, Oh LS, Cofield RH. Total shoulder replacement for osteoarthritis in patients 80 years of age and older. J Bone Joint Surg Br. 2010;92(7):970–4.
16. Bohsali KI, Bois AJ, Wirth MA. Complications of shoulder arthroplasty. J Bone Joint Surg (Am Vol). 2017;99(3):256–69.
17. Godenèche A, Boileau P, Favard HJC, Lévigne C, Nové-Josserand L, et al. Prosthetic replacement in the treatment of osteoarthritis of the shoulder: early results of 268 cases. J Shoulder Elb Surg. 2002;11:11–8.
18. Edwards TB, Boulahia A, Kempf J. The influence of rotator cuff disease on the results of shoulder arthroplasty for primary osteoarthritis. J Bone Joint Surg Am. 2006;88:2258.
19. Young AA, Walch G, Pape G, Gohlke F, Favard L. Secondary rotator cuff dysfunction following total shoulder arthroplasty for primary glenohumeral osteoarthritis: results of a multicenter study with more than five years of follow-up. J Bone Joint Surg Am. 2012;94:685.
20. Klemt C, Prinold JA, Morgans S, Smith SHL, Nolte D, Reilly P, et al. Analysis of shoulder compressive and shear forces during functional activities of daily life. Clin Biomech. 2018;54:34–41.
21. Nyffeler RW. Measurement of glenoid version: conventional radiographs versus computed tomography scans. J Shoulder Elb Surg. 2003;12:493.
22. Walch G, Moraga C, Young A, Castellanos-Rosas J. Results of anatomic nonconstrained prosthesis in primary osteoarthritis with biconcave glenoid. J Shoulder Elb Surg. 2012;21:1526–33.
23. Ho JC. Glenoid component retroversion is associated with osteolysis. J Bone Joint Surg Am. 2013;95:e82.
24. Malhas A, Rashid A, Copas D, Bale S, Trail I. Glenoid bone loss in primary and revision shoulder arthroplasty. Shoulder Elbow. 2016;8(4):229–40.
25. Jobe CM, Iannotti JP. Limits imposed on glenohumeral motion by joint geometry. J Shoulder Elb Surg. 1995;4:281–5.
26. Trail IA. Design of Polyethylene Glenoid Components. In: Textbook of shoulder surgery. Springer; 2019. p. 213–21.
27. Sabesan VJ, Lima DJL, Whaley JD, Pathak V, Zhang L. The effect of glenohumeral radial mismatch on different augmented total shoulder arthroplasty glenoid designs: a finite element analysis. J Shoulder Elb Surg. 2019;28(6):1146–53.
28. Sabesan VJ, Ackerman J, Sharma V, Baker KC, Kurdziel MD, Wiater JM. Glenohumeral mismatch affects micromotion of cemented glenoid components in total shoulder arthroplasty. J Shoulder Elb Surg. 2015;24(5):814–22.
29. Pinkas D, Wiater B, Wiater JM. The glenoid component in anatomic shoulder arthroplasty. J Am Acad Orthop Surg. 2015;23(5):317–26.
30. Nho SJ, Nam D, Ala OL, Craig E, Warren RF, Wright TM. Observations on retrieved glenoid components from total shoulder arthroplasty. J Shoulder Elb Surg. 2009;18:371–8.
31. Walch G, Edwards TB, Boulahia A, Boileau P, Mole D, Adeleine P. The influence of glenohumeral prosthetic mismatch on glenoid radiolucent lines: results of a multicenter study. J Bone Joint Surg Am. 2002;84:2186.
32. Raiss P, Schmitt M, Bruckner T. Results of cemented total shoulder replacement with a minimum follow-up of ten years. J Bone Joint Surg Am. 2012;94:e171.

33. Young A, Walch G, Boileau P, Favard L, Gohlke F, Loew M, et al. A multicentre study of the long-term results of using a flat-back polyethylene glenoid component in shoulder replacement for primary osteoarthritis. J Bone Joint Surg Br. 2011;93:210.
34. Anglin C, Wyss UP, Nyffeler RW, Gerber C. Loosening performance of cemented glenoid prosthesis design pairs. Clin Biomech. 2001;16:144.
35. Vavken P, Sadoghi P, von Keudell A, Rosso C, Valderrabano V, Müller AM. Rates of radiolucency and loosening after total shoulder arthroplasty with pegged or keeled glenoid components. JBJS. 2013;95(3):215–21.
36. Nuttall D, Haines JF, Trail IA. A study of the micromovment of pegged and keeled glenoid components compared using radio Stereometric analysis. J Shoulder Elb Surg. 2007;16(3 Suppl):S65–70.
37. Kilian CM, Press CM, Smith KM, O'Connor DP, Morris BJ, Elkousy HA, et al. Radiographic and clinical comparison of pegged and keeled glenoid components using modern cementing techniques: midterm results of a prospective randomized study. J Shoulder Elb Surg. 2017;26(12):2078–85.
38. Page RS, Alder-Price AC, Rainbird S, Graves SE, de Steiger RN, Peng Y, et al. Reduced revision rates in total shoulder arthroplasty with crosslinked polyethylene: results from the Australian Orthopaedic Association National Joint Replacement Registry. Clin Orthop Relat Res. 2022;480(10):1940–9.
39. Page RS, Pai V, Eng K, Bain G, Graves S, Lorimer M. Cementless versus cemented glenoid components in conventional total shoulder joint arthroplasty: analysis from the Australian Orthopaedic Association national joint replacement registry. J Shoulder Elb Surg. 2018;27(10):1859–65.
40. Chin PY, Sperling JW, Cofield RH, Schleck C. Complications of total shoulder arthroplasty: are they fewer or different? J Shoulder Elb Surg. 2006;15:19–22.
41. Anglin C, Tolhurst P, Wyss UP, Pichora DR. Glenoid cancellous bone strength and modulus. J Biomech. 1999;32(10):1091–7.
42. Nyffeler RW, Sheikh R, Atkinson TS, Jacob HA, Favre P, Gerber C. Effects of glenoid component version on humeral head displacement and joint reaction forces: an experimental study. J Shoulder Elb Surg. 2006;15:625–9.
43. Moskal MJ, Duckworth D, Matsen FA. An analysis of 122 failed shoulder arthroplasties. J Shoulder Elb Surg. 1999;8:554.
44. Büchler P, Ramaniraka NA, Rakotomanana LR, Iannotti JP, Farron A. A finite element model of the shoulder: application to the comparison of normal and osteoarthritic joints. Clin Biomech. 2002;17(9–10):630–9.
45. Glennie RA, Giles JW, Johnson JA, Athwal GS, Faber KJ. An in vitro study comparing limited to full cementation of polyethylene glenoid components. J Orthop Surg Res. 2015;17:142.
46. Clavert P, Bouchaïb J, Kling A, Kempf JF. Does the cement mantle thickness influence the glenoid loosening in anatomic total shoulder arthroplasty? An experimental study. J Orthop Sci. 2019;24(1):81–6.
47. Marcheggiani Muccioli GM, Fratini S, Rinaldi VG, Cammisa E, Alesi D, et al. Anatatomic shoulder arthroplasty: causes and indications to surgery. In: Shoulder arthroplasty. Springer; 2020. p. 47–52.
48. Nuttall D, Haines JF, Trail IA. The effect of the offset humeral head on the micromovement of pegged glenoid components: a comparative study using radiostereometric analysis. J Bone Joint Surg Br. 2009;91:757.
49. Bohsali KJ. Complications of total shoulder arthroplasty. J Bone Joint Surg Am. 2006;88:2279.
50. Torchia ME. Total shoulder arthroplasty with the Neer prosthesis: long-term results. J Shoulder Elb Surg. 1997;6:6.
51. Sanchez-Sotelo J, Wright TW, O'Driscoll SW, Cofield RH, Rowland CM. Radiographic assessment of uncemented humeral components in total shoulder arthroplasty. J Arthroplast. 2001;16:180.
52. Raiss P, Edwards TB, Deutsch A. Radiographic changes around humeral components in shoulder arthroplasty. J Bone Joint Surg Am. 2014;96:e54.
53. Uy M, Wang J, Horner NS, Bedi A, Leroux T, Alolabi B, et al. Cemented humeral stem versus press-fit humeral stem in total shoulder arthroplasty: a systematic review and meta-analysis. Bone Joint J. 2019;101(9):1107–14.
54. Godenèche A, Garret J, Barth J, Michelet A, Geais L. Comparison of revision rates and radiographic observations of long and short, uncoated and coated humeral stem designs in total shoulder arthroplasty. EFORT Open Rev. 2019;4(2):70–6.
55. Willems JIP, Hoffmann J, Sierevelt IN, van den Bekerom MPJ, Alta TDW, van Noort A. Results of stemless shoulder arthroplasty: a systematic review and meta-analysis. EFORT Open Rev. 2021;6(1):35–49.
56. Dillon MT, Ake CF, Burke MF, Singh A, Yian EH, Paxton EW, et al. The Kaiser Permanente shoulder arthroplasty registry: results from 6,336 primary shoulder arthroplasties. Acta Orthop. 2015;86(3):286–92.
57. Harryman DT, Sidles JA, Harris SL, Lippitt SB, Matsen FA. The effect of articular conformity and the size of the humeral head component on laxity and motion after glenohumeral arthroplasty. A study in cadavera. J Bone Joint Surg Am. 1995;77:555–63.
58. Griffiths EJ, Trail IA, Walch G. Design of humeral stems. In: Textbook of shoulder surgery. Springer; 2019. p. 223–31.
59. Walton M, Makki D, Brookes-Fazakerley S. Complications of shoulder arthroplasty. In: Textbook of shoulder surgery. Springer; 2019. p. 367–81.
60. Dunn R, Joyce CD, Bravman JT. Comparison of subscapularis management and repair techniques. J Shoulder Elb Arthroplast. 2019;3:247154921984815.
61. Bohsali KI, Bois AJ, Wirth MA. Complications of shoulder arthroplasty. [review]. J Bone Joint Surg Am. 2017;99:256–69.
62. Beazley JCS, Evans JP, Furness ND, Smith CD. Comparative learning curves for early complica-

tions in anatomical and reverse shoulder arthroplasty. Ann R Coll Surg Engl. 2018;100(6):491.
63. Hammond JW, Queale WS, Kim TK, McFarland EG. Surgeon experience and clinical and economic outcomes for shoulder arthroplasty. J Bone Joint Surg Am. 2003;85:2318–24.
64. Dodson CC, Craig E, Cordasco FA, Dines DM, Dines JS, DiCarlo E, et al. Propionibacterium acnes infection after shoulder arthroplasty: a diagnostic challenge. J Shoulder Elb Surg. 2010;19(2):303–7.
65. Bixby EC, Boddapati V, Anderson MJJ, Mueller JD, Jobin CM, Levine WN. Trends in total shoulder arthroplasty from 2005 to 2018: lower complications rates and shorter lengths of stay despite patients with more comorbidities. JSES Int. 2020;4(3):657–61.
66. Matsen FA, Russ SM, Vu PT, Hsu JE, Lucas RM, Comstock BA. What factors are predictive of patient-reported outcomes? A prospective study of 337 shoulder arthroplasties. Clin Orthop Relat Res. 2016;474(11):2496–510.
67. Leschinger T, Raiss P, Loew M, Zeifang F. Total shoulder arthroplasty: risk factors for intraoperative and postoperative complications in patients with primary arthritis. J Shoulder Elb Surg. 2017;26:e71–7.
68. Fu MC, Boddapati V, Dines DM, Warren RF, Dines JS, Gulotta L, v. The impact of insulin dependence on short-term postoperative complications in diabetic patients undergoing total shoulder arthroplasty. J Shoulder Elb Surg. 2017;26(12):2091–6.
69. Vajapey SP, Cvetanovich GL, Bishop JY, Neviaser AS. Psychosocial factors affecting outcomes after shoulder arthroplasty: a systematic review. J Shoulder Elb Surg. 2020;29(5):e175–84.
70. Craig RS, Lane JCE, Carr AJ, Furniss D, Collins GS, Rees JL. Serious adverse events and lifetime risk of reoperation after elective shoulder replacement: population based cohort study using hospital episode statistics for England. BMJ. 2019;364:l298.
71. Singh JA, Sperling JW, Cofield RH. Revision surgery following total shoulder arthroplasty: analysis of 2588 shoulders over three decades (1976 to 2008). J Bone Joint Surg Br. 2011;93:1513–7.
72. Bekerom MP, Geervliet PC, Somford MP, Borne MP, Boer R. Total shoulder arthroplasty versus hemiarthroplasty for glenohumeral arthritis: a systematic review of the literature at long-term follow-up. Int J Shoulder Surg. 2013;7:110–5.
73. Papadonikolakis A, Matsen FA. Metal-backed glenoid components have a higher rate of failure and fail by different modes in comparison with all-polyethylene components: a systematic review. J Bone Joint Surg Am. 2014;96:1041.
74. Tyrrell Burrus M, Cancienne JM, Boatright JD, Yang S, Brockmeier SF, Werner BC. Shoulder arthroplasty for humeral head avascular necrosis is associated with increased postoperative complications. HSS J. 2018;14(1):2–8.
75. Khan A, Bunker TD, Kitson JB. Clinical and radiological follow-up of the Aequalis third-generation cemented total shoulder replacement: a minimum ten-year study. J Bone Joint Surg B. 2009;91(12):1594–600.
76. Levy O, Tsvieli O, Merchant J, Young L, Trimarchi A, Dattani R, et al. Surface replacement arthroplasty for glenohumeral arthropathy in patients aged younger than fifty years: results after a minimum ten-year follow-up. J Shoulder Elb Surg. 2015;24:1049–60.
77. Schoch B, Schleck C, Cofield RH, Sperling JW. Shoulder arthroplasty in patients younger than 50 years: minimum 20-years follow-up. J Shoulder Elb Surg. 2015;24:705–10.
78. Sperling JW, Cofield RH, Rowland CM. Minimum fifteen-year follow-up of Neer hemiarthroplasty and total shoulder arthroplasty in patients aged fifty years or younger. J Shoulder Elbow Surg. 2004;13(6):604–13.
79. Tammachote N, Sperling JW, Vathana T, Cofield RH, Harmsen WS, Schleck CD. Long-term results of cemented metal-backed glenoid components for osteoarthritis of the shoulder. J Bone Joint Surg A. 2009;91(1):160–6.

Why Reverse Shoulder Arthroplasties Fail

2

Robert Z. Tashjian and Christopher D. Joyce

2.1 Introduction

Reverse shoulder arthroplasty (RSA) has become the standard of care to treat patients with rotator cuff tear arthropathy in an elderly patient population with limited function. Similarly, over the course of the past 20 years, since the Food and Drug Administration (FDA) approved the usage of RSA in the United States in 2003, the indications for RSA have expanded to include the treatment of osteoarthritis, failed total shoulder arthroplasty, acute proximal humeral fractures and fracture sequelae, inflammatory arthritis, massive irreparable rotator cuff tears without arthritis, and tumors [1]. With expanding indications, the volume of RSAs performed has risen exponentially with a 191.3% increase in cases performed between 2011 and 2017, with 63,845 cases performed in 2017 based upon the National Inpatient Sample database [2]. Based upon Poisson modeling to predict future growth, a 353% increase in growth is expected to occur with a total number of RSAs approaching 289,000 by 2025 [2]. As a consequence of increasing primary shoulder arthroplasty, revision shoulder arthroplasty burden will increase as well [3]. In an analysis using the Nationwide Inpatient Sample from 1993 to 2007, the burden of revision shoulder arthroplasty increased from 4.5% between 1993 and 1995 to approximately 7% after 2004 [3]. In another study utilizing the same dataset using data from 1988 to 2017, it was noted that the prevalence of individuals living with a shoulder replacement in the United States had risen from 0.031% in 1995 to 0.258% in 2017 [4]. Finally, the number of revision arthroplasties has risen, resulting from an increase in primary arthroplasty volume from 2216 cases in 2002 to 10,290 in 2017 [4]. In attempts to reduce the overall increasing revision procedures, understanding why and how shoulder arthroplasty fails can improve our ability to potentially limit the rise of revisions despite the exponential growth in shoulder arthroplasty in general.

RSA and anatomic total shoulder arthroplasty (aTSA) have some common and unique complications that are specific to the procedures. Some of these complications are early, whereas others are late, resulting in early and late failures, respectively. Infections and non-implant-related complications are the most common early reasons for failure and have been highlighted in several large registry studies evaluating both aTSA and RSA. Infection, loosening, and polyethylene wear remain the common late reasons for both RSA and aTSA failures. The unique reasons for early failure of an RSA, which are rarely seen after an aTSA, include instability and acromial

R. Z. Tashjian (✉) · C. D. Joyce
Department of Orthopaedics, University of Utah School of Medicine, Salt Lake City, UT, USA
e-mail: Robert.Tashjian@hsc.utah.edu; Christopher.Joyce@hsc.utah.edu

F. Franceschi et al. (eds.), *Revision Shoulder Arthroplasty*,
https://doi.org/10.1007/978-3-031-45944-3_2

fracture, whereas the unique reasons for late failure after an RSA include a functional decline of well-fixed, noninfected implants.

Several studies have evaluated the overall failure rates as well as the etiologies of failure after an RSA. Gauci et al. reviewed the epidemiology, etiology, and revision options for failed shoulder arthroplasties at two centers [5]. At an average of 8.7 years postoperatively, the top four etiologies of implant failure include instability (32% of all implant failures), infection (24%), glenoid loosening (24%), and humeral loosening (10%). [5] Fracture only accounted for 3% of all failures in this series [5]. Zumstein et al. reviewed the problems, complications, and revisions after an RSA [1]. The authors performed a systematic review on articles published between 1995 and 2008 and noted a global postoperative complication rate of 24%, with the top complications including instability occurring in 4.7% of cases, infection in 3.8% of cases, aseptic glenoid loosening in 3.5% of cases, scapula or acromial fractures in 1.5% of cases, and humeral loosening in 1.3% of cases [1]. Most complications had a negative impact on the final functional outcomes [1]. Comparing the overall complications, Zumstein et al.'s data are highly comparable to those of Gauci et al. [1, 5]. Both datasets reflect an earlier learning curve (prior to 2008) associated with RSAs. Kang et al. have reviewed a more recent experience with RSA by reviewing 1659 RSAs performed between 2009 and 2015 with an average follow-up of 2.5 years and reported a reoperation rate of 2.37% [6]. Reviewing the top reasons for reoperation after an RSA, 0.55% of patients were reoperated for infection, 0.55% for instability, 0.3% for glenoid loosening, and 0.24% for humeral loosening [6]. In comparison with Zumstein et al.'s data, which reflect older data, greater experience appears to reduce the rates of complication and reoperation after an RSA, although the overall types of failures have not changed.

Besides the learning curve associated with RSA, the diagnosis for which it is performed likely has a significant impact on complication and revision rates. Heifner et al. performed a systematic review of patients undergoing an RSA for primary osteoarthritis and reported a 3.8% risk of major complications and a 3.1% risk of revision, including infection, periprosthetic fracture, glenoid loosening, instability, and baseplate failure [7]. Petrillo et al. performed a systematic review of patients undergoing an RSA for massive irreparable rotator cuff tears and rotator cuff arthropathy [8]. The authors reported a 5.6% risk of the same complications reported by Heifner et al. and a 7.3% overall risk of revision, suggesting an increased risk of complications and revisions in the setting of RSA for cuff arthropathy compared to osteoarthritis [7, 8]. Risks of instability (1.2% vs. 0.4%) and acromial fracture (3.4% vs. 0%) appear to be higher for patients treated for rotator cuff arthropathy compared to those treated for osteoarthritis [7, 8]. The highest rates of revisions were confirmed by Gauci et al. and are seen in patients treated with an RSA for fracture sequelae and cuff tear arthropathy compared to fracture or osteoarthritis [5].

2.2 Comparison in Failure Types and Rates between Anatomic Total Shoulder Arthroplasty and RSA

With the expansion of indications of RSA beyond rotator cuff arthropathy, a consideration needs to be made regarding the failure mechanisms between RSA and aTSA. RSA is being utilized more and more for patients with milder amounts of glenoid bone loss, who would have previously been treated with aTSA with high side glenoid reaming, and for older patients with primary osteoarthritis with any glenoid wear pattern. The data are mixed in comparing the rates of complications between RSA and aTSA.

Parada et al. compared the types, incidence, and timing of complications between RSA and aTSA utilizing a large international database of a single platform stem shoulder arthroplasty system. The authors compared 2224 aTSAs and 4158 RSAs [9]. The overall complication rates between RSA and aTSA were 8.9% and 10.7% and the revision rates were 2.9% and 5.6%, respectively. The infection rates were similar between both implant types [9]. Aibinder et al. reported using the same database that suggested that while aTSA had a higher complication rate than RSA, aTSA had a much longer follow-up, which might suggest that some of the differences are due to the length of follow-up from the surgery [10].

Poondla et al. compared patients undergoing aTSA (482) and RSA (185) in a prospectively collected database between the ages of 50 and 89 and also compared the outcomes and revision rates at an average of 3.1 years postoperatively [11]. The authors determined no differences in functional outcome scores or pain, but the revision rates for RSA were significantly higher than those for aTSA (8.1% vs. 3.9%, respectively) [11]. Finally, Kiet et al. compared the outcomes of RSA and aTSA in a prospective, case-controlled study including 47 patients undergoing aTSA for osteoarthritis and 53 patients undergoing RSA for rotator cuff tear arthropathy [12]. At 2 years, there were no differences in complication rates (15% aTSA vs. 13% RSA) or revision surgeries (11% aTSA vs. 9% RSA) [12]. aTSA patients had greater external rotation at follow-up, but, otherwise, there was no difference in terms of outcomes.

Based upon the data, the relative chances for revision or complications in RSA versus aTSA are most likely comparable but have highly separate complication profiles. aTSA early failures typically result due to rotator cuff tearing or subscapularis repair failure, and RSA failures typically result from instability or scapula/acromion fractures. As a result, surgeons need to select the complication profile for their patients by understanding the potential benefits of each prosthesis and making a final decision based upon patient demographics and the disease process.

2.3 Early Etiologies for Implant Failure After an RSA

Early failures after an RSA (within 12 months) can be categorized as common to shoulder arthroplasty in general and unique to RSA. Common early failures include medical complications, intraoperative complications, and infections. Unique early complications related to RSA include acromial fracture and instability. Multiple large-scale database studies and multicenter studies have improved our understanding of patients at risk of intraoperative complications and early readmission as well as acromial fracture and shoulder instability after an RSA.

Aibinder et al. utilized the Exactech shoulder arthroplasty database to evaluate factors associated with intraoperative and early postoperative complications after aTSA and RSA [10]. The authors reported on 2964 aTSAs and 5616 RSAs. They reported no differences with regard to intraoperative complications between aTSA and RSA, although female sex and prior shoulder surgery were risk factors [10]. Regarding postoperative complications, younger age, rheumatoid arthritis, greater preoperative retroversion, larger humeral stem size, larger humeral liner thickness or offset, larger glenosphere, size, and greater blood loss were all identified as risk factors [10]. Based upon these data, if there is poor bone quality associated with older females or prior surgery, then care must be taken to avoid intraoperative fracture. Similarly in the setting of prior surgery, expectations need to be set with the patient for potential intraoperative or postoperative complications, as this can be predicted with more challenging surgery. Finally, the data would support that over-distalization or over-lateralization of RSA is associated with an increased risk of revision, so good judgment is required if these strategies are being utilized during an RSA.

Unplanned early readmissions after a shoulder arthroplasty are typically a result of both surgical and medical complications. Identifying the risk factors associated with early readmission will allow surgeons to optimize clinical care and also set expectations for patients undergoing an RSA. Burnett et al. evaluated 2805 aTSAs and 2605 RSAs for readmission within 90 days from primary aTSA or RSA drawn from 2 geographically diverse tertiary health-care systems [13]. The unplanned 90-day readmission rate was 3.2%. A total of 60% of indications for readmission were surgical and 40% were medical-related. Short inpatient stay was not associated with readmission, although RSA (in comparison with aTSA), discharge to a skilled nursing facility, revision surgery, and fracture were all associated with an increased risk of readmission [13]. Burns et al. performed an analysis of cost and length of stay data from a 7-hospital system evaluating 1317 shoulder arthroplasties [14]. Anemia, malnutrition, and obesity were all associated with increased charges, whereas anemia and malnutrition were associated with increased length of stay. The studies support that optimizing medical comorbidities, including anemia and malnutrition, as well as avoiding skilled nursing facilities can have a significant impact on short-term failure after an RSA.

Infection is the most frequent, common, early complication noted after both an RSA and aTSA. Park and colleagues performed a systematic review and meta-analysis of studies evaluating the risk factors for infection after shoulder arthroplasty [15]. The total cohort included patients from 8 studies with 420 infected cases and 28,464 controls [15]. The authors reported that male sex, a history of prior shoulder surgery, revision shoulder arthroplasty, acute trauma, and non-osteoarthritis as a diagnosis were all significantly associated with an elevated risk of infection [15]. In terms of medical comorbidities, diabetes, liver disease, alcohol abuse, anemia, and rheumatoid arthritis were all risk factors for prosthetic joint infection [15]. In a recent systematic review, they have identified a 2.4% risk of infection at a mean of 4.3 years after primary RSA and 2.6% at a mean of 3.8 years after revision RSA [16]. Higher rates of prosthetic joint infection (PJI) were noted for the treatment of fracture sequelae compared to rotator cuff tear arthropathy or acute fracture [16]. Alternate strategies should be considered in patients at a high risk of infection, including males, revisions, and patients with prior surgery like use of intraoperative local antibiotics, postoperative oral antibiotics, or preoperative benzoyl peroxide or intraoperative sterile betadine. Similarly, medical optimization, including improvement of glucose control in diabetics and treatment of anemia as well as reduction of alcohol usage, might have an impact on lowering infection rates postoperatively.

Early complications or failures associated with a shoulder arthroplasty that are, in general, unique to an RSA include shoulder instability and scapula spine or acromial fractures. While instability can occur with aTSA, the overall rates of instability have declined significantly with a better understanding of the limitations of aTSA in the setting of glenoid bone loss. Scapula spine or acromial fractures occur almost exclusively after an RSA. The ASES (American Shoulder and Elbow Surgeons) Complications of RSA Research Group published on the results of a multicenter retrospective analysis including 15 institutions and 21 surgeons evaluating 6755 RSAs with a minimum of 3 months follow-up to identify the incidence and risk factors associated with the development of scapula spine and acromial fractures [17]. At an average of 19 months follow-up, the overall stress fracture rate was 3.9% where acromial fractures accounted for 3% and scapula spine fractures 0.9% [17]. Fractures occurred at an average of 8 months follow-up with 21% resulting from trauma [17]. Patient factors predictive of acromial fracture were a diagnosis of a chronic dislocation, massive rotator cuff tear without arthritis, rotator cuff arthropathy, a self-report of osteoporosis, inflammatory arthritis, female sex, and older age [17]. Patient factors predictive of scapula spine fractures included osteoporosis, female sex, rotator cuff arthropathy, and inflammatory arthropathy [17]. Miller et al. also reported that inflammatory arthritis was shown to have a significant impact on the development of scapula spine and acromial fractures (18% with inflammatory arthritis versus 5% without inflammatory arthritis) [18]. In a recent systematic review, Shah et al. have reported a 2.6% acromial fracture or scapula spine fracture risk at a mean of 4.3 years after an RSA [19]. The primary risk factor identified was rheumatoid arthritis with no increased risk of a Grammont-style implant compared to other styles, and the rates have not changed since the report of Zumstein et al. [1, 19]. Understanding patients at risk of acromial fracture may improve our intraoperative decisions in these patients, including limitation of distalization and lateralization as well as consideration of less aggressive postoperative rehabilitation. Similarly, counseling these patients at a high risk may improve our ability to catch these injuries while they are still stress reactions and treat them with immobilization instead of allowing them to go on to complete fracture.

Instability is the other primary early postoperative complication after an RSA. Shah et al. reviewed a total of 9306 RSAs in a systematic review with a mean age of 72 with an overall instability rate of 3.3% at a mean follow-up of 3.2 years [19]. In all, 73% of dislocations required revision surgery, and 59% occurred within the first 90 days postoperatively. Dislocation rates were significantly lower for primary RSA at 2.5% compared to revision RSA at 5.7%. The Grammont-style implant had a higher instability rate compared to all other designs at 4% versus 1.3%. Overall, modern non-Grammont-style implants have a lower reported instability rate compared to those reported by Zumstein et al. [19] Other reported risk factors include male patients, revision surgery, increased body mass index (BMI), proximal humeral bone loss with loss of the greater tuberosity, and humeral shortening [20–23]. Based upon these data, surgeons should be aware of patient factors that may lead to instability, including large, male revision patients, and should consider restoring humeral length and proximal humeral bone loss at the same time as lateralization on the glenoid and/or the humerus to restore stability.

2.4 Late Etiologies of Implant Failure After an RSA

The two primary late complications or failures after an RSA include implant loosening and a late functional decline. Both glenoid and humeral loosening have been described and have different etiologies. In general, baseplate loosening is typically an early complication and has become increasingly uncommon if certain surgical principles are followed. Typically, baseplate loosening is a result of insufficient glenoid fixation, inappropriate glenoid component positioning, or the requirement for bone grafting, which may not get incorporated, thus resulting in baseplate loosening. Gutierrez et al. performed a biomechanical study confirming that an inferior tilt provides the most even distribution of forces, whereas a superior tilt results in uneven force distribution [24]. Ho et al. reported 25% bone graft resorption when an RSA was performed with glenoid bone grafting and 25% baseplate radiographic failure at an average of 8 months after the RSA [25]. Shah et al. reported on 30 studies and determined a 2.3% revision rate for baseplate loosening, which is lower than the rates reported by Zumstein et al. [1, 16]. These data emphasize the need for adequate initial baseplate fixation and positioning to achieve ingrowth and limit failure.

Humeral component loosening may result early from inadequate ingrowth due to poor ingrowth material, specifically grit-blasted stems. Late humeral loosening is the result of either osteolysis in cemented stems or stress shielding in uncemented stems. Morwood et al. compared humeral components with proximal humeral coating versus no-coating or grit blast and noted 20% radiolucencies with no loosening in the coated stems compared to 44% radiolucencies and 2.9% loosening in the uncoated stem group at an average of 27 months follow-up [26]. Lack of the proximal humeral bone, comparable to glenoid bone loss with baseplate loosening, is associated with humeral stem loosening as rotational forces are not controlled, thus resulting in stem loosening. Cuff et al. performed a biomechanical study determining the effect of proximal humeral bone loss on fixation of RSA implants [27]. The authors torsionally tested RSA implants in bone models in the setting of an intact humeral bone and 5 cm of proximal humeral bone loss [27]. They determined that there is a significant increase in micromotion of the implant and an inability to complete the testing protocol in the 5-cm proximal humeral bone loss group compared to the intact proximal humeral bone. Comparing cemented with uncemented stems, Melis et al. reviewed 122 RSAs at 10-year follow-up and reported 8.8% loose cemented stems and 2.9% loose uncemented stems [28]. Stress shielding and greater and lesser tuberosity resorption were noted to be greater in uncemented compared to cemented stems [28]. In contrast, Werthel et al. reported on the survivorship of shoulder arthroplasties without humeral loosening and 98% survivorship at 20 years for 1167 cemented stems and 91% survivorship at 20 years for 3469 cementless stems [29]. Shah et al. performed a systematic review of 26 studies and reported the need for revision due to humeral loosening at 1% [16]. These data support the need for restoration of proximal humeral bone loss and the use of coated ingrowth stems if cementless fixation is chosen. Cementless fixation is recommended to reduce loosening, but, if inadequate initial fixation is achieved, then cemented stems are recommended.

Finally, late functional decline has been reported by several authors as potentially a result of deltoid fatigue over time, which may occur progressively or as a late drop off. Multiple authors have reported decline in functional outcomes as determined by the Constant score overtime after an RSA. Bassens et al. reported on 126 primary Delta Xtend protheses and a 97% survivorship at an average of 8 years follow-up, although the Constant scores were significantly lower at the final follow-up as compared to the 5-year follow-up [30]. Guery et al. reported on 80 RSAs, and, at 120 months follow-up, there was 91% survivorship [31]. The authors reported that the survivorship as a Constant score greater than 30 was only 58% at 120 months, noting a significant decline in Constant scores at approximately 6 years postoperatively [31]. Bacle et al. reported long-term follow-up on 186 RSAs with a minimum follow-up of 10 years and noted a 93% survivorship at 10 years [32]. The authors also noted a significant decline in Constant scores in comparison with the authors of the earlier publication of the same cohort with a minimum of 2-year follow-up [32]. Schoch et al. evaluated the concept of deltoid fatigue by evaluating 165 RSAs over a 5-year period [33]. The authors reported a 0.8° loss of forward elevation and abduction per year starting at year 1 postoperatively without a significant drop at mid-term follow-up, thus supporting a progressive decline in function as opposed to a mid-term drop [33]. Irrespective of whether the decline occurs progressively or due to a mid-term drop, its etiology is unclear. Jang et al. performed a meta-analysis evaluating the impact of scapula notching on outcomes after RSA and determined that notching has a negative effect on Constant scores, ASES scores, and forward elevation and abduction [34]. Consequently, notching may have a direct impact on the long-term functionality of an RSA, and constructs should be chosen to limit notching to optimize long-term outcomes.

2.5 Conclusions

Multiple early and late complications can lead to failure after an RSA. Choosing between an aTSA and an RSA often means accepting different mechanisms of failure as opposed to one having an increased risk of failure compared to the other. Understanding patients at risk of failure is critical to optimizing success after an RSA. Patients with poor humeral bone and RSA after prior surgery are at a higher risk of failure, and, as such, they should be consulted regarding expectations. Optimizing medical comorbidities can have a significant impact on reducing early readmission and length of stay after an RSA. Infection, acromial fracture, instability, implant loosening, and late functional decline are all recognized etiologies of RSA failure. Understanding the risk factors for each of these factors will allow surgeons to optimize preventative treatments for each of these potential failure mechanisms to optimize outcomes.

References

1. Zumstein MA, Pinedo M, Old J, Boileau P. Problems, complications, reoperations, and revisions in reverse total shoulder arthroplasty: a systematic review. J Shoulder Elb Surg. 2011;20:146–57.
2. Wagner ER, Farley KX, Higgins I, Wilson JM, Daly CA, Gottschalk MB. The incidence of shoulder arthroplasty: rise and future projections compared with hip and knee arthroplasty. J Shoulder Elb Surg. 2020;29:2601–9.

3. Day JS, Lau E, Ong KL, Williams GR, Ramsey ML, Kurtz SM. Prevalence and projections of total shoulder and elbow arthroplasty in the United States to 2015. J Shoulder Elb Surg. 2010;19:1115–20.
4. Farley KX, Wilson JM, Kumar A, Gottschalk MB, Daly C, Sanchez-Sotelo J, Wagner ER. Prevalence of shoulder arthroplasty in the United States and the increasing burden of revision shoulder arthroplasty. JBJS Open Access. 2021;6(3):e20.00156.
5. Gauci MO, Cavalier M, Gonzalez JF, Holzer N, Baring T, Walch G, Boileau P. J Shoulder Elb Surg. 2020;29:541–9.
6. Kang JR, Dubiel MJ, Cofield RH, Steinmann SP, Elhassan BT, Morrey ME, Sperling JW, Sanchez-Sotelo J. Primary reverse shoulder arthroplasty using contemporary implants is associated with very low reoperation rates. J Shoulder Elb Surg. 2019;28(6S):S175–80.
7. Heifner JJ, Kumar AD, Wagner ER. Glenohumeral osteoarthritis with intact rotator cuff treated with reverse shoulder arthroplasty: a systematic review. J Shoulder Elb Surg. 2021;30(12):2895–903.
8. Petrillo S, Longo UG, Papalia R, Denaro V. Reverse shoulder arthroplasty for massive irreparable rotator cuff tears and cuff tear arthropathy: a systematic review. Musculoskelet Surg. 2017;101(2):105–12.
9. Parada AS, Flurin PH, Wright TW, Zuckerman JD, Elwell JHA, Roche CP, Friedman RJ. Comparison of complication types and rates associated with anatomic and reverse total shoulder arthroplasty. J Shoulder Elb Surg. 2021;30(4):811–8.
10. Aibinder W, Schoch B, Parsons M, Watling J, Ko JK, Gobbato B, Throckmorton T, Routman H, Fan W, Simmons C, Roche C. Risks factors for complications and revision surgery after anatomic and reverse total shoulder arthroplasty. J Shoulder Elb Surg. 2021;30(11):e689–701.
11. Poondla RK, Sheth MM, Heldt BL, Laughlin MS, Morris BJ, Elkousy HA, Edwards TB. Anatomic and reverse shoulder arthroplasty in patients 70 years of age and older: a comparison cohort at early to midterm follow-up. J Shoulder Elb Surg. 2021;30(6):1336–43.
12. Kiet TK, Feeley BT, Naimark M, Gajiu T, Hall SL, Chung TT, Ma CB. Outcomes after shoulder replacement: comparison between reverse and anatomic total shoulder arthroplasty. J Shoulder Elb Surg. 2015;24(2):179–85.
13. Burnett RA, Goltz DE, Levin JM, Wickman JR, Howell CB, Nicholson GP, Verma NN, Anakwenze OA, Lassiter TE Jr, Klifto CS, Garrigues GE. Characteristics and risk factors for 90-day readmission following shoulder arthroplasty. J Shoulder Elb Surg. 2022;31(2):324–32.
14. Burns KA, Robbins LM, LeMarr AR, Fortune K, Morton DJ, Wilson ML. Modifiable risk factors increase length of stay and 90-day cost of care after shoulder arthroplasty. J Shoulder Elb Surg. 2022;31(1):2–7.
15. Seok HG, Park JJ, Park SG. Risk factors for periprosthetic joint infection after shoulder arthroplasty: systematic review and meta-analysis. J Clin Med. 2022;11(14):4245.
16. Shah SS, Gaal BT, Roche AM, Namdari S, Grawe BM, Lawler M, Dalton S, King JJH, Helmkamp J, Garigues GE, Wright TW, Schoch BS, Flik K, Otto RJ, Jones R, Jawa A, McCann P, Abboud J, Horneff G, Ross G, Friedman R, Ricchetti ET, Boardman D, Tashjian RZ, Gulotta LV. The modern reverse shoulder arthroplasty and an updated systematic review for each complication: part I. JSES Int. 2020;4(4):929–43.
17. ASES Complications of RSA Research Group. Predictors of acromial and scapular stress fracture after reverse shoulder arthroplasty: a study by the ASES complications of RSA multicenter research group. J Shoulder Elb Surg. 2021;30(10):2296–305.
18. Miller M, Chalmers PN, Nyfeler J, Mhyre L, Wheelwright C, Konery K, Kawakami J, Tashjian RZ. Rheumatoid arthritis is associated with increased symptomatic acromial and scapular spine stress fracture after reverse total shoulder arthroplasty. JSES Int. 2020;5(2):261–5.
19. Shah SS, Roche AM, Sullivan SW, Gaal BT, Dalton S, Sharma A, King JJ, Grawe BM, Namdari S, Lawler M, Helmkamp J, Garrigues GE, Wright TW, Schoch BS, Flik K, Otto RJ, Jones R, Jawa A, McCann P, Abboud J, Horneff G, Ross G, Friedman R, Ricchetti ET, Boardman D, Tashjian RZ, Gulotta LV. The modern reverse shoulder arthroplasty and an updated systematic review for each complication: part II. JSES Int. 2020;5(1):121–37.
20. Padegimas EM, Zmistowski BM, Restrepo C, Abboud JÁ, Lazarus MD, Ramsey ML, Williams GR, Namdari S. Instability after reverse total shoulder arthroplasty: which patients dislocate? Am J Orthop (Belle Mead NJ). 2016;45(7):E444–50.
21. Kohan EM, Chalmers PN, Salazar D, Keener JD, Yamaguchi K, Chamberlain AM. Dislocation following reverse total shoulder arthroplasty. J Shoulder Elb Surg. 2017;26(7):1238–45.
22. Boileau P, Seeto BL, Clowez G, Gauci MO, Trojani C, Walch G, Chelli M. SECEC Grammont award 2017: the prejudicial effect of greater tuberosity osteotomy or excision in reverse shoulder arthroplasty for fracture sequelae. J Shoulder Elb Surg. 2020;29(12):2446–58.
23. Ladermann A, Williams MD, Melis B, Hoffmeyer P, Walch G. Objective evaluation of lengthening in reverse shoulder arthroplasty. J Shoulder Elb Surg. 2009;18(4):588–95.
24. Gutierrez S, Walker M, Willis M, Pupello DR, Frankle MA. Effects of tilt and glenosphere eccentricity on baseplate/bone interface forces in a computational model, validated by a mechanical model, of reverse shoulder arthroplasty. J Shoulder Elb Surg. 2011;20(5):732–9.
25. Ho JC, Thakar O, Chan WW, Nicholson T, Williams GR, Namdari S. Early radiographic failure of reverse total shoulder arthroplasty with structural bone graft for glenoid bone loss. J Shoulder Elb

Surg. 2020;29(3):550–60. https://doi.org/10.1016/j.jse.2019.07.035. Epub 2019 Oct 11.
26. Morwood MP, Johnston PS, Garrigues GE. Proximal ingrowth coating decreases risk of loosening following uncemented shoulder arthroplasty using mini-stem humeral components and lesser tuberosity osteotomy. J Shoulder Elb Surg. 2017;26(7):1246–52. https://doi.org/10.1016/j.jse.2016.11.041. Epub 2017 Jan 31.
27. Cuff D, Levy JC, Gutiérrez S, Frankle MA. Torsional stability of modular and non-modular reverse shoulder humeral components in a proximal humeral bone loss model. J Shoulder Elb Surg. 2011;20(4):646–51. https://doi.org/10.1016/j.jse.2010.10.026. Epub 2011 Jan 13.
28. Melis B, DeFranco M, Lädermann A, Molé D, Favard L, Nérot C, Maynou C, Walch G. An evaluation of the radiological changes around the Grammont reverse geometry shoulder arthroplasty after eight to 12 years. J Bone Joint Surg Br. 2011;93(9):1240–6. https://doi.org/10.1302/0301-620X.93B9.25926.
29. Werthel JD, Lonjon G, Jo S, Cofield R, Sperling JW, Elhassan BT. Long-term outcomes of cemented *versus* cementless humeral components in arthroplasty of the shoulder: a propensity score-matched analysis. Bone Joint J. 2017;99-B(5):666–73. https://doi.org/10.1302/0301-620X.99B5.BJJ-2016-0910.R1. Erratum in: Bone Joint J. 2018;100-B(9):1260.
30. Bassens D, Decock T, Van Tongel A, De Wilde L. Long-term results of the Delta Xtend reverse shoulder prosthesis. J Shoulder Elb Surg. 2019;28(6):1091–7. https://doi.org/10.1016/j.jse.2018.11.043. Epub 2019 Feb 1.
31. Guery J, Favard L, Sirveaux F, Oudet D, Mole D, Walch G. Reverse total shoulder arthroplasty. Survivorship analysis of eighty replacements followed for five to ten years. J Bone Joint Surg Am. 2006;88(8):1742–7. https://doi.org/10.2106/JBJS.E.00851.
32. Bacle G, Nové-Josserand L, Garaud P, Walch G. Long-term outcomes of reverse Total shoulder arthroplasty: a follow-up of a previous study. J Bone Joint Surg Am. 2017;99(6):454–61. https://doi.org/10.2106/JBJS.16.00223.
33. Schoch BS, Vigan M, Roche CP, Parsons M, Wright TW, King JJ, Werthel JD. Deltoid fatigue: a longitudinal assessment of reverse shoulder arthroplasty over time. J Shoulder Elb Surg. 2021;30(6):1375–83. https://doi.org/10.1016/j.jse.2020.08.038. Epub 2020 Sep 16
34. Jang YH, Lee JH, Kim SH. Effect of scapular notching on clinical outcomes after reverse total shoulder arthroplasty. Bone Joint J. 2020;102-B(11):1438–45. https://doi.org/10.1302/0301-620X.102B11.BJJ-2020-0449.R1.

Shoulder Hemiarthroplasties: How Do They Fail

3

Juan David Lacouture, Aníbal Debandi, and Pascal Boileau

3.1 Introduction

Primary shoulder hemiarthroplasty (HA) is commonly performed to treat various shoulder disorders, including glenohumeral arthritis, avascular necrosis, capsulorrhaphy arthropathy, and proximal humeral fractures [1]. HA is a treatment option for shoulder disorders, especially in younger and active patients who are difficult to treat because they have high physical demands and high expectations [2]. Additionally, they need pain relief to reduce restrictions when lifting objects using the operated upper extremity [3].

The increasing number of shoulder arthroplasties performed in the last decade is related to the number of revisions. In 2018, approximately 4000 cases of shoulder arthroplasties were performed in Germany, and this was equally observed in other countries regardless of the health-care systems [4, 5]. In total shoulder arthroplasty (TSA), more than one-third of reported complications are due to glenoid component loosening (37% of complications) and lead to a revision in 18% of the cases [6]. Regarding HA, different revision rates have been reported, ranging from 0 to 25% [1, 7]. The most frequent indications for HA revision are symptomatic erosion of the glenoid (Fig. 3.1), rotator cuff tear (mainly subscapularis tear; Fig. 3.2), and proximal humerus fracture sequelae or migration of the tuberosities (Fig. 3.3).

Heterogeneous data related to the indications for revision surgery for HA have been reported in the literature. Furthermore, no long-term comparative results on the use of associated procedures (glenoid reaming), different materials used (metal or pyrocarbon head), or the impact on the HA survival rate have been described.

This study aimed to perform a systematic review to (1) describe the overall revision rate, (2) identify indications for revision of shoulder HA, and (3) describe the overall revision rate in HA with glenoid reaming and HA with a pyrocarbon head.

We hypothesize that there will be a high rate of HA revisions caused by glenoid complications and a high rate of revisions to TSA.

J. D. Lacouture (✉)
ICR-Institut de Chirurgie Réparatrice – Groupe KANTYS, Institute for Sports & Reconstructive Surgery, Nice, France

Department of Orthopaedic Surgery, Hospital Serena del Mar, Cartagena, Serena del Mar, Colombia

A. Debandi
Department of Orthopaedic Surgery, Hospital Clínico Universidad de Chile, Santiago, Chile

Department of Orthopaedic surgery, Hospital Serena del Mar, Cartagena, Serena del Mar, Colombia
e-mail: anibal.debandi@meds.cl

P. Boileau
ICR-Institut de Chirurgie Réparatrice – Groupe KANTYS, Institute for Sports & Reconstructive Surgery, Nice, France
e-mail: pr.boileau@icr-nice.com

F. Franceschi et al. (eds.), *Revision Shoulder Arthroplasty*,
https://doi.org/10.1007/978-3-031-45944-3_3

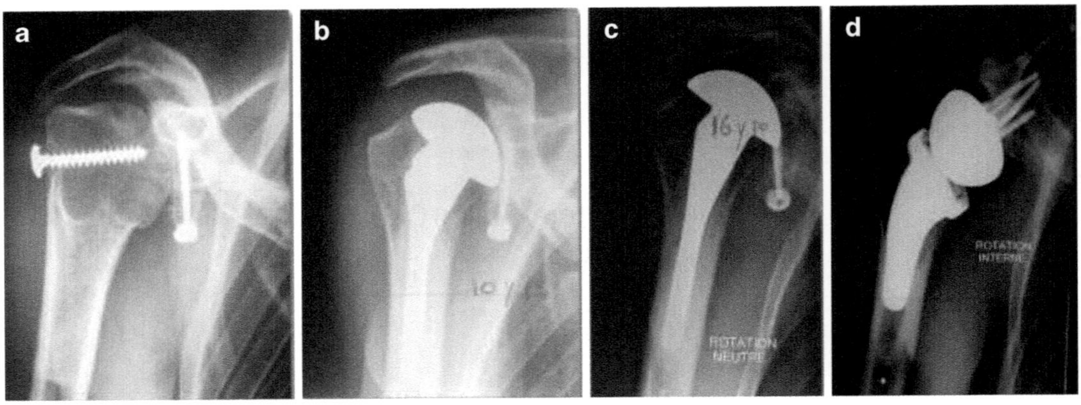

Fig. 3.1 (**a**) Post-instability arthritis of a 47-year-old patient. (**b**) A 10-year follow-up X-ray image of hemiarthroplasty. (**c**) Image of a 16-year follow-up, glenoid erosion Sperling type 4, in a patient with symptomatic glenoid erosion. (**d**) Reverse shoulder arthroplasty as the patient treatment

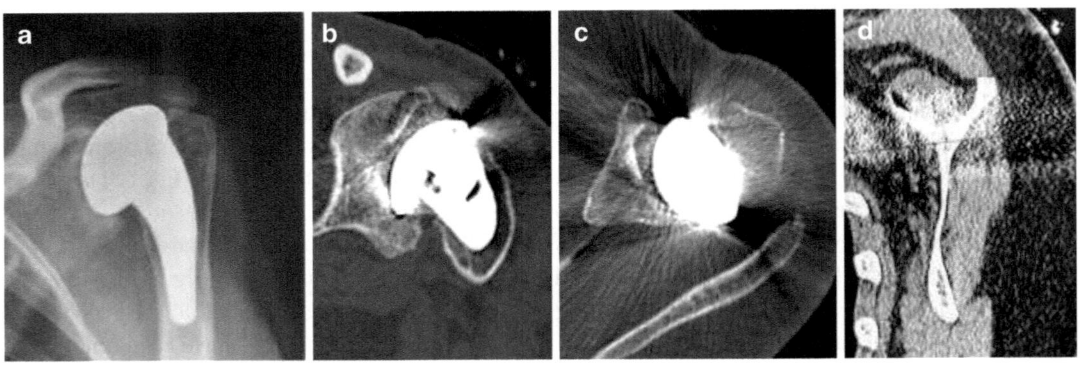

Fig. 3.2 (**a**) An X-ray image with a decreased acromiohumeral interval less than 7 mm, glenoid erosion Sperling classification type 4. (**b** and **c**) Severe glenoid erosion at the level of the base of the coracoid. (**d**) A sagittal view of the computed tomography (CT) scan image, muscle atrophy supraspinatus stage 3, and subscapularis stage 4

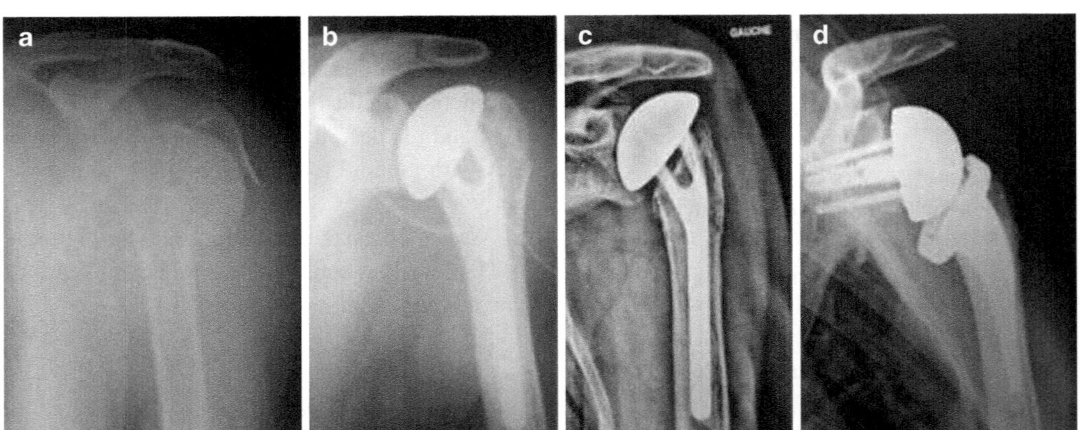

Fig. 3.3 (**a**) Proximal humerus fracture in three fragments of a 52-year-old patient. (**b**) A post-op X-ray image of hemiarthroplasty with tuberosity reconstruction. (**c**) Two years follow-up with tuberosity resorption in a patient with loss of elevation. (**d**) Reverse shoulder arthroplasty as the patient treatment

3.2 Methods

3.2.1 Study Design

A systematic review of HA complications was conducted to investigate the study hypothesis. The PRISMA (Preferred Reporting Items for Systematic Reviews and Meta-Analyses) guidelines were followed to evaluate and assess the study methodology [8].

3.2.2 Search Strategy

A systematic review was conducted by two independent reviewers according to the PRISMA guidelines [8]. On October 2, 2022, a literature search was conducted using the MEDLINE and EMBASE databases. The following field search terms were used based on the Boolean strategy: search ((Shoulder) AND (Complications) AND (Hemiarthroplasty)). The previous 20 years were specified as the time limit for publication. Any reference in the included studies that was missed by the initial search criteria was checked for potential inclusion.

3.2.3 Eligibility Criteria

Studies were included if they met the following criteria, as verified by two independent reviewers: (1) written in English, (2) available in full text, (3) cohort >18 years of age, (4) clinical studies of shoulder HA, and (5) reported complications as an outcome. The exclusion criteria were as follows: (1) comparative studies, (2) no report of complications, (3) acute proximal humerus fractures, and (4) biological interpositional HA.

3.2.4 Study Selection

The titles and abstracts returned from the initial database search were independently reviewed by two reviewers (J.D.L. and A.D.) against the inclusion and exclusion criteria. Based on the initial query, full-text articles were reviewed for those that met the inclusion criteria. In the event of a disagreement between the reviewers, a senior reviewer (P.B.) made the final decision. In studies with overlapping subject populations, the most recent publication was included for further analysis.

3.2.5 Definitions

A "revision" was defined as a procedure in which prosthetic components were entirely or partially exchanged or removed. A "reoperation" was defined as a surgical intervention without modification of the glenoid or humeral implant. A "reintervention" was either a revision or a reoperation [7].

3.2.6 Method of Review and Data Extraction

Complete versions of the selected publications were extracted by two authors and collected by reviewers using a predetermined datasheet. The study characteristics (year, authors, level of evidence, Methodological Index for Nonrandomized Studies (MINORS) [9]), patient demographic data (number of shoulders or patients, mean age, mean duration of follow-up), surgical technique (glenoid reaming), prosthesis characteristics, humeral head material, cemented or uncemented stem, reintervention surgery, reoperation surgery, indication for reoperation, revision surgery, indication for revision, and clinical outcomes were all tabulated.

3.2.7 Quality Assessment

The level of evidence for each study was evaluated based on the guidelines of the Oxford Centre for Evidence-Based Medicine [10]. The methodological quality of the articles included in this systematic review was assessed using the MINORS [9], a validated tool to discern the methodological quality of nonrandomized studies. The highest possible scores were 16 and 24 for non-comparative and comparative studies, respectively. Two authors independently applied MINORS, and the final score was determined by consensus.

3.2.8 Statistical Methods

Based on the heterogeneous nature of the studies included in this systematic review, according to techniques and outcome reporting, the studies with nonrandomized design and relatively low quality of their pooled statistics, including weighted means and standard deviations, were not reported to avoid describing potentially inaccurate conclusions. Ranges in objective outcomes (reinterventions, reoperations, and revision surgery) have been reported. Sub-analyses were performed to investigate the influence of the technique (reaming or non-reaming surgery) and the use of different humeral head materials in HA.

3.3 Results

3.3.1 Search Results

Of the 725 articles initially identified, 20 studies met the eligibility criteria. A PRISMA flow diagram detailing study identification, screening (title, abstract, and full text), and inclusion is provided in Fig. 3.4 [8]. Bias assessment was completed using the MINORS scoring criteria with a mean score of 11 ± 1.3 (7–15) [9].

3.3.2 Demographic Data

In the systematic review, we reported 920 patients (936 shoulders) that underwent surgery for HA. The age of the patients ranged from 32 to 72 years, with 369 males and 439 females, and the mean follow-up duration was 108 months (12–206 months) (Table 3.1). The main indications for HA were primary osteoarthritis (OA), cuff tear arthropathy, rheumatoid arthritis, and osteonecrosis (Table 3.2).

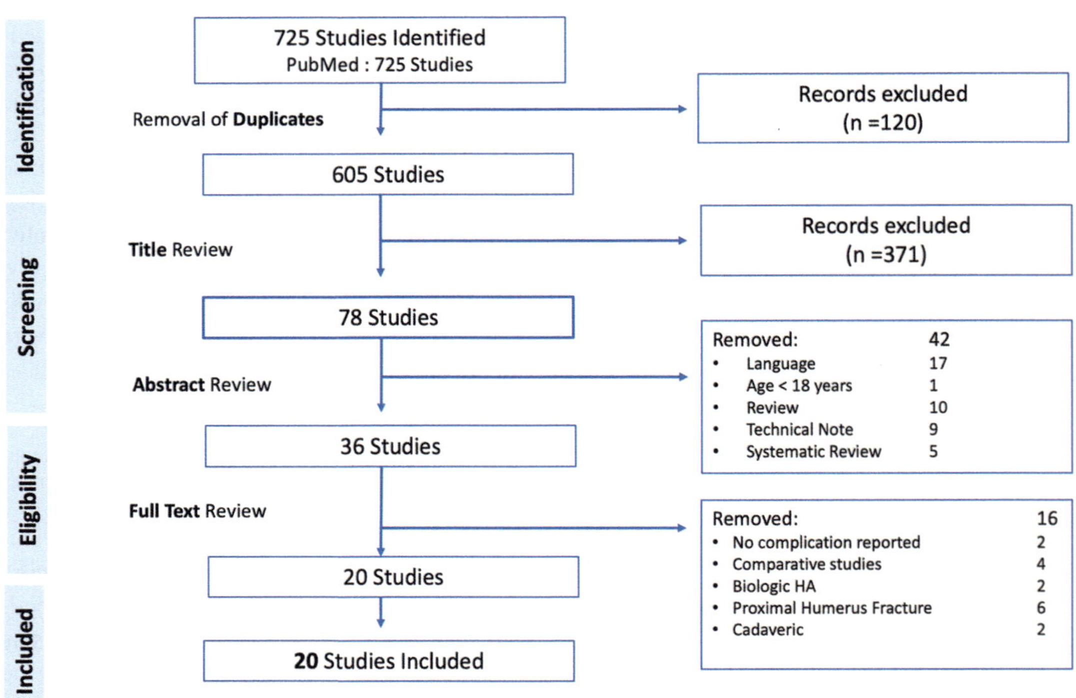

Fig. 3.4 Preferred Reporting Items for Systematic Review and Meta-Analyses (PRISMA) flow diagram

Table 3.1 Demographic and clinical data of included studies

Author	Year	LOE				Total cases		Follow-up		Age		Gender	
		1	2	3	4	Patients	Shoulders	Months	Range	Years	Range	Male	Female
Cointat et al. [13]	2022	0	0	0	1	62	64	33	24–60	53	25–60	20	44
Ibrahim et al. [14]	2018	0	0	0	1	11	14	125	70–167	36	19–49	2	13
Garret et al. [11]	2019	0	0	0	1	65	65	25.9		58.0	19–84		
Irlenbusch et al. [23]	2019	0	0	1	0	115	120	92.4	2.6–148.5	65.2	37.6–87.2	30	85
Tsitlakidis et al. [22]	2021	0	0	0	1	16	NS	24	10–36	53	29–65	7	9
Virk et al. [15]	2018	0	0	1	0	21	23	37		54	40–67	19	2
Robinson et al. [3]	2018	0	0	0	1	42	44	204	120–360	58	37–77	28	16
Getz et al. [16]	2017	0	0	0	1	23	24	44	28–59	50	32–62		
Leung et al. [24]	2017	0	0	1	0	92	97	12	NS	68.7	33–90	48	49
Herschel et al. [12]	2017	0	0	1	0	113	118	31	5–86	62	17–90	51	67
Levine et al. [17]	2012	0	0	0	1	30	31	206.4	156–252	51	26–81	15	15
Saltzman et al. [18]	2011	0	0	0	1	64	64	24	NS	46	27–55	59	6
Bonnevialle et al. [21]	2011	0	0	0	1	9	10	71	28–126	54	44–73	NS	NS
Rees et al. [28]	2010	0	0	1	0	72	72	36	72	69.9	27–88	12	60
Smith et al. [25]	2008	0	0	0	1	31	25	144	NS	49.4	25–86	9	23
Goldberg et al. [26]	2008	0	0	0	1	31	34	44.4	NS	72	48–90	12	22
Lynch et al. [19]	2007	0	0	0	1	37	38	32.4	24–48	57	35–80	31	3
Krepler et al. [29]	2006	0	0	0	1	35	35	72	24–216	62	29–87	NS	NS
Wirth et al. [20]	2006	0	0	0	1	43	50	44		63	44–78	25	18
Thomas et al. [27]	2005	0	0	0	1	8	8	72	59–89	32	25–50	1	7
Total		0	0	5	15	920	936	68.7		55.7		369	439

LOE level of evidence; *NS* nonsignificant

Table 3.2 Indications for hemiarthroplasty (HA)

	Indications								
Author	CTA	OA	Instability OA	Posttraumatic OA	FS	RA	Osteonecrosis	Juvenile idiopathic arthritis	Glenoid dysplasia
Cointat et al. [13]		20	15	13		3	13		
Ibrahim et al. [14]								11	
Garret et al. [11]		37				2	11		
Irlenbusch et al. [23]		60	19		16	17	8		
Tsitlakidis et al. [22]		10				2	4		
Virk et al. [15]		21							
Robinson et al. [3]		44							
Getz et al. [16]		23							
Leung et al. [24]	83					9			
Herschel et al. [12]						11			
Levine et al. [17]		9	4	7			10		
Saltzman et al. [18]		31	16	2		1			1
Bonnevialle et al. [21]									9
Rees et al. [28]	22	19				31			
Smith et al. [25]							32		
Goldberg et al. [26]	34								
Lynch et al. [19]		26	5	4					
Krepler et al. [29]		11		10		14	1		
Wirth et al. [20]	4	32					5		
Thomas et al. [27]								8	
Total	143	343	59	36	16	90	84	19	10

CTA cuff tear arthropathy; *OA* osteoarthritis; *FS* fracture sequalae; *RA* rheumatoid arthritis; *ON* osteonecrosis

3.3.3 Technique

Regarding technique, ten studies reported subscapularis management, mainly by peeling of the subscapularis, described in eight studies [11–20]. Regarding biceps management, five studies reported tenotomy or tenodesis of the biceps [11, 13–16]. Table 3.3 shows the prosthesis characteristics, humeral head material, cemented or uncemented status, and glenoid reaming.

3.3.4 Early vs. Late Complications

Among the patients in the included studies, 60% developed early complications (<24 months) and 40% developed late complications (>24 months). The early complications identified were pain (43%), stiffness (17%), rotator cuff injury (30%), and other causes (10%), whereas the late complications identified were pain (80%), posterior instability (10%), rotator cuff injury (5%), and stiffness (5%). Unfortunately, the etiology of pain was not classified between painful glenoid wear and unexplained severe pain in most of the included papers.

3.3.5 Revision Procedures

The overall revision rate after HA ranged from 0 to 25%, with a mean of 12.5%. The mean revision-free HA survival rate was 87.5% after 9 years. The major revisions were HA (16%), TSA (59%), and RSA (23%) (Table 3.4). Robinson et al., Getz et al., and Levine et al. reported higher revision rates of 22%, 25%, and 25.8%, respectively [3, 16, 17], and a longer follow-up (>2 years) in these studies. The indications for revision surgery were symptomatic glenoid erosion, rotator cuff tear (mainly subscapularis tear), and stiffness in 62%, 13%, and 8% of patients, respectively.

3.3.6 Reoperation Procedures

The overall reoperation rate after HA ranged from 0 to 14%, with a mean of 7%. The main reoperations performed were subacromial release (43%), repeated glenoid reaming (29%), and pectoralis major transfer (21%) (Table 3.5). Ibrahim et al. and Bonnevialle et al. reported higher reoperation rates of 14% and 10%, respectively [14, 21], with reoperation occurring within the first 6 months of surgery. The indications for reoperation surgery were symptomatic glenoid erosion (12%), impingement (12%), and subscapularis tear (12%). The indications for reoperation were not described in 60% of the cases (Table 3.5).

3.3.7 The Glenoid Reaming Procedure

Six studies reported glenoid reaming-associated outcomes [13, 15, 16, 18–20] and described revision rates ranging from 0 to 25% and reoperation rates ranging from 0 to 6.3%. A total of 14 studies did not use glenoid reaming and described revision rates ranging from 0 to 25.8% and reoperation rates ranging from 0 to 14.3% [3, 11, 12, 14, 17, 21–29]. Finally, no difference based on the indication of revision was found, with glenoid erosion being the main indication for both groups.

Regarding the head prosthesis material, three studies reported performing HA using pyrocarbon head material and reported revisions rates ranging from 4.6 to 7.8% and 0% reoperations.

Table 3.3 Prosthesis characteristics

Author	Prosthesis	Head		Stem		Reaming	
		Metal	PyC	Cemented	Uncemented	No	Yes
Cointat et al. [13]	Aequalis ascend flex stem (Tornier-Wright, Memphis, TN, USA)		1	1	1	1	1
Ibrahim et al. [14]	Copeland, Biomet	1			1	1	
Garret et al. [11]	Aequalis ascend flex stem (Tornier-Wright, Memphis, TN, USA)		1			1	
Irlenbusch et al. [23]	Affinis, Mathys, Bettlach, Switzerland	1		1	1	1	
Tsitlakidis et al. [22]	Aequalis ascend flex stem (Tornier-Wright, Memphis, TN, USA)		1		1	1	
Virk et al. [15]	DePuy global shoulder modular prosthesis	1					1
Robinson et al. [3]	25 Neer (3 M), 16 Cofield (Smith & Nephew), 3 Bimodular (Biomet)	1			1		
Getz CL et al. [16]	Tornier [14] and Depuy [10]	1			1		1
Leung AS et al. [24]	CTA hemiarthroplasty	1				1	
Herschel R et al. [12]	Zimmer anatomical shoulder system (Zimmer Inc., Warsaw, IN, USA)	1				1	
Levine et al. [17]	–	1					
Saltzman et al. [18]	DePuy global shoulder modular prosthesis	1			1		1
Bonnevialle et al. [21]	Four Neer II and six Neer 3 (Smith & Nephew, Memphis, TN)	1		1			
Rees et al. [28]	Corin, Cirencester, UK	1					
Smith et al. [25]	–	1				1	
Goldberg et al. [26]	–	1		1		1	
Lynch et al. [19]	DePuy global shoulder modular prosthesis	1					1
Krepler et al. [29]	Neer type (3 M, Switzerland)	1		1	1		
Wirth et al. [20]	DePuy global shoulder modular prosthesis	1		1			1
Thomas et al. [27]	Biomet Merck	1		1	1	1	
Total		17	3	7	9	10	6

PyC pyrocarbon

Table 3.4 Revision

	Follow-up						Revision					
Author	*n*	Months	Time (months)	Range (months)	Complications	Percentage (%)	*n*	Percentage (%)	Revision HA	Revisions to RSA	Revisions to TSA	Spacer
Cointat et al. [13]	64	33	24	15–37	5	7.8	5	7.8		4	1	
Ibrahim et al. [14]	14	125	6		2	14.3	0	0.0				
Garret et al. [11]	65	25.9	16		3	4.6	0	0.0				
Irlenbusch et al. [23]	120	92.4			16	13.3	11	9.2	6		5	
Tsitlakidis et al. [22]	16	24			1	6.3	1	6.3	1			
Virk et al. [15]	23	37			1	4.3	1	4.3			1	
Robinson et al. [3]	44	204	84		11	25.0	10	22.7	1		9	
Getz et al. [16]	24	44			6	25.0	6	25.0	1		5	
Leung et al. [24]	97	12	3		8	8.2	8	8.2		8		
Herschel et al. [12]	118	31			12	10.2	12	10.2	1	4	7	
Levine et al. [17]	31	206.4			8	25.8	8	25.8			8	
Saltzman et al. [18]	64	24	31	8–55	9	14.1	6	9.4		1	4	1
Bonnevialle et al. [21]	10	71	6		1	10.0		0.0				
Rees et al. [28]	72	36			0	0.0		0.0				
Smith et al. [25]	25	144			2	8.0	2	8.0			2	
Goldberg et al. [26]	34	44.4			2	5.9	1	2.9			1	
Lynch et al. [19]	38	32.4	8		1	2.6	0	0.0				
Krepler et al. [29]	35	72			5	14.3	2	5.7	2			
Wirth et al. [20]	50	44	24		4	8.0	1	2.0		0	1	
Thomas et al. [27]	8	72			1	12.5	0	0.0		0	0	
Total	952	68.7	22			0–25%	74	0–25%	12	17	44	1

HA hemiarthroplasty; *RSA* reverse shoulder arthroplasty; *TSA* total shoulder arthroplasty

Table 3.5 Reoperation

Author	Follow-up						Reoperation					
	n	Months	Time (months)	Range (months)	Complications	Percentage (%)	*n*	Percentage (%)	Pectoralis major transfer	Repeat reaming	Subacromial release	Resection of unwanted bone contact
Cointat et al. [13]	64	33	24	15–37	5	7.8	0	0.0				
Ibrahim et al. [14]	14	125	6		2	14.3	2	14.3			2	
Garret et al. [11]	65	25.9	16		3	4.6	3	4.6				
Irlenbusch et al. [23]	120	92.4			16	13.3	0	0.0				
Tsitlakidis et al. [22]	16	24			1	6.3	0	0.0				
Virk et al. [15]	23	37			1	4.3		0.0				
Robinson et al. [3]	44	204	84		11	25.0	1	2.3			1	
Getz et al. [16]	24	44			6	25.0		0.0				
Leung et al. [24]	97	12	3		8	8.2		0.0				
Herschel et al. [12]	118	31			12	10.2	0	0.0				
Levine et al. [17]	31	206.4			8	25.8	0	0.0				
Saltzman et al. [18]	64	24	31	8–55	9	14.1	4	6.3		2	1	1
Bonnevialle et al. [21]	10	71	6		1	10.0	1	10.0			1	
Rees et al. [28]	72	36			0	0.0		0.0				
Smith et al. [25]	25	144			2	8.0		0.0				
Goldberg et al. [26]	34	44.4			2	5.9	1	2.9		1		
Lynch et al. [19]	38	32.4	8		1	2.6	1	2.6		1		
Krepler et al. [29]	35	72			5	14.3	1	2.9	1			
Wirth et al. [20]	50	44	24		4	8.0	3	6.0	2		1	
Thomas et al. [27]	8	72			1	12.5	0	0.0				
Total	952	68.7	22			0–25%	17	0–14%	3	4	6	1

3.4 Discussion

The most important findings of this systematic review were as follows: (1) the overall revision rate of shoulder HA ranged from 0 to 25%, with a mean revision-free HA survivorship rate of 87.5% after 9 years. Approximately 59% of the cases revised to TSA, and (2) the main indication for revision was symptomatic glenoid erosion in 62% of the cases.

Three studies [3, 16, 17] showed higher revision rates of up to 25%. Robinson et al. [3] reported long-term outcomes (10-year minimum follow-up) with a revision rate of 22.7% predominantly for glenoid arthrosis, with moderate-to-severe glenoid erosion of 50% after 5 years, which increased to 59% after 15 years and to 88% after 20 years. They described glenoid wear as the leading cause of revision in long-term follow-up, with an implant survival rate of 75% after 20–25 years [3]. Levine et al. [17], in an average follow-up duration of 7.2 years, reported a revision rate of 25% and also that 25% of patients were satisfied after the procedure in the longest follow-up. The outcomes related to glenoid wear (with an average Neer score and Neer rating) for unrevised cases were significantly higher for concentric glenoid wear than for eccentric glenoid wear [17]. The studies by Robinson et al. [3] and Levine et al. [17] were the ones with the longest follow-up reporting revisions, with a mean clinical follow-up of 17 years and 17.2 years, respectively, which could explain the higher rate of revisions and decreased survival rate associated with longer follow-up.

Different conditions were related to the outcomes of glenoid erosion. Valgus positioning of the humeral component was associated with increased glenoid erosion, as reported by Herschel et al. [12]. Nevertheless, favorable conditions for resistance to erosion after HA were lack of glenoid cysts, intact glenoid cartilage, intact rotator cuff musculature, and fractures [12]. With regard to the position of the humeral head, studies have used different definitions for anatomic or nonanatomic reconstruction and how this has influenced the outcomes. Cointat et al. [13], in a case series, reported nonanatomic reconstruction of the proximal humerus (center of rotation of the prosthesis >3 mm from the anatomic center) in 29% of patients, which was associated with lower functional and subjective outcomes, more complications (subscapularis insufficiency and/or symptomatic glenoid erosion), and a higher risk of revision. They concluded that this nonanatomic reconstruction might be explained by the additional 1.5-mm thickness of the metal disc under the pyrocarbon head prosthesis used [13].

Techniques of concentric glenoid reaming have been reported, mainly based on orienting the reamer to the normalized glenoid centerline, enabling the surgeon to correct the pathological glenoid version and create a concentric and smooth glenoid surface as reported by Wirth et al. [20]. Other authors like Saltzman et al. [18], Virk et al. [15], and Lynch et al. [19] have described the denominated "ream and run procedure" revisions rates of 14.1%, 0%, and 2.6%, respectively. Regarding glenoid retroversion correction, Getz et al. [16] reported outcomes of concentric glenoid reaming in the B2 biconcave glenoid with revision rates of 25% after 2.7 years of follow-up. Cointat et al. [13] reported a 7.8% revision rate and concentric glenoid reaming in 36% of patients (28% type B or C glenoids), showing similar Constant scores and subjective shoulder values to those of the other patients and did not show more progression of glenoid wear. The use of associated reaming for creating a concentric glenoid and retroversion correction are options. However, a longer follow-up is needed to compare survival rates.

The pyrocarbon head prosthesis has been approved for clinical use in Europe and Australia; however, it is unavailable in the United States. The mechanical properties of the pyrocarbon-bearing surface material (moduli of elasticity and density) are similar to those of the cortical bone, which makes it ideal for implant-bone stress transfer [30]. The use of a pyrocarbon head prosthesis in HA was reported by Cointat et al. [13], who referred to five (8%) patients who underwent revision surgery mainly for cuff insufficiency or subscapularis tearing. Furthermore, Tsitlakidis et al. [22] and Garret et al. [11], in a short-term follow-up, reported the use of pyrocarbon head prosthesis in HA and described revision rates of 6.3% and 4.6%, respectively.

The use of this material may be an option for treating glenoid erosion. Nevertheless, longer follow-up and comparative studies are required.

Although TSA has a good survival rate in short- and long-term follow-ups [3], there are different conditions related to poor outcomes and complications (mainly related to the glenoid implant) in active and young patients or in case of a biconcave glenoid. HA may be the treatment of choice in this group of patients. However, associated procedures (i.e., glenoid reaming) and materials (i.e., pyrocarbon) should be studied to validate the improvement in outcomes, especially in symptomatic glenoid erosion.

3.4.1 Limitations

The low level of evidence in the analyzed studies suggests the need for prospective studies with comparative control groups. The heterogeneous population included in this systematic review of literature, which referred to different etiologies for HA, and the demographic differences among the included patients are the limitations of this review. Different radiographic definitions of glenoid erosion and medialization were used in relation to the outcome measures. The main technique used for follow-up was X-ray radiography and not computed tomography scanning.

3.5 Conclusions

Based on current data, our results show that the overall revision rate of shoulder HA ranges from 0 to 25%, with a mean revision-free HA survivorship rate of 87.5% after 9 years. Approximately 59% of the cases are revised to TSA. The indication for revision was mainly symptomatic glenoid erosion in 62% of the cases. Finally, our results suggest that different techniques for reducing revision due to glenoid erosion should be investigated.

References

1. Hackett DJ, Hsu JE, Matsen FA. Primary shoulder hemiarthroplasty: what can be learned from 359 cases that were surgically revised? Clin Orthop Relat Res. 2018;476(5):1031–40.
2. Essilfie AA, Gamradt SC. The role for shoulder hemiarthroplasty in the young, active patient. Clin Sports Med. 2018;37(4):527–35. https://doi.org/10.1016/j.csm.2018.05.004.
3. Robinson WA, Wagner ER, Cofield RH, Sánchez-Sotelo J, Sperling JW. Long-term outcomes of humeral head replacement for the treatment of osteoarthritis; a report of 44 arthroplasties with minimum 10-year follow-up. J Shoulder Elb Surg. 2018;27(5):846–52. https://doi.org/10.1016/j.jse.2017.10.017.
4. Kircher J, Ohly B, Fal MF, Magosch P, Mauch F. Analysis of revision shoulder arthroplasty in the German nationwide registry from 2014 to 2018. JSES Int. 2021;5(3):382–90.
5. Best MJ, Aziz KT, Wilckens JH, McFarland EG, Srikumaran U. Increasing incidence of primary reverse and anatomic total shoulder arthroplasty in the United States. J Shoulder Elb Surg. 2021;30(5):1159–66. https://doi.org/10.1016/j.jse.2020.08.010.
6. Weatherby PJ, Efejuku TA, Somerson JS. Complications after anatomic shoulder arthroplasty: revisiting leading causes of failure. Orthop Clin North Am. 2021;52(3):269–77. https://doi.org/10.1016/j.ocl.2021.03.002.
7. Gauci MO, Cavalier M, Gonzalez JF, Holzer N, Baring T, Walch G, et al. Revision of failed shoulder arthroplasty: epidemiology, etiology, and surgical options. J Shoulder Elb Surg. 2020;29(3):541–9.
8. Shamseer L, Moher D, Clarke M, Ghersi D, Liberati A, Petticrew M, et al. Preferred reporting items for systematic review and meta-analysis protocols (PRISMA-P) 2015: elaboration and explanation. BMJ. 2015;349:g7647. https://doi.org/10.1136/bmj.g7647.
9. Slim K, Nini E, Forestier D, Kwiatkowski F, Panis Y, Chipponi J. Methodological index for non-randomized studies (Minors): development and validation of a new instrument. ANZ J Surg. 2003;73(9):712–6.
10. Obremskey WT, Pappas N, Attallah-Wasif E, Tornetta P, Bhandari M. Level of evidence in orthopaedic journals. J Bone Jt Surg. 2005;87(12 I):2632–8.
11. Garret J, Harly E, Le Huec JC, Brunner U, Rotini R, Godenèche A. Pyrolytic carbon humeral head in hemi-shoulder arthroplasty: preliminary results at 2-year follow-up. JSES Open Access. 2019;3(1):37–42.
12. Herschel R, Wieser K, Morrey ME, Ramos CH, Gerber C, Meyer DC. Risk factors for glenoid erosion in patients with shoulder hemiarthroplasty: an analysis of 118 cases. J Shoulder Elb Surg. 2017;26(2):246–52. https://doi.org/10.1016/j.jse.2016.06.004.
13. Cointat C, Raynier JL, Vasseur H, Lareyre F, Raffort J, Gauci MO, et al. Short-term outcomes and survival

of pyrocarbon hemiarthroplasty in the young arthritic shoulder. J Shoulder Elb Surg. 2022;31(1):113–22.
14. Ibrahim EF, Rashid A, Thomas M. Resurfacing hemiarthroplasty of the shoulder for patients with juvenile idiopathic arthritis. J Shoulder Elb Surg. 2018;27(8):1468–74. https://doi.org/10.1016/j.jse.2018.02.041.
15. Virk M, Thorsness RJ, Griffin JW, Kim J, Aiyash S, Marissa Malaret AAR. Short-term clinical outcomes of hemiarthroplasty with concentric glenoid reaming: the ream and run procedure. Orthopedics. 2018;41(6):854–60.
16. Getz CL, Kearns KA, Padegimas EM, Johnston PS, Lazarus MD, Williams GR. Survivorship of hemiarthroplasty with concentric glenoid reaming for Glenohumeral arthritis in young, active patients with a biconcave glenoid. J Am Acad Orthop Surg. 2017;25(10):715–23.
17. Levine WN, Fischer CR, Nguyen D, Flatow EL, Ahmad CS, Bigliani LU. Long-term follow-up of shoulder hemiarthroplasty for glenohumeral osteoarthritis. J Bone Jt Surg. 2012;94(22):1–7.
18. Saltzman MD, Chamberlain AM, Mercer DM, Warme WJ, Bertelsen AL, Matsen FA. Shoulder hemiarthroplasty with concentric glenoid reaming in patients 55 years old or less. J Shoulder Elb Surg. 2011;20(4):609–15. https://doi.org/10.1016/j.jse.2010.08.027.
19. Lynch BJR, Franta AK Jr, WHM, Lenters TR, Mounce D, III FAM. Shoulder hemiarthroplasty with concentric glenoid reaming. J Bone Jt Surg Am. 2007;89(6):1284–92.
20. Wirth MA, Tapscott RS, Southworth C, Rockwood CA. Treatment of glenohumeral arthritis with a hemiarthroplasty: a minimum five-year follow-up outcome study. J Bone Jt Surg. 2006;88(5):964–73.
21. Bonnevialle N, Mansat P, Mansat M, Bonnevialle P. Hemiarthroplasty for osteoarthritis in shoulder with dysplastic morphology. J Shoulder Elb Surg. 2011;20(3):378–84. https://doi.org/10.1016/j.jse.2010.07.006.
22. Tsitlakidis S, Doll J, Westhauser F, Wolf M, Hetto P, Maier M, et al. Promising results after hemi-shoulder arthroplasty using pyrolytic carbon heads in young and middle-aged patients. Orthop Traumatol Surg Res. 2021;107(4):102896. https://doi.org/10.1016/j.otsr.2021.102896.
23. Irlenbusch U, Zenz P, Blatter G, Berth A. Adjustable stemmed shoulder hemiarthroplasty: ten-year results of a prospective multicentre study. Orthop Traumatol Surg Res. 2019;105(2):229–36. https://doi.org/10.1016/j.otsr.2018.09.017.
24. Leung AS, Hippe DS, Ha AS. Cuff tear arthropathy shoulder hemiarthroplasty: a radiographic outcome study. Skelet Radiol. 2017;46(7):909–18.
25. Smith RG, Sperling JW, Cofield RH, Hattrup SJ, Schleck CD. Shoulder hemiarthroplasty for steroid-associated osteonecrosis. J Shoulder Elb Surg. 2008;17(5):685–8.
26. Goldberg SS, Bell JE, Han JK, Bak SF, Levine WN, Bigliani LU. Hemiarthroplasty for the rotator cuff-deficient shoulder. J Bone Jt Surg. 2008;90(3):554–9.
27. Thomas S, Price AJ, Sankey RA, Thomas M. Shoulder hemiarthroplasty in patients with juvenile idiopathic arthritis. J Bone Jt Surg - Ser B. 2005;87(5):672–6.
28. Rees JL, Dawson J, Hand GCR, Cooper C, Judge A, Price AJ, et al. The use of patient-reported outcome measures and patient satisfaction ratings to assess outcome in hemiarthroplasty of the shoulder. J Bone Jt Surg - Ser B. 2010;92(8):1107–11.
29. Krepler P, Wanivenhaus AH, Wurnig C. Outcome assessment of hemiarthroplasty of the shoulder: a 5-year follow-up with 4 evaluation tools. Acta Orthop. 2006;77(5):778–84.
30. Mosillo G, Basso MA, Balato G, Bernasconi A, Coviello A, Tamborini F, et al. Adaptive proximal scaphoid implant (APSI): a systematic review of the literature. Orthop Rev (Pavia). 2022;14(1):1–8.

Part II

Planning and Operative Technique

4 Management of a Painful Shoulder Arthroplasty

Sumit Raniga and Antonio Arenas-Miquelez

4.1 Introduction

A shoulder arthroplasty, including anatomic total shoulder arthroplasty (aTSA) and reverse shoulder arthroplasty (RSA), is a common and successful definitive surgical solution for a number of conditions where nonoperative management fails [1, 2]. The most common indications for a shoulder arthroplasty include glenohumeral joint osteoarthritis, rotator cuff tear arthropathy, selected functionally irreparable rotator cuff arthropathy, inflammatory arthropathy, osteonecrosis, and certain proximal humerus fractures and their sequelae [2, 3]. A shoulder arthroplasty is an effective treatment that provides pain relief, improved range of motion, and better quality of life.

Although the number of shoulder arthroplasty procedures is still small compared to hip and knee arthroplasties [4], the past few decades have seen a significant rise in the number of primary and revision shoulder arthroplasty cases. In the United States, between 2012 and 2017, the population-adjusted incidence of primary aTSA increased from 9.5 to 12.5 procedures per 100,000 and that of RSA increased from 7.3 to 19.3 procedures per 100,000 for a total surgical procedure volume in 2017 of well more than 100,000 procedures per year [5]. This increase in the number of shoulder arthroplasties performed is mainly due to an aging population, better diagnostic modalities, improvement in implant material and design, expanded indications, and more widespread surgical training in shoulder replacement surgery [6–8]. The utilization of hemiarthroplasties continues to fall drastically, whereas that of reverse total shoulder arthroplasty has been increasing yearly since its introduction to the US market in 2004 [9, 10].

Although shoulder arthroplasty provides good outcomes with predictable pain relief [11–14], pain after the procedure is not uncommon. Deshmukh et al. [15] reported on 320 aTSA patients at a minimum of 10 years follow-up and, despite low revision rates (6.9%), reported some level of persistent pain in 32% of patients. A painful shoulder is consistently cited as the most common reason for a revision shoulder arthroplasty [16]. Hasan et al. [17] reviewed 141 patients with shoulder arthroplasties, who were evaluated for unsatisfactory results, and found that 82% had pain and 74% had stiffness.

Increasing utilization and expanding indications of total shoulder arthroplasty, especially in younger patients [18], are going to increase the burden and, possibly, the complexity of revision arthroplasty in the future [7, 19, 20]. Because of

S. Raniga (✉)
Faculty of Medicine, Health and Human Sciences, Macquarie University, Sydney, Australia
e-mail: sumit.raniga@mqhealth.org.au

A. Arenas-Miquelez
Hospital Quironsalud Valle del Henares, Hospital Quironsalud San Jose, Madrid, Spain

F. Franceschi et al. (eds.), *Revision Shoulder Arthroplasty*,
https://doi.org/10.1007/978-3-031-45944-3_4

the projected revision burden, a good understanding of the appropriate workup, accurate diagnosis, and evidence-based management of a painful shoulder arthroplasty is important for the shoulder surgeon caring for this complex patient population. This chapter will provide an evidence-based overview of the etiology, diagnosis, and early management of a painful shoulder arthroplasty.

4.2 The Etiology of a Painful Shoulder Arthroplasty

Although having pain in the early postoperative phase is expected, persistent pain or development of new pain after an uneventful recovery from surgery is considered abnormal and warrants further investigation. Persistent pain after a shoulder arthroplasty may be due to multiple factors [21]. Some may be extrinsic to the shoulder joint, whereas others may be intrinsic. Furthermore, certain intrinsic causes of pain after a shoulder arthroplasty are specific to either aTSA or RSA implants, whereas other causes are common for both implant styles (Table 4.1).

The causes of a painful shoulder arthroplasty may vary based on patient demographics, the primary etiology for surgery, and the type of implant (Fig. 4.1a–d) (Table I). Glenoid erosion is the most common cause of failure of hemiarthroplasty for osteoarthritis [17], whereas tuberosity nonunion or malunion is the most common cause of failure after hemiarthroplasty for proximal humerus fracture [22]. In the aTSA scenario, glenoid loosening and stiffness are the most common causes of failure [16], whereas in RSA, instability is the number one cause of

Table 4.1 Possible causes of pain after a shoulder arthroplasty (see Hagedorn et al. (2022), page 2, Table I [86])

	Intrinsic			EXTRINSIC
	Both anatomic and reverse	Reverse	Anatomic	
Prostheses	• Loosening • Wear with particulate-induced synovitis and/or osteolysis • Metal allergy	• Humeral bearing overhang/protrusion • Component disassociation or fracture		• ACJ, SCJ, and periscapular conditions • Cervical spine conditions • Complex regional pain syndrome • Vascular conditions • Psychiatric conditions • Fibromyalgia • Narcotic dependence
Bone	• Periprosthetic fractures	• Acromion or scapular spine fracture • Coracoid impingement • Scapular notching	• Glenoid erosion/ pain after hemiarthroplasty	
Soft tissues	• Dislocation • Capsular contracture/ stiffness • Heterotopic ossification	• Deltoid dehiscence • Excessive deltoid stretching/pain • Conjoint tendon impingement/pain	• Cuff insufficiency, subscapularis failure • Biceps tenosynovitis/pain	
Infection	• Deep periprosthetic joint infection (PJI) • Superficial (incisional) infection			
Other	• Brachial plexopathy • Axillary nerve injury • Neuroma • Recurrent hemarthrosis or seroma • Neoplasm	• Suprascapular nerve injury by screw		

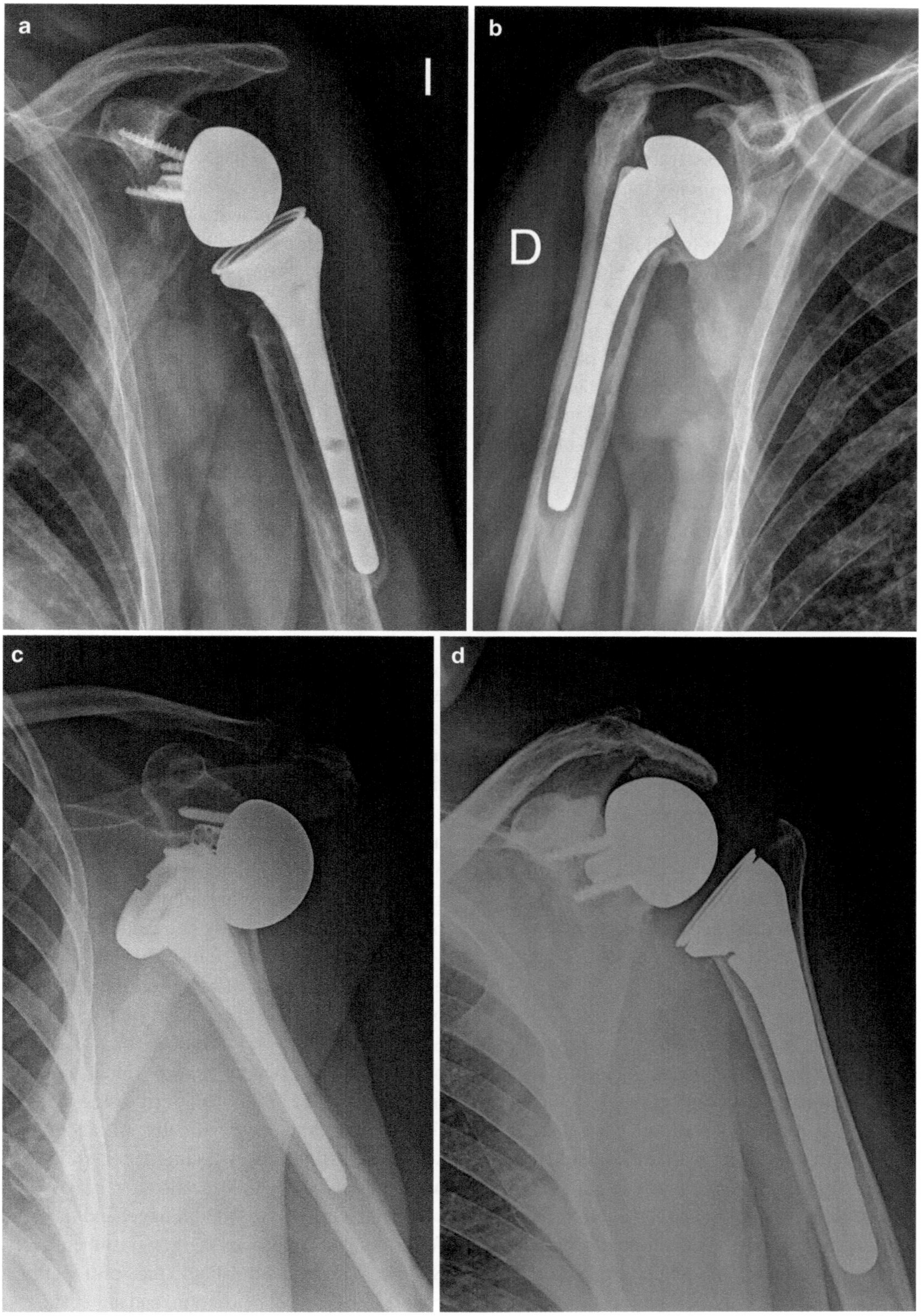

Fig. 4.1 (**a**) Reverse shoulder arthroplasty with a loose cemented humeral component. (**b**) Hemiarthroplasty with humeral stem loosening and glenoid erosion. (**c**) Dislocated reverse total shoulder arthroplasty. (**d**) Reverse total shoulder arthroplasty with acromion fracture

revision [23]. Interestingly, Bohsali et al. [24] reviewed the complication rates after shoulder arthroplasty in the past decade and reported that the overall rate of complications is trending down from 14.7% to 11.0%. Some etiologies such as scapular stress fracture are unique to reverse TSA and commonly happen in osteoporotic female patients [25].

Evaluation of a painful shoulder arthroplasty typically involves a thorough history, physical examination, and a careful review of sequential radiographs and diverse imaging studies. Investigations for possible deep periprosthetic joint infection (PJI) often include blood laboratory analyses and joint aspiration with subsequent culture and laboratory analyses of the fluid. Additional investigations may include computed tomography (CT), ultrasound (US), magnetic resonance (MR), scintigraphy, and electromyography (EMG) with nerve conduction studies. Occasionally, diagnostic injections are considered, trying to avoid the use of corticosteroids as it entails the risk of iatrogenic infection. Diagnostic arthroscopy may play a role. Surgeons should adopt an individualized approach to the evidence-based workup of painful shoulder arthroplasties to take into account all aforementioned available tools to develop the best strategy for the management of each patient.

4.3 Evaluation of a Painful Shoulder Arthroplasty

4.3.1 History

A thorough but focused history is probably the most important part of evaluating a painful shoulder arthroplasty. It is imperative to delineate the nature, severity, and anatomic location of the pain, its relationship with movement, and the timing of symptoms in relation to surgery.

The severity of pain and the overall impact on daily activities may be quantitated using a visual analogue scale and the subjective shoulder value (SSV), respectively [26]. The location of pain is important, especially with regard to excluding the extrinsic causes of pain (i.e., cervical spine pain may manifest at the neck or over the trapezius region, whereas intrinsic pain is typically centered around the deltoid region). The presence of numbness, tingling, hyperesthesia, or weakness in the whole upper extremity may also talk in favor of cervical spine origin. Other extrinsic causes are brachial plexopathy and complex regional pain syndrome that also produce pain in the whole upper extremity.

The temporal course of pain with the index procedure provides important insights as well. If the pain never improved after the arthroplasty, particularly if the pain is in the same location and has the same characteristics, then extrinsic causes could be the reason for persistent pain, but infection, persistent glenoid pain after hemiarthroplasty, painful capsular contracture, iatrogenic brachial plexopathy, and other nerve injuries may also follow the same temporal relationship. On the contrary, implant loosening or wear and chronic infection typically manifest years after the procedure. Stress fractures of the scapular spine and acromion classically manifest as acute onset of pain a few months after an RSA [27]. Any correlation between pain and activity is important too: pain at rest may be indicative of an infection or neuropathic pain, whereas pain at the time of activity may be related to mechanical causes such as implant loosening or painful glenoid erosion after hemiarthroplasty. Any associated symptoms, including stiffness, mechanical symptoms of clicking and popping, and a sense of instability are all highly relevant.

The details of the surgical procedure are extremely important. How severe was the pain before surgery? Did the patient undergo one or more procedures or corticosteroid injections before surgery? Although the typical signs of infection are rare in shoulder periprosthetic infection, patients should specifically ask about constitutional symptoms, including fever, chills, and night sweats, weight loss and any issues with wound healing, excessive drainage, and the need for prolonged antibiotics therapy postoperatively. Specific information about the postoperative course, rehabilitation program, and any history of a fall or direct trauma to the shoulder or upper extremity are highly valuable. A copy of the operative report should be carefully reviewed to determine how the biceps tendon and subscapularis muscles were managed. Components implanted should be noted because some may have a poor track record with known instances of early unexpected failure [28].

Relevant past medical history, including diabetes mellitus, smoking, osteoporosis, coagulopathy, and prior infection, should be obtained. A medication history, including the use of certain medications, such as chronic antibiotics, corticosteroids, systemic immunosuppressors, and anticoagulant medication, will also help reach a diagnosis. Previous surgical history, both before and after the index arthroplasty, recent dental work, urological or gastrointestinal procedure, and details of each surgery such as date, name of the surgeon, and hospital should all be collected.

4.3.2 Examination

Inspection is the first step and requires complete exposure of the shoulder girdle. The examiner should look for asymmetry, muscle wasting, bruising, deltoid detachment and locations of prior incisions, delayed wound healing, and signs of infection (erythema, swelling, or drainage). The deltoid, rotator cuff, and biceps should be inspected for deformity or atrophy. Gross shoulder deformity may be present in cases of anterosuperior escape after an anatomic arthroplasty or dislocation after a reverse arthroplasty.

Palpation is the next step and involves an assessment for tenderness around the incision, the glenohumeral joint, the acromioclavicular and sternoclavicular joints, the bicipital groove, the acromion and superomedial pole of the scapular spine, and the periscapular muscles. The cervical spine should also be palpated for tenderness if the history suggests a cervicogenic cause. A thorough range of motion evaluation in all planes, particularly combined multiplanar functional range of motion (abduction and external rotation; adduction and internal rotation), should be conducted. Particular attention should be paid to assess whether passive range of motion and active range of motion are equal to one another. If passive range of motion and active range of motion are equally limited, then the possible causes include extensive scar formation or mechanical impingement from the implant or bony abnormalities. If passive motion is preserved but active motion is limited, then disorders of the musculotendinous unit and its nerve supply need to be considered—muscle weakness, tendon rupture, or nerve deficit. The strength of the deltoid (activation of the three portions of the muscle under resisted abduction) and rotator cuff should be assessed with manual testing and performance of dedicated tests (Gerber's lift off, belly press, bear hug; external rotation lag sign and Hornblower's test; Jobe and Whipple's tests). Patients should be asked to reproduce mechanical symptoms such as palpable or audible crepitation, clicking, or locking, if possible.

A thorough neurovascular examination should be performed to assess both peripheral and central nerve functions and vascular perfusion of the upper extremity. A thorough neurovascular examination of the upper extremity should be completed to identify evidence of radiculopathy, brachial plexopathy, nerve injuries, or complex regional pain syndrome. Finally, the scapulothoracic region and the cervical spine should be evaluated as potential sources of referred pain.

4.3.3 Imaging

Imaging plays an integral role in evaluating a painful shoulder arthroplasty. The goal of imaging is to assess the bone, implants, surrounding soft tissue, and their relationships [29]. Plain X-rays and computed tomography (CT) scanning are the ideal modalities for assessing bone quality, bone lucencies, the presence of fractures, tuberosity healing, implant positioning, dislocation, and loosening. When it comes to soft tissue assessment, ultrasound (US) and CT arthrograms are the modalities of choice to assess soft tissue reaction, fluid collection, and integrity of the rotator cuff tendons and other muscles around the shoulder. The utility of magnetic resonance imaging (MRI) in assessing the soft tissues is limited in this setting due to the artifacts caused by the metallic implant, even with metal artifact subtraction sequences.

4.3.4 Radiographs

Image evaluation of a painful shoulder arthroplasty should always begin with radiographs. Plain X-rays are inexpensive, readily available in most clinical settings, and provide information about the bone, soft tissue, and implants [21, 30]. The requested series should, at minimum, include anteroposterior (AP), true AP or Grashey, and axillary views. Images should be taken in such a manner that ensures that the glenohumeral joint, the medial border of the scapula, and the entire implant, including the humeral stem, are all visible.

The AP and true AP views allow evaluation of the overall bone quality, focal bone resorption, fracture or notching, and the presence of heterotopic ossification. On the humeral side, implant alignment, humeral head size, tuberosity height, cement mantle, and osteolysis are evaluated for "overstuffing" [31] (Fig. 4.2), possible stem loosening, or subsidence. The axillary view is useful to assess the glenoid version, anteroposterior relationship of the implant to the glenoid, and implant subluxation or dislocation. It is also useful to assess the position and possible displacement of the lesser tuberosity osteotomy. Sometimes the interface between the implant and surrounding bone or cement is best visualized when radiographs are obtained under fluoroscopic positioning. In some patients, radiographs may clearly reveal the problem (bone or component fracture, dislocation, and gross loosening), and certain degrees of component malposition can be a source of persistent pain. However, many painful shoulder arthroplasties look well-positioned and well-fixed on radiographs.

Generally, pathological changes of interest are subtle and not noticeable in a single radiograph, and, therefore, comparisons between serial radiographs over time enhance the examiner's ability to discern bone loss and implant loosening or migration [30]. Radiographic assessment of glenoid component fixation after anatomic shoulder arthroplasties using all-polyethylene components, for example, may be extremely difficult to assess unless sequential radiographs that have been obtained over time are compared [32]. Radiolucent lines and change in component position are commonly used to identify component loosening.

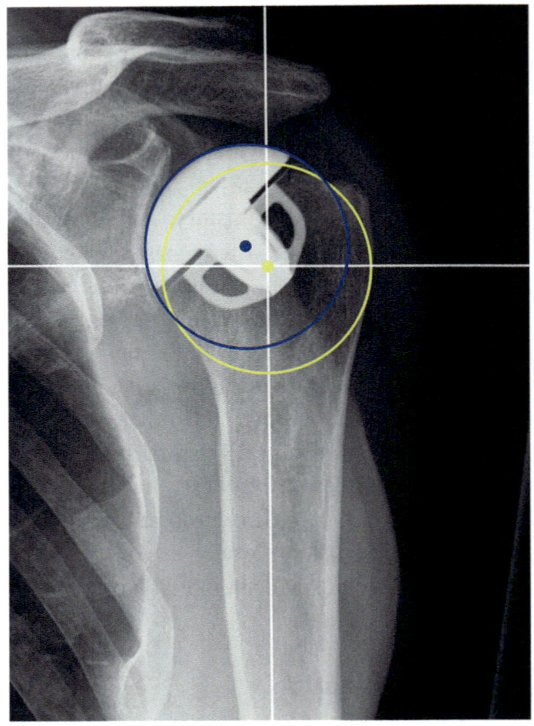

Fig. 4.2 Overstuffed stemless anatomic total shoulder arthroplasty; the best-fit circle of the proximal humerus (yellow circle) and the prosthetic COR (blue circle)

Fractures of the acromion and spine RSA may also be difficult to visualize on radiographs [33]. The examiner should specifically look for them in a painful RSA and compare preoperative and postoperative radiographs for evidence of acromion and/or scapular spine displacement. Radiographs are also an important tool for preoperative planning for revision surgery. Bilateral full-length arm X-rays with a scale included in the image is an objective preoperative tool to accurately measure arm lengthening and optimize soft tissue tensioning [34].

4.3.5 Computed Tomography

CT scanning plays an integral role as an advanced imaging modality in the evaluation of a painful shoulder arthroplasty. It provides a detailed assessment of bone stock, implant loosening, and migration (Fig. 4.3) [35]. Computed tomography is also useful to assess for fractures of the spine of the scapula or acromion after a reverse arthroplasty and to determine whether any of the screws used for baseplate fixation is in dangerous proximity to the suprascapular nerve (SSN). It can also be used to assess the degree of muscle atrophy and fatty infiltration of the rotator cuff and other muscles and also to identify wear, notching, and osteolysis. CT arthrograms may be particularly helpful to identify cuff failure, subscapularis insufficiency, or glenoid loosening after an anatomic arthroplasty [36]. However, Mallo et al. [37] found that CT arthrograms can underestimate glenoid loosening and cautioned against their use. The use of CT scans to quantify glenoid loosening in anatomic TSA was limited due to the metal artifact generated by the humeral head implant [38].

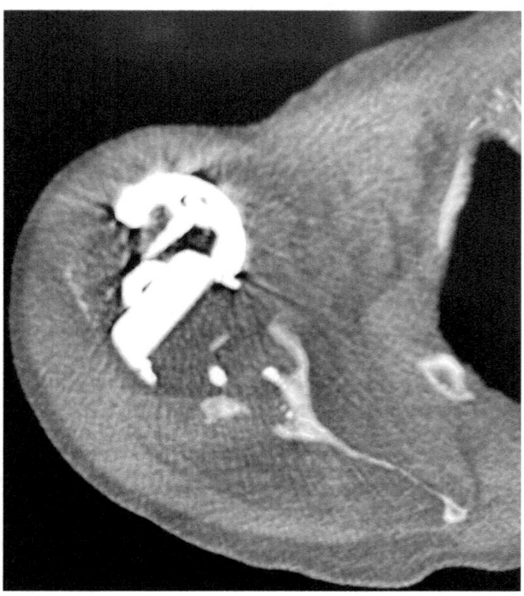

Fig. 4.3 A CT scan image of a reverse total shoulder arthroplasty with catastrophic baseplate failure, glenosphere disengagement, and glenoid bone loss

New metal artifact reduction protocols have improved the quality of CT images that can be obtained [39] and, along with simple patient positioning techniques [35], have made reproducible evaluation of glenoid loosening possible [40]. However, metal artifact reduction sequences have limitations, and, although they visually create better images with less streaking, they can affect the sizing of the metal implant and the quality of trabecular bone images [41, 42]. In recent years, three-dimensional (3D) reconstruction of CT images has become a powerful tool for preoperative planning for revision surgery.

4.3.6 Ultrasound

Ultrasound is a relatively low-cost imaging modality that allows detailed evaluation of soft tissue derangements, including rotator cuff tear, muscle detachment or atrophy, and fluid collections around the implant after a shoulder arthroplasty [43]. The significant advantage of ultrasound in the setting of a painful shoulder arthroplasty is that it is not affected by the metal artifact from the implant and allows dynamic evaluation of the joint [21]. The utility of ultrasound in evaluating posterior–superior rotator cuff tears or subscapularis failure in a shoulder arthroplasty has been well-established [29, 43]. Ultrasound is also extremely useful to assist in guided diagnostic aspiration of a painful shoulder arthroplasty. The major limitations of ultrasonography is its dependence on the experience and skill of the operator, difficulty in interpreting by the orthopedic surgeon, difficulty in patients with large body habitus, and the inability to assess bone and implant loosening.

4.3.7 Magnetic Resonance Imaging

Although MRI is considered by many to be the most useful advanced imaging modality for a painful native shoulder, MRI evaluation after arthroplasty is much less useful because of the presence of a metal artifact, even when dedicated metal subtraction techniques are used [44]. An

MRI has high soft tissue resolution, but, given its high cost and vulnerability to metal artifacts, its use has been limited in the evaluation of a painful shoulder arthroplasty [29]. The main advantage of MRI in the setting of arthroplasty, especially if metal artifact reduction protocols are applied, [45] is its ability to assess for rotator cuff tearing, rotator cuff muscle atrophy, brachial plexus injury, and surrounding soft tissue injury [46]. Sperling et al. [47] reported that, despite a metal artifact, MRI was able to correctly identify 10 out of 11 cases that had a full-thickness rotator cuff tear and 8 of 10 that did not have a rotator cuff tear after a shoulder arthroplasty. With these findings, selective application of MRI with metal artifact reduction protocols in patients who are at a high risk of a rotator cuff tear in the setting of anatomic total shoulder arthroplasty or hemiarthroplasty may play a role. Recently, the new advanced metal artifact reduction sequence-magnetic resonance imaging (MARS-MRI) has been prospectively tested and has demonstrated a high accuracy and reliability for the diagnosis of periprosthetic infection [48].

4.3.8 Nuclear Medicine

Application of nuclear medicine in the workup of a painful shoulder arthroplasty has focused on prosthetic joint infection, assessment of implant loosening, and occult fracture [29]. Radiographs are usually negative in the early stages of infection, implant loosening, and stress fracture, and their ability to detect a biological response is valuable and can lead to early diagnosis. The challenges of a conventional technetium bone scan are its lack of specificity in diagnosing prosthetic shoulder infection [21]. Technetium-99m [99mTc]-bisphosphonate (BP) bone scan (single-photon emission computed tomography (SPECT)) is credited with high sensitivity but plagued with poor specificity [49]. The specificity of BP SPECT is low because the imaging findings in aseptic loosening may overlap with the other implant-related disorders, such as post-operative bone remodeling, infection, and periprosthetic fracture [21].

Single-photon emission computerized tomography in combination with conventional computer tomography (SPECT/CT) pairs a high-resolution anatomic 3D CT with a functional single-photon emission tomography (SPECT) [50, 51]. Its specificity is improved by analyzing the uptake pattern and coupled CT anomalies. The specificity of SPECT/CT is higher in older prostheses. Increased postoperative uptake due to normal bone remodeling may be present at the arthroplasty site up to 1 year after surgery [52]. Good osseointegration of orthopedic implants results in a decrease of post-operative remodeling [53]. Using SPECT/CT, Berth et al. demonstrated that the primary osseointegration of a stemless shoulder prosthesis is completed almost 3 months after implantation [54]. Hirschmann et al. showed that SPECT/CT is useful for determining humeral and glenoidal component loosening in patients with shoulder prosthesis [51].

In the case of glenoiditis in hemiarthroplasty, bone scintigraphy shows a focally increased uptake of the glenoid, often with chondral erosion. The scintigraphic pattern of aTSA loosening is a more focal uptake and is more evident in the delayed phase images [55]. The interpretation criterion is the presence of an increased periprosthetic tracer uptake at the border and the bone–prosthesis interface with the increased border uptake affecting at least four contiguous zones around the polyethylene. In RSA, glenoid loosening can be highlighted with bone scintigraphy. A stage 3 notch corresponds to an increased border uptake around the screws, and a stage 4 notch corresponds to an increased uptake around the center block. According to Sirveaux et al.'s scoring system [56], a humeral implant is to be considered at risk when the bone scintigraphy discloses an increased uptake at the bone–prosthesis interface in at least three contiguous zones. The presence of a 2-mm or more radiolucent line on CT can help confirm the diagnosis.

In the case of infection, three-phase bone scan imaging is a highly sensitive test for diagnosis in patients with normal radiographs but provides low specificity, considering that an abnormal uptake may overlap with diverse anomalies such as mechanical loosening or osteolysis [21]. SPECT/CT is often employed because the technique is available, inexpensive, easy-to-perform, and exhibits high sensitivity, with a low radiation burden for the patient. A bone scintigraphy without abnormal uptake foci rules out infection with high confidence [55].

Labeling white blood cells (WBCs) with [99mTc] hexamethylpropyleneamine oxime is well-suited for diagnosing infected prostheses since, as shown by Love et al., [57] in the absence of an infection, WBCs basically do not accumulate at sites of increased bone mineral turnover. The specificity of labeled leukocyte imaging can be enhanced when interpreted alongside [99mTc]-sulfur colloid bone marrow (BM) imaging [58]. Many investigators have reported that paired WBC and BM scans bear extremely high sensitivity and specificity and may be the nuclear imaging modality of choice for diagnosing prosthetic joint infections [57–59]. Palestro and Love contended that labeled WBC imaging combined with BM imaging demonstrated the highest accuracy (90%) for diagnosing arthroplasty infections [58, 60]. The accumulation of labeled WBCs should mismatch with a photopenic area on the BM scan. In addition, the SPECT/CT combination allows the identification of radiological signs of infection that may improve specificity: widening of the periprosthetic lucency (2 mm or more), the presence of geodes, ill-defined osteolysis, the presence of granuloma, abscess or effusion, and florid periosteal reaction [29].

4.3.9 Laboratory Investigations

Infection is the number one differential diagnoses to rule out in any painful shoulder arthroplasty. Laboratory investigations, including white blood cell (WBC) count and inflammatory markers such as erythrocyte sedimentation rate (ESR) and C-reactive protein (CRP), should be requested at the outset to screen for infections. Unfortunately, most periprosthetic shoulder infections are caused by indolent organisms responsible for low-grade infection, and laboratory markers are commonly normal [61, 62]. There is a poor correlation between positive intraoperative cultures and elevated laboratory markers in failed arthroplasty cases [63]. When an infection is suspected, articular fluid (typically obtained under ultrasound guidance) may be analyzed for cell count with cell differential and sent for cultures.

It has been shown that WBC count has poor sensitivity and only predicts 7% of cases with positive cultures [64]. In a cohort of 193 revision shoulder arthroplasties, Pottinger et al. [65] showed that only 17% of patients with a positive culture for *Propionibacterium acnes* had elevated ESR levels. Furthermore, Grosso et al. [66] reported 33% sensitivity for CRP in detecting positive cultures in revision shoulder arthroplasty. Preoperative inflammatory markers and WBC count are commonly normal in a painful shoulder arthroplasty, but positive results are useful and, in most cases, should be taken seriously. Chalmers et al. looked at a large national insurance database and identified patients who developed infection 1 year following revision shoulder arthroplasty and found that besides male gender (odds ratio (OR) = 3.8, $P < 0.001$), elevated preoperative ESR significantly increased the odds of developing infection following revision arthroplasty (OR = 2.4, $P < 0.05$) [67].

It must be noted that a significant percentage of deep infections after a shoulder arthroplasty are caused by *Cutibacterium acnes*. This is a slow-growing bacterium that oftentimes will not lead to elevated serum inflammatory markers or elevated articular fluid cell counts. In addition, *Cutibacterium acnes* is more difficult to isolate in culture and may require extended 14 days of incubation. To reach a consensus on the diagnosis of infection complicating shoulder arthroplasty, the International Consensus Meeting on Orthopedic Infections published criteria for the definition of a periprosthetic shoulder infection, including a scoring system for definite, probably, possible, and unlikely infection (Table 4.2) [68]. Culture of sonicated fluid from explanted pros-

Table 4.2 Definition of infection according to the International Consensus Meeting on Orthopedic Infections [7]

The major criteria that define definite periprosthetic shoulder infection (meeting one of these criteria is diagnostic)
• The presence of a sinus tract from the skin surface to the prosthesis • Gross intraarticular pus • Two positive tissue cultures with phenotypically identical virulent organisms
The minor criteria to be considered for the scoring system below
• Unexpected wound drainage: 4 points • A single positive tissue culture with virulent organisms: 3 points • A single positive tissue culture with low-virulence organisms: 1 point • A second positive tissue culture (identical low-virulence organisms): 3 points • Humeral loosening: 3 points • A positive frozen section (5 Polymorphonuclear neutrophils (PMNs) in > high-power fields): 3 points • A positive preoperative aspirate culture (low- or high-virulence): 3 points • An elevated synovial neutrophil percentage (>80%)*: 2 points • An elevated synovial WBC count (>3000 cells/mL)*: 2 points • An elevated ESR (>30 mm/h)*: 2 points • An elevated CRP level (>10 mg/L)*: 2 points • An elevated synovial α-defensin level: 2 points • Cloudy fluid: 2 points
Probable infection
• Organisms identified in at least one culture and 6 or more points
Possible infection
• A single positive culture with virulent organisms • In all, 6 or more points with no organisms identified • In all, 2 positive cultures with low-virulence organisms
Unlikely infection
• Less than 6 points and negative cultures or only a single culture with low-virulence organisms

theses may provide additional diagnostic value as well [69].

Cytokine profiles analysis of the serum and joint aspirate such as interleukin-6 (IL-6) and α-defensin has shown promising results [70–72], but their applications are limited due to cost, lack of sensitivity toward blood samples [62], limited availability, and lack of clear, well-developed algorithms to interpret results.

4.3.10 Joint Aspiration

Aspiration of joint fluid can be an effective method of collecting fluid for culture from a painful shoulder arthroplasty, but its utility for diagnosis of periprosthetic infection has not yet been established. Blind aspiration of a shoulder arthroplasty may fail due to distorted anatomy and postoperative scar formation [73], but image-guided aspiration may have better success rates in targeting loculated fluid around the implant and can also lavage the joint in cases of a dry tap. Even when aspirations are successful, it is unclear whether they correlate with tissue cultures [74]. Dilisio et al. [75] compared the results of fluoroscopically guided joint aspiration with arthroscopically obtained tissue biopsies in 19 patients with a painful shoulder arthroplasty and showed a sensitivity of 16.7% and negative predictive values of 58.3%. Preoperative aspiration may be attempted under sterile conditions in all patients with an atraumatic, painful shoulder arthroplasty. Although the majority of arthroplasty aspirations will result in a dry tap or a negative result, a positive aspiration has a high specificity for infection. Most importantly, a negative aspiration cannot rule out infection in the setting of a painful shoulder arthroplasty.

4.3.11 Reconnaissance Shoulder Arthroscopy and Tissue Biopsy

The diagnosis of periprosthetic joint infection after a shoulder arthroplasty may prove elusive. It does require cultures from tissue samples and diagnostic arthroscopy to obtain multiple tissue biopsies, and synovial fluid may be considered for certain painful shoulder arthroplasties with no alternative, clear explanation for ongoing pain [76]. Samples obtained arthroscopically have been reported to be of a high diagnostic value [75]. Arthroscopy also allows assessment of glenoid component fixation, polyethylene wear, synovitis, and the condition of the rotator cuff and the long head of the biceps tendon [77].

In 1993, Bonutti et al. [78] were the first investigators to describe the use of arthroscopy in patients with a painful shoulder arthroplasty. They identified three patients without any obvious preoperative cause of pain and used arthroscopic evaluation to diagnose glenoid loosening in them. In a series of 19 patients, Dilisio et al. [75] found a 100% correlation between arthroscopic biopsy and open biopsy for the purposes of identifying PJI. All of the patients who had positive arthroscopic biopsy results had correlating positive biopsy results during the open procedure. All patients who had negative arthroscopic biopsy results had correlating negative biopsy results with the subsequent open procedure. The results of a recent study by Guild et al. [79] have been consistent with those of Dilisio et al. [75]; they also found a high correlation (100%) between cultures obtained arthroscopically and those obtained via open surgery. Tashjian et al. [80], in their analysis of 17 patients with failed shoulder arthroplasty, showed that sensitivity and specificity of pre-revision biopsies taken arthroscopically or open in predicting final cultures at the time of revision were 90% and 86%, respectively. Furthermore, assessment of implant stability through shoulder arthroscopy is more accurate than CT arthrograms [37]. In 2015, Mallo et al. [37] reported a series of 14 anatomic total shoulders yielding only 70% sensitivity and 75% specificity for glenoid loosening with CT arthrograms.

Reconnaissance shoulder arthroscopy allows for tissue biopsy with a high correlation of culture results when compared with open biopsy. In addition, arthroscopy allows the orthopedic surgeon to evaluate the rotator cuff complex and establish the presence of any glenoid loosening or implant failure in patients with painful shoulder arthroplasty without PJI (Table 4.3).

4.3.12 Examination Under Anesthesia

Examination under anesthesia in the setting of a painful shoulder arthroplasty can provide useful information about mechanical issues such as

Table 4.3 Diagnostic algorithm for painful shoulder arthroplasty

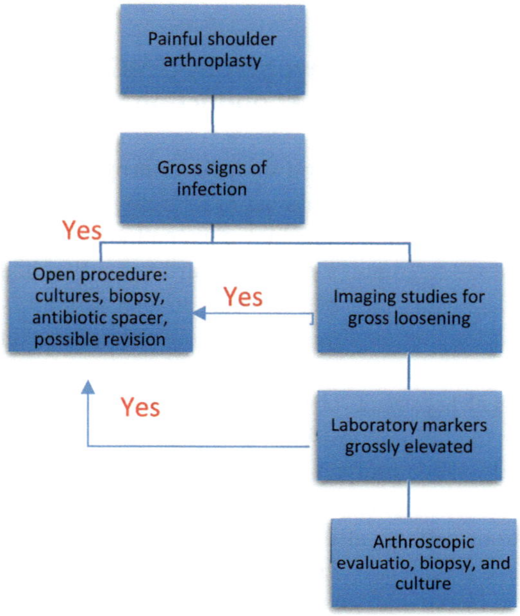

implant loosening, frank or subclinical instability, and possible bony and soft tissue impingement. Live fluoroscopy can help gain a better understanding of the stability of the implant prior to undertaking an arthroscopic or open surgery. Gee et al. [81] reported cases of posterior instability after TSA, which failed conservative management, were evaluated with examination under anaesthesia (EUA), and addressed through arthroscopic capsular imbrication. The surgeon should be mindful of the possibility of iatrogenic periprosthetic fracture, dislocation, or nerve injury during manipulation of a stiff or unstable shoulder arthroplasty.

4.3.13 Diagnostic Injections

As a general rule, diagnostic injections into the glenohumeral joint space after an arthroplasty are not recommended for fear of iatrogenic infection. However, image-guided diagnostic injections of a local anesthetic may be useful to confirm physical and imaging findings that may suggest an alternative painful structure, such as the acromioclavicular joint, the sternoclavicular joint, or the tendon of the long head of the biceps. However, the use of diagnostic injections after a shoulder arthroplasty remains controversial.

4.3.14 Electromyography (EMG) and Nerve Conduction Studies

Persistent pain after a shoulder arthroplasty may be secondary to a number of neurological conditions, including brachial plexopathy and complex regional pain syndrome. Brachial plexopathy may be secondary to a stretch injury during surgery, present as a complication of nerve blockade (secondary to the toxicity of a local anesthetic or mechanical injury), or occur in the form of postsurgical inflammatory plexopathy. Electromyography and nerve conduction studies may aid in the diagnosis of these conditions and can also be used to assess for severity and possibility of recovery.

Nerve injury is reported in 0.1–4.3% of shoulder arthroplasties, with the majority involving the axillary nerve. There is a high rate of spontaneous recovery in the first 3 months postoperatively [82, 83]. Involvement of the brachial plexus, the radial nerve, and the ulnar nerve has also been reported in the literature but with far less frequency [16]. In an RSA, excess arm lengthening >2 cm and placement of the arm in extreme positions during the surgery may stretch the brachial plexus and lead to nerve injury [28, 84]. Ladermann et al. [85] reported that the prevalence of nerve injury detected by EMG at 3.6 weeks was 10.5 times higher after a reverse than an anatomic TSA. If neurological recovery does not start by 12 weeks after surgery, then an EMG study should be requested to assess the integrity and function of the nerves.

4.4 Summary

Because of the projected revision burden of a shoulder arthroplasty, a good understanding of the appropriate workup, accurate diagnosis, and evidence-based management of a painful shoulder arthroplasty is important for the shoulder and elbow surgeon caring for this complex patient population. A patient with a painful shoulder arthroplasty may suffer from a wide range of pathologies with a long list of etiologies. There is little consensus in the literature on how these complex patients should be evaluated and what set of imaging studies, laboratory investigations, or diagnostic procedures should be requested in order to reach an accurate diagnosis. Moreover, it is common that the majority, if not all, of the investigations are negative, leaving surgeons without a clear explanation for a patient's continued pain and dysfunction. This chapter provides an evidence-based overview of the diagnostic approaches to a painful shoulder arthroplasty. The diagnostic evaluation includes a comprehensive history, physical examination, imaging, and laboratory investigations. The chapters that follow will further evaluate the causes of pain and dysfunction after a shoulder arthroplasty with a focus on diagnostic algorithms and management.

References

1. Kang JR, et al. Primary reverse shoulder arthroplasty using contemporary implants is associated with very low reoperation rates. J Shoulder Elb Surg. 2019;28(6S):S175–80.
2. Sanchez-Sotelo J. Total shoulder arthroplasty. Open Orthop J. 2011;5:106–14.
3. Sanchez-Sotelo J. Reverse total shoulder arthroplasty. Clin Anat. 2009;22(2):172–82.
4. Jain NB, et al. Trends in the epidemiology of total shoulder arthroplasty in the United States from 1990-2000. Arthritis Rheum. 2006;55(4):591–7.
5. Best MJ, et al. Increasing incidence of primary reverse and anatomic total shoulder arthroplasty in the United States. J Shoulder Elb Surg. 2021;30(5):1159–66.
6. Kim SH, et al. Increasing incidence of shoulder arthroplasty in the United States. J Bone Joint Surg Am. 2011;93(24):2249–54.
7. Schwartz BE, et al. National trends and perioperative outcomes in primary and revision total shoulder arthroplasty: trends in total shoulder arthroplasty. Int Orthop. 2015;39(2):271–6.
8. Dillon MT, et al. Yearly trends in elective shoulder arthroplasty, 2005-2013. Arthritis Care Res (Hoboken). 2017;69(10):1574–81.
9. Trofa D, Rajaee SS, Smith EL. Nationwide trends in total shoulder arthroplasty and hemiarthroplasty for osteoarthritis. Am J Orthop (Belle Mead NJ). 2014;43(4):166–72.

10. Jain NB, Yamaguchi K. The contribution of reverse shoulder arthroplasty to utilization of primary shoulder arthroplasty. J Shoulder Elb Surg. 2014;23(12):1905–12.
11. Walch G, et al. Results of a convex-back cemented keeled glenoid component in primary osteoarthritis: multicenter study with a follow-up greater than 5 years. J Shoulder Elb Surg. 2011;20(3):385–94.
12. Lo I. Quality-of-life outcome following hemiarthroplasty or Total shoulder arthroplasty in patients with osteoarthritis. A prospective, randomized trial. J Bone Joint Surg. 2005;87(10):2178–85.
13. Torchia ME, Cofield RH, Settergren CR. Total shoulder arthroplasty with the Neer prosthesis: long-term results. J Shoulder Elb Surg. 1997;6(6):495–505.
14. Hawkins RJ, Bell RH, Jallay B. Total shoulder arthroplasty. Clin Orthop Relat Res. 1989;242:188–94.
15. Deshmukh AV, et al. Total shoulder arthroplasty: long-term survivorship, functional outcome, and quality of life. J Shoulder Elb Surg. 2005;14(5):471–9.
16. Franta AK, et al. The complex characteristics of 282 unsatisfactory shoulder arthroplasties. J Shoulder Elb Surg. 2007;16(5):555–62.
17. Hasan SS, et al. The distribution of shoulder replacement among surgeons and hospitals is significantly different than that of hip or knee replacement. J Shoulder Elb Surg. 2003;12(2):164–9.
18. Raniga S, Arenas-Miquelez A, Bokor DJ. Anatomic total shoulder arthroplasty in patients under 50 and over 80 years of age. Part 1, vol. 17. Obere Extremität; 2022. p. 259.
19. Bansal A, Khatib ON, Zuckerman JD. Revision total joint arthroplasty: the epidemiology of 63,140 cases in New York state. J Arthroplast. 2014;29(1):23–7.
20. Day JS, et al. Prevalence and projections of total shoulder and elbow arthroplasty in the United States to 2015. J Shoulder Elb Surg. 2010;19(8):1115–20.
21. Wiater BP, Moravek JE Jr, Wiater JM. The evaluation of the failed shoulder arthroplasty. J Shoulder Elb Surg. 2014;23(5):745–58.
22. Boileau P, et al. Tuberosity malposition and migration: reasons for poor outcomes after hemiarthroplasty for displaced fractures of the proximal humerus. J Shoulder Elb Surg. 2002;11(5):401–12.
23. Boileau P. Complications and revision of reverse total shoulder arthroplasty. Orthop Traumatol Surg Res. 2016;102(1 Suppl):S33–43.
24. Bohsali KI, Bois AJ, Wirth MA. Complications of shoulder arthroplasty. J Bone Joint Surg Am. 2017;99(3):256–69.
25. Otto RJ, et al. Scapular fractures after reverse shoulder arthroplasty: evaluation of risk factors and the reliability of a proposed classification. J Shoulder Elb Surg. 2013;22(11):1514–21.
26. Gilbart M, Gerber C. Comparison of the subjective shoulder value and the constant score. J Shoulder Elb Surg. 2007;16(6):717–21.
27. Neyton L, et al. Grammont award 2018: scapular fractures in reverse shoulder arthroplasty (Grammont style): prevalence, functional, and radiographic results with minimum 5-year follow-up. J Shoulder Elb Surg. 2019;28(2):260–7.
28. Barco R, et al. Complications in reverse shoulder arthroplasty. EFORT Open Rev. 2016;1(3):72–80.
29. Gyftopoulos S, et al. ACR appropriateness criteria imaging after shoulder arthroplasty. J Am Coll Radiol. 2016;13(11):1324–36.
30. Sheridan BD, et al. Shoulder arthroplasty. Part 2: normal and abnormal radiographic findings. Clin Radiol. 2012;67(7):716–21.
31. Alolabi B, et al. Radiographic assessment of prosthetic humeral head size after anatomic shoulder arthroplasty. J Shoulder Elb Surg. 2014;23(11):1740–6.
32. McLendon PB, et al. Survival of the pegged glenoid component in shoulder arthroplasty: part II. J Shoulder Elb Surg. 2017;26(8):1469–76.
33. Chakravarthy K, et al. Review of recent advances in peripheral nerve stimulation (PNS). Curr Pain Headache Rep. 2016;20(11):60.
34. Ladermann A, et al. Objective evaluation of lengthening in reverse shoulder arthroplasty. J Shoulder Elb Surg. 2009;18(4):588–95.
35. Gregory T, et al. A CT scan protocol for the detection of radiographic loosening of the glenoid component after total shoulder arthroplasty. Acta Orthop. 2013;85:91.
36. Arican P, et al. The role of bone SPECT/CT in the evaluation of painful joint prostheses. Nucl Med Commun. 2015;36(9):931–40.
37. Mallo GC, et al. Assessment of painful total shoulder arthroplasty using computed tomography arthrography. J Shoulder Elb Surg. 2015;24(10):1507–11.
38. Yian EH, et al. Radiographic and computed tomography analysis of cemented pegged polyethylene glenoid components in total shoulder replacement. J Bone Joint Surg Am. 2005;87(9):1928–36.
39. Pessis E, et al. Reduction of metal artifact with dual-energy CT: virtual Monospectral imaging with fast Kilovoltage switching and metal artifact reduction software. Semin Musculoskelet Radiol. 2015;19(5):446–55.
40. Vidil A, et al. CT scan evaluation of glenoid component fixation: a prospective study of 27 minimally cemented shoulder arthroplasties. Eur J Orthop Surg Traumatol. 2013;23(5):521–5.
41. Huang JY, et al. An evaluation of three commercially available metal artifact reduction methods for CT imaging. Phys Med Biol. 2015;60(3):1047–67.
42. Shim E, et al. Metal artifact reduction for orthopedic implants (O-MAR): usefulness in CT evaluation of reverse Total shoulder arthroplasty. AJR Am J Roentgenol. 2017;209(4):860–6.
43. Sofka CM, Adler RS. Original report. Sonographic evaluation of shoulder arthroplasty. AJR Am J Roentgenol. 2003;180(4):1117–20.
44. Nwawka OK, et al. Magnetic resonance imaging of shoulder arthroplasty: review article. HSS J. 2014;10(3):213–24.
45. Jungmann PM, et al. Advances in MRI around metal. J Magn Reson Imaging. 2017;46(4):972–91.

46. Petscavage-Thomas J. Preoperative planning and postoperative imaging in shoulder arthroplasty. Semin Musculoskelet Radiol. 2014;18(4):448–62.
47. Sperling JW, et al. Magnetic resonance imaging of painful shoulder arthroplasty. J Shoulder Elb Surg. 2002;11(4):315–21.
48. Meshram P, et al. Can metal artifact reduction sequence magnetic resonance imaging (MARS-MRI) help in the diagnosis of periprosthetic shoulder infection? J Shoulder Elb Surg. 2022;31(3):e149–50.
49. Gnanasegaran G, et al. Patterns, variants, artifacts, and pitfalls in conventional radionuclide bone imaging and SPECT/CT. Semin Nucl Med. 2009;39(6):380–95.
50. Bybel B, et al. SPECT/CT imaging: clinical utility of an emerging technology. Radiographics. 2008;28(4):1097–113.
51. Hirschmann MT, et al. Combined single photon emission computerized tomography and conventional computerized tomography: clinical value for the shoulder surgeons? Int J Shoulder Surg. 2011;5(3):72–6.
52. Bockisch A, et al. Hybrid imaging by SPECT/CT and PET/CT: proven outcomes in cancer imaging. Semin Nucl Med. 2009;39(4):276–89.
53. Ogunsalu C, et al. Comparative study of the osteoblastic activity of two implant systems (Endopore versus Entegra) utilizing single photon emission computed tomography (SPECT): experimental study in pigs model. West Indian Med J. 2013;62(2):145–8.
54. Berth A, et al. SPECT/CT demonstrates the osseointegrative response of a stemless shoulder prosthesis. J Shoulder Elb Surg. 2016;25(4):e96–103.
55. Vaz S, et al. Bone scan usefulness in patients with painful hip or knee prosthesis: 10 situations that can cause pain, other than loosening and infection. Eur J Orthop Surg Traumatol. 2017;27(2):147–56.
56. Sirveaux F, et al. Grammont inverted total shoulder arthroplasty in the treatment of glenohumeral osteoarthritis with massive rupture of the cuff. Results of a multicentre study of 80 shoulders. J Bone Joint Surg Br Vol. 2004;86(3):388–95.
57. Love C, Marwin SE, Palestro CJ. Nuclear medicine and the infected joint replacement. Semin Nucl Med. 2009;39(1):66–78.
58. Palestro CJ, Love C. Role of nuclear medicine for diagnosing infection of recently implanted lower extremity arthroplasties. Semin Nucl Med. 2017;47(6):630–8.
59. Love C, et al. Diagnosing infection in the failed joint replacement: a comparison of coincidence detection 18F-FDG and 111In-labeled leukocyte/99mTc-sulfur colloid marrow imaging. J Nucl Med. 2004;45(11):1864–71.
60. Palestro CJ. Nuclear medicine and the failed joint replacement: past, present, and future. World J Radiol. 2014;6(7):446–58.
61. Dodson CC, et al. Propionibacterium acnes infection after shoulder arthroplasty: a diagnostic challenge. J Shoulder Elb Surg. 2010;19(2):303–7.
62. Shields MV, Abdullah L, Namdari S. The challenge of Propionibacterium acnes and revision shoulder arthroplasty: a review of current diagnostic options. J Shoulder Elb Surg. 2016;25(6):1034–40.
63. Topolski MS, et al. Revision shoulder arthroplasty with positive intraoperative cultures: the value of preoperative studies and intraoperative histology. J Shoulder Elb Surg. 2006;15(4):402–6.
64. Villacis D, et al. Serum interleukin-6 as a marker of periprosthetic shoulder infection. J Bone Joint Surg Am. 2014;96(1):41–5.
65. Pottinger P, et al. Prognostic factors for bacterial cultures positive for Propionibacterium acnes and other organisms in a large series of revision shoulder arthroplasties performed for stiffness, pain, or loosening. J Bone Joint Surg Am. 2012;94(22):2075–83.
66. Grosso MJ, et al. Sensitivity of frozen section histology for identifying Propionibacterium acnes infections in revision shoulder arthroplasty. J Bone Joint Surg Am. 2014;96(6):442–7.
67. Chalmers PN, Sumner S, Romeo AA, Tashjian RZ. Do elevated inflammatory markers associate with infection in revision shoulder arthroplasty? J Shoulder Elb Arthroplast. 2018;2:2.
68. Garrigues GE, et al. Proceedings from the 2018 international consensus meeting on orthopedic infections: the definition of periprosthetic shoulder infection. J Shoulder Elb Surg. 2019;28(6S):S8–S12.
69. Piper KE, et al. C-reactive protein, erythrocyte sedimentation rate and orthopedic implant infection. PLoS One. 2010;5(2):e9358.
70. Frangiamore SJ, et al. Alpha-defensin as a predictor of periprosthetic shoulder infection. J Shoulder Elb Surg. 2015;24(7):1021–7.
71. Frangiamore SJ, et al. Alpha-defensin accuracy to diagnose periprosthetic joint infection-Best available test? J Arthroplast. 2016;31(2):456–60.
72. Berbari E, et al. Inflammatory blood laboratory levels as markers of prosthetic joint infection: a systematic review and meta-analysis. J Bone Joint Surg Am. 2010;92(11):2102–9.
73. Ince A, et al. One-stage exchange shoulder arthroplasty for peri-prosthetic infection. J Bone Joint Surg Br. 2005;87(6):814–8.
74. Coste JS, et al. The management of infection in arthroplasty of the shoulder. J Bone Joint Surg Br Vol. 2004;86-B(1):65–9.
75. Dilisio MF, et al. Arthroscopic tissue culture for the evaluation of periprosthetic shoulder infection. J Bone Joint Surg Am. 2014;96(23):1952–8.
76. Sanchez-Sotelo J. Periprosthetic shoulder infections are less elusive to diagnostic arthroscopy: commentary on an article by Matthew F. Dilisio, MD, et al.: "arthroscopic tissue culture for the evaluation of periprosthetic shoulder infection". J Bone Joint Surg Am. 2014;96(23):e197.
77. Doherty C, et al. Arthroscopy of the symptomatic shoulder arthroplasty. J Shoulder Elb Surg. 2019;28(10):1971–6.
78. Bonutti PM, Hawkins RJ, Saddemi S. Arthroscopic assessment of glenoid component loosening after total shoulder arthroplasty. Arthroscopy. 1993;9(3):272–6.

79. Guild T, et al. The role of arthroscopy in painful shoulder arthroplasty: is revision always necessary? Arthroscopy. 2020;36(6):1508–14.
80. Tashjian RZ, Granger EK, Zhang Y. Utility of prerevision tissue biopsy sample to predict revision shoulder arthroplasty culture results in at-risk patients. J Shoulder Elb Surg. 2017;26(2):197–203.
81. Gee AO, et al. Shoulder instability after total shoulder arthroplasty: a case of arthroscopic repair. HSS J. 2014;10(1):88–91.
82. Gonzalez JF, et al. Complications of unconstrained shoulder prostheses. J Shoulder Elb Surg. 2011;20(4):666–82.
83. Lynch NM, et al. Neurologic complications after total shoulder arthroplasty. J Shoulder Elb Surg. 1996;5(1):53–61.
84. Ladermann A, et al. Influence of arm lengthening in reverse shoulder arthroplasty. J Shoulder Elb Surg. 2012;21(3):336–41.
85. Ladermann A, et al. Prevalence of neurologic lesions after total shoulder arthroplasty. J Bone Joint Surg Am Vol. 2011;93(14):1288–93.
86. Hagedorn JM, Pittelkow TP, Bendel MA, Moeschler SM, Orhurhu V, Sanchez-Sotelo J. The painful shoulder arthroplasty: appropriate work-up and review of interventional pain treatments. JSES Rev Rep Tech. 2022;2:269–76.

5 Preoperative Planning for Revision Arthroplasty: Imaging, Instruments, and Implants

Giuseppe Porcellini, Matilde Delvecchio, Andrea Giorgini, Gian Mario Micheloni, and Luigi Tarallo

5.1 Introduction

A successful revision shoulder replacement surgery is based on four fundamentals: knowledge of the implant to be explanted, good preoperative planning, choice of materials, and analysis of possible complications.

Preoperative evaluation should start with first-level imaging: radiographs. Second-level examinations, such as computed tomography (CT), magnetic resonance imaging (MRI), and bone scintigraphy, will be chosen based on the diagnostic suspicion. Imaging may not be diriment due to the presence of artifacts. In some cases, musculotendinous ultrasound, for evaluation of the soft tissues, especially the subscapularis tendon, and electromyography, especially for evaluation of the axillary nerve, may also be helpful.

It is necessary to exclude the presence of infection at the first instance with laboratory tests (complete blood count with white blood cell count, erythrocyte sedimentation rate (ESR), C-reactive protein (CRP)). To this end, a diagnostic arthrocentesis with culture and physical–chemical examination of joint fluid may also be useful.

G. Porcellini · M. Delvecchio (✉) · A. Giorgini · G. M. Micheloni · L. Tarallo
Orthopedic and Traumatology Department, University of Modena and Reggio Emilia, Modena, Italy
e-mail: tarallo.luigi@policlinico.mo.it

A thorough patient history must be conducted, to know the previous surgical access or accesses, the implanted prosthesis (sizes and types of components), and to have the removal instrumentation and components available at the time of revision.

It is important to know the functional demand of the patient and, based on this, to share the goals and strategy of revision surgery because it often needs multiple surgical steps, long hospitalization, and compliance in rehabilitation and follow-up.

Prior to surgery, it is mandatory to explain to the patient the possibility of using possible grafts with the autologous bone (iliac crest harvesting) or allograft (donor bone).

For this reason, preoperative planning is the key step before entering the operating room with the correct diagnosis and all the necessary materials for the surgery to obtain a satisfactory result.

5.2 Clinical Diagnosis

A painful shoulder implant should be considered, until proven otherwise, to be infected. To rule this out, an evaluation of the patient's condition by careful objective examination, monitoring of body temperature, and blood chemistry tests with index of inflammation (leukocyte count, ESR, CRP, fibrinogen, alpha-2 glycoprotein), and, in some cases, a diagnostic arthrocentesis and

F. Franceschi et al. (eds.), *Revision Shoulder Arthroplasty*,
https://doi.org/10.1007/978-3-031-45944-3_5

related culture and physical–chemical examination must be performed.

A thorough objective examination of the patient may lead us to suspect a possible ongoing infection: pain in the operated shoulder, the surgical wound or surgical scar with signs of edema, rubor, dolor, calor, drainage, the presence of fistulae, joint effusion, and joint collections. This is particularly true for acute infections. In chronic infections, symptoms may be more nuanced or even almost absent.

In case of fever, to rule out bacteremia, it is useful to perform blood cultures looking for aerobic and anaerobic bacteria [1].

The diagnosis of periprosthetic infection can be guided not only by the above signs and symptoms but also by the diagnostic criteria suggested by the International Consensus Meeting on Orthopedic Infections: if fistula, intraarticular pus, or two separate cultures positive for the same pathogen are present, then an infection is undoubtedly present; in the case of less obvious clinical signs, it is useful to look for the lesser criteria, and a score of 6 has been agreed upon as an indicator of a higher probability of shoulder periprosthetic joint infection (PJI) [2].

As for hematochemical tests, the evaluation of ESR and CRP seems to be universally agreed upon, whereas procalcitonin value does not seem to be useful in the differential diagnosis of periprosthetic infections [3].

Instability of a prosthesis can also be a sign of an underlying infection. Therefore, in preoperative planning of an unstable reverse shoulder prosthesis revision, one must first rule out infection, as this can lead to instability in 50% of cases [4].

5.3 Imaging

Imaging is of course extremely useful for the study of the bone component; however, it should not be forgotten that in the case of a prosthetic revision, a key role is played by the soft tissue.

Radiographic investigation is the starting point as far as the diagnostic hypothesis is concerned (Figs. 5.1 and 5.2).

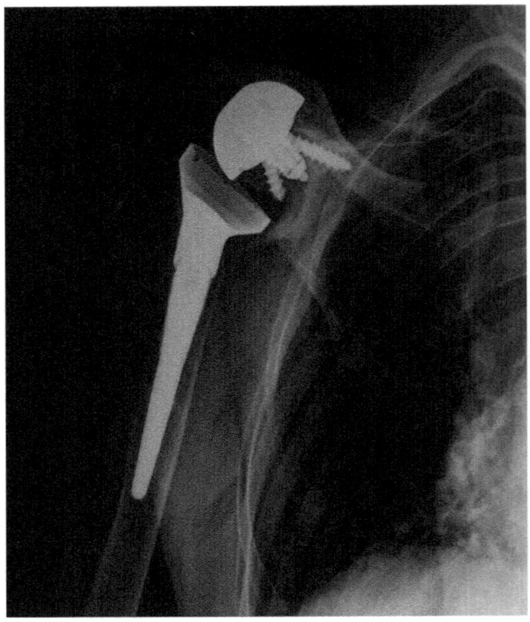

Fig. 5.1 Glenoid mobilization in a reverse shoulder arthroplasty (RSA) implant

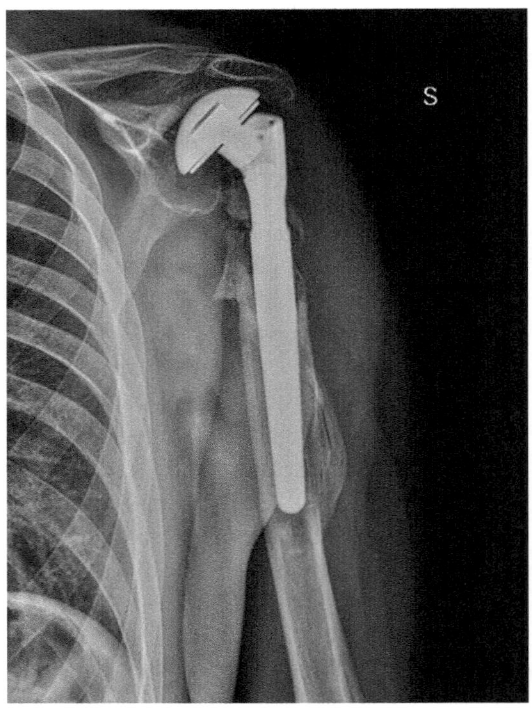

Fig. 5.2 Superior migration of endoprosthesis with humeral bone reabsorption

Not only are radiographs in the three conventional projections essential but also are those prior to prosthetic replacement surgery and those of the contralateral shoulder that can be compared with the radiographs of the already operated shoulder to be revised. Comparison of radiographs is useful to assess native metrics, humeral shortening following osteotomy, and the amount of bone loss in the proximal humerus.

A comparative analysis of radiographs is performed on a millimeter scale to quantify the humeral defect in shortening according to Lädermann et al. [5]; anteroposterior (AP) radiographs in neutral rotation are useful to quantify excessive humeral or/and glenoid medialization, so measuring the distance between the lateral border of the acromion and the humeral endomedullary axis is recommended [6].

CT remains the main examination during preoperative planning of shoulder prosthesis revisions, especially CT with artifact subtraction. We can distinguish three different situations:

- In case of trauma, it allows us to identify possible fractures at the level of either the humeral stem or the glenoid.
- In case of aseptic loosening of the prosthesis, it allows us to evaluate the prosthesis–bone interface: at the level of the humerus the orientation and height of the osteotomy, inclination, and version, and at the level of the glenoid inclination, version, and medialization.
- In case of infection or septic loosening, it allows to identify collections and study the prosthesis–bone interface (Figs. 5.3 and 5.4).

In total prosthesis revision (one or two stages), the glenoid and humeral bone stock should be evaluated (Fig. 5.5).

CT for this purpose is extremely useful, although the best characterization of bone loss occurs intraoperatively, once the components have been removed and after debridement of the fibrous tissue [7].

CT scanning with artifact subtraction is always useful in the presence of a metallic component in the field.

MRI remains a useful investigation to be applied when revising anatomic prostheses in a reverse shoulder arthroplasty (RSA) (evaluation of the rotator cuff and subscapularis) and for studying the nature of periprosthetic collections.

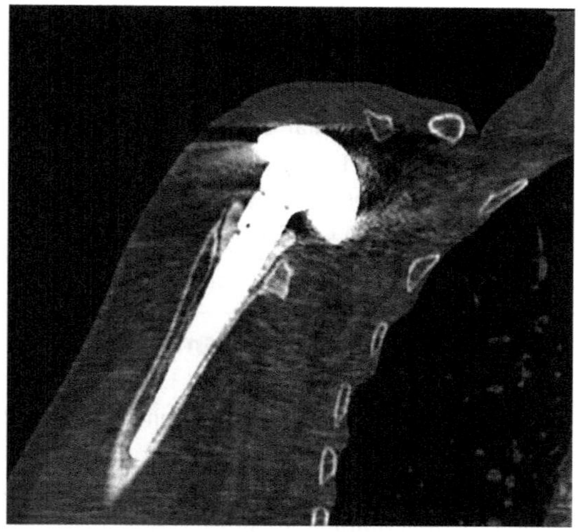

Fig. 5.3 Radiolucent lines between the cement and humeral bone

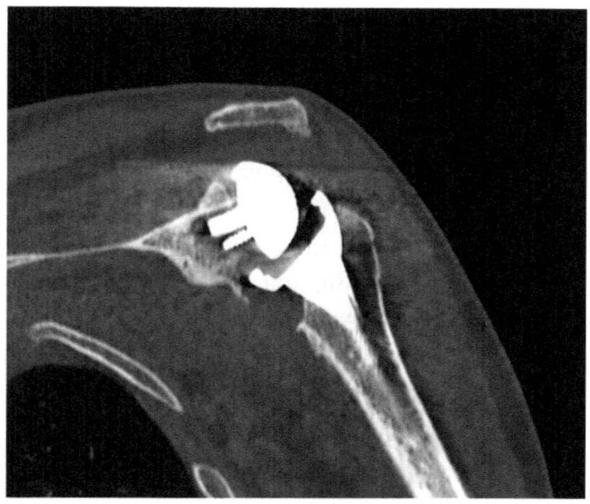

Fig. 5.4 Radiolucent lines between the metal back and glenoid bone

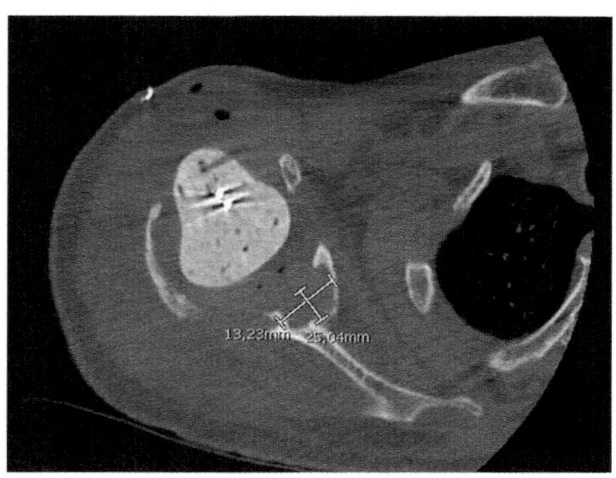

Fig. 5.5 Glenoid bone loss in a CT scan before two-stage revision

When diagnostic doubts remain unclear, it is advisable to perform a scintigraphy with labeled leukocytes: this exam is not indeed recommended by the last International Congress on PJI but is making a comeback in clinical practice in cases of suspected infection, as it is characterized by high sensitivity and specificity [8].

5.4 Soft Tissue Assessment

Patients who have already undergone a shoulder prosthesis surgery often have altered anatomy. In the case of revisions of anatomic prostheses, it is necessary to combine imaging (MRI and CT) with a thorough clinical evaluation of the rotator cuff to establish its integrity to improve implant stability.

Ultrasonography is a diagnostic adjunct examination, useful for studying the extent, morphology, and consistency of any periprosthetic collections.

In order to study the musculature, electromyography (EMG) and the study of nerve conduction may be useful; in particular, evaluation of axillary nerve conduction and deltoid muscle function is useful. Axillary nerve injury and deltoid dysfunction are a relative contraindication to revision shoulder replacement.

5.5 Instruments: Software

Correct positioning of the glenoid component is critical during shoulder prosthesis revisions; the accuracy of glenoid component insertion can be improved with appropriate preoperative and intraoperative assessment of glenoid morphology. CT is the gold standard for measuring glenoid version and inclination.

The evolution of three-dimensional (3D) imaging has enabled the development of virtual planning software that, based on CT images, allows simulation of the positioning of the glenoid component of the implant. Subsequently, computer-assisted intraoperative navigation has enabled important integration of such software into shoulder prosthetic surgery [9] (Figs. 5.6, 5.7, 5.8, 5.9, and 5.10).

This technology allows intraoperative monitoring and more accurate positioning of the glenoid component, but it is not without problems, including significantly increased operative time, associated costs, increased soft tissue exposure, and iatrogenic fractures. In addition, to achieve correct and accurate positioning of the glenoid component, patient-specific instrumentation (PSI) has been introduced and can be used (Figs. 5.11 and 5.12).

Several studies have evaluated the ability of PSI to accurately reproduce the preoperative 3D virtual plane, but large-scale studies of patients and with long-term follow-up will be needed to justify the use of these devices [10, 11].

As the severity of the glenoid deformity increases during revisions, it becomes more difficult to achieve the desired position of the glenoid implant. 3D planning can help learn more about glenoid morphology, calibrate glenoid version correction and inclination, measure the size of glenoid implants, and localize peripheral peg perforation and subchondral bone boundaries during reaming and glenoid preparation, when studying the baseplate–bone interface [12].

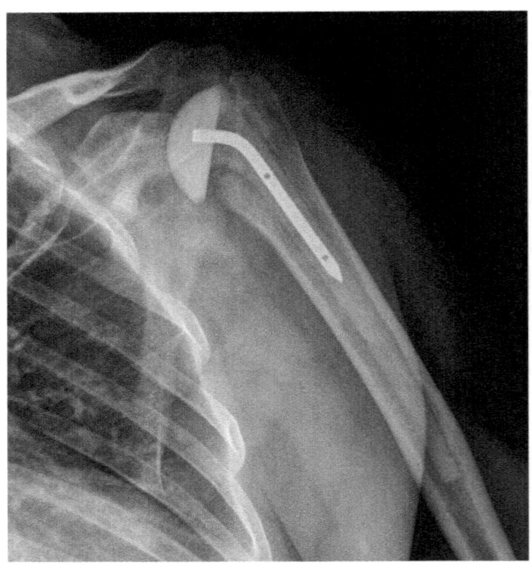

Fig. 5.6 An X-ray examination shows an antibiotic-loaded cement spacer after an RSA infection

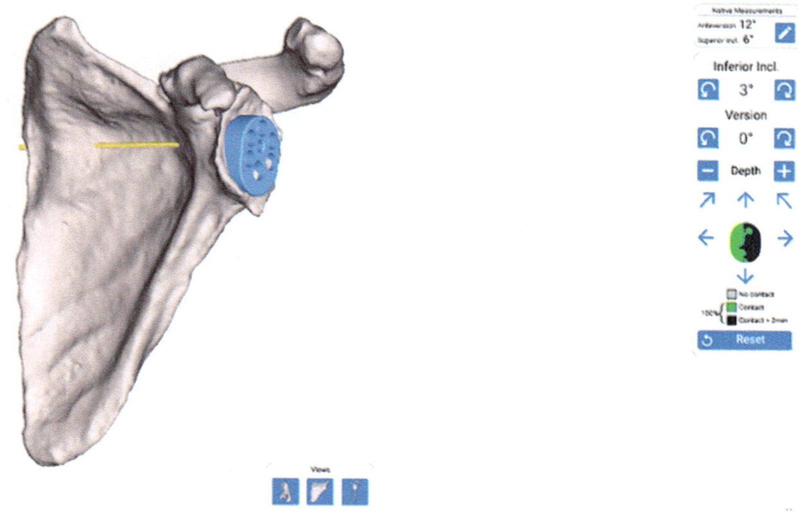

Fig. 5.7 3D planning of a staged revision (second stage after spacer implantation)

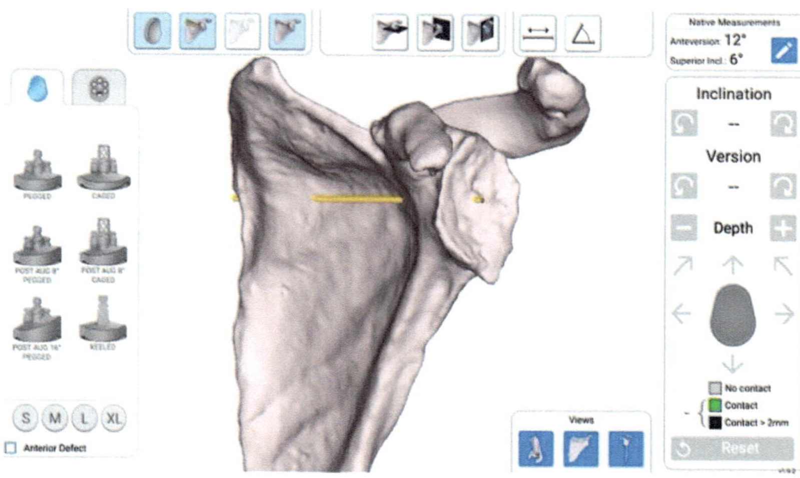

Fig. 5.8 3D planning of a staged revision (second stage after spacer implantation)

Currently, the use of planning software and intraoperative navigation in prosthesis revision cases appears to be not widely used. Companies are making great efforts in order to gain the availability of software planning even in the presence of artifacts and, so, in the case of revision surgery.

There are cases in which software does not always correctly represent the patient's anatomy and/or the patient's anatomy does not always allow proper placement of PSI instruments. In these cases, the surgeon's experience is essential to achieve a stable and long-lasting implant.

In the future, decreasing costs and the spread of the aforementioned technologies will lead to greater availability and utilization, then to greater accuracy of virtual preoperative planning and implantation of the glenoid components, and, ultimately, to better clinical outcomes of shoulder arthroplasty.

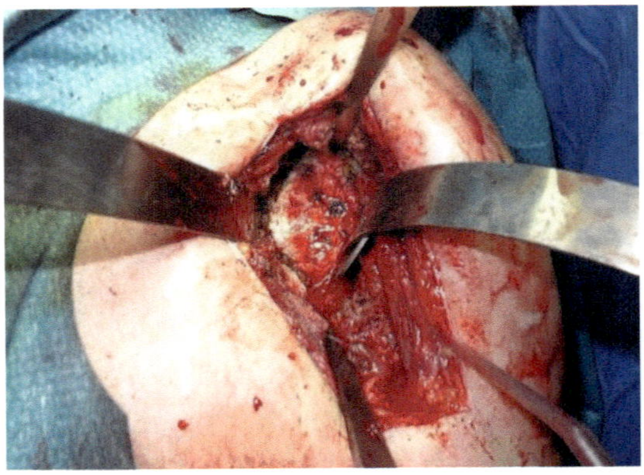

Fig. 5.9 Intraoperative glenoid bone stock after spacer removal

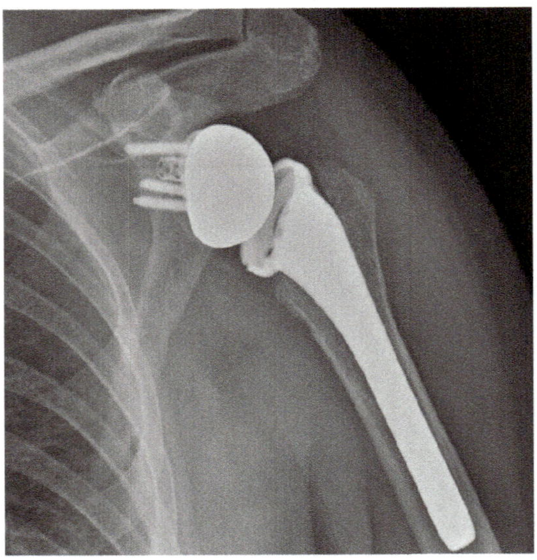

Fig. 5.10 Postoperative X-ray image after the second stage (performed with Global Positioning System (GPS)-aided navigation)

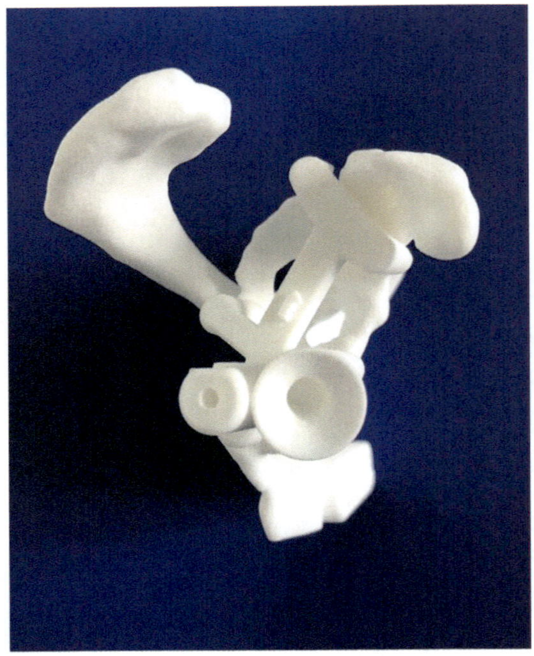

Fig. 5.11 PSI 3D-printed trials of a custom-made revision implant

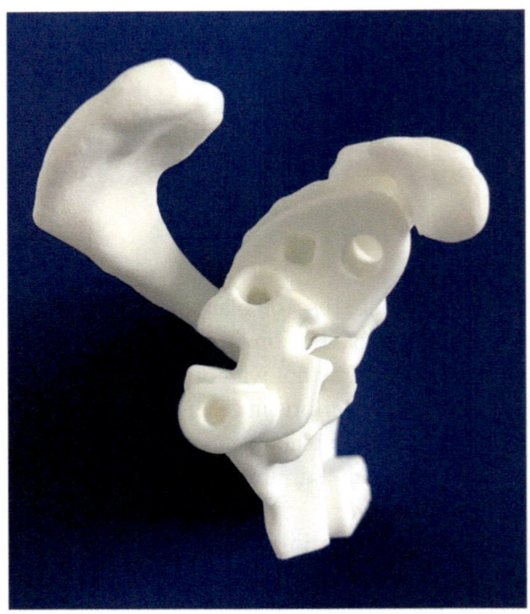

Fig. 5.12 PSI 3D-printed trials of a custom-made revision implant

5.6 Implants

The choice of prosthetic implant is one of the features on which the long-term success of revision prosthetic surgery is based.

During preoperative planning, it is necessary to know whether the prosthetic implant to be revised is cemented or uncemented, as removal of a cemented humeral stem is complex and can result in increased bone loss, risk of intraoperative fracture, blood loss, and increased operative time [13].

It is necessary to have dedicated chisels and drills available in the operating room to minimize bone loss. However, in cases of significant humeral bone loss or poor-quality bone tissue, one can avail oneself of the option of using revision implants with long, modular stems that allow a distal metaepiphyseal socket of the humerus.

In cases of revision of the glenoid component only, it should be made sure that the bearing is compatible with the preexisting humeral stem. In these cases, it is necessary for the humeral implant to be well-positioned and stable.

In the case of revision anatomic prosthesis, one may decide to keep the stem in place and convert the implant to an inverse prosthesis: at present, many systems are convertible (Stryker, Lima, etc.).

An absolute prerequisite for retaining the convertible primary stem is that it is well-placed and well-secured [14, 15].

Regarding the glenoid component, there are implants that allow endoprosthesis to be converted to reverse prosthesis without removing the metal-backed glenoid baseplate (MBG); in these cases, the polyethylene insert is removed, leaving the metal back in place, on which the revision metal ball will be placed.

Retaining one of the primary prosthetic components allows for reduced operative time, less impact on the soft tissue, and less aggression on the bone tissue.

Unfortunately, good stability of the stem is not enough to retain the humeral component: if there is malpositioning (i.e., excessive shortening of the humerus or wrong inclination of the baseplate), then it is necessary to go for a complete revision even of the fixed components..

In cases of severe humeral bone loss, it may be necessary to use an allograft with a cadaver humerus fragment [16] (Figs. 5.13 and 5.14).

Because of the high risk of allograft bone resorption, mainly related to the lack of muscle insertions, it is advisable to fix the graft to the native bone with a plate and screws.

A bone allograft, similar to BioRSA, or a metal back with augment can also be used in cases of glenoid bone loss (Figs. 5.15, 5.16, 5.17, and 5.18).

In cases of severe glenoid bone loss, however, it will be necessary to use custom-made implants prepared for the patient in order to preserve the native glenoid and implant a stable component (Figs. 5.19 and 5.20).

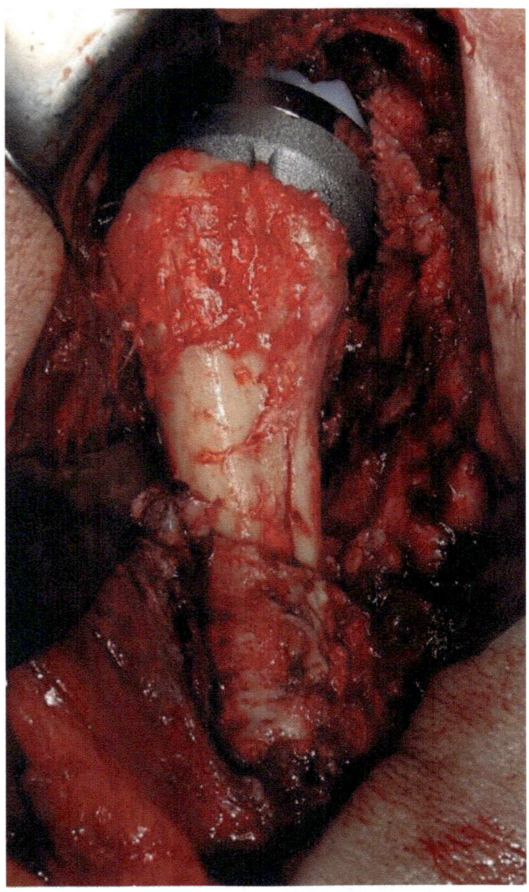

Fig. 5.13 Intraoperative severe humeral bone loss treated with an RSA and bone allograft

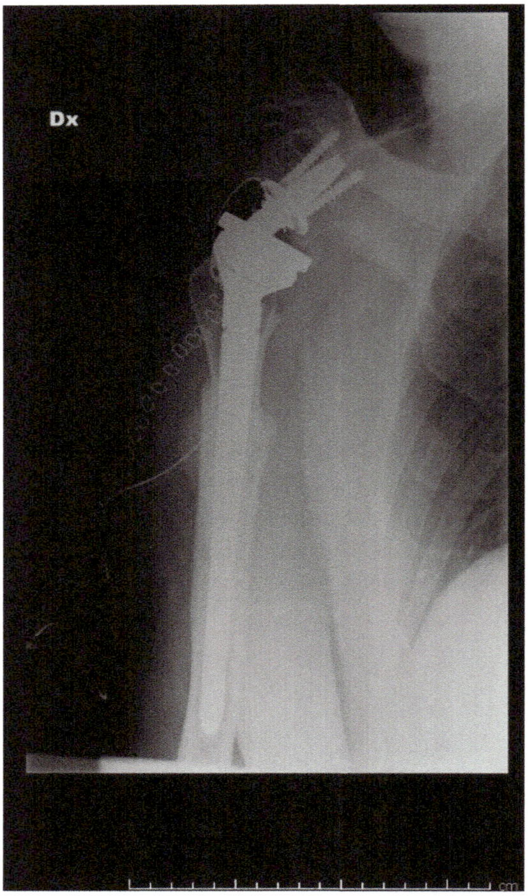

Fig. 5.14 A postoperative X-ray image of an RSA with a bone allograft

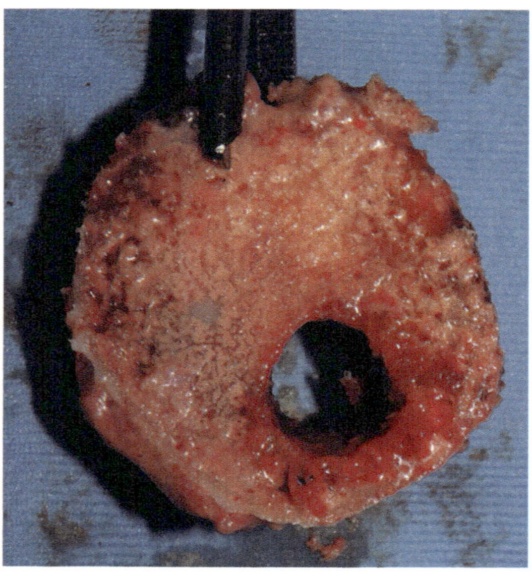

Fig. 5.15 A bone allograft prepared for glenoid bone loss

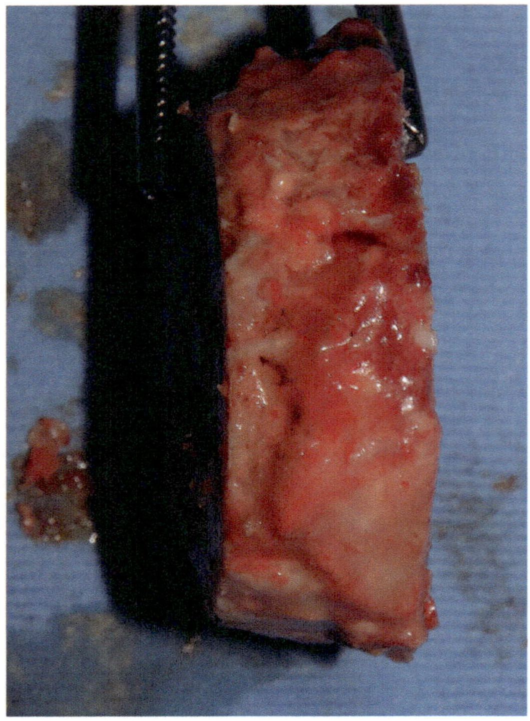

Fig. 5.16 A bone allograft prepared for glenoid bone loss

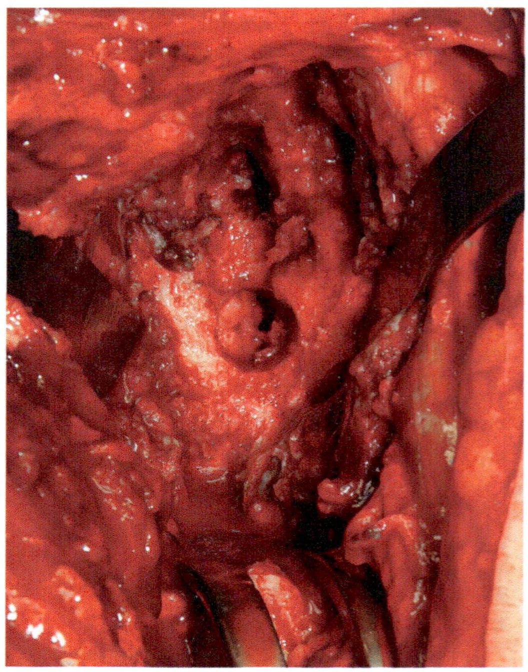

Fig. 5.17 Intraoperative glenoid bone loss before and after graft positioning

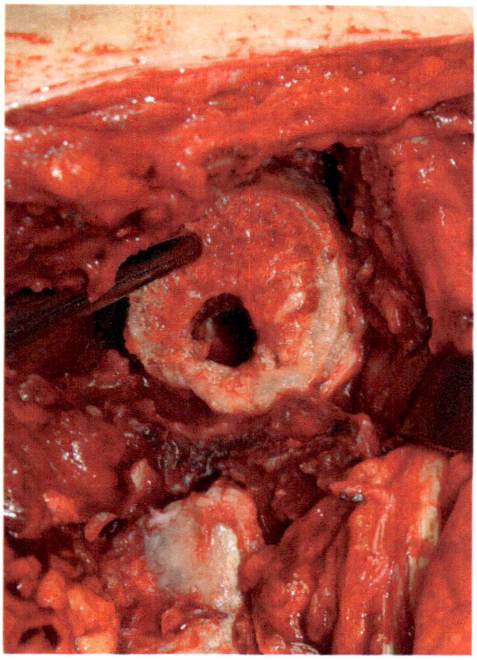

Fig. 5.18 Intraoperative glenoid bone loss before and after graft positioning

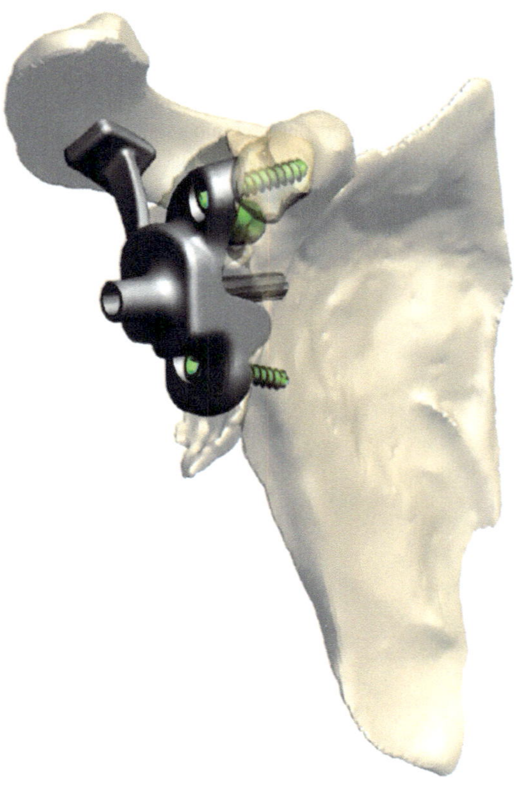

Fig. 5.19 3D planning of a glenoid custom-made implant

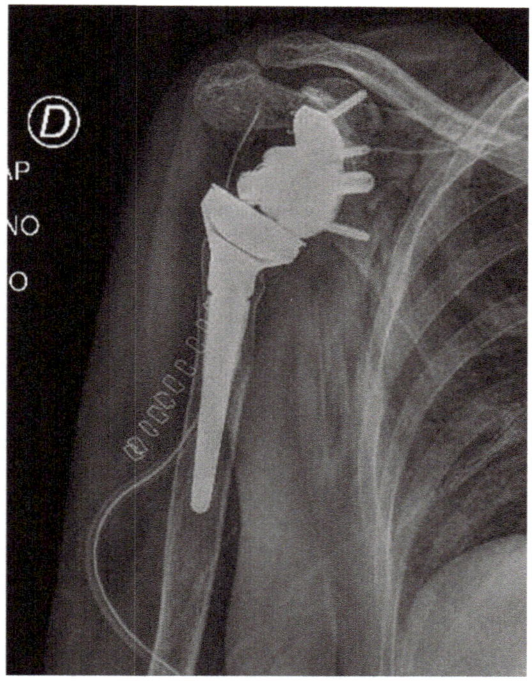

Fig. 5.20 Postoperative X-ray of revision RSA with a glenoid custom-made implant

Early results with these implants are encouraging, but further long-term follow-up studies are required to assess their efficacy and survivorship [17].

References

1. Osmon DR, Berbari EF, Berendt AR, Lew D, Zimmerli W, Steckelberg JM, Rao N, Hanssen A, Wilson WR. Infectious Diseases Society of America. Diagnosis and management of prosthetic joint infection: clinical practice guidelines by the Infectious Diseases Society of America. Clin Infect Dis. 2013;56(1):e1–e25. https://doi.org/10.1093/cid/cis803. Epub 2012 Dec 6.
2. Garrigues GE, Zmistowski B, Cooper AM, Green A, ICM Shoulder Group. Proceedings from the 2018 international consensus meeting on orthopedic infections: the definition of periprosthetic shoulder infection. J Shoulder Elb Surg. 2019;28(6S):S8–S12. https://doi.org/10.1016/j.jse.2019.04.034.
3. Busch A, Jäger M, Engler H, et al. Is Procalcitonin (PCT) a reliable biomarker for preoperative diagnosing of low grade periprosthetic joint infection? A prospective study. BMC Musculoskelet Disord. 2020;21:257. https://doi.org/10.1186/s12891-020-03266-6.
4. Gallo RA, Gamradt SC, Mattern CJ, Cordasco FA, Craig EV, Dines DM, Warren RF, Sports Medicine and

Shoulder Service at the Hospital for Special Surgery, New York, NY. Instability after reverse total shoulder replacement. J Shoulder Elb Surg. 2011;20(4):584–90. https://doi.org/10.1016/j.jse.2010.08.028. Epub 2010 Dec 16.
5. Lädermann A, Williams MD, Melis B, Hoffmeyer P, Walch G. Objective evaluation of lengthening in reverse shoulder arthroplasty. J Shoulder Elbow Surg. 2009;18(4):588–95. https://doi.org/10.1016/j.jse.2009.03.012. Epub 2009 May 28. PMID: 19481476.
6. Boileau P. Complications and revision of reverse total shoulder arthroplasty. Orthop Traumatol Surg Res. 2016;102:S33. https://doi.org/10.1016/j.otsr.2015.06.031.
7. Antuna SA, Sperling JW, Cofield RH, Rowland CM. Glenoid revision surgery after total shoulder arthroplasty. J Shoulder Elb Surg. 2001;10(3):217–24. https://doi.org/10.1067/mse.2001.113961.
8. Trevail C, Ravindranath-Reddy P, Sulkin T, Bartlett G. An evaluation of the role of nuclear medicine imaging in the diagnosis of periprosthetic infections of the hip. Clin Radiol. 2016;71(3):211–9. https://doi.org/10.1016/j.crad.2015.10.026. Epub 2015 Dec 17.
9. Verborgt O, De Smedt T, Vanhees M, Clockaerts S, Parizel PM, Van Glabbeek F. Accuracy of placement of the glenoid component in reversed shoulder arthroplasty with and without navigation. J Shoulder Elb Surg. 2011;20(1):21–6. https://doi.org/10.1016/j.jse.2010.07.014.
10. Throckmorton TW, Gulotta LV, Bonnarens FO, Wright SA, Hartzell JL, Rozzi WB, et al. Patient-specific targeting guides compared with traditional instrumentation for glenoid component placement in shoulder arthroplasty: a multi-surgeon study in 70 arthritic cadaver specimens. J Shoulder Elb Surg. 2015;24(6):965–71. https://doi.org/10.1016/j.jse.2014.10.013.
11. Iannotti JP, Davidson IU, Ricchetti ET. Three-dimensional preoperative planning and patient-specific instrumentation for total shoulder arthroplasty. Semin Arthroplast. 2017;28(1):25–9. https://doi.org/10.1053/j.sart.2017.05.005.
12. Gauci MO, Boileau P, Baba M, Chaoui J, Walch G. Patient-specific glenoid guides provide accuracy and reproducibility in total shoulder arthroplasty. Bone Joint J. 2016;98-B(8):1080–5. https://doi.org/10.1302/0301-620X.98B8.37257.
13. Hsu SH. Implant removal in revision arthroplasty: a tour de force. Semin arthroplasty. 2012; 23:118-24. Duquin TR, Sperling J. Revision shoulder arthroplasty: how to manage the humerus. Operative techniques in orthopedics. J Shoulder Elb Surg. 2011;21:44–51.
14. Crosby LA, Wright TW, Yu S, Zuckerman JD. Conversion to reverse Total shoulder arthroplasty with and without humeral stem retention: the role of a convertible-platform stem. J Bone Joint Surg Am. 2017;99(9):736–42. https://doi.org/10.2106/JBJS.16.00683.
15. Magosch P, Lichtenberg S, Habermeyer P. Survival of stemless humeral head replacement in anatomic shoulder arthroplasty: a prospective study. J Shoulder Elb Surg. 2021;30(7):e343–55. https://doi.org/10.1016/j.jse.2020.09.034. Epub 2020 Nov 1.
16. Garver J, Mata-Fink A, Zhu D, Javier F, Gallacher S, Blaine TA. Revision strategies in reverse total shoulder arthroplasty. J Shoulder Elb Arthroplast. 2017:1. https://doi.org/10.1177/2471549217695259.
17. Porcellini G, Micheloni GM, Tarallo L, Paladini P, Merolla G, Catani F. Custom-made reverse shoulder arthroplasty for severe glenoid bone loss: review of the literature and our preliminary results. J Orthop Traumatol. 2021;22(1):2. https://doi.org/10.1186/s10195-020-00564-6.

PSI, Navigation, AR, and MR in Revision Shoulder Arthroplasty

6

Jessica L. Churchill, Conner Paez, Jason C. Ho, Vahid Entezari, Joseph P. Iannotti, and Eric T. Ricchetti

6.1 Introduction

Revision total shoulder arthroplasty (TSA) brings unique challenges. Patient anatomy is often distorted by bone loss and abnormal soft tissue tension, which can impact component placement and lead to malposition or inadequate fixation. Proper implant positioning is necessary to avoid postoperative complications such as scapular notching, instability, decreased function, brachial plexus injury, and implant loosening and failure. The challenge in the revision setting can be achieving the optimal balance between ideal implant position and optimal implant fixation. Bone loss and soft tissue tension may impact the ability to place a glenoid baseplate to restore version, inclination, and joint line while also achieving adequate baseplate contact with the native glenoid bone. The emergence of new technologies now allows for three-dimensional (3D) preoperative surgical planning, intraoperative patient-specific instrumentation (PSI) or navigation, and the potential for use of intraoperative augmented reality (AR) or mixed reality (MR), all based off 3D computed tomography (CT). These tools can help surgeons achieve optimal component placement in revision TSA; however, challenges still exist in the use of these emerging technologies in the revision setting because of the presence of metal artifacts from the existing implant.

Preoperative planning with 3D CT imaging helps the surgeon choose the optimal implant size and position in patients with significant glenoid bone loss or reduced scapular neck length and can also help decide whether bone graft or implant augmentation is necessary to achieve these goals. Intraoperative PSI and navigation offer further customization to help the surgeon transfer information from the preoperative planning software to the patient during surgery. While virtual reality (VR) is an emerging technology that can be utilized for surgical simulation or training prior to surgery, AR and MR are cutting-edge new technologies that can be directly used at the time of surgery to further guide the surgeon with accurate implant placement. At present, most of the literature involving these new technologies examine primary TSA, with limited studies including a mix of primary and revision cases. Therefore, the findings must be extrapolated to revision TSA. As the worldwide rate of primary shoulder arthroplasty rises, there will be a compensatory increase in revision cases, making technologies such as preoperative planning, PSI, intraoperative navigation, and AR, and MR more relevant and useful in this setting.

J. L. Churchill · C. Paez · J. C. Ho · V. Entezari · J. P. Iannotti · E. T. Ricchetti (✉)
Department of Orthopaedic Surgery, Orthopaedic and Rheumatologic Institute, Cleveland Clinic, Cleveland, OH, USA
e-mail: churchj6@ccf.org; paezc@ccf.org; hoj@ccf.org; entezav@ccf.org; iannotj@ccf.org; ricchee@ccf.org

F. Franceschi et al. (eds.), *Revision Shoulder Arthroplasty*,
https://doi.org/10.1007/978-3-031-45944-3_6

Examining the results of these innovations in primary arthroplasty and applying them to revision TSA represents an important frontier in shoulder arthroplasty.

This chapter is divided into four sections. The first section briefly discusses preoperative planning. The second section discusses PSI as a way of improving execution of a preoperative plan for revision TSA. This section explores custom guides for placement of the glenoid baseplate, both single-use and reusable, as well as custom glenoid components. The third section discusses intraoperative navigation. The fourth section discusses the emerging technologies of AR and MR. The application of these technologies in reverse TSA will be the focus, as this is the predominant implant choice in revision TSA.

6.2 Preoperative Planning

Implant positioning can be straightforward in patients with minimal glenoid bone loss but becomes more challenging with significant glenoid bone loss or reduced scapular neck length, both of which are common in the revision setting. Multiple studies in the literature have shown that 3D CT more accurately assesses glenoid pathology, including version, inclination, and bone loss, compared to standard X-rays and two-dimensional (2D) CT, both from the ability to allow for 3D measurement and the elimination of measurement error due to the plane of image acquisition [1–5]. This has led to the widespread development of preoperative planning software in shoulder arthroplasty that utilizes 3D CT technology and allows for quantifying glenoid version, inclination, and bone loss accurately in a 3D coordinate system defined by the planes of the glenoid and scapula to guide surgical decision-making [6–11]. Each of the commercially available preoperative planning software has unique features that can assist the surgeon in determining the optimal position and size of the glenoid baseplate and glenosphere, including several with tools to allow for assessment of premorbid anatomy. The glenoid vault model, for example, has been extensively studied and validated as an imaging method to determine premorbid version, inclination, and joint line from pathological glenoid anatomy, allowing for a better understanding of the extent of glenoid bone loss prior to surgery [12–17] (Fig. 6.1). Other software methods have more recently reported use of statistical modeling of the entire scapula to define premorbid scapular and glenoid anatomy from pathological anatomy [18–20].

The ability to assess premorbid anatomy can be important in revision TSA when glenoid bone loss is significant; however, these tools have not been fully validated for use in the revision setting. Preoperative planning with 3D CT imaging also provides useful information about the surface anatomy of the glenoid, such as indentations or surface defects as well as osteophytes, which can be used as landmarks for the superior–inferior and/or anterior–posterior location of the central post or screw of the glenoid baseplate. Additionally, these surface irregularities may be helpful for determining the proper position or rotational orientation of PSI guides.

When using 3D preoperative planning in the revision setting, virtual templating allows the surgeon to determine the implant size and location that achieves the best balance of optimal component position and bony fixation based on the pattern of glenoid bone loss that is present. The surgeon must be aware that the position of the glenoid baseplate may be constrained by the bone loss pattern, with the central post or screw placed in a location with adequate glenoid bone stock for fixation. Glenoid bone grafting, augmented glenoid baseplates, eccentric glenospheres, and glenospheres of different diameter sizes and/or lateral offset have the ability to choose a contained location for the central post or screw in the bone while positioning the glenosphere in the desired location. In revision cases with more advanced glenoid bone loss, the remaining glenoid vault may be too shallow to contain the central post or screw completely in the native bone in any location. In these cases, preoperative planning software can be used to determine the exact size and location of a bone graft or baseplate augment to allow for appropriate baseplate fixation or to determine whether a custom implant is

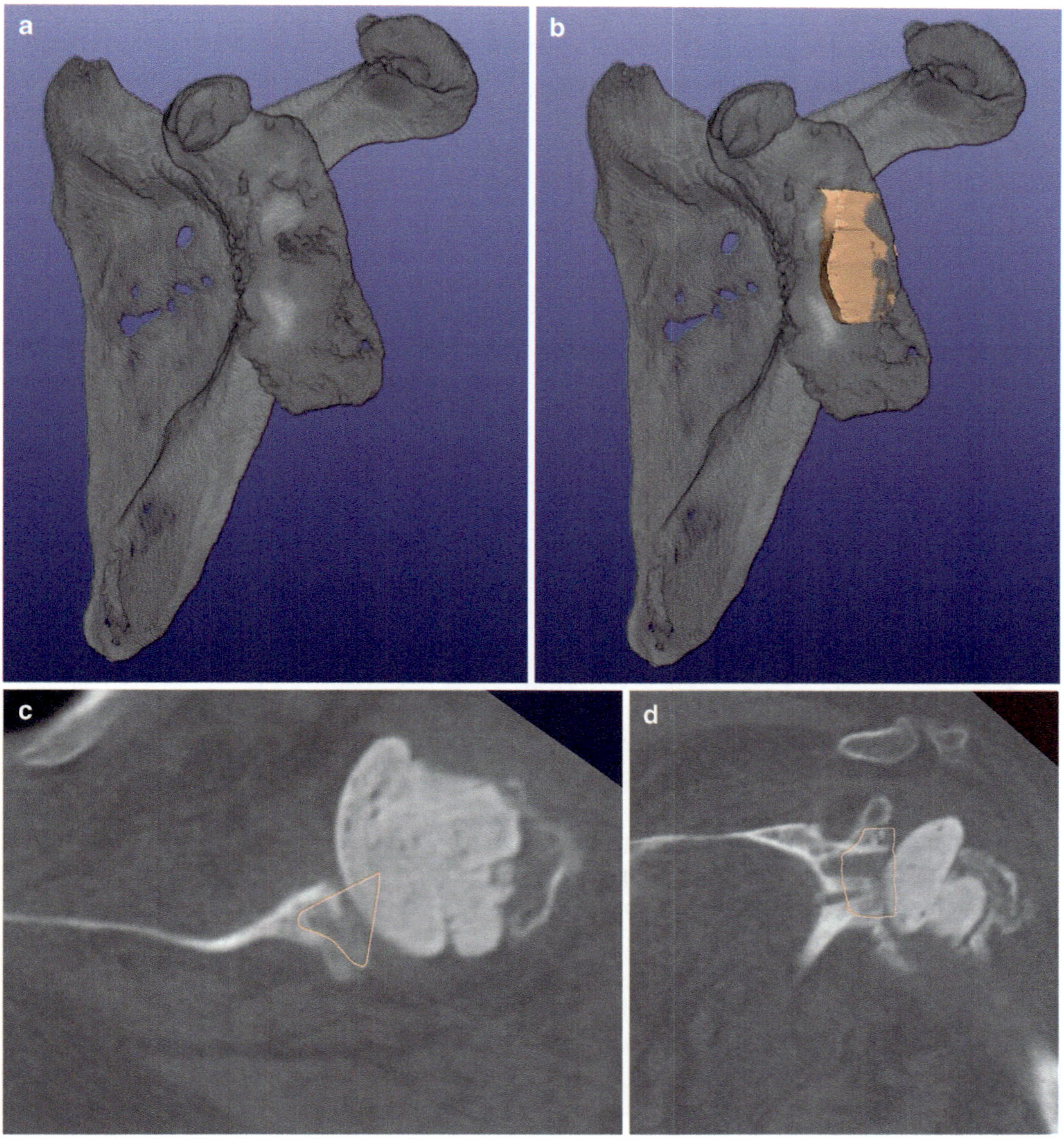

Fig. 6.1 Preoperative planning with three-dimensional (3D) computed tomography (CT) planning software (OrthoVis Research, Cleveland Clinic, Cleveland, OH) prior to second-stage reimplantation of a previously infected reverse total shoulder arthroplasty. The 3D reconstruction of the patient's scapula shows significant anterior and central glenoid bone loss with inferior osteophyte formation from prior scapular notching (**a** and **b**). Three points on the glenoid and scapula are selected to determine the planes of the glenoid (green) and scapula (blue). The software uses this information to automatically calculate glenoid version (+15.8°) and inclination (+3.1°). The vault model (orange) has been positioned and sized to match the inner cortex of the glenoid in the axial, sagittal, and coronal planes (**b**–**d**). The lateral extent of the vault model represents the premorbid joint line, highlighting the anterior and central glenoid bone loss on the 3D reconstruction (**b**) as well as the axial (**c**) and coronal (**d**) cross sections. The software calculates vault version (°), inclination (°), and sagittal plane roll (°) as well as implant version (°), inclination (°), and sagittal plane roll (°)

needed due to inadequate fixation even with a bone graft or standard augment.

Three important considerations that may limit the ability to use 3D preoperative planning software as accurately in the revision setting when compared to primary shoulder arthroplasty are: (1) the abnormal soft tissue tension that may be present at the time of surgery, (2) metal artifacts that may be generated by the existing implant on the 3D CT imaging, and (3) difficulty predicting the final bony anatomy after implant removal, as this may be altered during surgery by the implant, cement, and fibrous/reactive tissue that are taken out. Abnormal soft tissue tension can occur in the revision setting because of rotator cuff and other soft tissue deficiency as well as soft tissue contractures or adhesions. This impacts implant stability and cannot be completely assessed on 3D preoperative planning; therefore, the final glenosphere size may need to be adjusted intraoperatively based on the patient's soft tissue tension and implant stability. Metal artifacts from the existing implant can cause image distortion on the preoperative 3D CT or make bony segmentation of the humerus and scapula difficult, both of which can affect the accuracy of the preoperative planning software. This has been the primary limitation to employing preoperative planning software in the revision setting, with only limited published studies to date and limited availability in commercial software. The decreased ability to preoperatively plan because of this has subsequently limited the ability to reliably and consistently utilize PSI, navigation, or AR and MR technologies to date in revision cases, as they are based off of the preoperative planning software. Metal artifact reduction (MAR) techniques have been developed to address this limitation, however, and are expected to allow for increased use of preoperative planning software in the revision setting in the future. These novel techniques for CT acquisition, reconstruction, and analysis have been shown to allow for accurate and reliable measurement of postoperative implant position and can make preoperative planning of revision cases possible by reducing streak artifacts and capturing details near the metal–bone interface more clearly to avoid image distortion and allow for appropriate bony segmentation [9, 10, 21–30].

Currently, the revision cases that allow the most accurate preoperative planning with MAR techniques are those in which the amount of metal within the bony glenoid is minimized, including revision of hemiarthroplasties, anatomic TSAs with all-polyethylene glenoid components, or those with an antibiotic spacer present in the setting of two-stage revision. Preoperative planning may still be challenging even with MAR techniques in cases with extensive metal present in the bony glenoid, including revision of reverse TSAs or anatomic TSAs with metal-back glenoid components. Despite these advances in MAR technology that can allow for preoperative planning in the revision setting, it is important to keep in mind that the final bony anatomy after implant removal can still be difficult to predict, as this may be altered further during surgery by the implant, cement, and fibrous/reactive tissue that are taken out. Therefore, the preoperative plan may need to be adjusted intraoperatively based on the patients' true anatomy.

In reviewing the current literature, studies in primary shoulder arthroplasty have shown that 3D CT imaging with virtual implant templating provides superior accuracy over standard 2D CT imaging without virtual planning with regard to glenoid component position [6, 7, 9, 10]. Iannotti et al. compared 3D CT templating to standard 2D CT imaging in placing the guide pin with standard instrumentation for anatomic TSA in nine sawbone models from patients with a variety of glenohumeral arthritis [7]. They found that standard instrumentation with 2D imaging produced a mean deviation from the planned component position of 11.1° ± 7.3° in version, 10.7° ± 5.8° in inclination, and 2.9 ± 1.6 mm in position. The use of 3D preoperative planning with standard instrumentation improved the mean deviation from plan to 6.7° ± 5.9° in version, 9.3° ± 5.6° in inclination, and 2.4 ± 1.3 mm in location. Iannotti et al. followed up their work with a randomized clinical trial of 46 patients as well as a larger prospective study of 173 patients, undergoing primary anatomic TSA with and without different PSI guides and found that use of 3D templating with either standard instrumentation or different PSI guides was superior to standard instrumentation with 2D CT imaging and no preoperative planning with regard to accuracy of glenoid component placement [9, 10]. The cases not undergoing 3D CT preoperative planning had a significantly higher rate of malpositioned glenoid implants.

There are currently no published studies on the accuracy of glenoid component placement with 3D CT preoperative planning software in the setting of revision TSA. The findings in studies performed in primary TSA should be cautiously extrapolated to revision TSA cases for the reasons discussed above.

6.3 Patient-Specific Instrumentation

Patient-specific instrumentation (PSI) is another technology used to help facilitate accurate baseplate and glenosphere placement in revision TSA. PSI involves creating a custom guide based on a 3D CT preoperative plan that references and fits to the patient's bony glenoid to place the guide pin in the planned location, version, and inclination at the time of surgery. Revision TSA cases can be complicated by glenoid bone loss after implant removal, making guide pin placement based on conventional anatomic landmarks difficult. PSI presents a unique opportunity to more directly translate a preoperative plan into surgical reality in severe bone loss cases. There are two types of commercially available PSI guides: single-use and reusable. At present, all manufacturers of PSI guides provide preoperative planning software that allow the surgeon to template their implants based on a preoperative 3D CT. Many of these systems also provide a sterile 3D-printed model of the patient's glenoid and guide pin position based off of the preoperative plan that can be referenced intraoperatively (Fig. 6.2). In systems with reusable PSI guides, the guide is adjusted based off of the preoperative planning software with or without the use of a 3D-printed bone model or a reusable, adjustable base at the time of surgery.

There are limited published studies on the accuracy of glenoid component placement with PSI in the setting of revision TSA. We will review some of the relevant studies of the different PSI guides performed in primary TSA but again acknowledge that the findings should be cautiously extrapolated to the revision setting, as the presence of a metal artifact may alter the accuracy of PSI or preclude the ability to use it in certain cases.

6.3.1 PSI: Single-Use PSI in the Literature

Reverse TSA is the most common implant choice in revision TSA cases, and, while there is a paucity of literature on use of PSI in revision TSA specifically, multiple studies have investigated the accuracy of single-use PSI in primary reverse TSA. In a cadaveric study, Levy et al. used 3D planning software and PSI to place a baseplate in 14 shoulders [31]. The location and trajectory of the guide pin were then evaluated with 3D CT imaging and compared with the preoperative plan. The authors demonstrated accuracy in version of 2.6° ± 1.7°, inferior tilt of 1.2° ± 1.2°, and starting point location of 1.2 ± 0.7 mm. Additionally, Subramanya et al. presented a case series using 3D planning software and PSI to perform reverse TSA in seven patients [32]. The authors defined the "ideal position" of the glenosphere baseplate on the preoperative planning software and compared this position to the glenosphere baseplate placement at the time of surgery using PSI. The use of 3D planning software and PSI resulted in a high level of accuracy with the mean deviation from planned version measuring 0.04° ± 0.71° and the mean deviation from planned inclination measuring 0.04° ± 0.26°. More recently, Kwak et al. have examined 39 patients undergoing reverse TSA, 20 with conventional instrumentation and 19 with PSI [33]. The mean differences between the planned and postoperative length and angle of the baseplate screws in the PSI group were significantly less than those in the conventional group. The mean difference in baseplate rotation between the

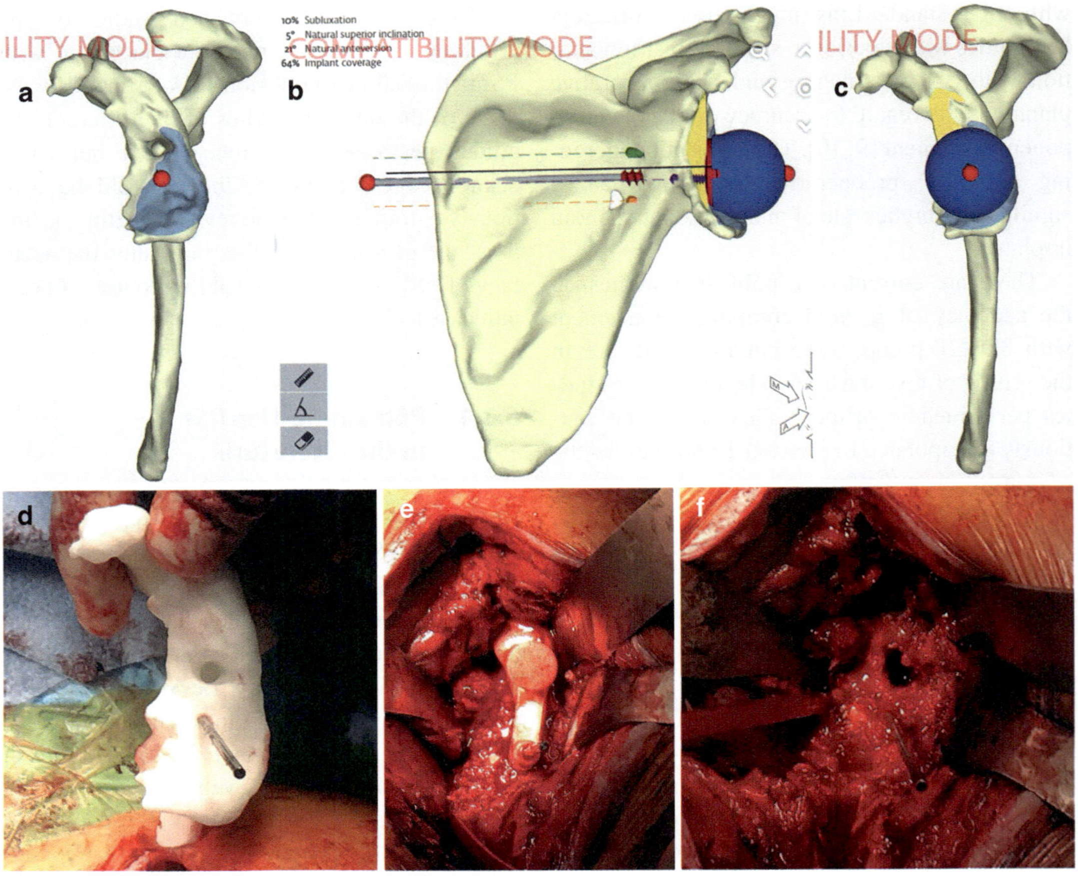

Fig. 6.2 Preoperative planning and patient-specific instrumentation (PSI) of the patient in Fig. 6.1 used for second-stage reimplantation of a previously infected reverse total shoulder arthroplasty. The commercially available preoperative planning software allows for definition of the bony defect (**a**) as well as planning of the central guide pin (**a**) and implant position and areas of planned bone grafting (**b** and **c**, bone graft area in yellow). Many systems provide a sterile three-dimensional (3D) model of the patient's glenoid and guide pin position (**d**) based off of the preoperative plan that can be referenced intraoperatively. A single-use PSI guide was used in the case (**e**), with the intraoperative defect and guide pin position (**f**) matching the 3D model (**d**) preoperative plan (**a**) following use of the PSI guide

planned and postoperative measurements in the PSI group was also significantly lower than that in the conventional group (4.5° vs. 10.6°).

6.3.2 PSI: Reusable PSI in the Literature

Reusable PSI may offer cost advantages to single-use devices because it does not require fabrication of a custom guide for each patient. The previously mentioned 3D templating studies by Iannotti et al. examined the effectiveness of a patient-specific reusable guide (Intelligent Reusable Instrument IRI™) to assist with guide pin placement in primary anatomic TSA. In the sawbones study, the authors found that use of 3D CT preoperative planning with standard instrumentation produced a mean deviation from plan of 6.7° ± 5.9° in version, 9.3° ± 5.6° in inclination, and 2.4 ± 1.3 mm in location. 3D CT templating with the reusable PSI improved the mean deviation from plan to 3.1° ± 2.6° in version, 2.8° ± 2.1° in inclination, and 1.2 ± 0.7 mm in location [7]. Their randomized clinical trial of 46 patients compared patients undergoing 3D CT

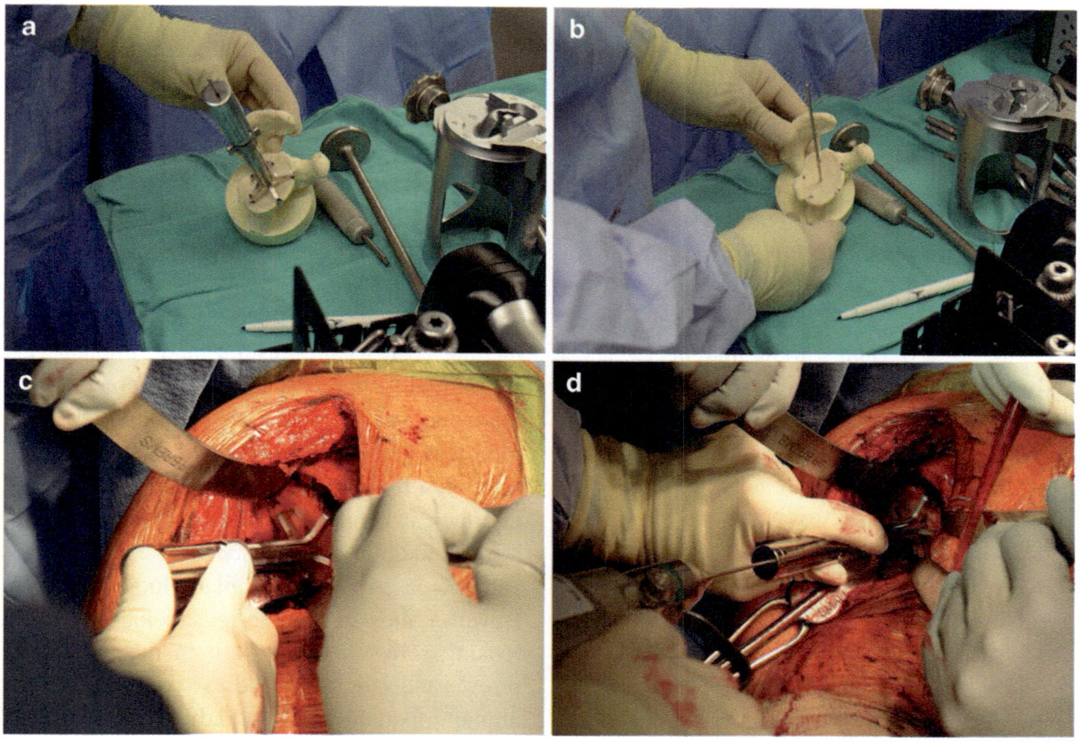

Fig. 6.3 Intelligent Reusable Instrument IRI™. The patient-specific reusable guide is placed onto a three-dimensional (3D) model of the patient's glenoid. The 3D model is made with a drill hole that positions the guide pin in the location and orientation determined by the preoperative plan, and the surgeon marks the location of the guide feet on the model (**a** and **b**). These marks are used to reference rotational alignment when placing the guide on the patient's glenoid intraoperatively (**c**). The guide pin is then inserted through the reusable guide, and the surgeon confirms the pin's position and orientation relative to the model (**d**). Reprinted from Donohue, K.W., Ricchetti, E.T., El-Telbany, A.S., Iannotti, J.P. Patient-Specific Instruments and Implants in Reverse Shoulder Arthroplasty. In: Dines, D., Dines, J., Edwards, T.B. (Eds.), Reverse Shoulder Arthroplasty: A Practical Approach. New York: Thieme Publishers, 2017, pp. 173–186

preoperative planning with use of standard instrumentation (n = 21) or a reusable PSI guide (n = 21) for glenoid component placement [10] (Fig. 6.3). The larger clinical trial of 173 patients compared patients undergoing 3D CT preoperative planning across three groups: use of standard instrumentation (n = 64), a reusable PSI guide (n = 68), or a single-use PSI guide (n = 41) for glenoid component placement [9]. In both of these clinical studies, Iannotti et al. found no significant differences in the accuracy of component placement overall across the studied groups, suggesting that virtual templating with 3D CT preoperative planning software was the most important tool for accurate component placement at the time of surgery. However, the authors did find some evidence that there was a significantly higher frequency of outliers for glenoid component position for cases with preoperative glenoid retroversion of >15° when using standard instrumentation rather than PSI guides. This finding has also been reported in other studies of PSI in primary anatomic and reverse TSA and may suggest that PSI is especially useful in patients with more glenoid deformity, such as those undergoing revision TSA [6, 34]. The lack of difference in accuracy between the reusable and single-use PSI in this study also suggests that multiple, different PSI options can be utilized to improve the accuracy of glenoid component placement at the time of surgery and underlines the importance of surgeons selecting the instrumentation with which they are the most comfortable.

Lewis et al. performed a study that examined the use of a reusable six-pin array guide on bone models from nine patients with varying amounts of glenohumeral arthritis planned for anatomic TSA [35]. The authors compared pin placement with PSI and 3D templating to two groups where the pin was placed by a freehand technique without instrumentation. In the groups without instrumentation, the surgeon either used no imaging or was assisted by a 3D preoperative plan. The authors found that PSI with 3D templating significantly reduced version errors (3° ± 2°), when compared to the freehand technique with 3D planning (8° ± 6°) and without imaging (9° ± 7°). PSI with 3D templating also significantly decreased inclination errors (3° ± 2°), when compared to the freehand technique without imaging (9° ± 6°).

6.3.3 Patient-Specific Implants: Customized Glenoid Components

Glenoid implant position and fixation are arguably the most challenging aspects of revision TSA due to the prevalence of large bony defects in revision cases. Custom-made implants can be used in cases of severe, complex glenoid defects if standard techniques will not provide adequate fixation. These custom components are metal-augmented implants that are specially produced for a certain defect utilizing a preoperative 3D CT and CAD/CAM (computer-aided design/computer-aided manufacturing) planning software and design (Fig. 6.4). Some software identify the extent of missing glenoid bone and the original joint line by defining native anatomy through the aid of premorbid statistical shape modeling [36]. As discussed above, MAR techniques should be utilized with preoperative 3D CT to allow for appropriate planning and design of the custom implant. Revision cases, in which the amount of metal within the bony glenoid is minimized, are the most ideal, including revision of hemiarthroplasties, anatomic TSAs with all-polyethylene glenoid components, or those with an antibiotic spacer present in the setting of two-stage revision. It is also important to be aware of the timeline to plan and manufacture these implants, as this may require a 6–8-week period or longer. A recent CT should be utilized for the planning and design of the implant to avoid any risk of changes in the bony anatomy at the time of surgery from further bony erosion.

Once designed, the custom components come with intraoperative models and PSI guides based off of the 3D CT preoperative plan to facilitate accurate placement at the time of surgery, including planning for screw direction and length [37]. The drawbacks to custom glenoid implants include cost, as the custom-made implants are substantially more expensive than conventional implants, and the potential increase in shearing forces. A greater distance between the center of rotation of the implant and the bone/implant interface, in combination with decreased bone for implant fixation, may cause more shearing forces and increased risk of implant loosening [38]. However, most custom designs include increased locking screw fixation, both in the number of screws and length, to address the concerns for implant fixation in these advanced bone loss cases.

Ortmaier et al. examined 10 patients with shoulders with severe glenoid defects who underwent revision reverse TSA using a custom-made glenoid implant [38]. The pre- and postoperative Constant–Murley Score (CMS), the University of California, Los Angeles (UCLA) score, and Subjective Shoulder Value (SSV) were assessed, with significant postoperative increases of 51.7 ($p < 0.001$), 22.9 ($p < 0.001$), and 52.0 ($p < 0.001$), respectively, at a mean follow-up of 23.1 months. There were no signs of loosening of implants or scapular notching, and no revisions were necessary at the latest follow-up. This study is particularly notable as only revision TSA cases were examined.

Several other studies have reported on mixed patient groups of both primary and revision reverse TSA with custom glenoid implants. Bodendorfer et al. looked at 12 shoulders, 7 primary and 5 revision cases, treated with custom glenoid baseplates [39]. They found significant improvements in patient-reported outcomes Single Assessment Numeric Evaluation (SANE) 43 points, American Shoulder and Elbow Surgeons (ASES) score 45 points, Penn Shoulder

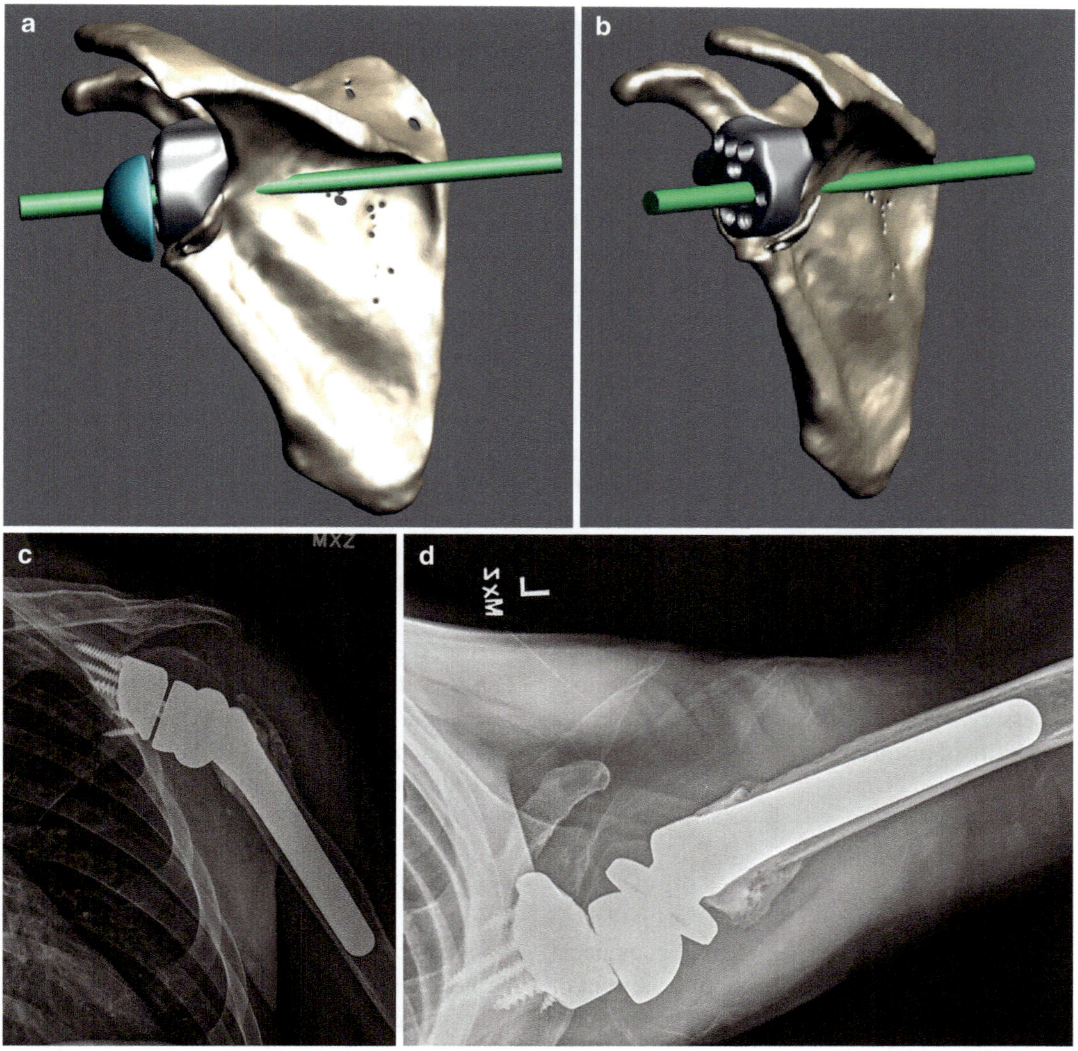

Fig. 6.4 Three-dimensional (3D) preoperative planning with a custom glenoid component, the Comprehensive Vault Reconstruction System (VRS) by Zimmer-Biomet, for a revision reverse total shoulder with advanced glenoid bone loss performed as a second-stage reimplantation of a previously infected hemiarthroplasty (**a** and **b**). These custom components are metal-augmented implants that are specially produced for a certain defect utilizing a preoperative 3D CT and CAD/CAM (computer-aided design/computer-aided manufacturing) planning software and design. Postoperative radiographs of the patient showing the custom metal augment matching the glenoid defect on the anteroposterior (**c**) and axillary (**d**) views

Score 49 points) and statistically significant improvements in the median range of motion measurements (forward elevation 20°, external rotation 40°, internal rotation 2 spinal levels) at a mean follow-up of 30 months. All implants were radiographically stable without loosening at the latest follow-up. Similarly, Rangarajan et al. examined 19 patients with severe glenoid bone deficiency, 9 primary and 10 revision cases, treated with the same custom glenoid component [40]. They also found significant improvement in patient-reported outcomes and active shoulder motion, including mean active forward flexion (53° ± 27° to 124° ± 23°), mean active abduction (42° ± 17° to 77° ± 15°), and mean external rotation (17° ± 19° to 32° ± 24°) at a mean follow-up of 18 months. No radiographic evidence of component loosening, scapular notching, or hardware failure was observed at the last follow-up. Complications occurred in four patients (21%) unrelated to the custom implant, including a nondisplaced greater tuberosity fracture treated conservatively, an intraoperative cortical perforation during humeral cement removal treated with an allograft strut, recurrent instability and hematoma formation treated with humeral component revision, and a postoperative periprosthetic joint infection treated with implant removal and antibiotic spacer placement.

Overall, PSI guides have been shown in the literature to increase surgeon accuracy for glenoid component placement at the time of surgery, although the clinical significance of these results remains unclear regarding whether this increased accuracy leads to improved long-term clinical outcomes. Similarly, the preliminary results of revision TSAs using patient-specific, custom glenoid implants to manage severe glenoid bone deficiency are promising, but longer follow-up is necessary to determine implant longevity and durability of results.

6.4 Navigation

Intraoperative navigation has been suggested to aid with implantation of the glenoid component in the revision setting, again due to the extent of glenoid bone loss and lack of normal anatomic landmarks that commonly occurs [41]. Intraoperative navigation utilizes an optical tracking system to determine the orientation of the glenoid guide pin relative to landmarks on the bony glenoid and scapula. This technique requires intraoperative calibration of the tracking system relative to a preoperative 3D CT scan of the patient's scapula, with the goal of using the intraoperative navigation to achieve a preoperative plan made with virtual planning. It also provides the surgeon with real-time feedback during surgery of reaming and baseplate placement as well as screw placement.

Navigation in shoulder arthroplasty is an emerging technology. As such, there is no current literature examining its use in revision TSA. There is a small body of literature examining navigation use in primary reverse TSA that we will review but again acknowledge that the findings should be cautiously extrapolated to the revision setting, as the presence of a metal artifact may alter the accuracy of navigation or preclude the ability to use it in certain cases. Stubig et al. performed an in vitro study on 3D-navigated implantation of the glenoid component in reverse TSA [42]. They evaluated the accuracy of 27 implantations using a Kirschner wire (12 cases) placed freehand based on a preoperative plan or a navigated drill (15 cases). They found no significant difference between groups with respect to the glenoid drilling distance and inferior tilt; however, they found significantly higher accuracy in the navigated group with regard to pin placement in the axial plan. The authors concluded that accurate positioning of the glenoid baseplate may be improved in the axial plane using navigation [42].

Hones et al. reviewed 200 primary reverse TSAs, with 100 performed prior to computer navigation compared to 100 performed using computer navigation [43]. They found that the total number of screws used without computer navigation was 414, whereas the total number used in the computer navigation cases was 344, with significantly fewer screws per case (3.4 screws vs. 4.1 screws) and significantly greater average screw length (35.0 mm vs. 32.6 mm) in the navigation cases. They postulated that computer navigation appears to assist with better screw placement, potentially saving glenoid bone stock by decreasing the number of screws needed to achieve adequate fixation, avoiding potential glenoid stress risers, and decreasing operative time. Similarly, Sprowls et al. compared 51 patients who underwent navigated primary reverse TSA with 63 control cases [44]. They also found that intraoperative navigation resulted in the use of significantly longer individual screws (36.7 mm vs. 30 mm), greater composite screw length (84 mm vs. 76 mm), and fewer screws (2.5 ± 0.7 vs. 2.8 ± 1), suggesting that navigation may lead to more optimal screw placement and fixation. Finally, Nashikkar et al. compared 27 patients undergoing reverse TSA using navigation and 23 control patients in a case–control study and found that the median screw purchase length was significantly longer in the navigation group for both anterior (20 mm vs. 15 mm) and posterior screws (20 mm vs. 13 mm) [45]. The navigation group also displayed significantly lower incidences of inadequate screw purchase (<22 mm) for the anterior (64.7% vs. 95.2%) and posterior (70.6% vs. 100%) screws. The navigation group further displayed significantly lower incidence of central cage perforation (17.7% vs. 52.4%).

Although the evidence for improved accuracy with intraoperative navigation is promising, the potential downsides to this technology include concerns for increased operative time and substantial cost for the system without a clear clinical benefit. Several clinical studies have reported that intraoperative navigation has increased operative time by approximately 30 min and that technical problems have required abandoning the technology up to 37.5% of the time [46, 47]. However, Wang et al. have recently examined the learning curve of a single surgeon performing computer navigation of glenoid implant placement in primary reverse TSA and found that the total surgical time was 77.3 min in the navigated cohort versus 78.5 min in the non-navigated group [48]. Additionally, they noted a significant decrease in the total surgical time ($p = 0.038$) in the navigated cohort, which flattened after eight cases, indicating that prior training can flatten the learning curve with this technology [47]. These data may suggest that intraoperative computer navigation will not require substantially increased operating times compared with standard surgical techniques.

6.5 Augmented and Mixed Reality

While PSI and navigation are already commercially available methods to potentially improve the accuracy of glenoid component placement at the time of revision TSA, augmented reality (AR) and mixed reality (MR) are emerging technologies that may promise similar results with lower cost and ease of use. Currently with AR and MR, the preoperatively planned component position can be superimposed for viewing within the surgical field via a head-mounted display worn at the time of surgery. The preoperative plan can be manipulated for visualization in 3D through the head-mounted display, but it is not directly linked to the surgical anatomy for true intraoperative navigation at the time of surgery. At this time, AR and MR technologies are not yet able to digitize the 3D surgical anatomy and register it to the surgical site in the absence of traditional optical tracking that uses contact-based mapping. These technologies are new to shoulder arthroplasty; therefore, little data exist in the shoulder arthroplasty literature on their use at the time of publication, either in the primary or revision setting. Despite this, there are several studies exploring the theoretical viability of AR and MR.

Kriechling et al. performed a feasibility study by 3D printing 10 models from cadaver scapulae and superimposing a hologram of the planned glenoid guidewire position from a head-mounted display worn by the surgeon [49]. After placement of the central guidewires, CT imaging of the models was recorded and deviation from the planned versus executed central guide pin trajectory and entry point was analyzed. They calculated the 3D angular error and found that the mean deviation from the planned trajectory was $2.7° \pm 1.3°$ and that the mean deviation from the planned entry point measured 2.3 mm ± 1.1 mm. This novel technology and method yielded acceptable applicability and high accuracy in the placement of the glenoid guidewire in this study. Kriechling et al. then performed a follow-up cadaveric study with a head-mounted MR display [50]. In all, 12 cadaver shoulders were CT-scanned, and baseplate positioning was preoperatively planned using modeling software. During surgery, a hologram showing the preoperative plan was superimposed using a head-mounted display and the central glenoid guidewire was placed using the display to achieve the preplanned entry point and trajectory (Fig. 6.5). Postoperative CT scans were performed, and the deviation from plan was calculated. They found that the mean deviation of the entry point was 3.5 mm ± 1.7 mm and that the 3D

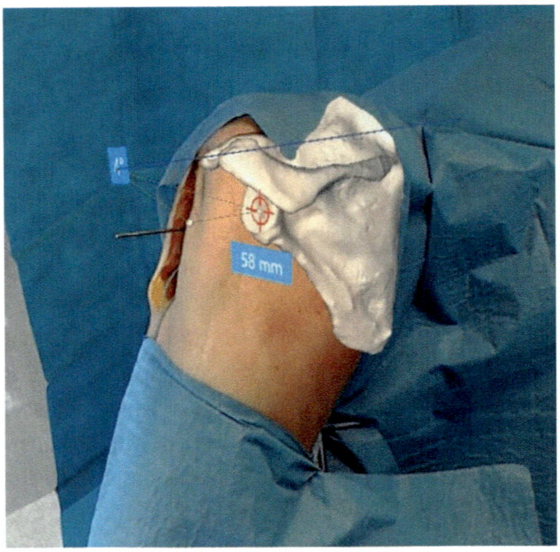

Fig. 6.5 The surgeon's view obtained from an augmented (AR) and mixed reality (MR) head-mounted display camera, Microsoft Head-Mounted Display HoloLense Version 1 (Microsoft, Redmond, WA, USA), used in a cadaveric study to show proof of concept. The superimposed AR and MR hologram shows the scapula with the planned guide pin entry point and the deviation in millimeters. The planned trajectory of the guide pin and the current deviation is displayed in degrees. Reprinted from Kriechling P, Loucas R, Loucas M, Casari F, Fürnstahl P, Wieser K. Augmented reality through head-mounted display for navigation of baseplate component placement in reverse total shoulder arthroplasty: a cadaveric study. *Arch Orthop Trauma Surg*. 2021 Jul 2

angular error from the actual to planned trajectory was 3.8° ± 1.7° [50].

Although still in the proof-of-concept phase, AR and MR present important technological developments for both primary and revision shoulder arthroplasties. Achieving the planned component positioning is particularly difficult in cases with significant glenoid bone loss, and these emerging technologies have the potential to aid in this execution without the need for physical guides or trackers.

6.6 Conclusions

With the increasing use of shoulder arthroplasty and its expanding indications, surgeons today are facing a larger volume of revision arthroplasty cases with reconstructive challenges and the goal of still providing the patient with a good clinical outcome. Advanced glenoid bone loss is commonly encountered in the revision setting and presents a challenge to the surgeon during glenoid component positioning. The surgeon must place the implant in a location and orientation that attempts to maximize implant fixation, soft tissue stability, and shoulder function. In order to address this, surgeons can look to the use of 3D imaging and technology in order to better understand each patient's pathology and successfully execute a surgical plan. The greatest current limitation for use of this technology in the revision setting is metal artifacts, which can limit the ability to accurately define the bony anatomy before the implant is removed and the ability to know the bony anatomy after implant removal. In spite of these limitations, the use of virtual planning has improved the ability to arrive in the operating room with a surgical plan in order to better address the deformity present. This can help in determining whether glenoid bone grafting, eccentric reaming, or the use of augmented or even custom components is the best choice for addressing bony deformity and maximizing soft tissue stability and function. Furthermore, with the advent and continued refinement of PSI and intraoperative navigation, the surgeon has the means to translate the preoperative plan into the operating room with increased accuracy. This improved accuracy has been demonstrated in primary shoulder arthroplasty, but further study of the technology in revision TSA is needed. Increased use of patient-specific implants and AR and MR technologies in the future may also further enhance the ability of surgeons to successfully execute a preoperative plan. Although there are still limited studies on the use of these technologies in the revision setting, with continued improvements in imaging techniques and MAR technology, the application of these tools in revision shoulder arthroplasty will continue to grow.

References

1. Bryce CD, Pennypacker JL, Kulkarni N, et al. Validation of three-dimensional models of in situ scapulae. J Shoulder Elb Surg. 2008;17:825–32.
2. Bryce CD, Davison AC, Lewis GS, Wang L, Flemming DJ, Armstrong AD. Two-dimensional glenoid version measurements vary with coronal and sagittal scapular rotation. J Bone Joint Surg Am. 2010;92:692–9.
3. Budge MD, Lewis GS, Schaefer E, Coquia S, Flemming DJ, Armstrong AD. Comparison of standard two-dimensional and three-dimensional corrected glenoid version measurements. J Shoulder Elbow Surg. 2011;20:577–83.
4. Chalmers PN, Salazar D, Chamberlain A, Keener JD. Radiographic characterization of the B2 glenoid: the effect of computed tomographic axis orientation. J Shoulder Elb Surg. 2017;26:258–64.
5. Kwon YW, Powell KA, Yum JK, Brems JJ, Iannotti JP. Use of three-dimensional computed tomography for the analysis of the glenoid anatomy. J Shoulder Elb Surg. 2005;14:85–90.
6. Hendel MD, Bryan JA, Barsoum WK, Rodriguez EJ, Brems JJ, Evans PJ, et al. Comparison of patient-specific instruments with standard surgical instruments in determining glenoid component position: a randomized prospective clinical trial. J Bone Joint Surg Am. 2012;94(23):2167–75.
7. Iannotti J, Baker J, Rodriguez E, Brems J, Ricchetti E, Mesiha M, Bryan J. Three-dimensional preoperative planning software and a novel information transfer technology improve glenoid component positioning. J Bone Joint Surg Am. 2014;96:e71. (1–8).
8. Iannotti JP, Greeson C, Downing D, Sabesan V, Bryan JA. Effect of glenoid deformity on glenoid component placement in primary shoulder arthroplasty. J Shoulder Elb Surg. 2012;21:48–55.
9. Iannotti JP, Walker K, Rodriguez E, Patterson TE, Jun BJ, Ricchetti ET. Accuracy of 3-dimensional planning, implant templating, and patient-specific instrumentation in anatomic Total shoulder arthroplasty. J Bone Joint Surg Am. 2019;101(5):446–57.
10. Iannotti JP, Weiner S, Rodriguez E, Patterson TE, Jun BJ, Ricchetti ET. Three dimensional imaging and templating improve glenoid implant positioning. J Bone Joint Surg Am. 2015;97:651–8.
11. Scalise JJ, Codsi MJ, Bryan J, Brems JJ, Iannotti JP. The influence of three-dimensional computed tomography images of the shoulder in preoperative planning for total shoulder arthroplasty. J Bone Joint Surg Am. 2008;90:2438–45.
12. Codsi MJ, Bennetts C, Gordiev K, Baeck DM, Kwon Y, Brems J, Powell K, Iannotti JP. Normal glenoid vault anatomy and validation of a novel glenoid implant shape. J Shoulder Elb Surg. 2008;17:471–8.
13. Ganapathi A, McCarron JA, Chen X, Iannotti JP. Predicting normal glenoid version from the pathologic scapula: a comparison of 4 methods in 2- and 3-dimensional models. J Shoulder Elb Surg. 2011;20:234–44.
14. Iannotti JP, Jun BJ, Patterson TE, Ricchetti ET. Quantitative measurement of osseous pathology in advanced glenohumeral osteoarthritis. J Bone Joint Surg Am. 2017;99:1460–8.
15. Ricchetti ET, Hendel MD, Collins DN, Iannotti JP. Is premorbid glenoid anatomy altered in patients with glenohumeral osteoarthritis? Clin Orthop Relat Res. 2013;471:2932–9.
16. Scalise JJ, Bryan J, Polster J, Brems JJ, Iannotti JP. Quantitative analysis of glenoid bone loss in osteoarthritis using three-dimensional computed tomography scans. J Shoulder Elb Surg. 2008;17:328–35.
17. Scalise JJ, Codsi MJ, Bryan J, Iannotti JP. The three-dimensional glenoid vault model can estimate normal glenoid version in osteoarthritis. J Shoulder Elb Surg. 2008;17:487–91.
18. Plessers K, Vanden Berghe P, Van Dijck C, Wirix-Speetjens R, Debeer P, Jonkers I, Vander Sloten J. Virtual reconstruction of glenoid bone defects using a statistical shape model. J Shoulder Elb Surg. 2018;27:160–6.
19. Plessers K, Verhaegen F, Van Dijck C, Wirix-Speetjens R, Debeer P, Jonkers I, Vander Sloten J. Automated quantification of glenoid bone defects using 3-dimensional measurements. J Shoulder Elb Surg. 2020;29:1050–8.
20. Verhaegen F, Plessers K, Verborgt O, Scheys L, Debeer P. Can the contralateral scapula be used as a reliable template to reconstruct the eroded scapula during shoulder arthroplasty? J Shoulder Elb Surg. 2018;27:1133–8.
21. Gregory T, Hansen U, Taillieu F, et al. Glenoid loosening after total shoulder arthroplasty: an in vitro CT-scan study. J Orthop Res. 2009;27:1589–95.
22. Iannotti JP, Ricchetti ET, Rodriguez EJ, Bryan JA. Development and validation of a new method of 3-dimensional assessment of glenoid and humeral component position after total shoulder arthroplasty. J Shoulder Elb Surg. 2013;22:1413–22.
23. Iannotti JP, Jun BJ, Derwin KA, Ricchetti ET. Stepped augmented glenoid component in anatomic total shoulder arthroplasty for B2 and B3 glenoid pathology: a study of early outcomes. J Bone Joint Surg Am. 2021;103:1798–806.
24. Jun BJ, Ricchetti ET, Haladik J, Bey MJ, Patterson TE, Subhas N, et al. Validation of a 3D CT imaging method for quantifying implant migration following anatomic total shoulder arthroplasty. J Orthop Res. 2022;40:1270–80.
25. Ricchetti ET, Jun BJ, Cain RA, Youderian A, Rodriguez EJ, Kusin D, Subhas N, Patterson TE, Iannotti JP. Sequential 3-dimensional computed tomography analysis of implant position following total shoulder arthroplasty. J Shoulder Elb Surg. 2018;27:983–92.
26. Ricchetti ET, Jun BJ, Jin Y, Ho JC, Patterson TE, Dalton JE, et al. Relationship between glenoid component shift and osteolysis after anatomic total

shoulder arthroplasty: three-dimensional computed tomography analysis. J Bone Joint Surg Am. 2021;103:1417–30.
27. Subhas N, Polster JM, Obuchowski NA, Primak AN, Dong FF, Herts BR, Iannotti JP. Imaging of arthroplasties: improved image quality and lesion detection with iterative metal artifact reduction, a new CT metal artifact reduction technique. AJR Am J Roentgenol. 2016;207:378–85.
28. Subhas N, Primak AN, Obuchowski NA, Gupta A, Polster JM, Krauss A, Iannotti JP. Iterative metal artifact reduction: evaluation and optimization of technique. Skelet Radiol. 2014;43(12):1729–35.
29. Veldkamp WJ, Joemai RM, van der Molen AJ, Geleijns J. Development and validation of segmentation and interpolation techniques in sinograms for metal artifact suppression in CT. Med Phys. 2010;37:620–8.
30. Verburg JM, Seco J. CT metal artifact reduction method correcting for beam hardening and missing projections. Phys Med Biol. 2012;57:2803–18.
31. Levy JC, Everding NG, Frankle MA, Keppler LJ. Accuracy of patient-specific guided glenoid baseplate positioning for reverse shoulder arthroplasty. J Shoulder Elb Surg. 2014;23(10):1563–7.
32. Subramanya S, Herald J. Reverse shoulder arthroplasty with patient-specific glenoid implant positioning guides. Tech Should Elbow Surg. 2014;15(4):122–9.
33. Kwak JM, Jeon IH, Kim H, Choi S, Lee H, Koh KH. Patient-specific instrumentation improves the reproducibility of preoperative planning for the positioning of baseplate components with reverse total shoulder arthroplasty: a comparative clinical study in 39 patients. J Shoulder Elb Surg. 2022;31(7):1488–98. https://doi.org/10.1016/j.jse.2021.12.012.
34. Throckmorton TW, Vogt W, Wasmaier J, Hurst JM, Frostick SM, Sperling JW. Patient-specific targeting guides for glenoid component placement in shoulder arthroplasty: technique and initial clinical experience. Tech Should Elbow Surg. 2014;15(4):103–8.
35. Lewis GS, Stevens NM, Armstrong AD. Testing of a novel pin array guide for accurate three-dimensional glenoid component positioning. J Shoulder Elb Surg. 2015;24(12):1939–47.
36. Salhi A, Burdin V, Boutillon A, Brochard S, Mutsvangwa T, Borotikar B. Statistical shape modeling approach to predict missing scapular bone. Ann Biomed Eng. 2020;48:367–79.
37. Porcellini G, Micheloni GM, Tarallo L, Paladini P, Merolla G, Catani F. Custom-made reverse shoulder arthroplasty for severe glenoid bone loss: review of the literature and our preliminary results. J Orthop Traumatol. 2021;22:2.
38. Ortmaier R, Wierer G, Gruber MS. Functional and radiological outcomes after treatment with custom-made glenoid components in revision reverse shoulder arthroplasty. J Clin Med. 2022;11(3):551.
39. Bodendorfer BM, Loughran GJ, Looney AM, Velott AT, Stein JA, Lutton DM, Wiesel BB, Murthi AM. Short-term outcomes of reverse shoulder arthroplasty using a custom baseplate for severe glenoid deficiency. J Shoulder Elb Surg. 2021;30(5):1060–7.
40. Rangarajan R, Blout CK, Patel VV, Bastian SA, Lee BK, Itamura JM. Early results of reverse total shoulder arthroplasty using a patient-matched glenoid implant for severe glenoid bone deficiency. J Shoulder Elb Surg. 2020;29(7S):S139–48.
41. Sadoghi P, Vavken J, Leithner A, Vavken P. Benefit of intraoperative navigation on glenoid component positioning during total shoulder arthroplasty. Arch Orthop Trauma Surg. 2015;135(1):41–7.
42. Stubig T, Petri M, Zeckey C, Hawi N, Krettek C, Citak M, et al. 3D navigated implantation of the glenoid component in reversed shoulder arthroplasty. Feasibility and results in an anatomic study. Int J Med Robot Comput Assist Surg. 2013;9:480–5.
43. Hones KM, King JJ, Schoch BS, Struk AM, Farmer KW, Wright TW. The in vivo impact of computer navigation on screw number and length in reverse total shoulder arthroplasty. J Shoulder Elb Surg. 2021;30(10):e629–35.
44. Sprowls GR, Wilson CD, Stewart W, Hammonds KAP, Baruch NH, Ward RA, Robin BN. Intraoperative navigation and preoperative templating software are associated with increased glenoid baseplate screw length and use of augmented baseplates in reverse total shoulder arthroplasty. JSES Int. 2020;5(1):102–8.
45. Nashikkar PS, Scholes CJ, Haber MD. Role of intraoperative navigation in the fixation of the glenoid component in reverse total shoulder arthroplasty: a clinical case-control study. J Shoulder Elb Surg. 2019;28(9):1685–91.
46. Edwards TB, Gartsman GM, O'Connor DP, Sarin VK. Safety and utility of computer-aided shoulder arthroplasty. J Shoulder Elb Surg. 2008;17(3):503–8.
47. Kircher J, Wiedemann M, Magosch P, Lichtenberg S, Habermeyer P. Improved accuracy of glenoid positioning in total shoulder arthroplasty with intraoperative navigation: a prospective-randomized clinical study. J Shoulder Elb Surg. 2009;18(4):515–20.
48. Wang AW, Hayes A, Gibbons R, Mackie KE. Computer navigation of the glenoid component in reverse total shoulder arthroplasty: a clinical trial to evaluate the learning curve. J Shoulder Elb Surg. 2020;29(3):617–23.
49. Kriechling P, Roner S, Liebmann F, Casari F, Fürnstahl P, Wieser K. Augmented reality for base plate component placement in reverse total shoulder arthroplasty: a feasibility study. Arch Orthop Trauma Surg. 2021;141(9):1447–53.
50. Kriechling P, Loucas R, Loucas M, Casari F, Fürnstahl P, Wieser K. Augmented reality through head-mounted display for navigation of baseplate component placement in reverse total shoulder arthroplasty: a cadaveric study. Arch Orthop Trauma Surg. 2023;143(1):169–75.

Surgical Approach in Shoulder Arthroplasty Revision

7

Arnaud Godenèche, Joris Tiercelin, Jérôme Garret, and Thais Dutra Vieira

7.1 Introduction

The advent of shoulder prosthesis and its increasing indications, together with the population's longer survival, has also led to an increase in complications related to this surgery and a consequent increase in the number of revision surgeries.

Often multifactorial, the complications of arthroplasties seem more generally related to an implant problem (loosening, notching, and material rupture), to the soft tissues (infection, rotator cuff injury, and instabilitý), or to the bony framework (fractures), [1] leading to a high revision rate [2–4].

However, the clinical outcomes of these revision surgeries are often inferior to primary arthroplasties [5–7] with a higher complication rate [8, 9].

The major technical difficulties are due to the presence of numerous scar adhesions and the need for sometimes extensive excision. The soft tissue management represents the main challenge, both to ensure exposure to allow for correct placement of the implants and to avoid problems of instability.

Major structures have to be preserved, both musculotendinous (deltoid and rotator cuff) and nervous (musculocutaneous nerve and axillary nerve), guaranteeing a good postoperative functional result.

7.2 Pre-operative Assessment

Shoulder arthroplasty revision should only be considered after a complete preoperative evaluation, which should identify any problems that may be present in the choice and procedure of the approach.

It should review the history of the patient's disease, i.e., the primary indication for the prosthesis and the reasons for its revision, the patient's history (medical but especially surgical on the operated shoulder), as well as a complete clinical evaluation (mobilities, cuff testing, deltoid tone, stiffness, instability, and local skin condition).

All previous patient's surgical reports must be retrieved not only to plan the necessary equipment but also to obtain important information about the approach (subscapularis management (SS), possible musculotendinous transfers, and integrity of landmarks in anatomical position such as the coracoid and the conjoint tendon (CT)).

A. Godenèche (✉) · T. D. Vieira
Centre Orthopédique Santy, FIFA Medical Center of Excellence, Hôpital Privé Jean Mermoz, Groupe GDS-Ramsay, Lyon, France

J. Tiercelin
CHU de Toulouse, Hôpital Riquet, Toulouse, France

J. Garret
Clinique du Parc, Lyon, France
e-mail: j.garret@cliniqueduparclyon.com

F. Franceschi et al. (eds.), *Revision Shoulder Arthroplasty*,
https://doi.org/10.1007/978-3-031-45944-3_7

A complete imaging workup is mandatory: front and profile X-rays (associated if necessary with a contralateral comparative X-ray to measure humeral length), CT-scan (version of the implants, bone stock, and rotator cuff), and also MRI, even if less informative due to artifacts related to the prosthesis.

Any suspicion infection will require a complete biological workup (blood workup (CBC, CRP) or puncture aspiration with analysis min >21 days); this will mostly direct the surgeon toward a revision through the primary approach, samples collection for culture and bacterioscopy added to a more extensive excision of the soft tissues.

Evaluation of any nerve damage should be performed and explored by ENMG if necessary.

In case of foreseeable risk of vascular injury, skin covering procedure, difficult neurolysis, consultation, and coordination with other surgical specialties (vascular, plastic) must be organized so that a multidisciplinary approach can be planned.

Since shoulder arthroplasty revision is a high-risk procedure, particularly for neurological injury, nerve monitoring should be used intraoperatively.

The case can be discussed academically to ensure the best strategy, and it will also be important to communicate the revision surgery strategy with all the assistants and operating room nurses present during the surgery.

Finally, one must give the patient clear, fair, and appropriate information, in particular on the expected benefits but especially on the possible risks (intraoperative fracture, nerve damage, infections, and also the possibility iliac crest bone graft harvesting).

7.3 Surgical Technique [10–14]

The installation of the patient is paramount. This is preferably done in a 45° beach-chair position with the hips and knees in flexion, with the head in a straight position with the trunk (to avoid any vascular and neurological complications), and with the use of a pneumatic articulated arm.

Skin preparation of the entire upper extremity is performed with alcoholic betadine, and the operative area is covered after draping with an anti-microbial Ioban-type adhesive (3 M™ Ioban™ 2). If grafting is required, the same procedure is applied to the iliac crest area.

The choice of the surgical approach is crucial, two main techniques are described:

1. **Deltoid splitting approach (superolateral, anteromedial, and anterolateral)**

   A cleavage plan between the middle/anterior deltoid is performed and possible detachment of the previously fixed anterior deltoid [15–17]. The theoretical advantages are: access to the posterior rotator cuff, reduced stress on the humerus in osteopenic bone or in cases of proximal bone lysis, better visibility of the tuberosities, no retraction of the anterior deltoid muscle, and easier glenoid preparation in complex cases. The disadvantages are: non-anatomical dissection, possible damage to the anterior deltoid muscle (significant postoperative functional impact), risk of axillary nerve injury, and limited exposure of the inferior border of the glenoid and humerus. In practice, if this was the primary approach, its reuse may be of interest in the event of the need for a procedure on the posterior rotator cuff or a unipolar change of the humeral head or insert.
2. **Deltopectoral**

   This approach is preferred by the authors, as it allows full exposure of the joint (in particular the lower part of the glenoid) and the humeral shaft, as well as associated structures (better visibility and, if necessary, better exposure of the axillary nerve) [11]. It can be used even in the case of anterior approach scars, and if necessary, simultaneous use is possible because the region has good skin vascularization with a low risk of scarring disorders.

Its description is the main object throughout this book chapter.

With the arm in a slightly abduction and external rotation position, the incision is made along a line from the coracoid to the outer aspect of the

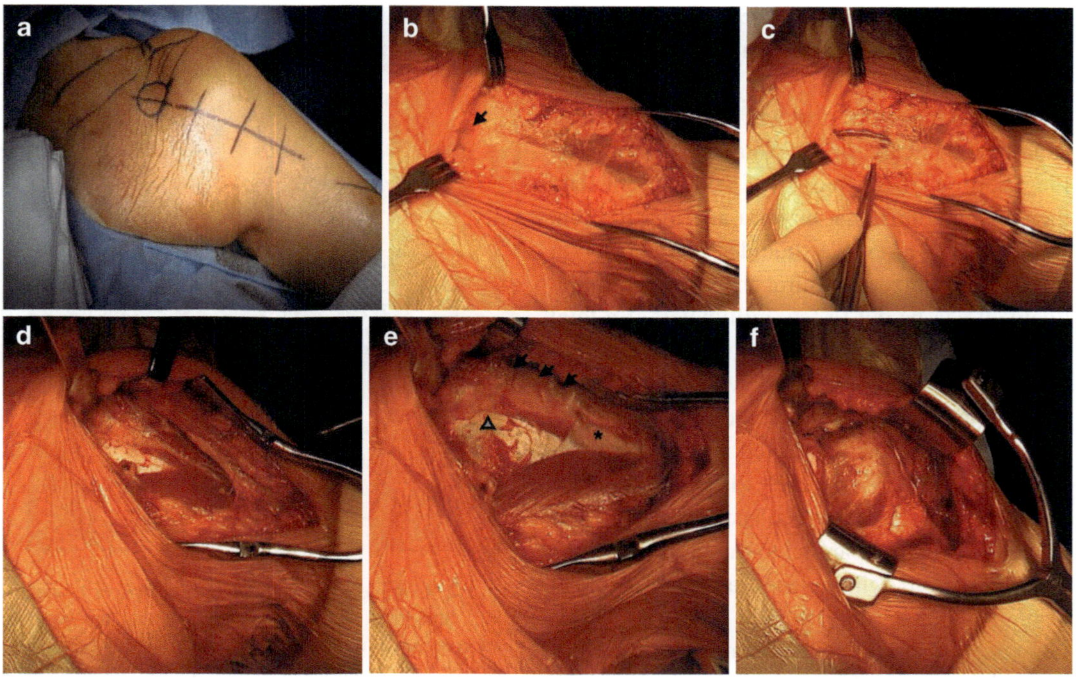

Fig. 7.1 (**a**) Skin marking of the approach: line from the coracoid to the deltoid V. (**b**) Location of Mohrenheim's fossa (arrow), and (**c**) the cephalic vein in order to identify the deltopectoral groove. (**d**) Location of the coracoid with placement of an Hohmann-type retractor. (**e**) Subdeltoid release (arrows) and excision of the clavipectoral fascia to identify the conjoint tendon (triangle) and the Pectoralis major muscle tendon (star) which will be sectioned. (**f**) Placement of a valve retractor to expose the subscapularis

arm opposite the deltoid "V" (Fig. 7.1a). If there is a previous surgery scar, it is necessary to widen proximally and distally to find healthy non-scar tissue; distally, this will also allow a humeral osteotomy to be performed if necessary.

The first step is to find the deltopectoral groove. Very often scarred, dissection in the right plan is important to avoid damage to part of the anterior deltoid muscle (impact on postoperative clinical results) [16], with all the interest in extending the scar proximally in order to find a fatty triangle (Mohrenheim's fossa). Finding the cephalic vein can be challenging, it is often sheathed in fibrosis: if possible, dissection is performed medially (fewer collaterals), otherwise a ligation is performed in order to obtain optimal control of bleeding (Fig. 7.1b, c). At the proximal level, there is a risk of bleeding due to the presence of branches of the thoracoacromial artery.

The second major step is to find the coracoid bone, which is the surgeon's guide. A Mayo-type chisel is slid over it to push back the soft tissue, and then a Hohmann-type retractor is positioned to obtain better visibility and allow identification of the coracoid tubercle (CT) (Fig. 7.1d).

The third step aims to liberate three essential spaces: subdeltoid, subacromial, and perisubscapular.

After exposing the deltopectoral groove, the clavipectoral fascia is excised, taking the superior acromiocoracoid ligament, the lateral border of the coracobrachial tendon, and the medial border of the deltoid as limits (Fig. 7.1e). Throughout the subsequent release step, rotation of the arm can help differentiate the fibrosis of the muscle.

Exposure is continued by releasing the adhesions between the deltoid and the humerus: start proximally at the level of the interval, or distally by sectioning the pectoralis major (PM) tendon over 1 cm, which will allow to expose the latissimus dorsi tendon posteriorly and the biceps laterally in its groove. Its repair will be ensured at the end of the operation by means of tendon stitches while performing a tenodesis of the biceps at the same time. The positioning of a Beckmann-type retractor under the deltoid facilitates the release.

Subacromial work plan will allow the identification and release of the rotator interval. The long portion of the biceps, if still present, can then be tenotomized at its intra-articular portion. In the case of a reverse shoulder arthroplasty, in order to optimize exposure, the coracoacromial ligament can be cut (a few millimeters if a total anatomical prosthesis is used), or the supraspinatus can be carefully excised without damaging the external rotators. In extreme cases, the anterior deltoid may be disinserted with a transosseous suture [15] or the clavicle may be osteotomized (Redfern–Wallace technique: curvilinear osteotomy parallel to the insertion of the anterior deltoid with reinsertion with a thread using five nice knots) [18, 19].

Except in special cases, the dissection is continued lateral to the CT (musculocutaneous nerve medial to the CT) and there are often adhesions between the latter and the deep surface of the PM: the position of the arm in anterior elevation and flexion of the elbow makes it possible to relax the joint tendon and facilitate exposure.

The release of these spaces allows identification of the subscapularis (SS), if it is still present (usefulness of the operative report and of preoperative imaging) (Fig. 7.1f). Additional release of the anterior aspect of the subscapularis under the CT is continued, without extending beyond the medial border of the latter, allowing positioning of a valve retractor which will then be removed to expose the glenoid (risk of traction of the musculocutaneous nerve). At this point, if the subscapularis tendon is still present, all the landmarks are visible: the upper border is posterior to the tip of the coracoid, the bicipital groove is at the lateral edge, and the tendon of the latissimus dorsi is at the lower edge (Fig. 7.2). Ligation or cauterization of the “three sisters” (anterior humeral circumflex artery and its venae comitantes) is performed at its inferior border.

The SS is then managed using one of the four techniques, with no demonstrated superiority of one over the others: tenotomy, peel-off, lesser tuberosity osteotomy, and split [20]. In the case of tenotomy or peel-off, it is useful to position traction wires on the SS to facilitate sectioning of the humeral attachments and then its medial release, with dissection limited to the “safe zone” (located at the anterior aspect of the SS, below the CT) or at most 1.5 cm from the medial edge of the glenoid. The risk of injury to the subscapularis branches is higher if the arm is in external rotation or if traction is performed on a retracted SS [21].

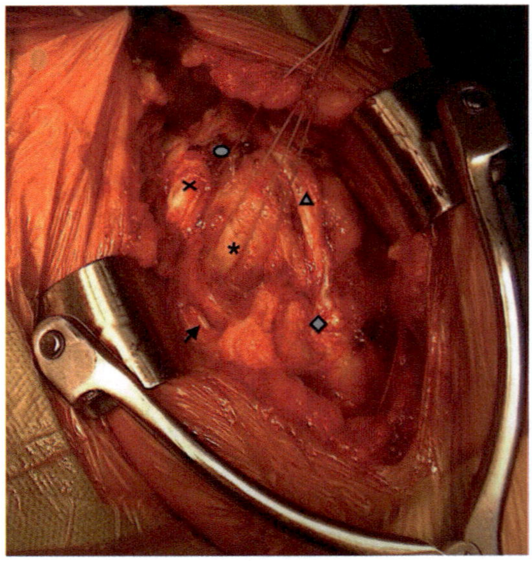

Fig. 7.2 Complete release of the three spaces (subacromial, subdeltoid, and perisubcapular) with the conjoint tendon reclined (cross) allowing identification of the limits of the subscapularis (star): rotator cuff interval (circle), long head of the biceps tendon (triangle), and latissimus dorsi tendon (diamond). The identification of the axillary nerve (arrow) will be done by following the deep layer of the subscapularis

In some particular cases (insufficient glenoid exposure, impossibility of implant reduction, instability due to inferior cam effect, and major adhesions), extensive excision of scar tissue must be performed and it will then be necessary to explore the axillary nerve or even perform a complete neurolysis: with the arm in neutral rotation and slight anterior elevation, it is possible to identify the musculocutaneous nerve located between the PM and the medial border of the CT (magnifying glass, neurostimulator [22]) and to dissect distally the branches for the biceps, and then proximally to find the axillary artery. This artery is a real guide and will allow the identification of the posterior cord of the brachial plexus behind it and to dissect this cord distally to identify the axillary nerve [23].

Even if it has no real use in practice, the "Tug test" can also be used to ensure the continuity of the axillary nerve: by hooking the nerve to the finger at the level of the SS and the deep face of the deltoid, a traction is then transmitted from one finger to the other if the nerve continuity is preserved [24].

If, however, the exposure is still not enough, it is possible to section the conjoined tendon at the level of its coracoid insertion. Its reinsertion is not required at the end of the procedure [23].

This extensive dissection of the plexus and axillary nerve is only performed in complex cases, but in the majority of cases a careful dissection (with the use of the electric scalpel in section mode) going straight to the bone and remaining close to it is the most prudent attitude.

The next major step is exposure of the glenoid. This can be done immediately after exposure of the humerus, without removal of the primary stem, or after extraction of the stem, but care must be taken to ensure that a provisional stem is left in good press fit to avoid any risk of fracture during the glenoid preparation phase.

A Hohmann-type retractor is placed in the joint at the medial border of the humerus and another in the subacromial space at the level of the humeral neck, and the arm is then brought into extension-external rotation in order to dislocate the prosthesis. If dislocation is not possible, further release of adhesions in the lower capsule along the humerus is required. External hyperrotation then allows exposure and progressive debridement of the landmarks around the implant. Humeral extraction is then performed using various techniques described in another chapter of this book.

To retract the humerus and begin exposure, a Favard-type retractor is placed at the posteroinferior edge of the glenoid. The first capsulotomy is performed on the superior border of the SS and then on its deep surface in order to free it and push it back (wrapped in a compress) into the subscapular fossa. A Hohmann-type retractor is placed on its deep surface at the anteroinferior edge of the glenoid to protect the axillary nerve, and two others are placed at the posterior and superior edges. Periglenoid debridement is then performed, progressing from superior to inferior border and anterior to posterior to 6 o'clock. Additional capsular release of the deep aspect of the subscapularis ensures complete excursion, and a link-type retractor is placed at the anteroinferior border of the glenoid to ensure optimal exposure.

If necessary, a more complete exposure can be performed at the posterior edge.

Thus, based on the authors' experience, the deltopectoral approach provides complete exposure of both the humerus and the glenoid, allowing the safest possible revision of the implants.

7.4 Conclusion

Shoulder arthroplasty revision is complex, and its demand will increase in the years to come. Its planning requires a precise preoperative evaluation indicating the causes of failure, orienting the approach and the gestures that will be associated during the revision surgery. The exposure must follow a series of systematic steps, identifying the key anatomical elements, while remaining as close as possible to the bone structures, in order to avoid any complication and thus ensure the best possible functional result.

References

1. Petersen SA, Hawkins RJ. Revision of failed total shoulder arthroplasty. Orthop Clin North Am. 1998;29(3):519–33.
2. Zumstein MA, Pinedo M, Old J, Boileau P. Problems, complications, reoperations, and revisions in reverse total shoulder arthroplasty: a systematic review. J Shoulder Elb Surg. 2011;20(1):146–57.
3. Gauci MO, Cavalier M, Gonzalez JF, Holzer N, Baring T, Walch G, et al. Revision of failed shoulder arthroplasty: epidemiology, etiology, and surgical options. J Shoulder Elb Surg. 2020;29(3):541–9.
4. Knowles NK, Columbus MP, Wegmann K, Ferreira LM, Athwal GS. Revision shoulder arthroplasty: a

systematic review and comparison of north American vs. European outcomes and complications. J Shoulder Elb Surg. 2020;29(5):1071–82.
5. Bacle G, Nové-Josserand L, Garaud P, Walch G. Long-term outcomes of reverse total shoulder arthroplasty: a follow-up of a previous study. J Bone Jt Surg. 2017;99(6):454–61.
6. Wall B, Nové-Josserand L, O'Connor DP, Edwards TB, Walch G. Reverse total shoulder arthroplasty: a review of results according to etiology. J Bone Jt Surg. 2007;89(7):1476–85.
7. Antoni M, Barthoulot M, Kempf JF, Clavert P. Revisions of total shoulder arthroplasty: clinical results and complications of various modalities. Orthop Traumatol Surg Res. 2016;102(3):297–303.
8. Saltzman BM, Chalmers PN, Gupta AK, Romeo AA, Nicholson GP. Complication rates comparing primary with revision reverse total shoulder arthroplasty. J Shoulder Elb Surg. 2014;23(11):1647–54.
9. Boileau P. Complications and revision of reverse total shoulder arthroplasty. Orthop Traumatol Surg Res. 2016;102(1):S33–43.
10. Klein JS, Getz CL. Surgical exposure in revision shoulder arthroplasty. In: Tashjian RZ, editor. Complex and revision shoulder arthroplasty. Cham: Springer International Publishing; 2019. p. 215–23. https://doi.org/10.1007/978-3-030-02756-8_16.
11. Chalmers PN, Van Thiel GS, Trenhaile SW. Surgical exposures of the shoulder. J Am Acad Orthop Surg. 2016;24(4):250–8.
12. Abboud JA, Anakwenze OA, Hsu JE. Soft-tissue management in revision total shoulder arthroplasty. J Am Acad Orthop Surg. 2013;21(1):23–31.
13. Chalmers PN, Boileau P, Romeo AA, Tashjian RZ. Revision reverse shoulder arthroplasty. J Am Acad Orthop Surg. 2019;27(12):426–36.
14. Garver J, Mata-Fink A, Zhu D, Javier F, Gallacher S, Blaine TA. Revision strategies in reverse total shoulder arthroplasty. J Shoulder Elb Arthroplasty. 2017;1:247154921769525.
15. Gill DRJ, Cofield RH, Rowland C. The anteromedial approach for shoulder arthroplasty: the importance of the anterior deltoid. J Shoulder Elb Surg. 2004;13(5):532–7.
16. Groh GI, Simoni M, Rolla P, Rockwood CA. Loss of the deltoid after shoulder operations: an operative disaster. J Shoulder Elb Surg. 1994;3(4):243–53.
17. Foruria AM, Oh LS, Sperling JW, Cofield RH. Anteromedial approach for shoulder arthroplasty: current indications, complications, and results. J Shoulder Elb Surg. 2010;19(5):734–8.
18. Redfern TR, Wallace WA, Beddow FH. Clavicular osteotomy in shoulder arthroplasty. Int Orthop. 1989;13(1):61–3. https://doi.org/10.1007/BF00266725.
19. Verhofste BP, Van Tongel ACG, Van Den Broucke J, Willemot LB, De Wilde LF. Clavicular osteotomy in complicated revision of total shoulder arthroplasty: indications, surgical technique, and outcomes. Int Orthop. 2020;44(7):1341–52.
20. Lopez CD, Maier SP, Bloom ZJ, Shiu BB, Petkovic D, Jobin CM. Outcomes of lesser tuberosity osteotomy in revision anatomic shoulder arthroplasty. J Shoulder Elb Surg. 2018;27(7):e219–24.
21. Yung SW, Lazarus MD, Harryman DT. Practical guidelines to safe surgery about the subscapularis. J Shoulder Elb Surg. 1996;5(6):467–70.
22. Patel MS, Wilent WB, Gutman MJ, Abboud JA. Incidence of peripheral nerve injury in revision total shoulder arthroplasty: an intraoperative nerve monitoring study. J Shoulder Elb Surg. 2021;30(7):1603–12.
23. Rojas J, Familiari F, Borade AU, Joseph J, Deune EG, Ingari JV, et al. Exposure of the brachial plexus in complex revisions to reverse total shoulder arthroplasty. Int Orthop. 2019;43(12):2789–97.
24. Flatow EL, Bigliani LU. Tips of the trade. Locating and protecting the axillary nerve in shoulder surgery: the tug test. Orthop Rev. 1992;21(4):503–5.

Custom Glenoid Implants for Revision Shoulder Arthroplasty

8

Jay D. Keener, Ben Zmistowski, and Anand Murthi

8.1 Background

In the last decade, there has been significant growth in shoulder arthroplasty, especially reverse shoulder arthroplasty (RSA). Reverse shoulder arthroplasty provides a durable solution for a variety of clinical problems producing reliable results across most shoulder pathologies. With the increase in popularity of shoulder arthroplasty, we will likely see a growing number of failed arthroplasties requiring revision surgery. The burden of revision arthroplasty will, indeed, represent a significant challenge to the field of shoulder arthroplasty in the coming years.

Failed shoulder arthroplasty presents many challenges to the surgeon due to the presence of the variable degrees of bone and soft tissue deficiencies encountered. One consistent problem encountered is destruction of the native glenoid bone stock, which can be seen in failed shoulder hemiarthroplasty, anatomic and reverse shoulder arthroplasties, and fracture sequelae. The options for the management of a failed shoulder arthroplasty in the presence of a glenoid bone loss are highly dependent on the pattern of bone loss and the quantity and quality of the remaining glenoid bone stock. Due to the high prevalence of both soft tissue and bony defects, the majority of failed shoulder arthroplasties are managed with RSA. Reverse arthroplasty offers semiconstrained biomechanics to address soft tissue deficiencies and allows solid glenoid fixation in the presence of bone deficiency. The options for glenoid fixation include standard or augmented baseplates with or without glenoid bone grafting or custom glenoid baseplates. This chapter will discuss the expanding indications, options, and outcomes for the use of custom glenoid implants in revision RSA.

8.2 Classification and Incidence

There are several classification systems of glenoid bone loss that are descriptive but do not necessarily guide appropriate treatment strategies. More importantly, the relative indications to consider alternative implant fixation options such as the need for glenoid bone graft or a custom implant are not currently defined by these classification systems. Existing classification systems are based on bone loss patterns that are

J. D. Keener (✉)
Department of Orthopedic Surgery, Washington University, St. Louis, MO, USA
e-mail: keenerj@wustl.edu

B. Zmistowski
Department of Orthopaedic Surgery, Department of Orthopedic Surgery, Washington University, St. Louis, MO, USA
e-mail: bzmistowski@wustl.edu

A. Murthi
Georgetown University School of Medicine, MedStar Union Memorial Hospital, Baltimore, MD, USA

F. Franceschi et al. (eds.), *Revision Shoulder Arthroplasty*,
https://doi.org/10.1007/978-3-031-45944-3_8

somewhat—ill-defined and without consideration for the quality or density of the remaining bone. In the setting of glenoid bone erosion, CT scan imaging is recommended to localize and quantify bone loss and define the remaining bone available for implant fixation. Three-dimensional reconstructions of the glenoid vault are helpful to the surgeon by replicating the anatomy that will be encountered upon glenoid exposure. Two-dimensional images are very helpful to identify the depth of the remaining bone in the vault among the optional pathways (anatomic or alternative centerline axis) for implant fixation. CT scan analysis is somewhat hindered by the presence of implants in the revision setting but remains the gold standard for advanced imaging. In some cases, a staged revision with the removal of existing implants is needed if adequate subtraction of the existing implants is not possible.

The Antuna classification is most commonly used to classify glenoid bone loss and was described to characterize glenoid defects encountered with failed TSA cases (Fig. 8.1). Antuna described defects as central, peripheral, or combined and subdivided these into mild, moderate, or severe grades [1]. There are no clear proposed definitions of what qualifies the individual subgrades of bone loss severity. Goelke et al. proposed a 5-stage classification system based upon the pattern and severity of glenoid bone loss and the amount of glenoid vault that remains intact (Fig. 8.2) [2]. This system may be more helpful to direct treatment options but has not been studied to this effect. Goelke stage 4 and 5 glenoid defects are associated with severe medialization of the intact vault due to combined central and peripheral bone loss. The distinction between these stages is the depth of the remaining vault for baseplate anchorage. Stage 5 lesions have <10 mm of vault. According to Goelke, stage 5 defects should be treated with either 2 stage glenoid bone grafting or a custom glenoid implant. The difficulty remains in the quality of the bone in the vault both initially and after preparation. The question remains, will this vault support a standard or custom baseplate with excellent time zero fixation?

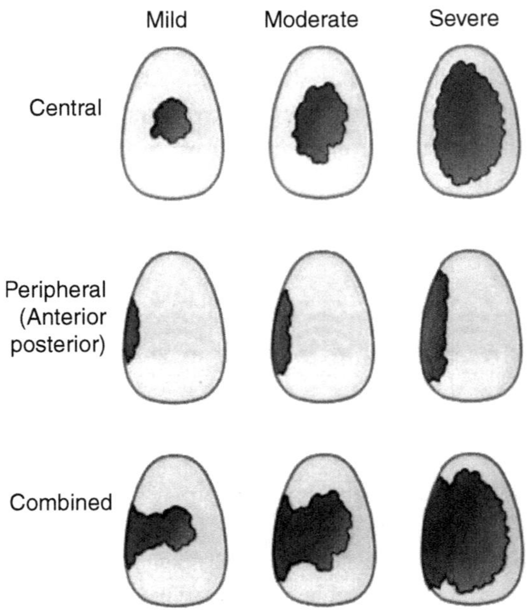

Fig. 8.1 Antuna classification for glenoid bone loss. Reprinted Fig. 8.1. J Shld Elbow Surg 2001;10 (3):217–224. Glenoid bone loss is described as central, peripheral, and combined. Each category is subdivided as mild, moderate, or severe

Severe glenoid bone loss can be seen in the primary or revision setting; however, the need for custom glenoid implants is most often seen in a revision setting. With revision surgery, the patterns and severity of glenoid bone loss will depend on the nature of the previous surgery. In comparing bone loss between shoulders with planned revision of hemiarthroplasty compared to anatomic TSA, Zmistowski et al. noted no difference in the complexity of glenoid bone loss, the degree of medialization, or the need for glenoid bone graft at the time of revision [3]. Although the incidence of complex glenoid lesions classified as combined central and peripheral was similar between groups (approximately 20%), the hemiarthroplasty group had a higher rate of eccentric or peripheral erosion compared to failed anatomic replacements.

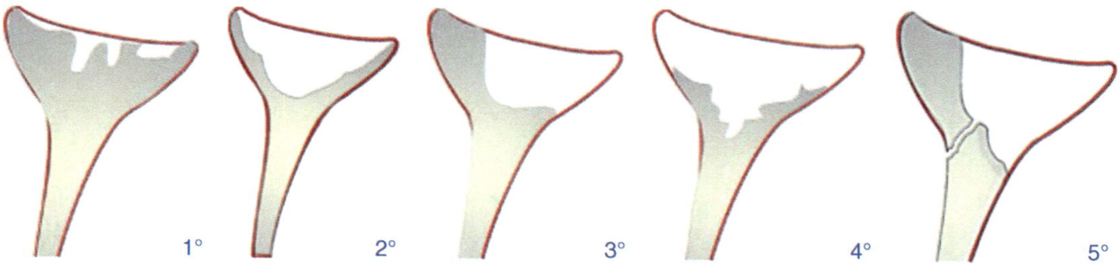

Fig. 8.2 Goelke classification for glenoid bone loss. Adapted from Table 1. Operative Orthopadie und Trauamtologie 2019;2:98–114. Stage 1—Mild central or peripheral bone loss. Less than 10° version, less than 40% loss of native glenoid surface. Stage 2—>40% glenoid loss of glenoid face but rim is intact. Stage 3—Severe eccentric bone loss >20° version or >50% glenoid width. Glenoid rim is broken or missing. Stage 4—Severe bone defect and moderate medialization below the coracoid base. Native vault allows at least the central peg to be fixed in >10 mm bone. Stage 5—Severe bone defect and deep medialization. Fatigue fracture up to glenoid neck. Less than 10 mm bone remains for central peg anchorage

8.3 Indications for Custom Glenoid Implant

The primary indication to consider a custom baseplate is situations where the bone loss is so severe that there is concern for inadequate initial glenoid construct fixation strength to allow standard joint loading bearing. In these cases, the options include either a 2-stage revision with a glenoid graft (autograft or allograft), a single-stage procedure with primary glenoid baseplate with or without supporting graft or a with custom glenoid baseplate. A popular option for addressing large defects in the glenoid vault includes placement of a structural graft. In the revision setting, this option is complicated by lack of native humeral autograft necessitating the use of either structural allograft or iliac crest graft. Although bone grafting remains a popular technique, this surgery is technically challenging and there remain concerns for graft healing and long-term implant fixation [4, 5]. The use of glenoid allograft in the revision RSA setting has been associated with a 18–25% risk of incomplete graft healing or graft failure and a 9–25% risk of baseplate loosening [6–10]. Furthermore, the utilization of the alternative center line with glenoid bone grafting in both contained and uncontained vaults has been used with some success [11, 12]. Ensuring adequate baseplate post compression into the native vault is paramount.

The most common situation to consider a custom baseplate includes revision cases with inadequate glenoid vault depth to allow central post or screw fixation in at least 10–12 mm of the native glenoid vault (Fig. 8.3). These cases often include variable amounts of peripheral or combined central and peripheral bone loss (Fig. 8.4). Custom baseplates should also be considered in primary cases with severe erosion such as end-stage inflammatory arthritis. The majority of primary or revision cases with at least 10-12 mm intact vault and some intact glenoid rim, thus allowing partial load bearing of the native glenoid face, can be managed with a glenoid allograft and a standard baseplate. It is not currently known how much of the baseplate face should be supported by the native glenoid in the presence of adequate vault depth, especially in a revision setting. The authors also prefer to use custom baseplate in cases with more than 10–12 mm of vault depth when combined severe rim deficiency (>70%) and/or poor remaining rim bone stock, i.e., cortical thinning. When contemplating a standard or custom baseplate not only should the vault fixation be studied but also the resulting geographic positioning on the sphere/baseplate face. If the desired inclination, lateralization, and offset of the glenoid cannot be reproduced by standard implants, one must consider custom designs.

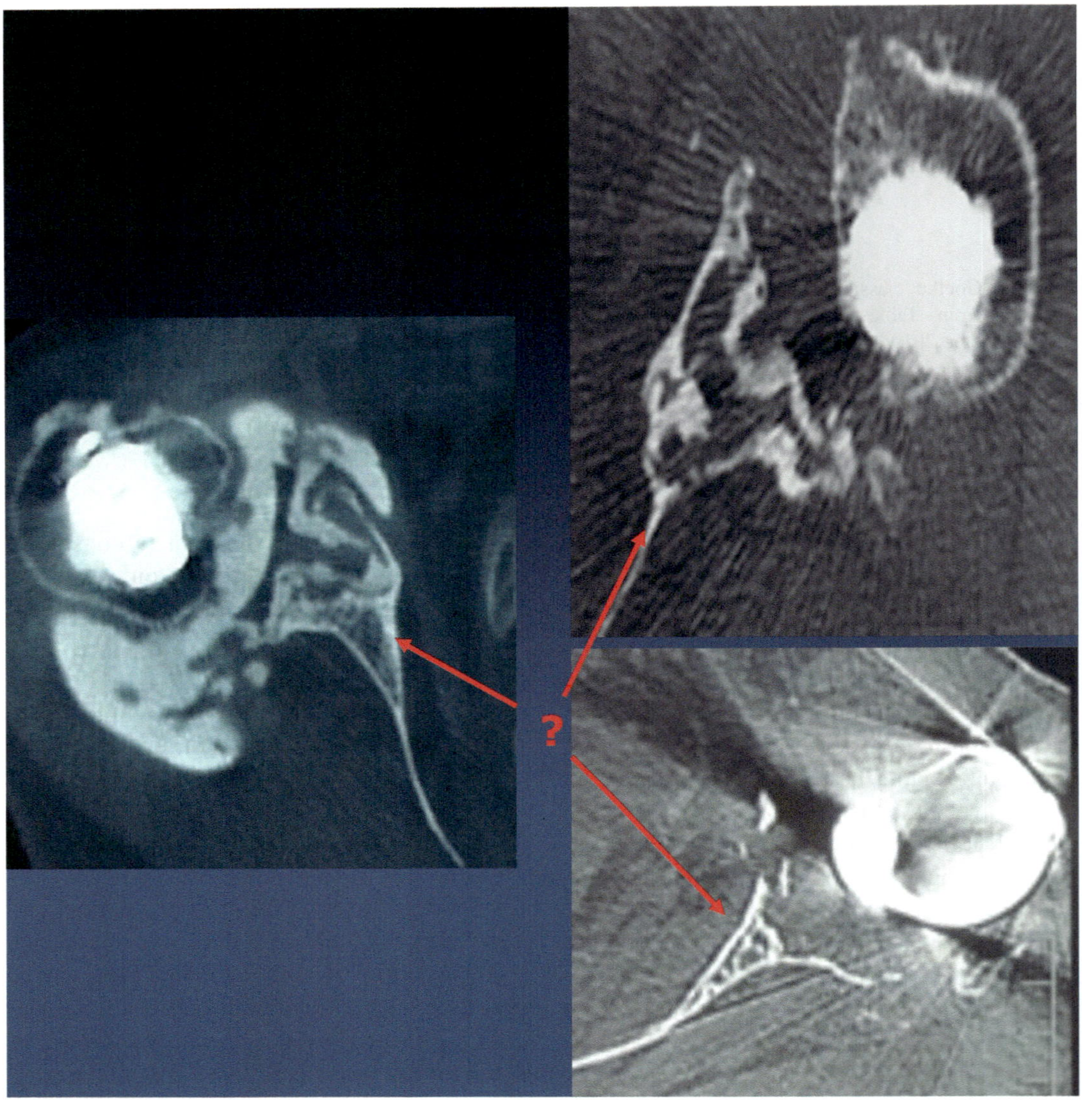

Fig. 8.3 Two-dimensional axial images glenoid bone loss. Three cases of failed anatomic total shoulder arthroplasty with large central bone defects, glenoid rim thinning, and less than 10 mm of remaining glenoid vault

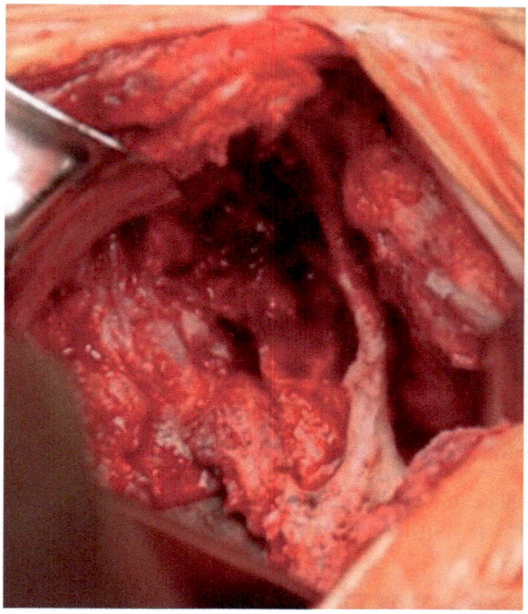

Fig. 8.4 Intraoperative image of complex glenoid bone loss. Right shoulder with failed glenoid implant (removed) showing combined central and peripheral bone loss

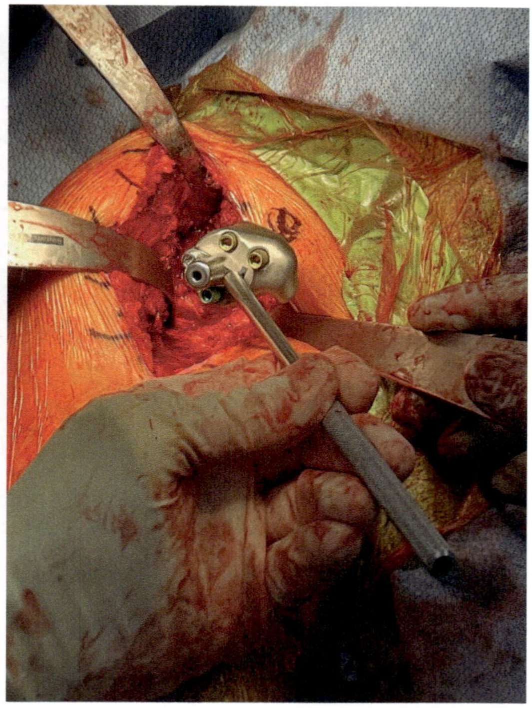

Fig. 8.5 Custom glenoid Implant. Intraoperative photograph of Biomet Vault Reconstruction System (Zimmer Biomet, Warsaw IN) baseplate and inserter. The implant is shaped to match the glenoid defect with porous metal on the backside of the implant

8.4 Design Rationale

Custom glenoid baseplates offer design features that improve initial construct fixation strength and backside baseplate support compared to conventional implants. This is achieved primarily in three manners—increased baseplate to vault contact area, alternative baseplate fixation points, and custom baseplate screw trajectories. Custom baseplates are contoured to match the unique pattern of glenoid vault deficiency from three-dimensional CT scan reconstructions of the vault. The baseplate is 3D printed to match the bone deformity and coated with a bony ingrowth/ongrowth material (Fig. 8.5). This serves to maximize baseplate support on the native bone and potentially allow bone ingrowth over a large contact area. The thickness of the baseplate can be customized in an effort to restore the native joint line. Alternative points of baseplate fixation can be accomplished by modifying the shape of the baseplate to achieve contact on areas of the scapula that does not normally support the baseplate such as the base of the scapular spine and/or the base of the coracoid (Fig. 8.6). Typically, these areas are preserved in cases of complex glenoid bone deformity and typically possess good bone density. Additionally, in the presence of rim deficiency, tabs or extensions of the baseplate can be placed that allow the baseplate to key into the vault by hooking around the remaining glenoid rim. These tabs can accommodate both compression and locked screw fixation. The varied morphology of the baseplate allows creation of custom screw trajectories to achieve compression of the baseplate in available bone (Fig. 8.7). The central fixation can be either a custom post or a large diameter screw. Stability is achieved with variably oriented peripheral compression and locking screws. Commercially available custom baseplates frequently come with surrogate sterile and nonsterile models to aid in three-dimensional orientation needed during glenoid exposure and preparation (Fig. 8.8). The process of implant fabrication is typically initiated by implant company engineers. Design programs

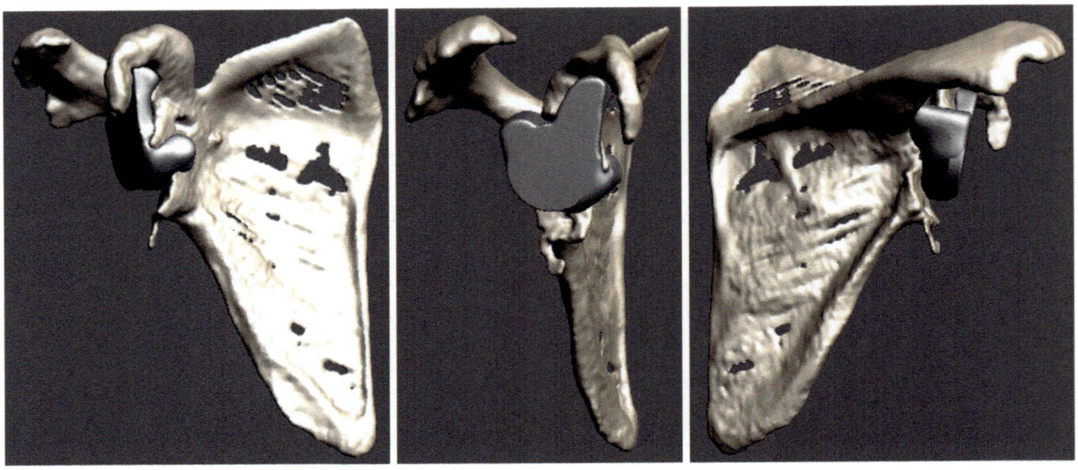

Fig. 8.6 Alternative fixation points of custom glenoid baseplate. CT guided planning images of custom baseplate. Alternative fixation points demonstrated include the coracoid base, scapular spine, and remaining anterior glenoid rim

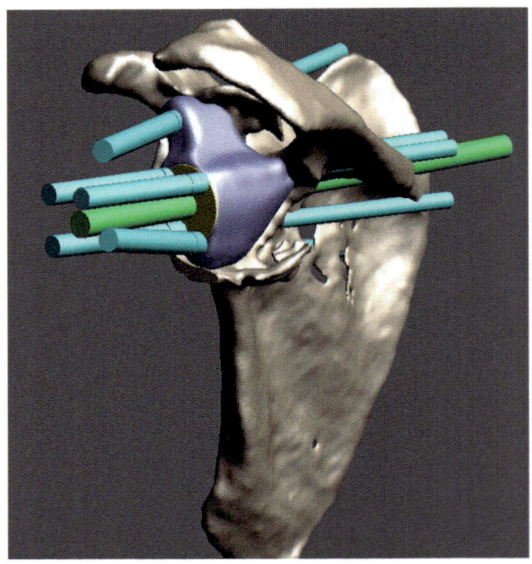

Fig. 8.7 Baseplate screw trajectories. The peripheral screws (aqua) are customized to achieve fixation in remaining bone. The central screw (green) is centered in the baseplate

exist to overlay the contralateral 3-dimensional glenoid with its premorbid condition to plan the custom glenoid. Special CT sequencing can provide information into bone quality and density in the glenoid vault and scapula to provide optimal screw post-trajectory (Fig. 8.9). The plan can be modified according to surgeon input. Once the plan is finalized, typically there is a manufacturing time period of 6–8 weeks before the implant is available.

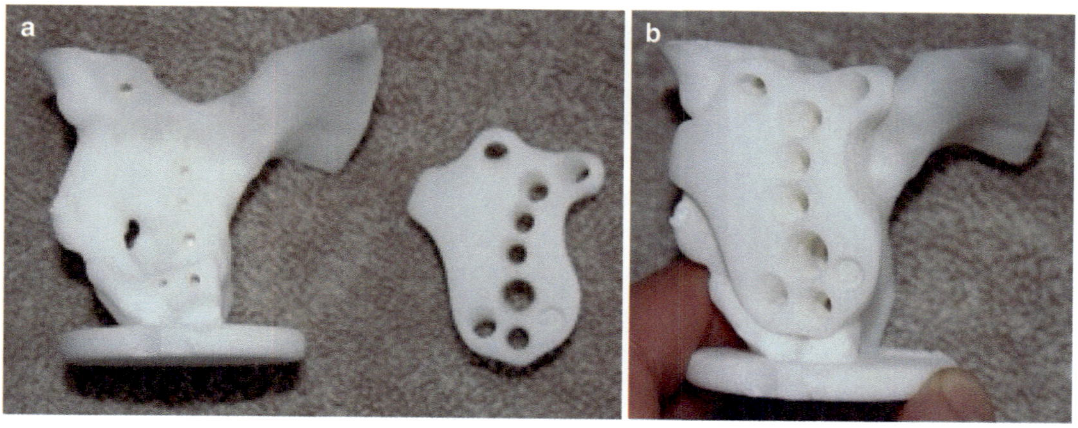

Fig. 8.8 Custom model of scapula and baseplate implant. Surrogate models of the glenoid defect (**a**) and custom baseplate (**b**) are fabricated to assist with intraoperative orientation of the glenoid and baseplate

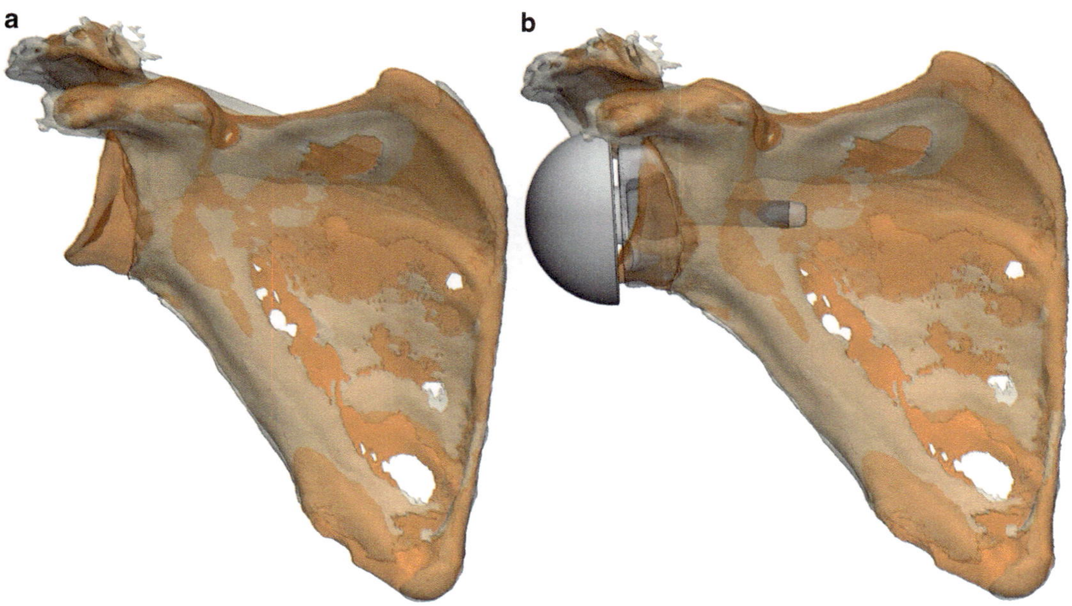

Fig. 8.9 Computer-generated model of scapula. (**a**) Model of deformed glenoid and calculated premorbid bony anatomy. (**b**) Model of custom glenoid baseplate and glenosphere

8.5 Case Examples

Case 1

Seventy-three year old female with a failed anatomic shoulder arthroplasty due to glenoid loosening. The original implant was placed 10 years ago. She reports 6 months of pain and progressive stiffness. Radiographs and CT scan show a loose hybrid anatomic glenoid with severe medialization of the glenoid (Figs. 8.10 and 8.11). Three-dimensional reconstructions of the glenoid/scapula show a complex glenoid deformity with severe central erosion and partial anterior and posterior glenoid rim deficiency (Fig. 8.12). Figure 8.13a, b demonstrating custom VRS glenoid implant with 1 central and 3 peripheral screw trajectories. Note custom flange around anterior glenoid rim. Intraoperative

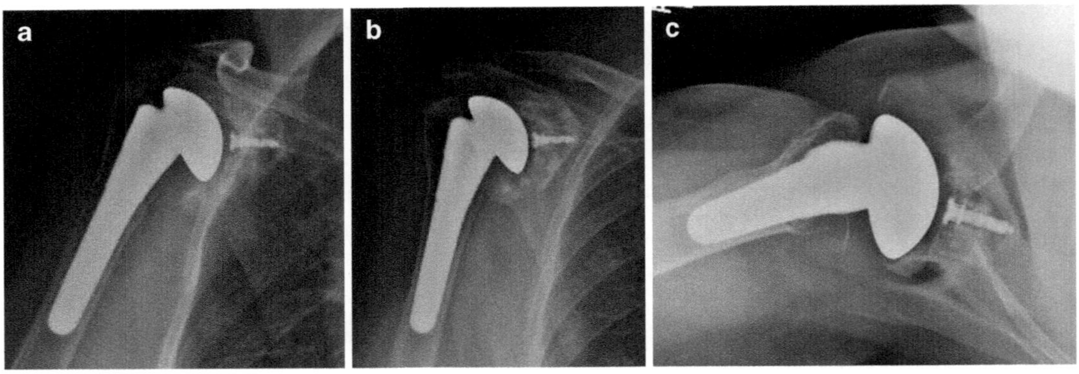

Fig. 8.10 Radiographs for Case 1. Anteroposterior, (**a**) Grashey (**b**), and axillary (**c**) views of failed anatomic arthroplasty with glenoid loosening and severe implant medialization

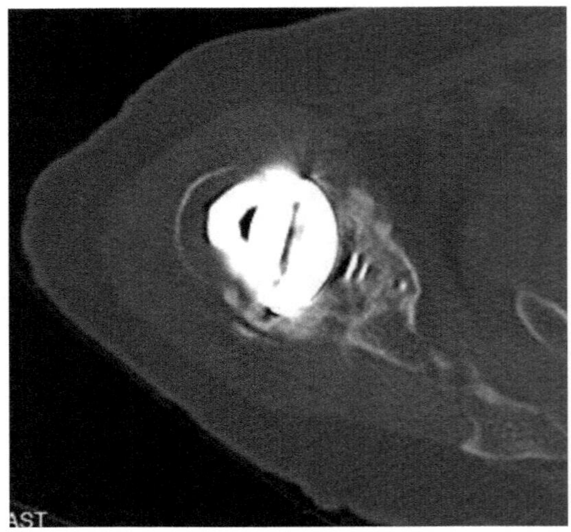

Fig. 8.11 CT scan Case 1. 2D axial CT scan slice showing loose glenoid implant and severe medialization into the glenoid vault

photos of glenoid exposure including glenoid removal, bone surrogate models, and final position of custom glenoid baseplate (Fig. 8.14). Post-operative radiographs are shown in Fig. 8.15.

Case 2

Seventy-nine year old 20 years s/p limited open reduction and internal fixation of right proximal humerus fracture. Patient did well initially but now has 10 years of progressive pain and loss of function. Preoperative radiographs showing post-traumatic osteoarthritis, humeral head collapse, and severe glenoid bone loss and medialization (Fig. 8.16). Axial two-dimensional CT images demonstrating severe glenoid medialization with compromise of medial vault depth and severe thinning of the glenoid rim (Fig. 8.17). Figure 8.18 demonstrates a custom 3D printed baseplate (Restor3D, Durham NC) to match glenoid deformity with a central post positioned in the remaining vault and custom screw trajectories. Figure 8.19 demonstrates with planned and actual patient-specific guides around which the implant is placed. Images of planned and actual implanted custom baseplate are shown in Fig. 8.20. Glenosphere options demonstrate modularity choices to optimize implant position (Fig. 8.21). Postoperative radiograph for case 2 (Fig. 8.22).

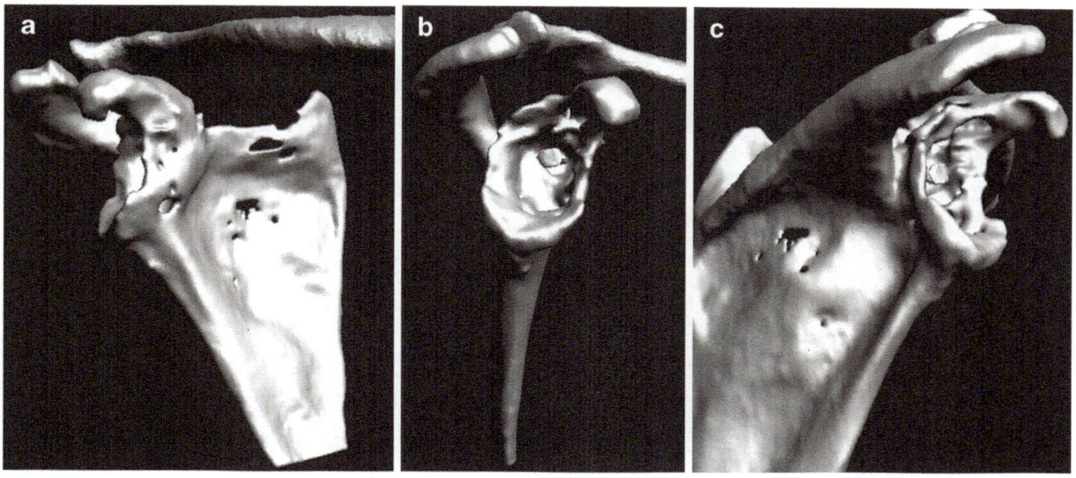

Fig. 8.12 Three-dimensional reconstruction images for Case 1. Anterior, (**a**) central (**b**), and posterior (**c**) views of complex glenoid bone defect for Case 1. There is severe medialization and anterior and posterior glenoid rim deficiency. Erosion into the coracoid base is noted

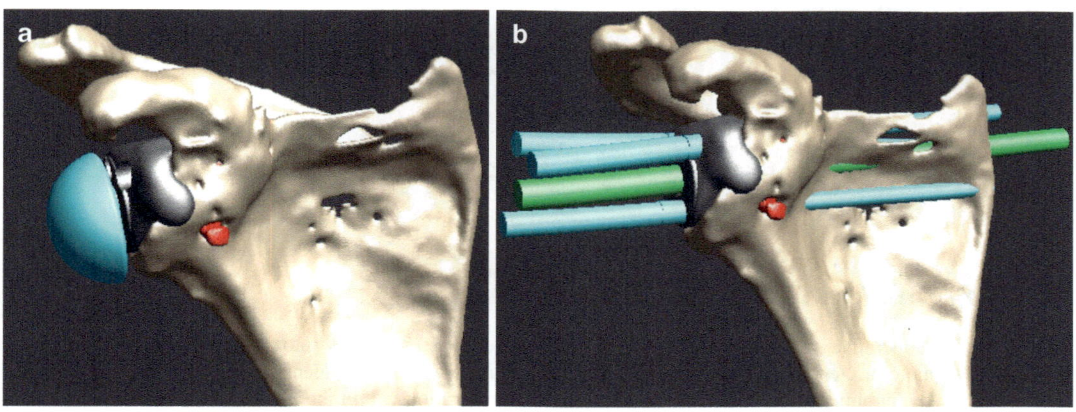

Fig. 8.13 Custom VRS glenoid implant. (**a**) Custom baseplate model with modular glenosphere. (**b**) VRS custom glenoid implant model demonstrating screw trajectories

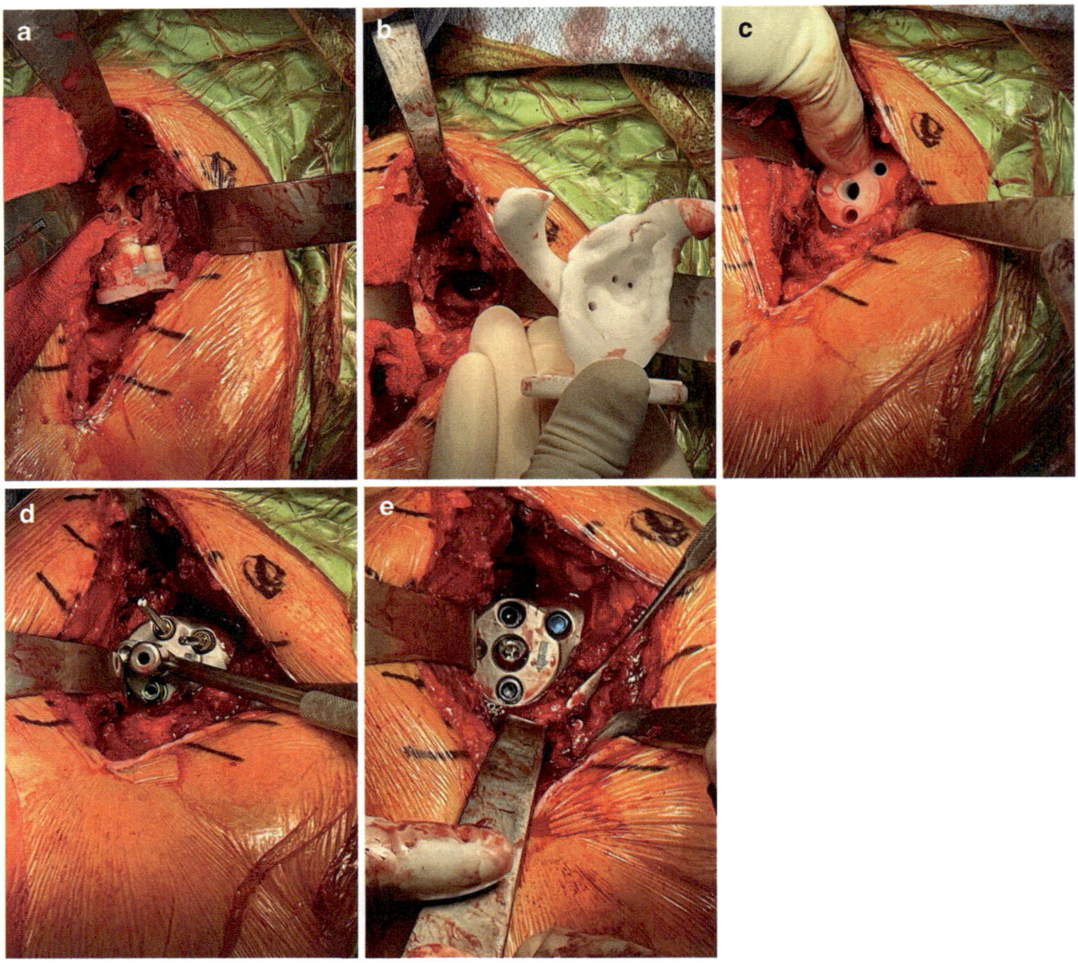

Fig. 8.14 Intraoperative photos of Case 1. (**a**) Intraoperative photo of glenoid vault and glenoid component removal. (**b**) Intraoperative photo of bone surrogate model matching the intraoperative appearance of the glenoid defect. (**c**) Intraoperative photo of baseplate surrogate VRS model fits into glenoid defect assuring good contact with native glenoid. (**d**) VRS baseplate pinned into position within the glenoid. (**e**) Final baseplate fixation with central and peripheral screws

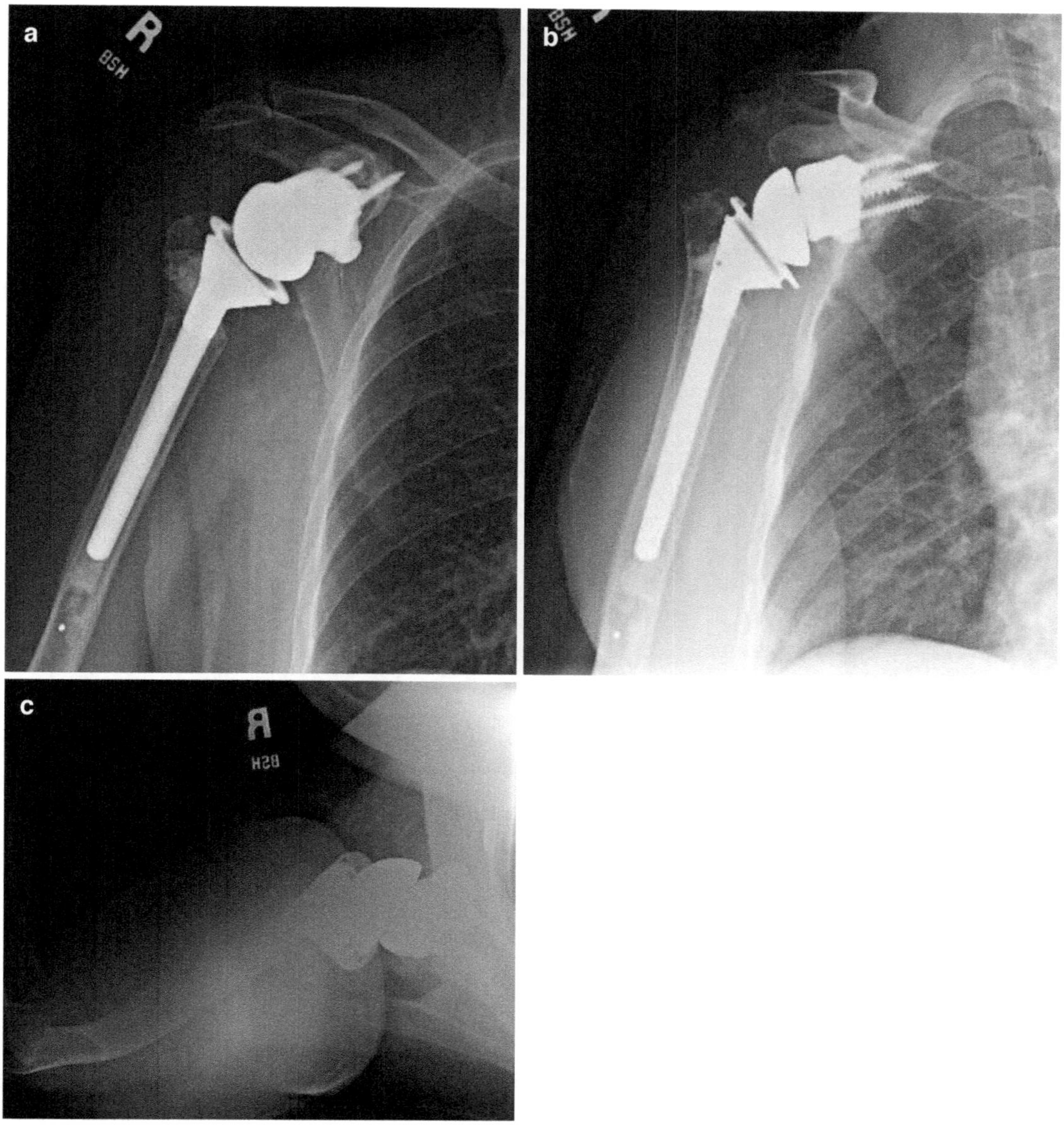

Fig. 8.15 Postoperative radiographs for Case 1. Postoperative anteroposterior (**a**), Grashey (**b**), and axillary (**c**) radiographs

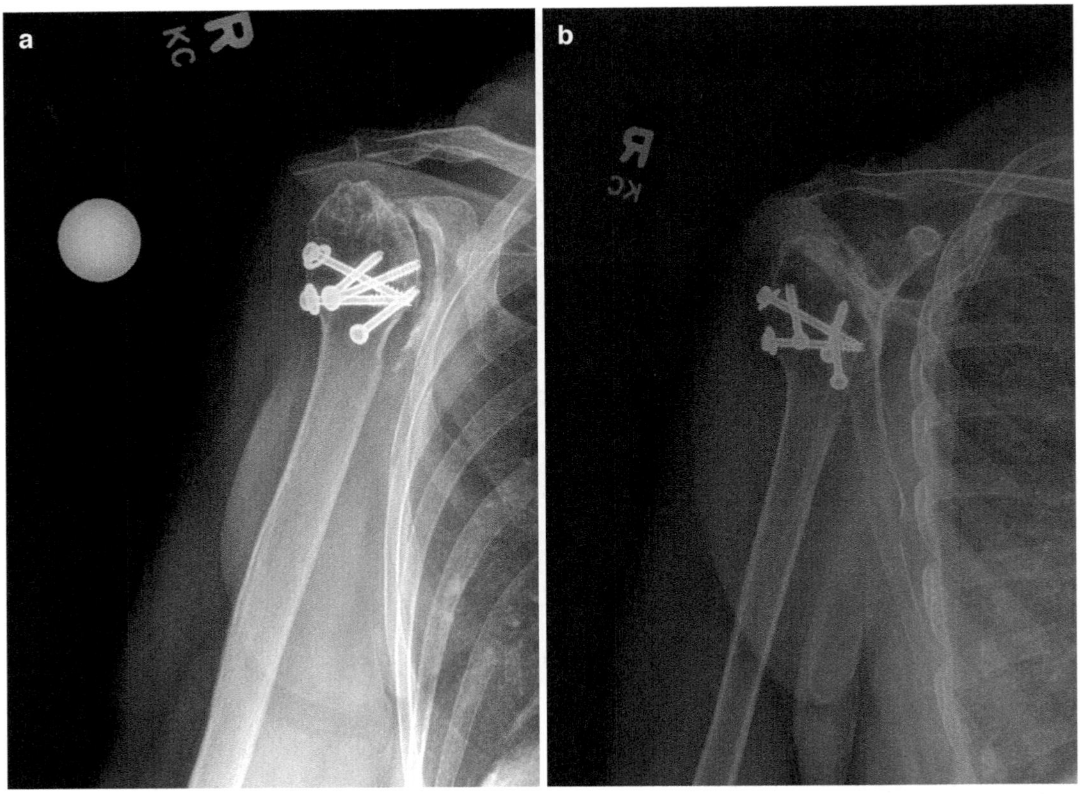

Fig. 8.16 Preoperative radiographs for Case 2. Preoperative anteroposterior (**a**) and Y-view (**b**) radiographs

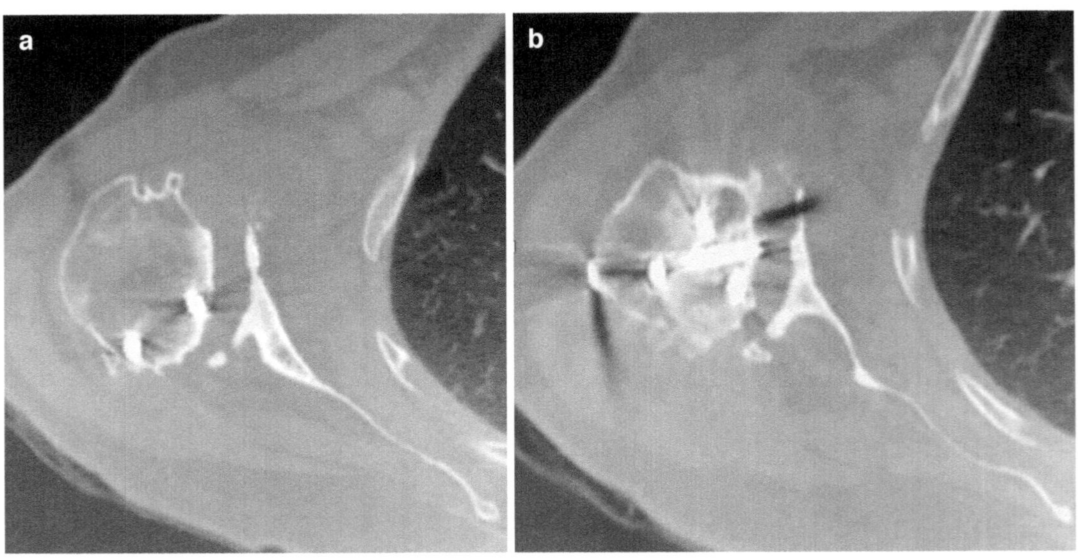

Fig. 8.17 Two-dimensional CT scan images for Case 2. Two axial CT scan slices (**a** and **b**) demonstrating severe glenoid medialization with glenoid rim thinning. The glenoid vault depth is severely compromised

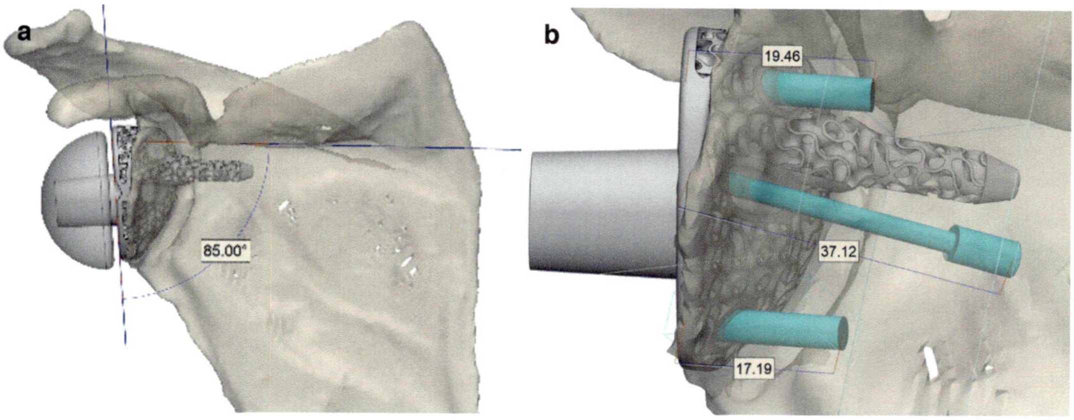

Fig. 8.18 Custom baseplate plan for Case 2. (**a**) CT based custom 3D printed baseplate (Restor3D, Durham NC) with central post in glenoid vault/scapular body. (**b**) Screw trajectories for custom baseplate

Fig. 8.19 Custom glenoid guide for Case 2. (**a**) Planned glenoid guide. (**b**) Actual glenoid guide placed on surrogate model

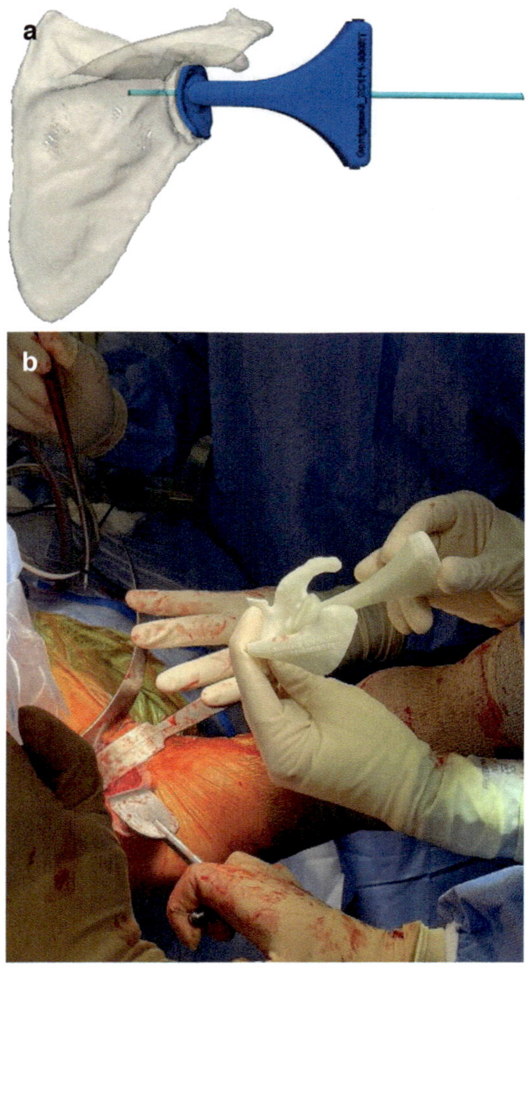

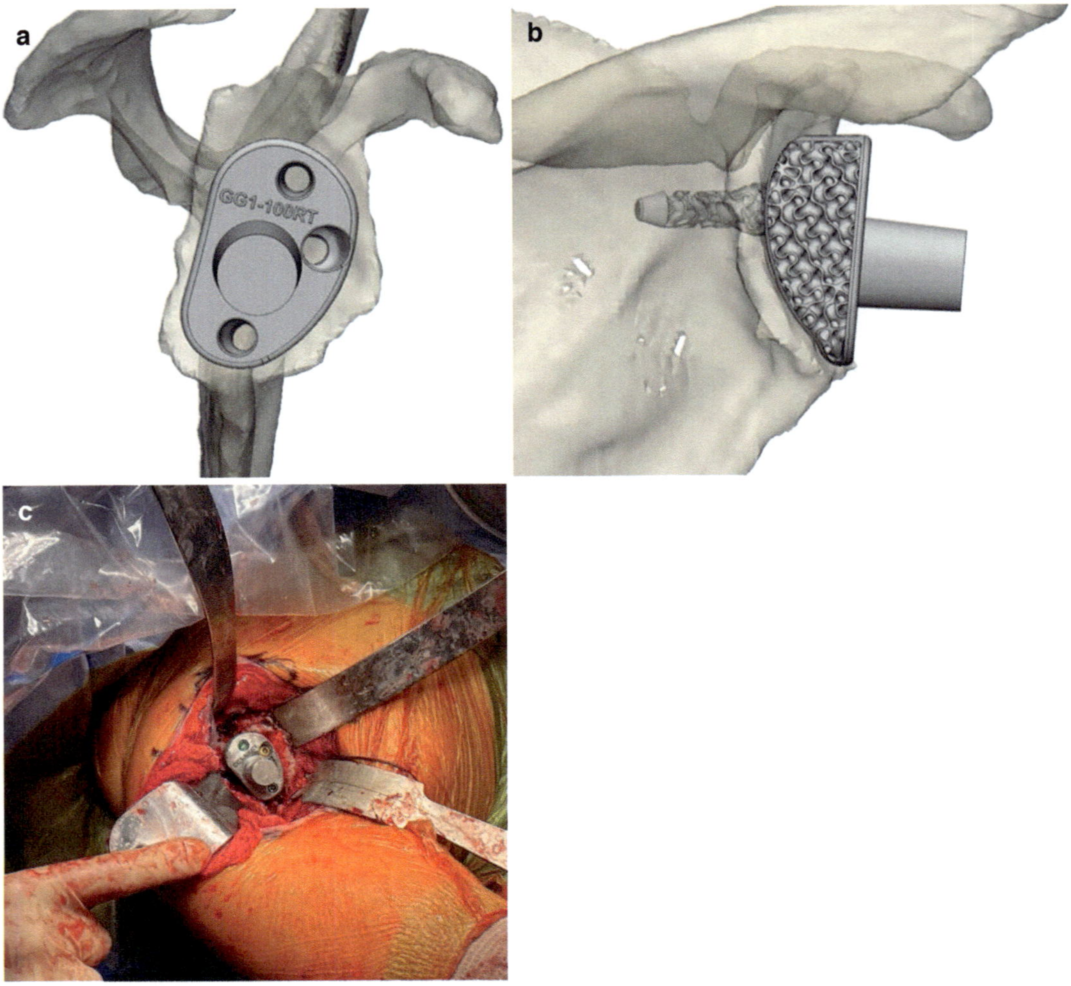

Fig. 8.20 Custom baseplate implant for Case 2. (**a**) Lateral planned view of implanted baseplate. (**b**) Posterior planned view of implanted baseplate. (**c**) Intraoperative view of implanted baseplate

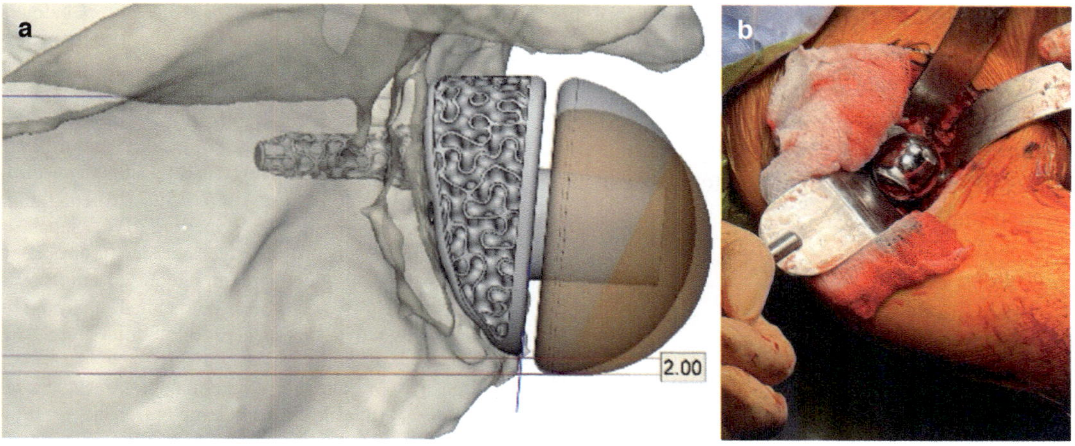

Fig. 8.21 Glenosphere placement for Case 2. (**a**) Glenosphere modularity options to optimize implant position. (**b**) Intraoperative view of implanted glenosphere

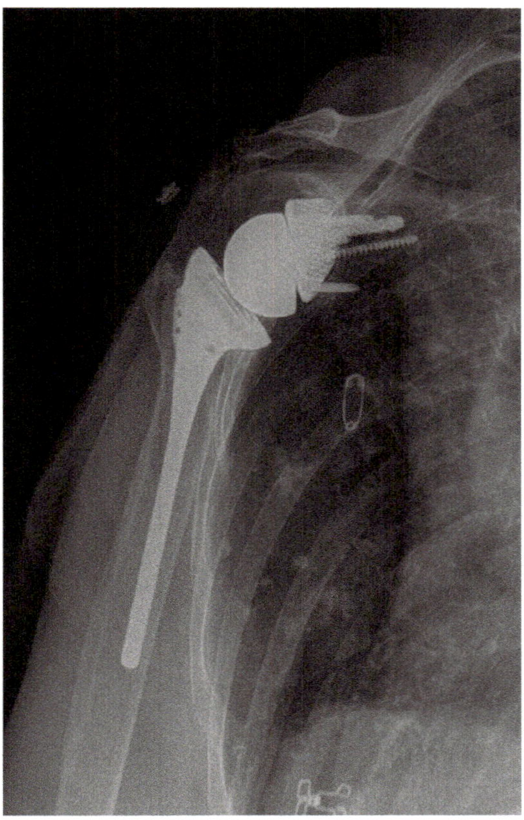

Fig. 8.22 Postoperative Grashey view for Case 2

8.6 Outcomes

There are few studies reporting outcomes of custom glenoid baseplates in RSA. Rangarajan et al. reported the results of 19 shoulders treated with the Comprehensive Vault Reconstruction System (VRS, Zimmer Biomet, Warsaw, IN) [13]. Nine cases were primary, and 10 were revision surgeries. Significant improvement in clinical outcomes was reported at a mean of 18 months, showing a mean ASES and Constant score improvements preoperative to postoperative from 32 to 79 and 24 to 60, respectively. There were significant improvements in active range of motion and no cases of hardware loosening or failure. Four patients had complications including 1 case of each of the following; instability, intraoperative greater tuberosity fracture, intraoperative humeral cortical bone perforation, and infection. Bodenfor et al. reported short-term results of the same VRS implant in 12 shoulders with a mean of 30 months follow-up [14]. Significant improvements in numeric pain score (7 points), SANE score (43%), ASES score (45 points), and Penn Score (49 points) were noted with no revision surgeries or instances of implants loosening.

The early results of custom glenoid baseplates are promising, but longer follow-up is needed to better define implant performance, longevity, and complications over time. Long-term survivorship of the implants will be contingent on bony ingrowth on the face and/or custom post of the glenoid implant.

References

1. Antuna SA, Sperling JW, Cofield RH, Rowland CM. Glenoid revision surgery after total shoulder arthroplasty. J Shoulder Elb Surg. 2001;10(3):217–24.
2. Gohlke F, Werner B, Wiese I. Glenoidrekonstruktion bei Wechseloperationen an der Schulter. Operative Orthopadie und Traumatologie. 2018;31:98–114.
3. Zmistowski B, Hill JR, Aleem AW, Chamberlain AM, Keener JD. Glenoid bone quality in revision of anatomic shoulder arthroplasty: the impact of prior glenoid resurfacing. J Shoulder Elbow Surg. 2022.
4. Iannotti JP, Frangiamore SJ. Fate of large structural allograft for treatment of severe uncontained glenoid bone deficiency. J Shoulder Elb Surg. 2012;21(6):765–71.
5. Scalise JJ, Iannotti JP. Bone grafting severe glenoid defects in revision shoulder arthroplasty. Clin Orthop Relat Res. 2008;466(1):139–45.
6. Ho JC, Thakar O, Chan WW, Nicholson T, Williams GR, Namdari S. Early radiographic failure of reverse total shoulder arthroplasty with structural bone graft for glenoid bone loss. J Shoulder Elb Surg. 2020;29(3):550–60.
7. Tashjian RZ, Broschinsky K, Stertz I, Chalmers PN. Structural glenoid allograft reconstruction during reverse total shoulder arthroplasty. J Shoulder Elb Surg. 2020;29(3):534–40.
8. Wagner E, Houdek MT, Griffith T, Elhassan BT, Sanchez-Sotelo J, Sperling JW, et al. Glenoid bone-grafting in revision to a reverse Total shoulder arthroplasty. J Bone Joint Surg Am. 2015;97(20):1653–60.
9. Bartels DW, Marigi E, Sperling JW, Sanchez-Sotelo J. Revision reverse shoulder arthroplasty for anatomical glenoid component loosening was not universally successful: a detailed analysis of 127 consecutive shoulders. J Bone Joint Surg Am. 2021;103(10):879–86.
10. Jones RB, Wright TW, Zuckerman JD. Reverse total shoulder arthroplasty with structural bone grafting of large glenoid defects. J Shoulder Elb Surg. 2016;25(9):1425–32.
11. Colley R, Polisetty TS, Levy JC. Mid-term outcomes of reverse shoulder arthroplasty using the alternative center line for glenoid baseplate fixation: a case-controlled study. J Shoulder Elb Surg. 2021;30(2):298–305.
12. Frankle MA, Teramoto A, Luo ZP, Levy JC, Pupello D. Glenoid morphology in reverse shoulder arthroplasty: classification and surgical implications. J Shoulder Elb Surg. 2009;18(6):874–85.
13. Rangarajan R, Blout CK, Patel VV, Bastian SA, Lee BK, Itamura JM. Early results of reverse total shoulder arthroplasty using a patient-matched glenoid implant for severe glenoid bone deficiency. J Shoulder Elb Surg. 2020;29(7S):S139–S48.
14. Bodendorfer BM, Loughran GJ, Looney AM, Velott AT, Stein JA, Lutton DM, et al. Short-term outcomes of reverse shoulder arthroplasty using a custom baseplate for severe glenoid deficiency. J Shoulder Elb Surg. 2021;30(5):1060–7.

Part III

Glenoid

9 Classifying Bone Loss in Revision Arthroplasty

Khai Cheong Wong, Bryan H. G. Loh, and Denny T. T. Lie

9.1 Introduction

During primary shoulder arthroplasty, whether total shoulder arthroplasty (TSA) or reverse shoulder arthroplasty (RSA), implanting the prosthetic glenoid component can be difficult if the bony glenoid is deficient [1] or abnormal, as in Walch type B2 or C glenoid [2]. It is estimated that approximately 32% of shoulders with primary glenohumeral osteoarthritis are type B glenoid and 9% are type C glenoid [3]. Glenoid erosions are commonly seen in primary RSA. It has been estimated that around 40% of primary RSAs present with glenoid defects at the time of surgery [4]. This difficulty is made worse in revision shoulder arthroplasty where there is loss of the glenoid bone stock from erosion or osteolysis [5]. In revision shoulder arthroplasty, it is often the glenoid component that fails. The Australian Orthopaedic Association National Joint Replacement Registry estimated that 10.7% of all types of shoulder arthroplasty were revisions and 48% of these involved the glenoid component [6]. In performing revision shoulder arthroplasty, it is evident that an understanding of the bone loss and remnant bone stock in the glenoid is of critical importance to ensure success of the revision surgery.

There are many classifications of glenoid bone loss in the published literature, some of which are variations or modifications of the others. Some describe posterior glenoid bone loss, like the classic Walch classification [3], and others describe the severity of medial erosions and bone loss in specific monoplanar directions like superior or inferior (Hamada classification) [7]. This chapter is dedicated to a review of the many classifications available. Section 9.3 lists and describes the classifications of glenoid bone loss mainly seen in primary arthroplasty. This however does not mean that these patterns of bone loss are not seen in revision arthroplasty, only that they are often not as severe as those seen in revision cases. Classifications in primary arthroplasty can be sub-categorized by the pathology (primary OA, RA, cuff arthropathy, or dislocation arthropathy) or by the monoplanar directions (posterior, superior, or inferior). Classifications of more complex glenoid bone loss seen in revision cases, like those described by Antuna [8] and more recently by Kocsis [9], are described in detail, in Sect. 9.4. The key considerations in assessing and classifying glenoid bone loss in

K. C. Wong · B. H. G. Loh
Department of Orthopaedic Surgery, Division of Musculoskeletal Sciences, Singapore General Hospital, Singapore, Singapore

D. T. T. Lie (✉)
Department of Orthopaedic Surgery, Division of Musculoskeletal Sciences, Singapore General Hospital, Singapore, Singapore

Duke-National University of Singapore Medical School, Singapore, Singapore

F. Franceschi et al. (eds.), *Revision Shoulder Arthroplasty*,
https://doi.org/10.1007/978-3-031-45944-3_9

revision arthroplasty are *location of the defect, severity of the defect, and containment (integrity of both the glenoid rim and vault).*

9.2 Assessing Glenoid Bone Loss

Preoperative planning is crucial to assess glenoid bone loss and to plan for the type of bone grafting required. A thorough assessment of glenoid morphology (version, inclination, and depth) is also important to aid with implant positioning. This starts with obtaining full-length scaled radiographs of both humeri (**True anteroposterior view (Grashey view), axillary view, and Y scapular view**) to assess for humeral shortening and medialization. It also allows for a 2-dimensional assessment of glenoid bone stock and glenoid inclination.

Glenoid inclination is the angle of the glenoid in the plane of the scapula and is measured using the ***β*-angle** described by Maurer et al. [10]. It is defined as the angle between the floor of the supraspinatus fossa marked by a sclerotic line and the glenoid fossa line (Fig. 9.1). The glenoid inclination is useful when implanting a total shoulder arthroplasty (TSA) as it represents the global glenoid inclination. However, it is not appropriate for implanting a reverse shoulder arthroplasty (RSA) as most RSA base plates are seated at the lower part of the glenoid surface as illustrated in Fig. 9.2. A recent modification to this is the "reverse shoulder angle" described by Boileau et al. [11]. The **RSA angle** (Fig. 9.3) is defined as the angle between the inferior part of the glenoid fossa and perpendicular to the floor of the supraspinatus fossa. The RSA angle is useful to avoid placement of the baseplate in superior tilt which is associated with increased risk of scapular notching and component loosening [12, 13].

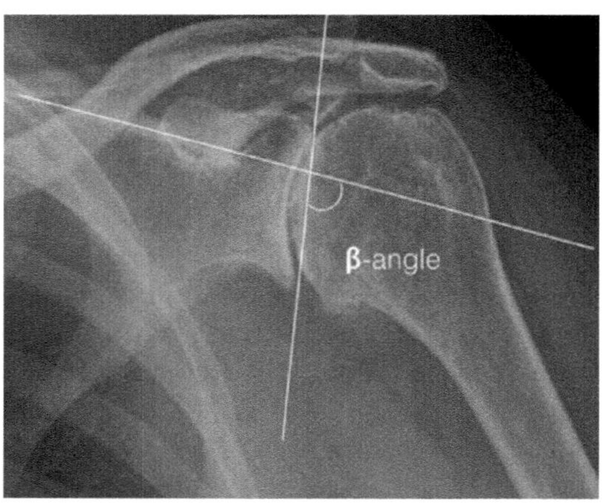

Fig. 9.1 The β-angle is formed between the floor of the supraspinatus fossa marked by a sclerotic line and the glenoid fossa line

Computed tomography (CT) provides the most detailed assessment of glenoid morphology. It allows precise measurements of the *vault, version, and depth* of the glenoid when 3-dimensional (3D) images are constructed together. **Glenoid version** is best determined using CT (axial) cuts along the plane of the scapula at the level of the coracoid tip as described by Friedman et al. [14]. The Scapular axis (A) is determined by a line drawn between the medial tip of the scapula to the midpoint of the glenoid. A second line (B) is drawn between the anterior and posterior margins of the glenoid rim. Glenoid version is the angle subtended between a perpendicular line to (A) and (B) (Fig. 9.4). **Glenoid depth** can be best measured in the horizontal plane using CT (axial) cuts using a method adapted from Hill and Norris [15]. Originally described using axillary radiographs, other authors have adapted its use for CT scan [2, 4]. The depth is measured by the maximum perpendicular distance between the posterior border of glenoid erosion (CF) and the glenoid reference line (AF). The ratio between CF/AF represents the percentage bone loss (Fig. 9.5).

The advent of 3D CT has led to the use of patient-specific instrumentation (PSI) for shoulder arthroplasty. It has been validated in both cadaveric and clinical studies [4, 16] and includes manufacturing of PSI cutting jigs, custom drill guides as well as patient-specific implants. This is especially pertinent in revision arthroplasty where there may be very little "real estate" left on the glenoid for implantation.

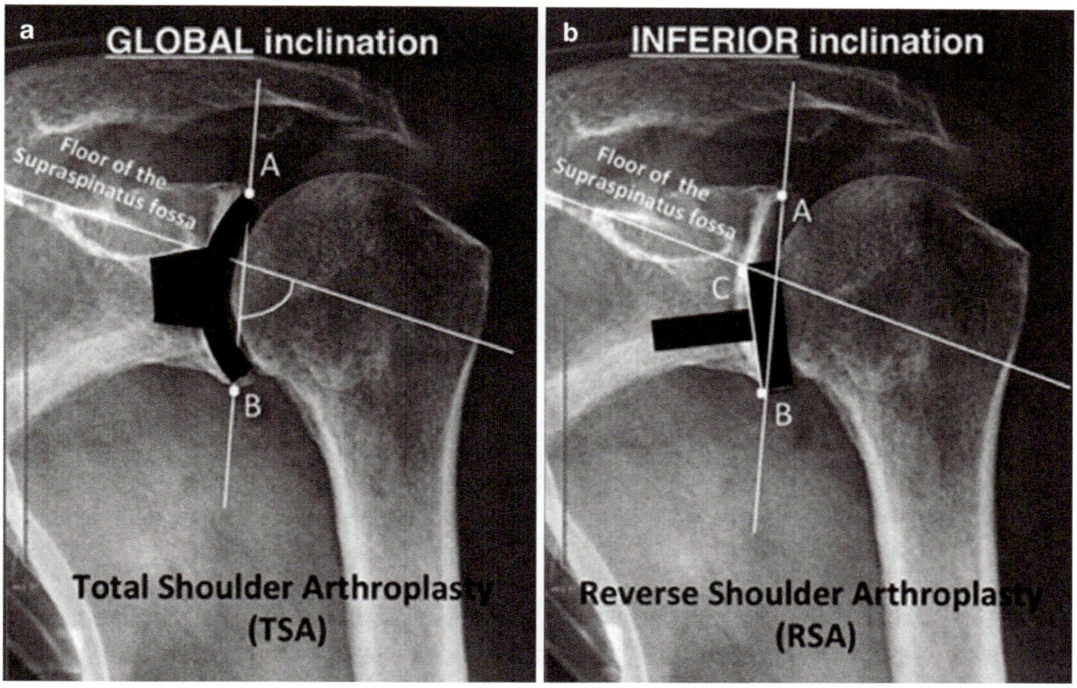

Fig. 9.2 (**a**) shows the global inclination in a TSA, while (**b**) shows the inferior inclination of the glenoid in an RSA

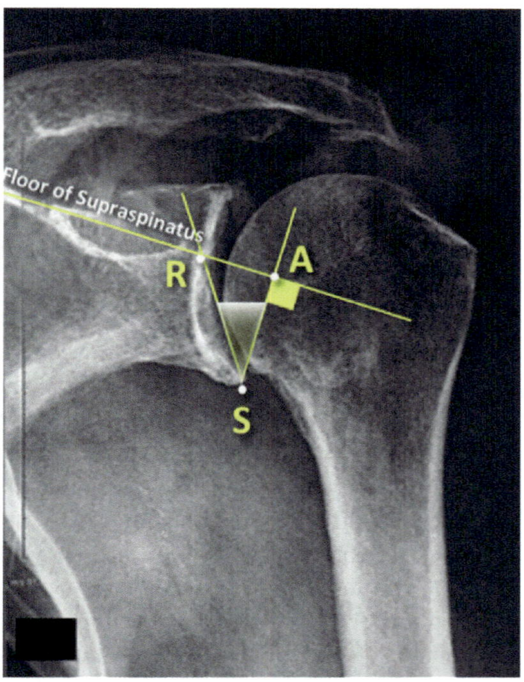

Fig. 9.3 The RSA angle is defined as the angle between the inferior part of the glenoid fossa and the perpendicular to the floor of the supraspinatus fossa

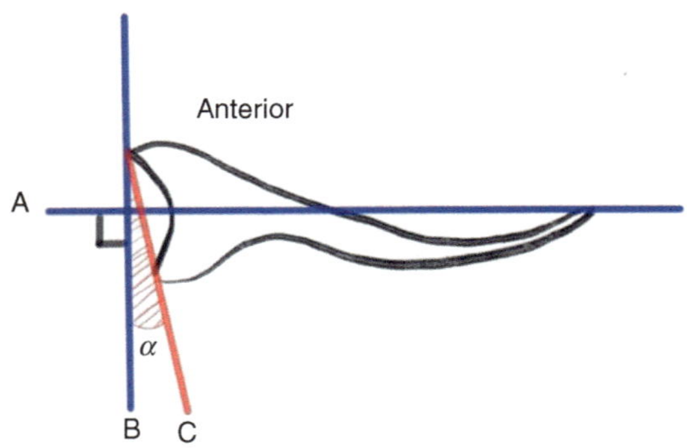

Fig. 9.4 The Scapular axis (A) is determined by a line drawn between the medial tip of the scapula to the mid-point of the glenoid. A perpendicular line (B) is drawn to the scapular axis. A third line (C) is drawn between the anterior and posterior margins of the glenoid rim. Glenoid version is the angle subtended between Line (B) and (C)

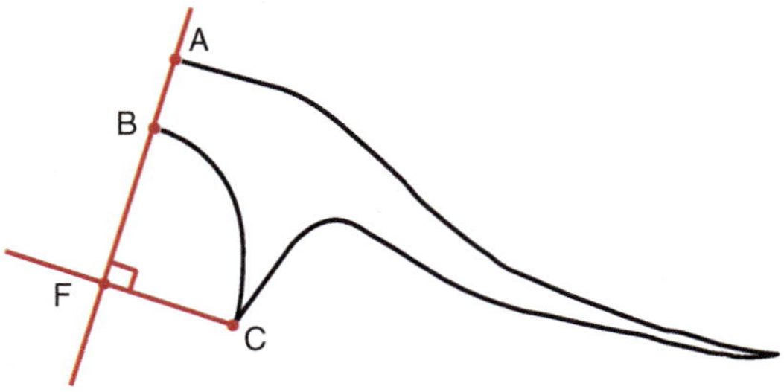

Fig. 9.5 The glenoid depth is measured by the maximum perpendicular distance between the posterior border of glenoid erosion (CF) and the glenoid reference line (AF). The ratio between CF/AF represents the percentage bone loss

9.3 Classification of Bone Loss in Primary Arthroplasty

Walch et al. [3] analyzed the types of glenoid morphology using pre-operative computed tomography (CT) scans of 133 shoulders with primary osteoarthritis of the glenohumeral joint. Parameters assessed included degree of glenoid retroversion (Fig. 9.4), pattern of erosion (central or posterior), and amount of humeral head subluxation with the patient in supine position. Patients were then categorized into 3 different types of glenoid morphology based on CT scan findings (Fig. 9.6). Central glenoid wear (Type A) made up 59% of the cohort, where the humeral head was centered. These had an average glenoid retroversion of 11.5°. The amount of glenoid erosion was further divided into minor (Type A1) and major (Type A2) where marked erosion resulted in a glenoid cupula. Type B (32%) consisted of posterior glenoid wear with the humeral head subluxed posteriorly. The average glenoid retroversion was 18°. These were then subdivided into Type B1 where there was narrowing of posterior joint space, subchondral sclerosis, and osteophytes, whilst Type B2 included glenoids with a posterior cupula resulting in a biconcave appearance. In extreme cases, the chronically subluxed humeral head may require more extensive soft tissue release and bony reconstruction intra-operatively to achieve stable implants with good range of motion. Type C (9%) included all glenoids with a retroversion of more than 25°, regardless of degree of erosion. Most of these glenoids were dysplastic in origin, with the humeral head either centered or slightly subluxed posteriorly. This group had an average retroversion of 35.7°. Good intraobserver reproducibility and interobserver reliability were achieved for this classification system with kappa index ranging from 0.65 to 0.70.

However, several authors have since critiqued Walch's classification, with Scalise et al. [17] reporting only fair agreement for interobserver and intraobserver assessments. Bercik et al. [18] highlighted that they did not assess the glenoid with the scapula as a free body using 3-dimensional reconstructions of CT scans, which is more accurate in the determination of version and degree of subluxation. Further, there were subtypes of glenoid morphologies not included in the original classification, and the type C glenoid was not clearly defined and led to mislabeling of type B2 glenoids with significant retroversion. Bercik et al. [18] suggested that the definition of a type A2 glenoid should be revised to one where a line drawn from the anterior to posterior rim of the native glenoid does not transect the humeral head (Fig. 9.7). Type C glenoids should also be defined as a dysplastic glenoid with at least 25° of retroversion "not caused by erosion." The authors also suggested the addition of a type B3 and a type D glenoid. A "type B3" glenoid is mono-concave and posteriorly worn with at least 15° of retroversion or at least 70% posterior humeral head subluxation, or both. The "type B3" glenoid is likely formed from either increased erosion of a B2 glenoid that completely destroys the paleo-glenoid, or persistent posterior subluxation preferentially eroding the posterior glenoid, leading to significant retroversion without an interval biconcave morphology. These values were based on previous studies which showed that eccentric reaming in glenoids with at least 15° of retroversion does not allow for proper implantation of an anatomic glenoid without perforating the glenoid walls, and posterior subluxation has been reported to be a risk factor for early glenoid loosening. A "type D" glenoid is one with any level of glenoid anteversion or with humeral head subluxation of less than 40% (i.e.,

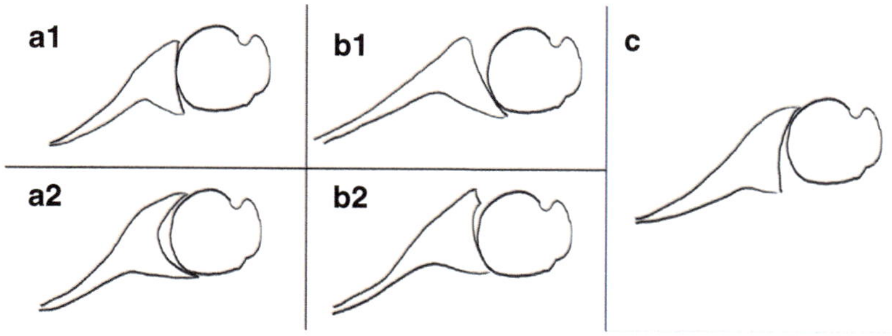

Fig. 9.6 Walch's morphologic types of glenoid in primary glenohumeral osteoarthritis

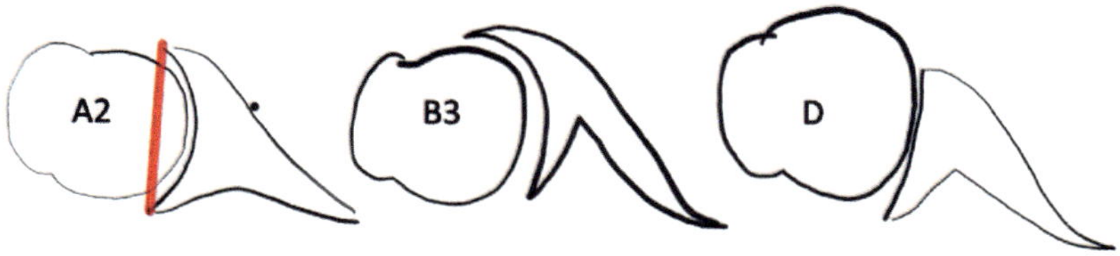

Fig. 9.7 Bercik's modification to Walch's classification

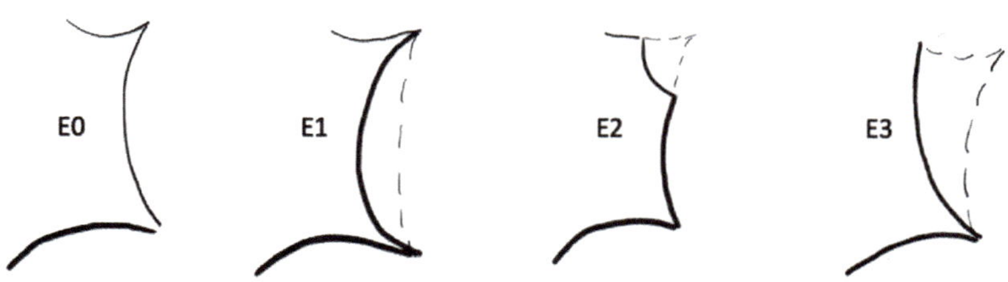

Fig. 9.8 Sirveaux's classification of glenoid erosion in rotator cuff arthropathy

anterior subluxation). This modification to the Walch's classification has been shown to achieve superior intraobserver and interobserver reliability.

Sirveaux et al. [19] followed up on 80 Grammont inverted total shoulder arthroplasties in 77 patients who suffered from rotator cuff arthropathy and performed clinical and radiological measurements pre- and postoperatively. Using the preoperative radiographic appearances of each glenoid, four main categories of glenoid erosion were defined (Fig. 9.8). Type E0 included shoulders with no erosion of the glenoid but with superior migration of the humeral head. Type E1 was defined by a concentric erosion of the glenoid. For type E2, there was erosion of the superior part of the glenoid. Lastly, type E3 was defined by a type E2 erosion extending to the inferior part of the glenoid. It is important to consider these subtypes of glenoid erosion, especially in types E2 and E3, as these may influence the surgeon to position the glenoid base plate incorrectly on the superior edge, with risks of impingement. Instead, it is recommended for the baseplate to be positioned on the inferior part of the glenoid with a slight tilt.

Habermeyer et al. [20] compared 100 patients with primary osteoarthritis with a control group and developed a classification system using true anteroposterior radiographs with the patient standing upright and the arm in neutral rotation to assess the glenoid morphology in the coronal plane, to complement Walch's classification of glenoid wear in the transverse plane. The glenoid inclination angle was measured with a line drawn along the superior and inferior glenoid rim (glenoid line) and another line drawn along the lateral base of the coracoid process from the superior glenoid perpendicular to the bottom margin of the radiograph (coracoid base line) (Fig. 9.9). A negative value indicates an inferiorly directed glenoid, whilst a positive value indi-

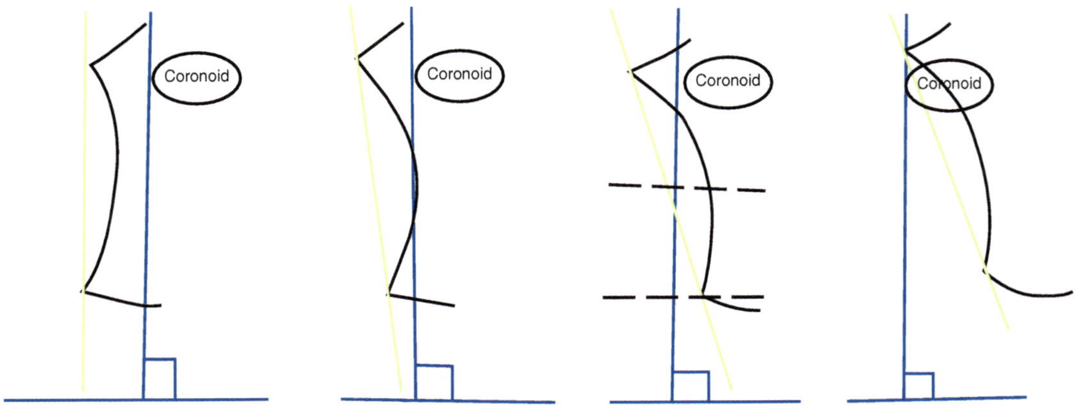

Fig. 9.9 Habermeyer's classification of glenoid inclination

cates a superiorly directed glenoid. Type 0 included normal glenoids, where the glenoid line and coracoid base line run parallel. Type 1 included glenoids where the lines intersect below the inferior glenoid rim. Type 2 included glenoids where the lines intersect between the inferior glenoid rim and the glenoid center. Type 3 included glenoids where the lines intersect above the coracoid base. In essence, this classification grades the extent of inferior inclination of the glenoid and their study found that more patients with osteoarthritis were found to have types 2 and 3 glenoids when compared to the control group. Moreover, no significant association between the glenoid morphology in the coronal plane and the glenoid morphology in the transverse plane was established in this study. The degree of inferior inclination not only depends on the amount of inferior glenoid wear but also the extent of superior glenoid wear, as it is a composite of both variables. Hence, inclination angle may not describe the degree of glenoid wear in the coronal plane adequately, and this is further limited by the confounding factor of scapular rotation on the chest on these anteroposterior radiographs.

Williams et al. [21] adopted a slightly different approach in assessing glenoid bone loss in shoulder arthroplasty, on the basis that glenoid components are designed to sit on the subchondral bone with fixation points drilled or burred through the subchondral plate into the cancellous bone of the glenoid vault. The normal glenoid consists of a subchondral surface (S) approximately 5 mm from the base of the coracoid, a vault (V), and a rim (R), the most lateral extension of the vault on which the subchondral surface rests. This gives rise to 8 potential combinations of the subchondral bone, glenoid rim, and glenoid vault: central defects that are contained (S + R + V+ and S-R + V+) and uncontained (S + R + V- and S-R + V-); peripheral defects that are symmetrical (S + R-V+ and S + R-V-) and asymmetrical (S + R-V+ and S + R-V-); and combined defects that are symmetrical (S-R-V+ and S-R-V-) and asymmetrical (S-R-V+ and S-R-V-). Mild and moderate central deficiencies could be managed with cancellous bone grafting and implantation of a surface-dependent glenoid component, whilst uncontained defects may require a cortical graft to address the vault defect if cementation is to be performed. Symmetrical peripheral defects can be treated with a thicker implant to mitigate the medial position of the joint line. Mild to moderate asymmetrical peripheral defects can be addressed with asymmetric reaming, bone grafting, or an augmented glenoid component, whilst severe asymmetric peripheral defects will require combined treatment for rim and vault with an augmented component or bone graft. Combined defects, depending on severity, may require a customized glenoid component, with or without augments, to fit within the glenoid vault.

9.4 Classification of Bone Loss in Revision Arthroplasty

Franklin et al. [22] examined 30 shoulders after total shoulder arthroplasty and developed a classification for lucency about the glenoid component. Class 0 included glenoids with no lucency. Class 1 was defined as lucency at the superior and/or inferior flange only, whilst class 2 was defined as incomplete lucency at the keel. Class 3 included those with complete lucency of up to 2 mm around the component, whilst those with more than 2 mm complete lucency were allocated to class 4. Class 5a was defined as component translated (for example, tipped or shifted), and class 5b was defined as component dislocated from the bone. Three patients in the cohort with class 4 glenoid lucency did not have additional surgery, whilst four patients with class 5 glenoid lucency had either removal of glenoid component, or removal of both glenoid and humeral components, or revision arthroplasty.

Later, Antuna et al. [8] studied 48 total shoulder arthroplasties that underwent glenoid component revision and developed an intra-operative classification based on location and severity, examining glenoid bone loss after removal of glenoid component, with suggested management strategies for each type of glenoid bone loss. This classification system is comprehensive but less specific, categorizing defects based on location (central, peripheral, or combined) and severity. Severity is further classified into mild (less than 1/3 of glenoid rim or surface), moderate (between 1/3 and 2/3), or severe (more than 2/3) (Fig. 9.10). When deficiencies are mild or moderate and not combined, implantation of a new glenoid component is amenable with options of concentric reaming, reconstructing with bone graft, or adding augments to the glenoid component. However, in severe central or combined deficiencies, patients were less likely to have a new glenoid component implanted and instead may often require bone grafting to increase bone stock for subsequent reconstruction. The main limitation of this classification system is that it is based on intraoperative findings of the appearance of the glenoid and cannot be used in pre-operative planning.

Subsequently, Page et al. [23] modified Antuna's classification to improve its use in planning for glenoid component revision. This modified classification is based on preoperative radiographic assessment of bone stock availability and degree of containment of the associated defects, as conventional CT scanning is impeded by scatter created by the adjacent humeral head prosthesis. Type I defects are contained within the face of the glenoid (Fig. 9.11). Type II defects involve the face of the glenoid and a portion of the anterior or posterior wall, with the glenoid rim remaining intact. Type II defects involve the glenoid face, wall, and rim to a varying degree. Each defect type is then sub-classified according to whether the bone loss is less than (A) or greater than (B) 50% of the total glenoid bone stock. Type I and II defects can be managed via impaction bone grafting, as they are either contained or convertible to a contained defect. Type I defects can be restored using cancellous bone graft, whilst type IIA defects require a mix of cortical, to restore the wall defect, and cancellous bone, to fill up the void in the glenoid body. Type IIB defects may require a mesh or prosthetic augment to contain and stabilize the defect, to allow cancellous bone impaction grafting. Type III defects, however, are not considered reconstructable by impaction grafting.

To further improve the classification of glenoid bone loss in revision arthroplasty, Kocsis et al. [9] developed a classification using anteroposterior and axial radiographs of the shoulder. If it is not possible to perform an axial view due to shoulder stiffness, a modified axial view or CT imaging can be performed. Instead of describing the area of bone loss in reference to the face of the glenoid, this classification system divides glenoid bone loss into three zones using two anatomical reference points: the most medial point of the spino-glenoid notch, and the most lateral edge of the base of the coracoid. A glenoid is classified as type 1 if the most medial/lowest point of the intact glenoid articular surface is at the level of or lateral to the base of the coracoid

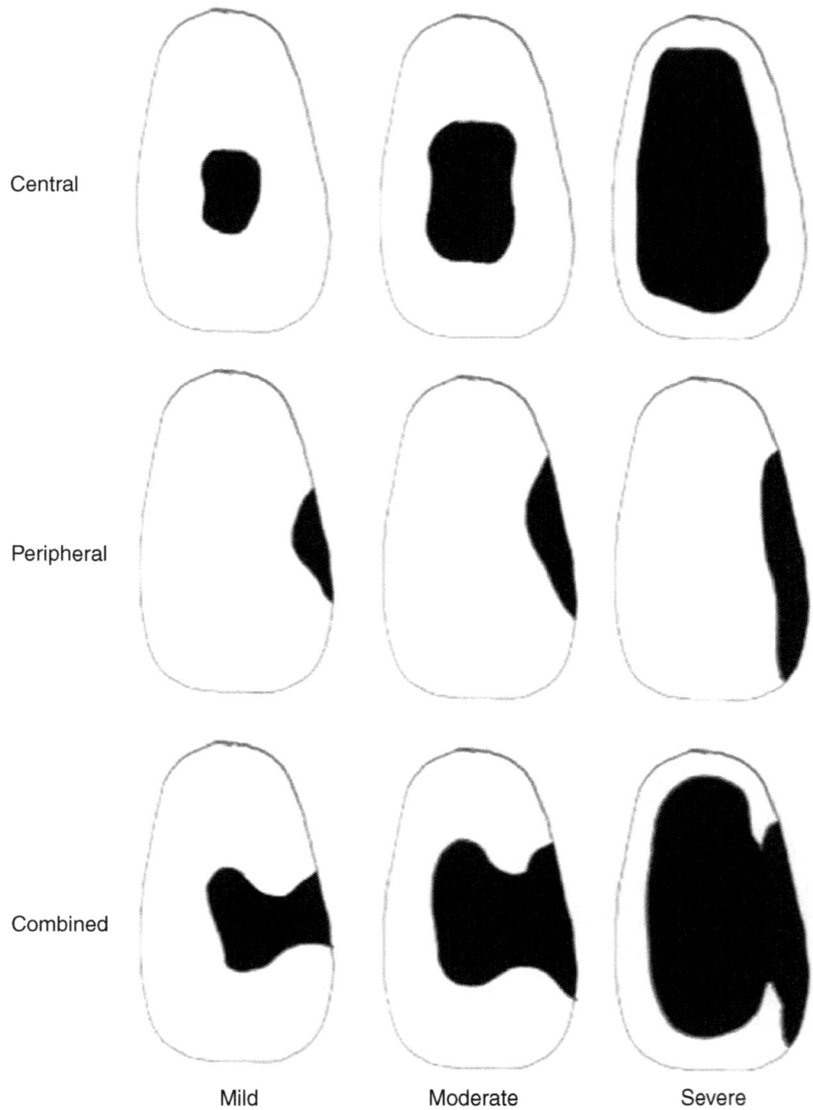

Fig. 9.10 Antuna's classification of glenoid bone loss after removal of glenoid component

(Zone 1) (Figs. 9.12 and 9.13). If the most medial/lowest point of the intact glenoid articular surface falls between the base of the coracoid and the most medial point of the spino-glenoid notch (Zone 2), the bony glenoid is classified as type 2. If the most medial/lowest point of the glenoid articular surface reaches the level of the spino-glenoid notch or is medial to it (Zone 3), the bony glenoid is classified as type 3. This classification system has been shown to have good interobserver reliability, and it is recommended to classify the glenoid as the worse of the two types when any uncertainty existed. The merits of this classification include allowing surgeons to choose the most appropriate surgical technique preoperatively and also decide if further imaging is required. A type 1 glenoid rarely requires further imaging, and the bony defect is usually correctable by preferential reaming. For a type 2 glenoid, further imaging is advised as bone grafting is often required. Structural bone grafting, glenoid component augments, or customized glenoid components should be considered as preferential reaming will likely result in over-medialization and further bone loss. Last, it is mandatory to perform further imaging for a type 3 glenoid, which often has too little bone stock for the safe and stable implantation of

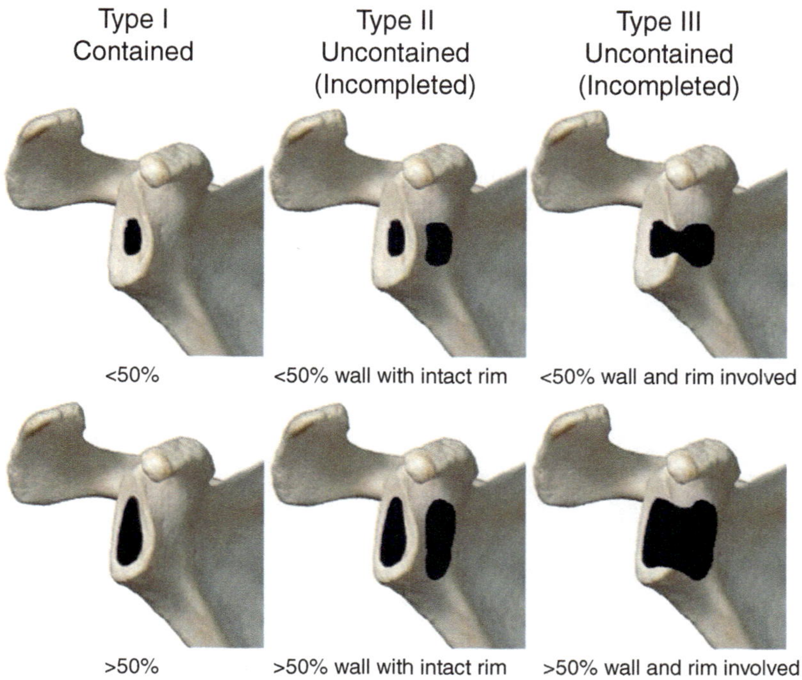

Fig. 9.11 Page's modification to Antuna's classification of glenoid bone loss

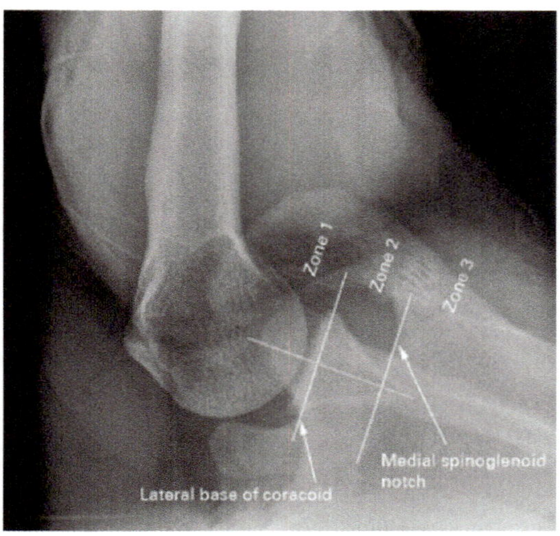

Fig. 9.12 Kocsis' Type 1 glenoid in an axial radiograph

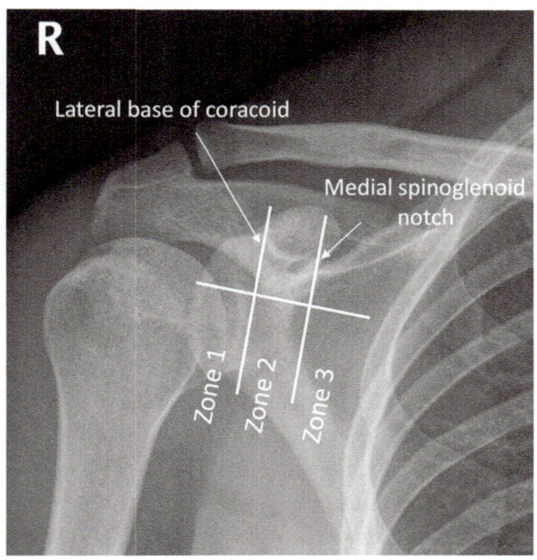

Fig. 9.13 Kocsis' Type 1 glenoid in an anteroposterior radiograph

available glenoid components, and surgeons should consider impaction bone grafting as a salvage procedure.

Sirveaux et al. [19] also classified glenoid bone loss in reverse shoulder arthroplasty, based on the degree of scapular notching seen on plain radiographs. Scapular notching refers to the bony defect in the inferior aspect of the glenoid component and Sirveaux's classification stratified the degree of bone loss into 4 various grades (Table 9.1 and Fig. 9.14). A defect confined to the pillar corresponded to grade 1. Defect is grade 2 when it is in contact with the lower screw, grade 3 when it is over the lower screw, and grade 4 when it extends under the baseplate. A clinical

Table 9.1 Sirveaux's classification of glenoid bone loss in revision arthroplasty

Grade	Description
1	A defect which is confined to the pillar.
2	The defect is in contact with the lower screw.
3	The defect is over the lower screw.
4	The defect extends under the base plate.

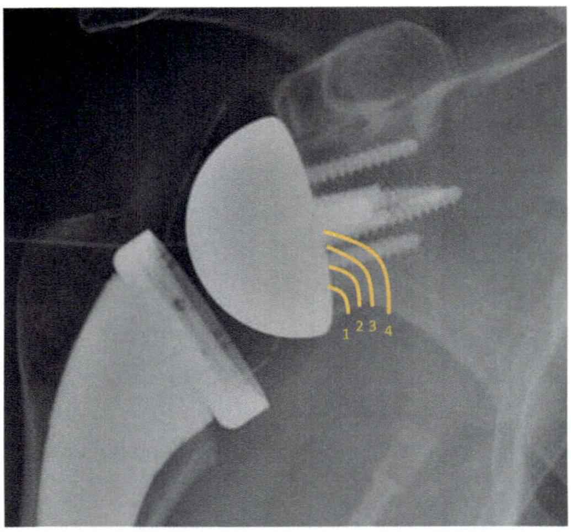

Fig. 9.14 Degree of scapular notching in Sirveaux's classification

study conducted by the authors found that the size of the defect was influenced by the type of glenoid erosion prior to the index surgery, and the presence of grade 3 and 4 notching significantly affected the Constant score. However, there are a few limitations of this classification system. First, it is descriptive with no suggestion of how such bone loss should be managed. Further, it is based on plain radiographs, only assessing the medial-lateral types of inferior glenoid bone loss and is not comprehensive in describing the 3-dimensional nature of such bone loss in revision shoulder arthroplasty.

Sauziere et al. [24] studied total shoulder arthroplasties requiring revision surgery and described a system to classify different types of glenoid bone deficiencies after removal of the glenoid component. Unlike Sirveaux's classification, Sauziere describes the types of glenoid bone loss in a 3-dimensional model based on 5 stages, depending on location of bone loss (central, anterior wall, posterior wall, or both) and severity (Fig. 9.15). A corresponding management strategy was also suggested for each stage (Table 9.2). For a Type A glenoid, the defect can be grafted with cancellous bone and this can be protected with cortico-cancellous bone covering. For a Type B or C glenoid, the metal back glenoid component allows the use of a screwed cortico-cancellous bone graft. For a Type D glenoid, a special revision implant with a longer central peg is required. For a Type E glenoid, total shoulder arthroplasty is contra-indicated. However, a shortfall of this classification is that it does not include the description of superior and inferior glenoid bone loss.

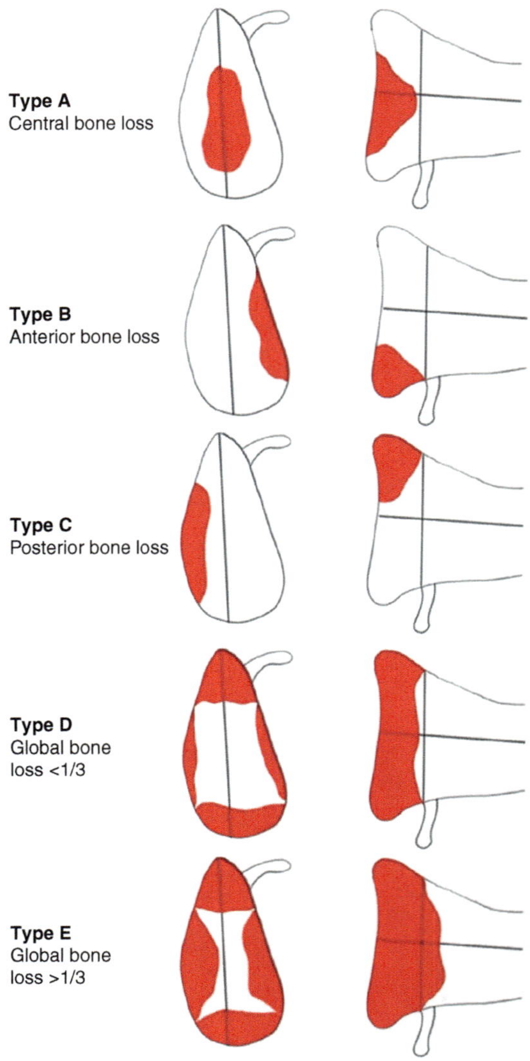

Fig. 9.15 Sauziere's classification of glenoid bone loss in revision arthroplasty

Table 9.2 Sauziere's classification of glenoid bone loss in revision arthroplasty

Type	Description	Management
A	Central loss respecting cortical bone	The glenoid can be grafted with cancellous bone and by protecting the grafts with a cortico-cancellous bone covering
B	Bone defect on the anterior wall of less than one-third of the length of the trumpet-shaped glenoid	The metal back glenoid component allows the use of a screwed cortico-cancellous bone graft
C	Bone defect on the posterior wall of less than one-third of the length of the trumpet-shaped glenoid	The metal back glenoid component allows the use of a screwed cortico-cancellous bone graft
D	Bone loss affecting both walls for at least one-third of the bony trumpet-shaped glenoid	This needs a special revision implant with a longer central peg
E	Bone defect for more than one-third	This is not an indication for a total shoulder arthroplasty

9.5 Approach to Glenoid Bone Loss

Managing glenoid bone loss remains a challenge in primary and revision shoulder arthroplasty and has been associated with poor outcomes in the short to midterm due to graft failure, component loosening, and malposition [25, 26]. Risk factors for poor outcome following revision surgery include age, BMI, and smoking which can result in glenoid lucency preoperatively. In addition, revision of hemiarthroplasty was associated with a lower failure rate than RSA [25]. The classifications of glenoid bone loss described earlier offer a guide to managing bone loss. For example, central bone defects tend to be contained and hence are amenable to impaction bone grafting. Neer et al. reported some success using cancellous impaction grafting to treat small central defects in 45 shoulders [27]. Neyton et al. described the use of iliac crest cortico-cancellous bone graft to fill a large central defect left by a previous cemented glenoid component [28].

On the other hand, peripheral bone defects represent a significant challenge to manage. It is often uncontained and commonly seen in Walch B2 type glenoids. Studies have reported high failure rates of up to 47% with bone grafting of these defects [15, 29]. One of the techniques described to deal with bone loss arose from a modification of the BIO (Bony-Increased-Offset) technique by Boileau et al. [30]. The BIO technique utilizes a circular bone graft threaded through the peg and then pinned with screws. This technique has been adopted by Amar et al. to deal with severe glenoid bone loss, and they have reported high rates of peg and graft integration [31]. However, this technique requires a minimum of 10 mm of vault depth to accommodate the peg and screws. Alternatives to this include a 2-stage procedure (graft then implant at a later stage) or the use of humeral hemiarthroplasty. In terms of the type of bone grafting, either autograft (humeral head or iliac crest) or allograft may be used with no differences in outcome [25, 31, 32].

In instances of significant glenoid destruction where conventional implants may not be technically achievable, use of augmented and custom-made implants may be considered. Advances in 3D printing technology have now made it possible to manufacture implants that are specific to the patient. Customized cutting jigs have also been developed and help to facilitate accuracy of glenoid component implantation [31]. While initial reports of these newer technologies are promising, there is a paucity of evidence to demonstrate improved patient outcomes and survivorship at the moment.

In conclusion, a systemic approach to glenoid bone loss is crucial when dealing with revision surgery. An algorithm proposed by Wagner et al. advocates achieving sufficient contact (30–50%) between host bone and prosthesis after reaming

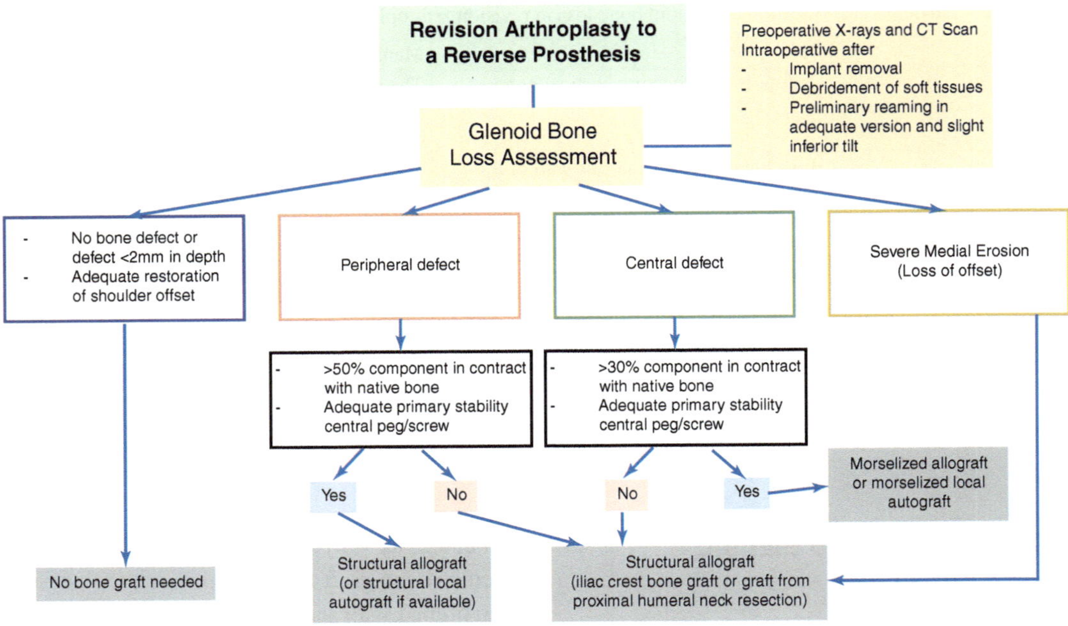

Fig. 9.16 Algorithm for glenoid bone-grafting in the setting of revision to a reverse shoulder arthroplasty

[25] (Fig. 9.16). Lesser defects may be managed with cancellous bone grafting, while larger defects require structural bone grafting.

References

1. Kany J, Katz D. How to deal with glenoid type B2 or C? How to prevent mistakes in implantation of glenoid component? Eur J Orthop Surg Traumatol. 2013;23:379–85.
2. Walch G, Moraga C, Young A, Castellanos-Rosas J. Results of anatomic non-constrained prosthesis in primary osteoarthritis with biconcave glenoid. J Should Elbow Surg. 2012;21:1526–33.
3. Walch G, Badet R, Boulahia A, Khoury A. Morphologic study of the glenoid in primary glenohumeral osteoarthritis. J Arthroplast. 1999;14:756–60.
4. Seidl AJ, Williams G, Boileau P. Challenges in reverse shoulder arthroplasty: addressing glenoid bone loss. Orthopedics. 2016;39:14–23.
5. Matsen FA, Clinton J, Lynch J, Bertelsen A, Richardson ML. Glenoid component failure in total shoulder arthroplasty. J Bone Joint Surg Am. 2008;90-A:885–96.
6. Australian Orthopaedic Association National Joint Replacement Registry. https://aoanjrr.sahmri.com/. Accessed 3 Feb 2016.
7. Hamada K, Fukuda H, Mikasa M, Kobayashi Y. Roentgenographic findings in massive rotator cuff tears. A long-term observation. Clin Orthop Relat Res. 1990;254:92–6.
8. Antuna SA, Sperling JW, Cofield RH, Rowland CM. Glenoid revision surgery after total shoulder arthroplasty. J Shoulder Elb Surg. 2001;10:217–24.
9. Kocsis G, Thyagarajan DS, Fairbairn KJ, Wallace WA. A new classification of glenoid bone loss to help plan the implantation of a glenoid component before revision arthroplasty of the shoulder. Bone Joint J. 2016;98-B(3).
10. Maurer A, Fucentese SF, Pfirrmann CW, Wirth SH, Djahangiri A, Jost B, Gerber C. Assessment of glenoid inclination on routine clinical radiographs and computed tomography examinations of the shoulder. J Shoulder Elb Surg. 2012;21(8):1096–103. https://doi.org/10.1016/j.jse.2011.07.010. Epub 2011 Oct 29.
11. Boileau P, Gauci MO, Wagner ER, Clowez G, Chaoui J, Chelli M, Walch G. The reverse shoulder arthroplasty angle: a new measurement of glenoid inclination for reverse shoulder arthroplasty. J Shoulder Elb Surg. 2019;28(7):1281–90.
12. Simovitch RW, Zumstein MA, Lohri E, Helmy N, Gerber C. Predictors of scapular notching in patients managed with the Delta III reverse total shoulder replacement. J Bone Joint Surg Am. 2007;89:934.
13. Zumstein MA, Pinedo M, Old J, Boileau P. Problems, complications, reoperations, and revisions in reverse total shoulder arthroplasty: a systematic review. J Shoulder Elb Surg. 2011;20:146–57.
14. Friedman RJ, Hawthorne KB, Genez BM. The use of computerized tomography in the measurement of glenoid version. J Bone Joint Surg Am. 1992;74(7):1032–7.
15. Hill JM, Norris TR. Long-term results of total shoulder arthroplasty following bone-grafting of the glenoid. J Bone Joint Surg Am. 2001;83(6):877–83.

16. Hendel MD, Bryan JA, Barsoum WK, Rodriguez EJ, Brems JJ, Evans PJ, Iannotti JP. Comparison of patient-specific instruments with standard surgical instruments in determining glenoid component position: a randomized prospective clinical trial. J Bone Joint Surg Am. 2012;94(23):2167–75.
17. Scalise JJ, Codsi MJ, Brems JJ, Iannotti JP. Inter-rater reliability of an arthritic glenoid morphology classification system. J Shoulder Elb Surg. 2008;17(4):575–7. https://doi.org/10.1016/j.jse.2007.12.006.
18. Bercik MJ, Kruse K 2nd, Yalizis M, Gauci MO, Chaoui J, Walch G. A modification to the Walch classification of the glenoid in primary glenohumeral osteoarthritis using three-dimensional imaging. J Shoulder Elb Surg. 2016;25(10):1601–6. https://doi.org/10.1016/j.jse.2016.03.010.
19. Sirveaux F, Favard L, Oudet D, Huquet D, Walch G, Molé D. Grammont inverted total shoulder arthroplasty in the treatment of glenohumeral osteoarthritis with massive rupture of the cuff. Results of a multicentre study of 80 shoulders. J Bone Joint Surg Br. 2004;86(3):388–95. https://doi.org/10.1302/0301-620x.86b3.14024.
20. Habermeyer P, Magosch P, Luz V, Lichtenberg S. Three-dimensional glenoid deformity in patients with osteoarthritis: a radiographic analysis. J Bone Joint Surg Am. 2006;88(6):1301–7. https://doi.org/10.2106/JBJS.E.00622.
21. Williams GR Jr, Iannotti JP. Options for glenoid bone loss: composites of prosthetics and biologics. J Shoulder Elb Surg. 2007;16(5 Suppl):S267–72. https://doi.org/10.1016/j.jse.2007.05.003.
22. Franklin JL, Barrett WP, Jackins SE, Matsen FA 3rd. Glenoid loosening in total shoulder arthroplasty. Association with rotator cuff deficiency. J Arthroplast. 1988;3(1):39–46. https://doi.org/10.1016/s0883-5403(88)80051-2.
23. Page RS, Haines JF, Trail I. Impaction bone grafting of the glenoid in revision shoulder arthroplasty: classification, technical description and early results. Shoulder Elbow. 2009;1(2):81–8. https://doi.org/10.1111/j.1758-5740.2009.00017.
24. Katz DC, Sauzières P, Valenti P, Kany J. The case for the metal-backed glenoid design in total anatomical shoulder arthroplasty. Eur J Orthop Surg Traumatol. 2011;22(1):9–16. https://doi.org/10.1007/s00590-011-0796-8.
25. Wagner E, Houdek MT, Griffith T, Elhassan BT, Sanchez-Sotelo J, Sperling JW, Cofield RH. Glenoid bone-grafting in revision to a reverse Total shoulder arthroplasty. J Bone Joint Surg Am. 2015;97(20):1653–60. https://doi.org/10.2106/JBJS.N.00732.
26. Frankle MA, Teramoto A, Luo ZP, Levy JC, Pupello D. Glenoid morphology in reverse shoulder arthroplasty: classification and surgical implications. J Shoulder Elb Surg. 2009;18(6):874–85. Epub 2009 May 30
27. Neer CS, Morrison DS. Glenoid bone-grafting in total shoulder arthroplasty. J Bone Joint Surg. 1988;70:1154–62.
28. Neyton L, Walch G, Nové-Josserand L, Edwards TB. Glenoid corticocancellous bone grafting after glenoid component removal in the treatment of glenoid loosening. J Shoulder Elb Surg. 2006;15(2):173–9. https://doi.org/10.1016/j.jse.2005.07.010.
29. Steinmann SP, Cofield RH. Bone grafting for glenoid deficiency in total shoulder replacement. J Shoulder Elb Surg. 2000;9:361–7.
30. Boileau P, Moineau G, Roussanne Y, O'Shea K. Bony increased-offset reversed shoulder arthroplasty: minimizing scapular impingement while maximizing glenoid fixation. Clin Orth Relat Res. 2011;469:2558–67.
31. Malhas A, Rashid A, Copas D, Bale S, Trail I. Glenoid bone loss in primary and revision shoulder arthroplasty. Shoulder Elbow. 2016;8(4):229–40. https://doi.org/10.1177/1758573216648601. Epub 2016 May 6.
32. Jones RB, Wright TW, Zuckerman JD. Reverse total shoulder arthroplasty with structural bone grafting of large glenoid defects. J Shoulder Elb Surg. 2016;25(9):1425–32.

The Convertible Glenoid in Revision Shoulder Arthroplasty

10

Riccardo Ranieri, Mario Borroni, Giacomo Delle Rose, Marco Maria Minelli, and Alessandro Castagna

10.1 Introduction

In the last two decades, shoulder arthroplasty incidence has dramatically increased [1, 2]. Since the introduction of the first-generation Total Shoulder Arthroplasty in 1974 [3], all-polyethylene (PE) glenoids have spread as the gold standard for total shoulder arthroplasty. Despite good clinical outcomes, two main issues still remain in the field of anatomical shoulder arthroplasty: (1) long-term survival and (2) revision procedures.

The main complications and revision causes following total shoulder arthroplasty appear to be glenoid loosening, accounting for 24–37.7% of all complications [4, 5] and soft tissue disorders (instability and rotator cuff tears) which represent 19–27% of the cases [4, 5]. Frequently, both these complications are present at the same time. Indeed, shoulder peculiar biomechanics and soft tissue primary role in shoulder stability make anatomical shoulder prostheses intrinsically vulnerable to these complications. Even if in the last decades, a better understanding of the pathology and technological development led to outcomes improvement, these issues are not completely solved yet. In fact, radiographic loosening has been reported to be 34% at 10 years [6], with some studies reaching almost half of the cases at longer follow-up times [7]. Radiolucent lines (RLLs) and symptomatic glenoid loosening occur at a rate of 7.3% per year and 1.2% per year, respectively [8], and glenoid wear appears to be a time-dependent issue [9]. Clinical function deteriorates with progression of RLL [10, 11]. Even more recent studies underlined that glenoid component failure still remains an unsolved issue [9]. Rotator cuff dysfunction rate was reported to be 17% at a mean follow-up of 8.6 years and appears to be linked to the duration of follow-up [12].

Revision of anatomic shoulder prostheses is a challenging procedure. Soft tissue failure is often impossible to address. Reimplantation of a loose cemented PE glenoid [13] or PE exchange following wear and dissociation of a metal back implant [14] is associated with a high risk of failure, complications, and low patient satisfaction.

In the 90s, the introduction of reverse shoulder arthroplasty (RSA) changed the world of shoulder arthroplasty. After good results in cuff tear

R. Ranieri (✉) · M. M. Minelli
Department of Biomedical Sciences, Humanitas University, Milan, Italy

M. Borroni · G. Delle Rose
Department of Orthopaedic and Trauma Surgery, Humanitas Clinical and Research Center – IRCCS, Milan, Italy
e-mail: giacomo.delle_rose@humanitas.it

A. Castagna
Department of Biomedical Sciences, Humanitas University, Milan, Italy

Department of Orthopaedic and Trauma Surgery, Humanitas Clinical and Research Center – IRCCS, Milan, Italy

F. Franceschi et al. (eds.), *Revision Shoulder Arthroplasty*,
https://doi.org/10.1007/978-3-031-45944-3_10

arthropathy, this procedure began to spread for other indications, becoming the most performed procedure in case of shoulder arthroplasty revision [15]. In this setting, whenever the soft tissues are deficient, a reverse design allows to recreate a stable joint, improving pain and mobility [16, 17]. However, the major issue to be addressed in the setting of TSA revision is the bone defect on the glenoid side, which can be found in the case of a loosened implant or may be the consequence of glenoid removal. These procedures often require the use of bone grafts, multiple stages, and custom-made implants [18, 19], and nonetheless clinical outcomes appear to be worse when compared to RSA, presenting a considerable rate of complications and glenoid failures [19–21]. A recent systematic review which analyzes loose glenoid component management after TSA concluded that the current optimal management of symptomatic glenoid loosening is still unclear. RSA provides better outcomes, but revision rate remains very high whatever revision arthroplasty procedure is chosen [22].

For all these reasons, convertible glenoid designs were introduced at the beginning of the 2000s.

10.2 The Convertible Glenoid

A convertible glenoid is a glenoid design which can support the implantation of an anatomical polyethylene component or a glenosphere. It is characterized by a metal-backed baseplate which should be theoretically retained in case conversion of TSA to RSA is needed. Potential advantages include revision procedure simplification, by making the operation quicker and avoiding the major issue of glenoid bone loss. The main drawback is represented by the fact that a metal-backed glenoid is required: higher revision rate is reported with this kind of implant [9, 23, 24] and, in case of polyethylene wear, metallic humeral head and baseplate contact lead to metallosis, making glenoid failure more symptomatic. Another criticism could be related to the fact that the glenoid position usually recommended for an anatomic implant (centered, respecting the joint line) should shift in a different position in case of RSA, in which glenoid is recommended to be positioned as low as possible with some amount of lateralization. However, with modern modular convertible platforms, lateralizing and/or eccentric glenosphere are available, allowing to correct this potential risk of malpositioning.

The value of platform system and convertibility during revision arthroplasty is well recognized for the humeral implant: converting a humeral stem without removal allows to decrease intraoperative humeral fracture rate, major complications, and blood loss [25–27]. On the other hand, less data are reported regarding convertible glenoid.

10.3 Outcomes for Revision with Convertible Glenoid

In 2013, Castagna et al. first reported the outcomes of TSA to RSA conversion retaining both humeral and glenoid implant in eight cases at 31 months of follow-up [27]. All patients improved in terms of range of motion and Constant score, and no radiolucency lines around glenoid were reported with CT scan showing good integration and no signs of loosening. No intraoperative or postoperative complications occurred. An example is provided in Fig. 10.1.

Kany et al. in a series including different implants reported the outcomes of 16 TSA to RSA revisions with a convertible glenoid implant [28]. Excluding two infected patients treated with explant, in 12 out of 14 cases, it was possible to convert the implant to a RSA without any metal-back revision; in two cases treated for a Walch B2 glenoid, the metal back had to be changed because of loosening. At a mean follow-up of 28 months, all clinical parameters were improved and no radiological glenoid or stem loosening, scapular notching, or complications were observed.

Weber-Spickschen et al. reported the outcomes of 13 consecutive modular TSA conversion, mainly for rotator cuff failure [29]. The conversion was performed at a mean of 9 months (6–14) after primary implantation, and intraop-

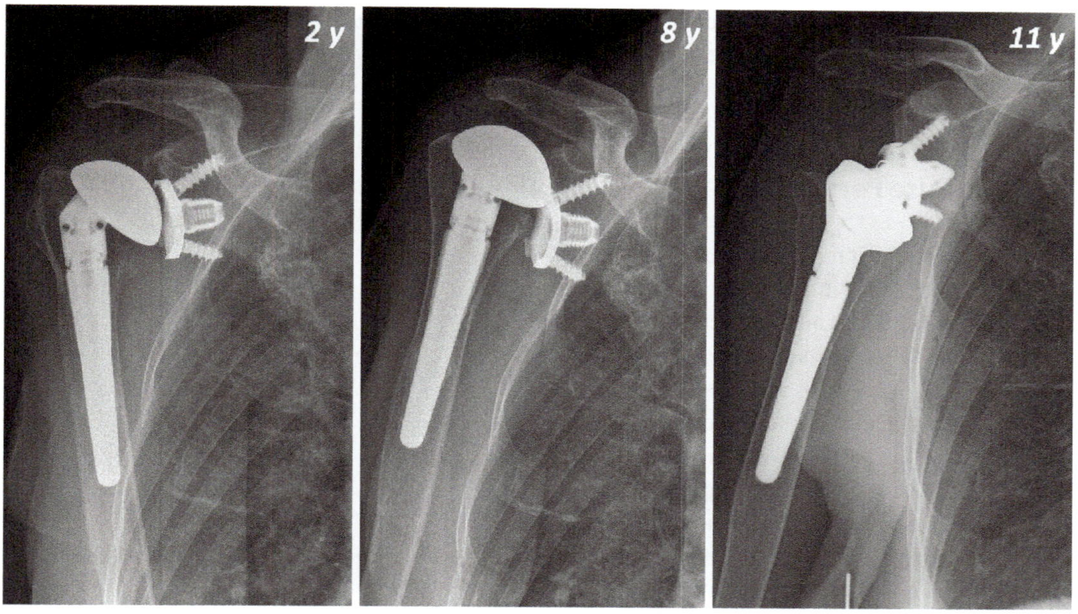

Fig. 10.1 Example of antero-superior rotator cuff failure in TSA after 8 years; conversion to RSA retaining both the humeral and the glenoid implant

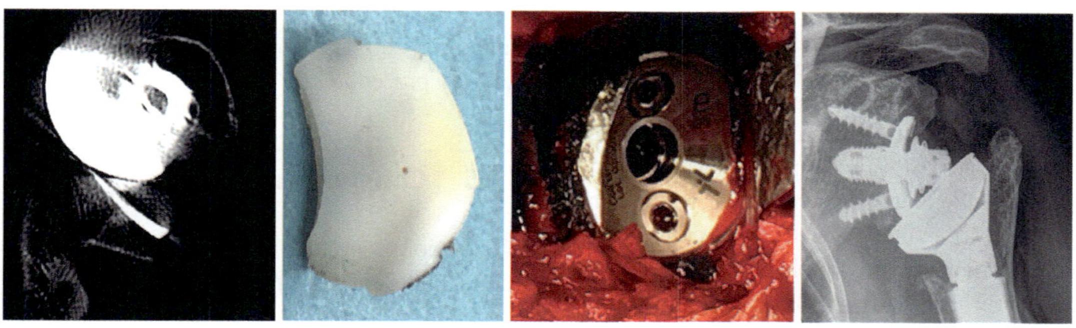

Fig. 10.2 An example of a conversion for chronic subscapularis rupture. Despite asymmetric anterior erosion of the polyethylene and the metal-back, the glenoid is stable and allows conversion to RSA without revising the glenoid

eratively all implants were found to be well-fixed, with no need to exchange implant position. At a mean follow-up of 43 months, all clinical scores improved significantly and no RLLs around the glenoid were observed. Four cases presented grade 1 scapular notching. A low rate (6.6%) of complications was reported, with only one patient experiencing a dislocation episode.

In 2018, Valenti et al. presented a series of 13 TSA to RSA conversions with a modular convertible glenoid [30]. Main causes for conversion included rotator cuff tear and dislocation. Mean time interval between primary TSA and revision was 15 months (range, 1–61 months). At a mean follow-up time of 22 months (range, 7–38 months) after revision, range of motion and clinical scores were improved and no intra- or post-operative complications were reported. No periprosthetic radiolucency or shift in components, no scapular notching were observed at the last follow-up visit.

Another important value of a platform system which includes a convertible glenoid is revision procedure simplification. No bone graft was required in all the previous series with a stable metal-backed baseplate (Fig. 10.2). All authors reported a mean surgical time of about 1 h, which is comparable to the surgical time for a primary RSA.

10.4 Future Perspectives

A perfect gold standard regarding glenoid replacement in TSA, similar to the acetabular cup in hip replacement, has not been reached yet [31]. All-PE glenoid designs have lower revision rate, but long-term loosening remains an unsolved issue. Modern metal-backed glenoid designs, even if they eliminate several implant-related complications, still present the main weakness of PE wear [32]. Given this background and considering the spread of RSA in revision setting, convertible glenoid may help surgeons to manage complicated situations, such as TSA revision for rotator cuff failure and/or instability, in a relatively easy way. Novel solutions may be represented by hybrid glenoid designs, which include a combination of PE and metal-back glenoid technology, trying to integrate the positive features and eliminate the negative ones of the two kinds of implants, maintaining the possibility of conversion to a reverse prosthesis. Recent designs replaced the metal-back baseplate with a central trabecular metal peg which can be connected to a PE component with peripheral cemented pegs in case of anatomic prosthesis or to a classic metal-backed baseplate in case of RSA [31] (Fig. 10.3). However, in view of the history of glenoid replacement in TSA, caution is warranted and studies with long-term follow-up are recommended before a generalized use of new glenoid implants.

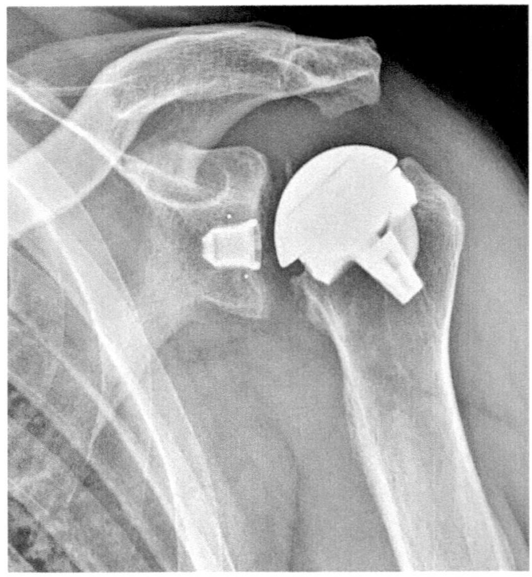

Fig. 10.3 An example of a modern convertible hybrid glenoid

Modularity will be another important field of innovation [25]. Indeed, conversion to RSA retaining the glenoid and/or the humerus forced the surgeon to accept the position of the previously implanted prosthesis, with risk of malpositioning. Given the better understanding of reverse shoulder design and biomechanics, a convertible platform should provide several options in terms of lateralization, distalization, and offset/version modification whenever a conversion to RSA is needed. In this way, the surgeon would have the opportunity to adapt the procedure to the single case, bypassing the limit of having a previously implanted glenoid baseplate or humeral stem, and optimizing functional results even in case of revision procedures.

10.5 Conclusion

The glenoid continues to be the weak link in anatomic total shoulder replacement. The conversion from TSA to RSA has been proved to be a safe procedure with low risk of complications, short surgical time, and good clinical results. Considering the risk of soft tissue failure and glenoid complications after TSA, a convertible modular glenoid offers significant versatility and several advantages in revision setting.

References

1. Longo UG, Papalia R, Castagna A, De Salvatore S, Guerra E, Piergentili I, et al. Shoulder replacement: an epidemiological nationwide study from 2009 to 2019. BMC Musculoskelet Disord. 2022;23:889.
2. Chalmers PN, Salazar DH, Romeo AA, Keener JD, Yamaguchi K, Chamberlain AM. Comparative utilization of reverse and anatomic total shoulder arthroplasty: a comprehensive analysis of a high-volume center. J Am Acad Orthop Surg. 2018;26:e504–10.

3. Neer CS. Replacement arthroplasty for glenohumeral osteoarthritis. J Bone Joint Surg Am. 1974;56:1–13.
4. Bohsali KI, Bois AJ, Wirth MA. Complications of shoulder arthroplasty. J Bone Joint Surg Am. 2017;99:256–69.
5. Gonzalez J-F, Alami GB, Baque F, Walch G, Boileau P. Complications of unconstrained shoulder prostheses. J Shoulder Elb Surg. 2011;20:666–82.
6. Bohsali KI, Wirth MA, Rockwood CA. Complications of total shoulder arthroplasty. J Bone Joint Surg Am. 2006;88:2279–92.
7. Walch G, Young AA, Melis B, Gazielly D, Loew M, Boileau P. Results of a convex-back cemented keeled glenoid component in primary osteoarthritis: multicenter study with a follow-up greater than 5 years. J Shoulder Elb Surg. 2011;20:385–94.
8. Papadonikolakis A, Neradilek MB, Matsen FA. Failure of the glenoid component in anatomic total shoulder arthroplasty: a systematic review of the English-language literature between 2006 and 2012. J Bone Joint Surg Am. 2013;95:2205–12.
9. Hsu JE, Hackett DJ, Vo KV, Matsen FA. What can be learned from an analysis of 215 glenoid component failures? J Shoulder Elb Surg. 2018;27:478–86.
10. Merolla G, Campi F, Paladini P, Lollino N, Fauci F, Porcellini G. Correlation between radiographic risk for glenoid component loosening and clinical scores in shoulder arthroplasty. Chir Organi Mov. 2009;93(Suppl 1):S29–34.
11. Collin P, Tay AKL, Melis B, Boileau P, Walch G. A ten-year radiologic comparison of two-all polyethylene glenoid component designs: a prospective trial. J Shoulder Elb Surg. 2011;20:1217–23.
12. Young AA, Walch G, Pape G, Gohlke F, Favard L. Secondary rotator cuff dysfunction following total shoulder arthroplasty for primary glenohumeral osteoarthritis: results of a multicenter study with more than five years of follow-up. J Bone Joint Surg Am. 2012;94:685–93.
13. Bonnevialle N, Melis B, Neyton L, Favard L, Molé D, Walch G, et al. Aseptic glenoid loosening or failure in total shoulder arthroplasty: revision with glenoid reimplantation. J Shoulder Elb Surg. 2013;22:745–51.
14. Cheung EV, Sperling JW, Cofield RH. Polyethylene insert exchange for wear after total shoulder arthroplasty. J Shoulder Elb Surg. 2007;16:574–8.
15. Knowles NK, Columbus MP, Wegmann K, Ferreira LM, Athwal GS. Revision shoulder arthroplasty: a systematic review and comparison of north American vs. European outcomes and complications. J Shoulder Elb Surg. 2020;29:1071–82.
16. Grammont PM, Baulot E. Delta shoulder prosthesis for rotator cuff rupture. Orthopedics. 1993;16:65–8.
17. Boileau P, Watkinson D, Hatzidakis AM, Hovorka I. Neer award 2005: the Grammont reverse shoulder prosthesis: results in cuff tear arthritis, fracture sequelae, and revision arthroplasty. J Shoulder Elb Surg. 2006;15:527–40.
18. Flurin P-H, Janout M, Roche CP, Wright TW, Zuckerman J. Revision of the loose glenoid component in anatomic total shoulder arthroplasty. Bull Hosp Jt Dis. 2013;2013(71 Suppl 2):68–76.
19. Melis B, Bonnevialle N, Neyton L, Lévigne C, Favard L, Walch G, et al. Glenoid loosening and failure in anatomical total shoulder arthroplasty: is revision with a reverse shoulder arthroplasty a reliable option? J Shoulder Elb Surg. 2012;21:342–9.
20. Austin L, Zmistowski B, Chang ES, Williams GR. Is reverse shoulder arthroplasty a reasonable alternative for revision arthroplasty? Clin Orthop Relat Res. 2011;469:2531–7.
21. Bartels DW, Marigi E, Sperling JW, Sanchez-Sotelo J. Revision reverse shoulder arthroplasty for anatomical glenoid component loosening was not universally successful: a detailed analysis of 127 consecutive shoulders. J Bone Joint Surg Am. 2021;103:879–86.
22. Sharareh B, Yao JJ, Matsen FA, Hsu JE. What is the optimal management of a loose glenoid component after anatomic total shoulder arthroplasty: a systematic review. J Shoulder Elb Surg. 2022;S1058-2746(22):00808–4.
23. Papadonikolakis A, Matsen FA. Metal-backed glenoid components have a higher rate of failure and fail by different modes in comparison with all-polyethylene components: a systematic review. J Bone Joint Surg Am. 2014;96:1041–7.
24. Australian Orthopaedic Association. Australian Orthopaedic Association National Joint Replacement Registry (AOANJRR). Hip, Knee & Shoulder Arthroplasty; 2021.
25. Werner BC, Dines JS, Dines DM. Platform systems in shoulder arthroplasty. Curr Rev Musculoskelet Med. 2016;9:49–53.
26. Crosby LA, Wright TW, Yu S, Zuckerman JD. Conversion to reverse total shoulder arthroplasty with and without humeral stem retention: the role of a convertible-platform stem. J Bone Joint Surg Am. 2017;99:736–42.
27. Castagna A, Delcogliano M, de Caro F, Ziveri G, Borroni M, Gumina S, et al. Conversion of shoulder arthroplasty to reverse implants: clinical and radiological results using a modular system. Int Orthop. 2013;37:1297–305.
28. Kany J, Amouyel T, Flamand O, Katz D, Valenti P. A convertible shoulder system: is it useful in total shoulder arthroplasty revisions? Int Orthop. 2015;39:299–304.
29. Weber-Spickschen TS, Alfke D, Agneskirchner JD. The use of a modular system to convert an anatomical total shoulder arthroplasty to a reverse shoulder arthroplasty: clinical and radiological results. Bone Joint J. 2015;97-B:1662–7.
30. Valenti P, Katz D, Kany J, Werthel J-D. Convertible glenoid components facilitate revisions to reverse shoulder arthroplasty easier: retrospective review of 13 cases. Am J Orthop (Belle Mead NJ). 2018:47.
31. Castagna A, Garofalo R. Journey of the glenoid in anatomic total shoulder replacement. Shoulder Elbow. 2019;11:140–8.
32. Castagna A, Delle Rose G, Borroni M, Gumina S, Garofalo R, Ranieri R. The glenoid: a weak link in total shoulder arthroplasty: metal backs as possible solutions and future perspectives. Obere Extremität Springer Medizin. 2022;17:59–66.

11 How to Remove a Well-Fixed Glenoid Component in a Failed Anatomic Total Shoulder Arthroplasty

Kristian Efremov and Andrew Jawa

11.1 Introduction

Glenoid loosening remains a very common cause of anatomic total shoulder arthroplasty (ATSA) revision and often coexists with other causes of revision including instability and rotator cuff failure [1–5]. Removing a loose glenoid can be a simple step in the case. Having to remove a well-fixed glenoid is less common and is usually encountered in revisions to reverse shoulder arthroplasty (RSA) for rotator cuff failure, humeral-sided failure, or periprosthetic fractures. Removal and reconstruction of a well-fixed glenoid component are easier than a loose one, which is often associated with significant bone loss. After careful removal of a well-fixed glenoid, there will be better glenoid bone stock to implant a baseplate compared to a loose implant, where glenoid defects and fibrous tissue increase the chance of baseplate failure [6, 7]. Therefore, the key to achieve good results in revisions with well-fixed glenoid components is to preserve the available bone stock.

11.2 Background

ATSA has shown great results in the treatment of glenohumeral osteoarthritis, but it comes with some significant potential complications. The most common of these is glenoid loosening, which occurs in 3.9% of all shoulder replacements, followed by instability and rotator cuff tears [8]. Glenoid loosening is reported as being between 20.4% and 37.7% of all complications and modes of failure [8, 9].

Before revising a failed ATSA to a RSA, it is helpful to establish whether the glenoid component is loose or not, as this can influence if the revision may require extensive glenoid reconstruction with graft, a custom baseplate or two stages. Workup for this includes radiographs (Grashey and Axillary) and CT scan with 3D reconstructions [6, 7]. CT arthrograms can be particularly helpful in determining if a glenoid component is loose. More recently, newer technology can create CT reconstructions with the removal of the glenoid component and delineation of the glenoid defect.

Unfortunately, standard radiographic workup can lead to both false positives and negatives. In a study of 79 revisions, Hernandez-Ortiz and colleagues [10] found that only 30 out of 47 components were loose intraoperatively which were classified as such based on radiographs. Conversely, six components that were classified as not loose ended up being so during surgery. It

K. Efremov (✉) · A. Jawa
Department of Orthopaedic Surgery, New England Baptist Hospital, Boston, MA, USA

F. Franceschi et al. (eds.), *Revision Shoulder Arthroplasty*,
https://doi.org/10.1007/978-3-031-45944-3_11

is, therefore, always crucial to prepare for encountering both possibilities during revision surgery.

The presence of a loose glenoid in a revision setting can influence the procedure in several ways. Franke et al. [6], in their series of 158 failed ATSA, did not find any difference in pre- or postoperative ASES scores in patients who had a loose or well-fixed glenoid. However, glenoid allograft was used more often in patients with loose glenoids (56%) compared to the well-fixed cases (34%). More importantly, 11 of 96 patients who underwent revision in the loose glenoid group had baseplate failure and underwent further revision. No baseplate failure was observed in the group that had a well-fixed glenoid. Similarly, Bartels et al. [7] reported a 17% baseplate failure rate in patients who had undergone a revision from ATSA to RSA for glenoid component loosening.

11.3 Technique

11.3.1 Implant Design

The first step in a successful removal of a well-fixed glenoid is knowing the implant design. The technique and instruments used for removal, as well as the ensuing reimplant, can vary based on whether the glenoid is an all-polyethylene implant (Fig. 11.1a), metal-backed implant (Fig. 11.1b), or hybrid design with metal pegs (Fig. 11.1c). Well-fixed metal-backed glenoids, in general, are harder to remove than all-polyethylene designs.

11.3.2 Exposure

Excellent exposure of the glenoid is fundamental for successful revisions and starts on the humeral side. The head/all modular implants should be removed when the stem is retained. Stems that are convertible to an RSA are advantageous as they lead to shorter surgeries, less bone loss, and fewer complications [11]. In cases where the humeral stem must be removed, it is recommended that this can be done after addressing the glenoid, as the stem protects the humeral bone from iatrogenic damage caused by the glenoid retractors. If the humeral component is loose or the decision is made to remove it beforehand, a plate protector or trial stem should be put in place to protect the humerus. Exposure is further improved with careful circumferential release of all capsule and scar tissue around the glenoid. Removal of inferior scar tissue is often critical but must be balanced with protection of the axillary nerve, which is facilitated with spiked-Hohmann retractor.

11.3.3 Removal

Once adequate exposure of the glenoid implant has been obtained, any scar tissue formed between the implant and bone needs to be meticulously removed using electrocautery and rongeurs (Fig. 11.2). The next step depends on the design of the implant being removed. All-polyethylene implants are perhaps the easiest to remove. The simplest and quickest technique involves separating the polyethene articulating surfaces from the underlying pegs. This can be done by using a sharp rigid osteotome, placing it at the anterior implant-bone interference and using tangential force to break the contact between the two parts of the implant (Fig. 11.3a, b). This will leave the cemented or ingrown pegs flush with the native bone, without any disruption of the glenoid bone stock (Fig. 11.3c). The glenoid can then be reamed, and the center hole drilled in preparation for baseplate implantation. This will cause any pegs that are in the way to become loose when they can easily be removed with a grasper (Fig. 11.3d, e). The center hole is then cleaned out with a curette of any remaining debris (Fig. 11.3f). The remaining pegs, whether they will be covered by the baseplate or not, can be left in place, as their involvement with bone-metal interference will be minimal. Similarly, in monoblock implants that do not require the drilling of a large central hole, the screw can usually be placed in native glenoid bone stock that will not be affected by the remaining pegs. In certain

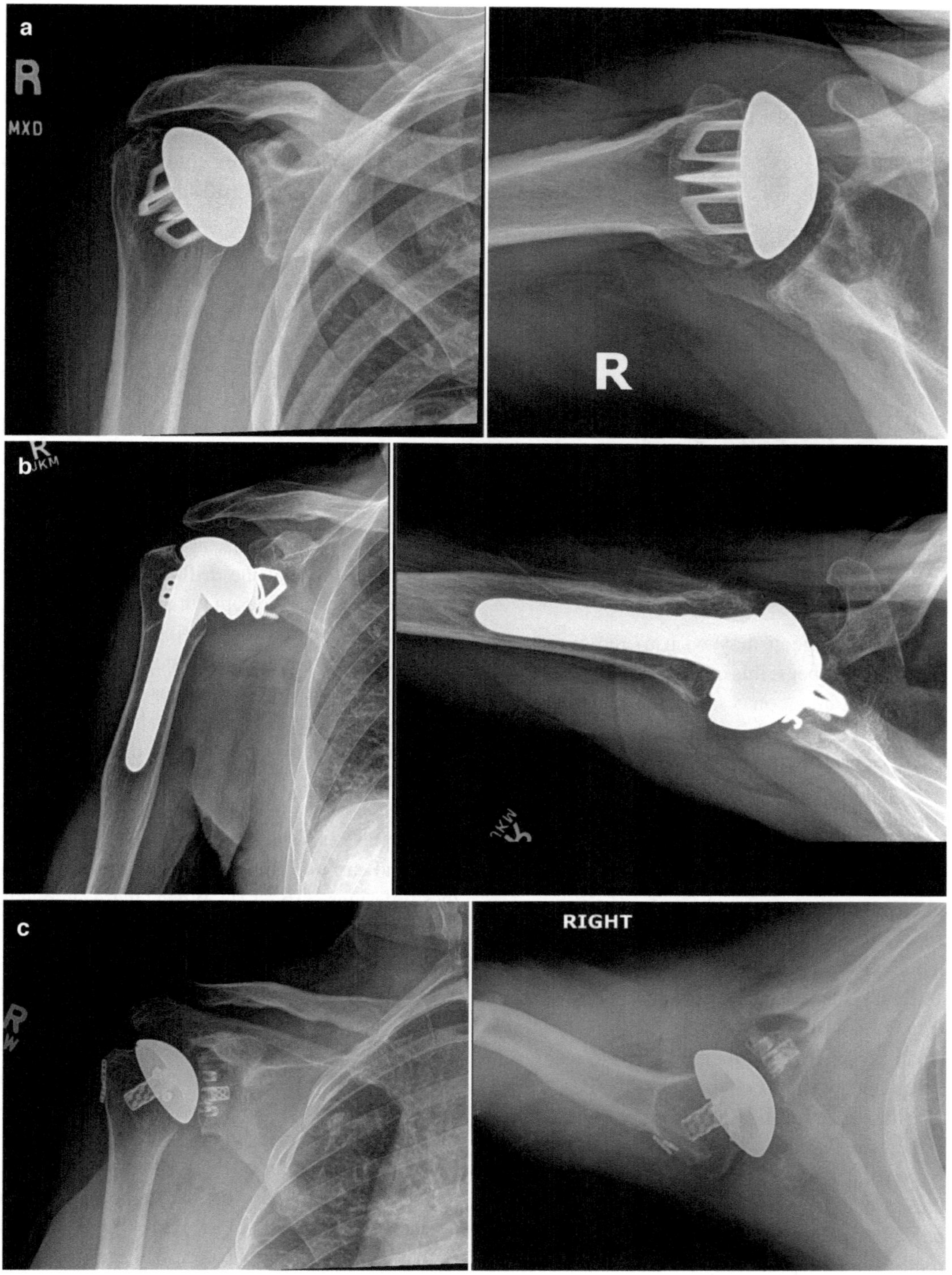

Fig. 11.1 Grashey and Axillary X-rays of TSAs with well-fixed glenoids. (**a**) An all-polyethylene glenoid model, (**b**) a metal back model, and (**c**) a hybrid design with metal pegs

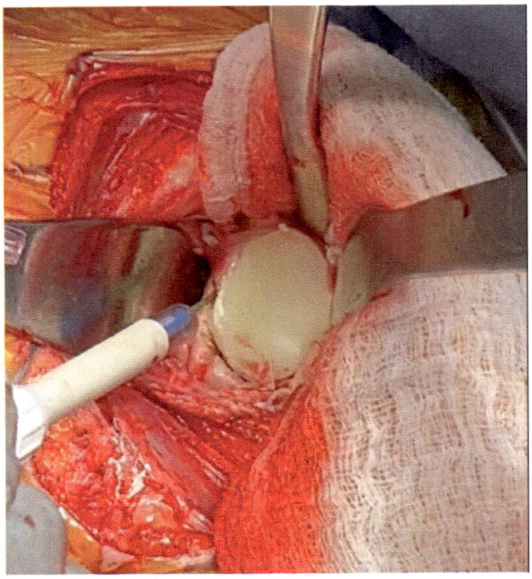

Fig. 11.2 Exposure of a well-fixed anatomic all poly glenoid. Electrocautery is being used to remove soft tissue around the implant before extraction

cases, the surgeon may wish to remove all the polyethylene pegs; this could be the case in which an indolent infection is suspected, and removal of all implant material is desired to allow for adequate debridement. In this case, the remaining pegs can be cleared out using a high-speed pencil tipped burr.

Sometimes, it might be impossible to bring the osteotome parallel to the glenoid, and a different technique needs to be used. In these cases, a small oscillating saw can be used to cut the glenoid implant with two horizontal and two vertical lines, in a checkerboard pattern (Fig. 11.4a, b). This will split the implant in nine small pieces that can then be grabbed using rongeurs and twisted out individually (Fig. 11.4c). The baseplate for the RSA can then be positioned as described above.

Several hybrid glenoid implants, either with only a central porous titanium post or all metal pegs, have been recently released. They are currently showing promising results, with loosening rates equivalent or better than those of all-polyethylene designs due to the bone in-growth in the metal pegs [12–15]. These models can require additional steps for removal. Osteotomes can be used to separate the polyethylene body from the metal pegs, in a similar manner to the all-polyethylene implants described previously. Unlike the polyethylene pegs however, the metal pegs should be removed in order to allow adequate room for the placement of a baseplate. To achieve this, a trephine drill should be used to cut all around the metal pegs. Knowing the length of the pegs is needed in order to not over drill the glenoid. If trephines of appropriate sizes are not available, this step can be achieved using a high-speed pencil tip burr to cut around the pegs, taking great care to remove as little bone as possible.

Some companies may have guides designed for glenoid removal. The trephine drill guide is placed onto the face of the implant, making sure that it is fully seated. The peg trephine drill is then used with the guide, at a slow to moderate speed to ensure that the drilling is on axis. The drill is designed to bottom out and then removed, with the polyethylene and peripheral peg remaining inside the trephine. This step is repeated on all peripheral pegs first. A larger trephine drill is then used to remove the central peg last. The remaining polyethylene body is then loose and can be taken off.

Metal-backed glenoids have fallen out of favor in over the years due to accelerated polyethylene wear and early revision surgery encountered with these designs [16, 17]. When these implants become loose, they cause a large amount of glenoid bone loss and require major bone grafting. When well-fixed, removing these implants is a longer and more arduous process than the other designs. To remove metal-backed glenoids, osteotomes and burrs are used to slowly break away the implant from the glenoid bone. A Neviaser or posterior portal can be useful in releasing the superior and posterior margin of the glenoid, respectively, which might otherwise be hard to reach through the normal approach (Fig. 11.5a). These designs will have significant bone ingrowth and will cause major bone loss when removed (Fig. 11.5b), which will need to be bone-grafted before a baseplate can be implanted. Newer designs which are convertible to RSA show promise.

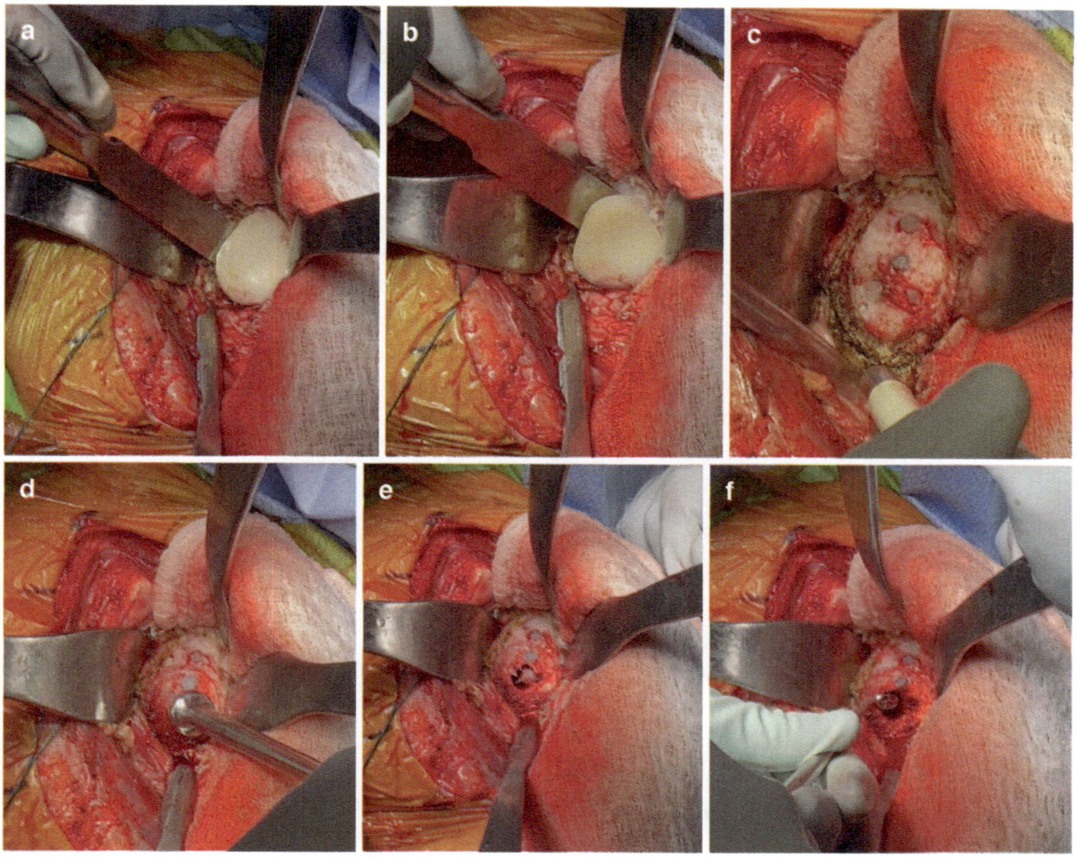

Fig. 11.3 Removal of an all-polyethylene glenoid. (**a**) An osteotome is placed between the implant and bone. (**b**) The osteotome will break the face of the implant from the pegs. (**c**) View of the glenoid with the polyethylene pegs in place. (**d**) The central drill for the RSA baseplate is used to drill with the pegs in place. (**e**) Any pegs that are in the way will become loose and can be easily removed. (**f**) A curette is used to remove any remaining polyethylene debris

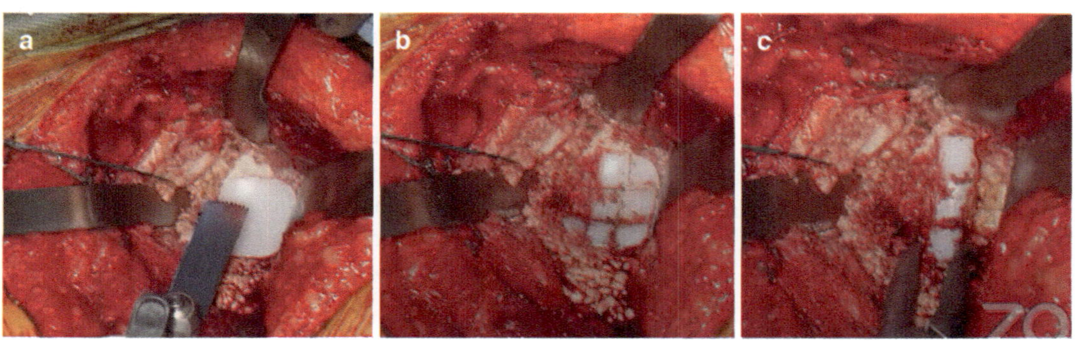

Fig. 11.4 (**a**) An oscillating saw is used to perform two vertical and two horizontal cuts across the glenoid implant. (**b**) The implant is divided into nine individual pieces, in a checkerboard pattern. (**c**) Each individual piece is the removed with a rongeur. (Courtesy of John Sperling)

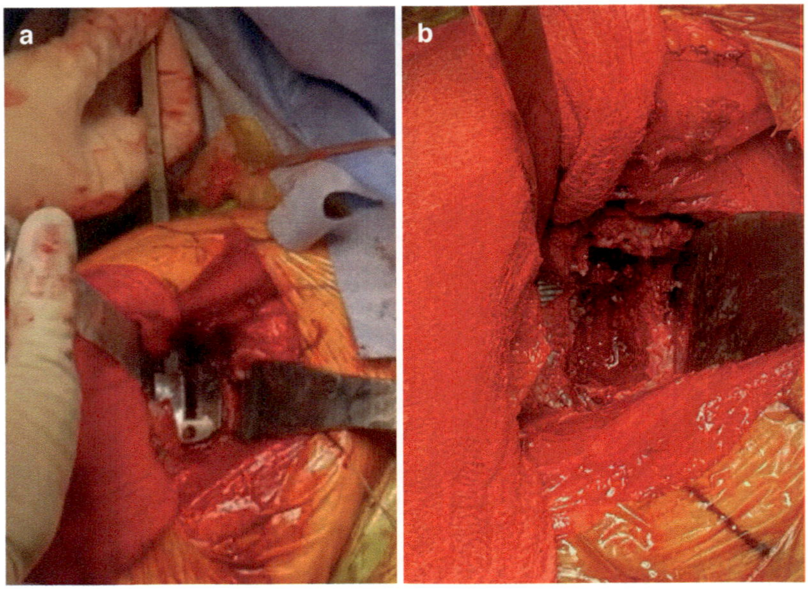

Fig. 11.5 View of a metal-backed glenoid after the articulating surface has been removed (**a**); an osteotome is inserted through portal of Neviaser to get behind the implant and release if from the glenoid. (**b**) Large glenoid bone defect after the removal of the implant, which requires bone grafting

11.4 Arthroscopic Removal

While most revision of failed ATSA, both with a loose and well-fixed glenoid, will involve conversion to RSA, sometimes the patient and surgeon may elect for a simpler procedure. Conversion to hemiarthroplasty has been described as a valid treatment for painful loose glenoid components, with good results [18]. In addition, this procedure can be indicated in patients with symptomatic glenoid wear, with rotator cuff tears to avoid further rocking horse phenomenon, or in cases with suspected low-grade infection.

O'Driscoll et al. [18] first described arthroscopic conversion of ATSA into hemiarthroplasty. Their series involved 5 patients with keeled glenoid. Cuts were performed using a 4 or 6 mm osteotome through the anterior portal, using the keel design to ensure the cut pieces remain in place until removal and are not lost within the joint. The first cut separates the superior-posterior third of the glenoid, leaving a small attachment to the keel. This is followed by a cut parallel to the glenoid to remove the implant from the keel to allow for it to be extracted. These two cuts are then repeated to remove the inferior-anterior third from the central part. A final cut is made to separate the middle third of the articulating surface from the keel. Each piece is removed with a grasper through the anterior portal, with the keel remaining in place (Fig. 11.6).

Removal of the entire loose implant as a single unit has been described as well [19]. This is done by first separating the implant from the glenoid by using a rasp, followed by carefully releasing all implant-bone scar tissue using electrocautery. Once the component is completely free, it can be removed using a robust forceps through the anterior portal through the rotator interval. In this case, the portal must be larger, at least 2 cm, than when the implant is cut into separate segments.

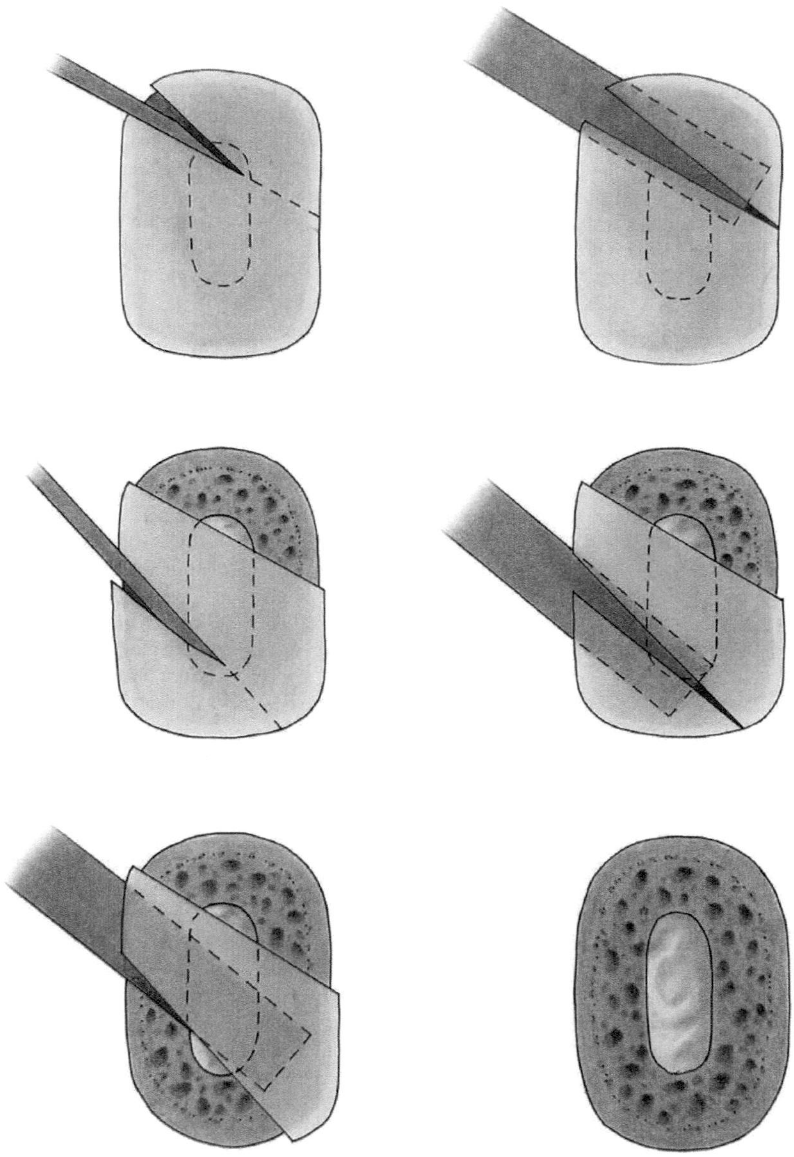

Fig. 11.6 Diagram showing the osteotome cuts required for arthroscopic removal of an all-polyethylene glenoid component. A transverse cut is made to separate the superior-posterior third of the glenoid from the rest of the implant, followed by a cut parallel to the glenoid. This step is repeated for the inferior-anterior third of the implant. A final parallel cut is made to remove the middle third [18]

11.5 Conclusion

Removing a well-fixed glenoid can be a challenging task; however, when done properly, it can be achieved with little bone loss. This can allow the revision to be performed in a single stage with immediate implantation of a baseplate, with little or no bone grafting. Due to this, outcomes after revising a well-fixed glenoid can be better than those after a loose one. Knowledge of the implant is critical before surgery to make sure all tools are available for the removal.

References

1. Gauci MO, Cavalier M, Gonzalez JF, Holzer N, Baring T, Walch G, Boileau P. Revision of failed shoulder arthroplasty: epidemiology, etiology, and surgical options. J Shoulder Elb Surg. 2020;29:541–9.
2. Pinkas D, Wiater B, Wiater JM. The glenoid component in anatomic shoulder arthroplasty. J Am Acad Orthop Surg. 2015;23:317–26.
3. Taunton MJ, McIntosh AL, Sperling JW, Cofield RH. Total shoulder arthroplasty with a metal-backed, bone-ingrowth glenoid component. Medium to long-term results. J Bone Joint Surg Am. 2008;90:2180–8.

4. Page RS, Pai V, Eng K, Bain G, Graves S, Lorimer M. Cementless versus cemented glenoid components in conventional total shoulder joint arthroplasty: analysis from the Australian Orthopaedic Association National Joint Replacement Registry. J Shoulder Elb Surg. 2018;27:1859–65.
5. Matsen FA 3rd, Clinton J, Lynch J, Bertelsen A, Richardson ML. Glenoid component failure in total shoulder arthroplasty. J Bone Joint Surg Am. 2008;90(4):885–96.
6. Franke KJ, Christmas KN, Simon P, Mighell MA, Frankle MA. The effect of glenoid bone loss and rotator cuff status in failed anatomic shoulder arthroplasty after revision to reverse shoulder arthroplasty. J Shoulder Elb Surg. 2021;30:844–9.
7. Bartels DW, Marigi E, Sperling JW, Sanchez-Sotelo J. Revision reverse shoulder arthroplasty for anatomical glenoid component loosening was not universally successful: a detailed analysis of 127 consecutive shoulders. J Bone Joint Surg Am. 2021;19(103):879–86.
8. Bohsali KI, Bois AJ, Wirth MA. Complications of shoulder arthroplasty. J Bone Joint Surg Am. 2017;99(3):256–69. https://doi.org/10.2106/JBJS.16.00935. Erratum in: J Bone Joint Surg Am 2017;21;99:e67
9. Somerson JS, Hsu JE, Neradilek MB, Matsen FA 3rd. Analysis of 4063 complications of shoulder arthroplasty reported to the US Food and Drug Administration from 2012 to 2016. J Shoulder Elb Surg. 2018;27:1978–86.
10. Hernandez-Ortiz EG, Christmas KN, Simon P, Diaz MA, Hess AV 2nd, O'Briain DE, McLendon PB, Mighell MA, Frankle MA. Improving preoperative planning of revision surgery after previous anatomic total shoulder arthroplasty. J Shoulder Elb Surg. 2019;28:S168–74.
11. Dilisio MF, Miller LR, Siegel EJ, Higgins LD. Conversion to reverse shoulder arthroplasty: humeral stem retention versus revision. Orthopedics. 2015;38:e773–9.
12. Marigi EM, Lenartowicz KA, Jennewine B, Throckmorton TW, Sperling JW. Clinical and radiographic outcomes of hybrid glenoid fixation with a central porous titanium post: analysis of 713 consecutive shoulders. J Shoulder Elb Surg. 2022;31:1524–32.
13. Friedman RJ, Cheung E, Grey SG, Flurin PH, Wright TW, Zuckerman JD, et al. Clinical and radiographic comparison of a hybrid cage glenoid to a cemented polyethylene glenoid in anatomic total shoulder arthroplasty. J Shoulder Elb Surg. 2019;28:2308–16.
14. Gulotta LV, Chambers KL, Warren RF, Dines DM, Craig EV. No differences in early results of a hybrid glenoid compared with a pegged implant. Clin Orthop Relat Res. 2015;473:3918–24.
15. Malahias MA, Kostretzis L, Gkiatas I, Chronopoulos E, Brilakis E, Antonogiannakis E. Total shoulder arthroplasty with hybrid fixation of glenoid components consisting of cementless porous metal pegs or cage along with cemented backside polyethylene surface: a systematic review. Musculoskelet Surg. 2020;104:229–36.
16. Boileau P, Moineau G, Morin-Salvo N, Avidor C, Godenèche A, Lévigne C, Baba M, Walch G. Metal-backed glenoid implant with polyethylene insert is not a viable long-term therapeutic option. J Shoulder Elb Surg. 2015;24:1534–43.
17. Boileau P, Avidor C, Krishnan SG, Walch G, Kempf JF, Molé D. Cemented polyethylene versus uncemented metal-backed glenoid components in total shoulder arthroplasty: a prospective, double-blind, randomized study. J Shoulder Elb Surg. 2002;11:351–9.
18. O'Driscoll SW, Petrie RS, Torchia ME. Arthroscopic removal of the glenoid component for failed total shoulder arthroplasty. A report of five cases. J Bone Joint Surg Am. 2005;87:858–63.
19. Venjakob AJ, Reichwein F, Nebelung W. Arthroscopic removal of a polyethylene glenoid component in total shoulder arthroplasty. Arthrosc Tech. 2015;6(4):e149–52.

Revising the Glenoid in Hemiarthroplasty

12

Giuseppe Sircana, Giovanni Merolla, and Paolo Paladini

12.1 Introduction

Shoulder hemiarthroplasty (HA) was the most common type of implant used at the end of the XX century, accounting for nearly half of the performed shoulder arthroplasties [1]. In 2017, in the USA, 0.258% of the general population has undergone shoulder arthroplasty and prevalence of HA was 0.061% [2]. The most common indications for its use were osteoarthritis and acute fractures of the proximal humerus [1]. Due to the popularization and wide adoption of the reverse shoulder arthroplasty (RSA), a dramatic decrease in the use of HA has been registered [1–4], especially in the last decade, with an estimated annual decrease of 16.5% in the USA [5] and with HA accounting for <10% of shoulder arthroplasties [1, 4, 6]. Predictions for the next 10 years implantations indicate a further decrease in the use of shoulder HA, which will account for 3.9% of implants in the general population and for 23.5% of implants in patients 55 years old or younger [5]. Furthermore, long-term survivorship of HA was demonstrated to be lower than that of reverse shoulder arthroplasty [1, 4] with 10 years failure rate ranging from 6.85 to 19.1% [1, 3, 4, 7–10]. Failure rate is dependent on preoperative diagnosis, with lower revision rates for fractures and highest after fracture sequelae [8].

The impact of the reduction of HA implantation on surgeons' expertise and, as a consequence, on outcomes, is still unknown, as surgeons less familiar with this kind of implants might be more prone to technical errors during implantation, thus reducing the expected survivorship of the implant. On the other hand, a reduction in implantation could restrict the range of indications to the most reliable ones, reducing disappointing results due to outdated indications.

Regardless of the reason, surgeons will have to face failed HA in whom revision surgery will be required. In the last two decades, revision shoulder arthroplasty showed a 39.2% increase [2] and revision surgery accounts for 12.6% of surgeries in high volume shoulder centers [11]; HA revision activity has overtaken primary HA implantation at the end of the first decade of this century [11].

The main causes of HA revision are rotator cuff failure and painful glenoid erosion [12, 13], but they include pain, decreased ROM, limited

G. Sircana (✉) · P. Paladini
UO Chirurgia Ortopedica della Spalla Romagna, Dipartimento Osteoarticolare, AUSL Romagna, Ospedale Cervesi, Cattolica, RN, Italy

G. Merolla
UO Chirurgia Ortopedica della Spalla Romagna, Dipartimento Osteoarticolare, AUSL Romagna, Ospedale Cervesi, Cattolica, RN, Italy

Biomechanics Laboratory, Cervesi Hospital, Cattolica—AUSL Romagna, Cattolica, Italy

International Doctorate School (PhD) in Clinical and Experimental Medicine, UNIMORE, Modena, Italy

F. Franceschi et al. (eds.), *Revision Shoulder Arthroplasty*,
https://doi.org/10.1007/978-3-031-45944-3_12

shoulder function, fracture, implant loosening, osteoarthritis, instability, infection, subluxation, avascular necrosis, dislocation, heterotopic ossification, malunion, greater tuberosity lysis or migration, technical errors (overstuffing, malposition), and implant migration, as well [10, 11, 13, 14]. Prevalence of revision causes proved to be different depending on the initial diagnosis: glenoid erosion and rotator cuff insufficiency are typical revision causes for HA implanted for primary osteoarthritis, while tuberosity migration, non-union, or malunion were the main causes of revision in HA implanted for fractures or fracture sequelae [11].

Risk of HA revision is increased by patients' age [10, 15]: younger patients tend to be more active, to have higher expectations of surgical results and greater demands; furthermore, they are less easily satisfied with their outcomes as measured by patient-reported outcome measures (PROMs). Various reasons for this have been proposed: on one side, higher activity level may lead to early prosthetic wear and glenoid erosion; on the other side, higher expectations could lower the threshold for revision. High BMI has been related to HA revision as well, while gender, ASA class, and Charlson index appeared not to be related [10, 15].

Early revision causes (<1 year from implantation) were analyzed on a large database population, resulting in dislocation (26.2%), rotator cuff disease (15.1%), loosening (13.4%), and infection (10.1%) being the main causes [16]. Risk factors associated with early revision were age younger than 65 years, smoking, and obesity [16].

Recent outcomes of a large cohort suggested that nowadays the implant of choice for HA revision is RSA, used in 58% of patients, whereas anatomic total shoulder arthroplasty (aTSA) accounts for 19% of revisions and HA accounts for 17%; resection arthroplasty and spacer positioning total 6% of revision cases [11].

12.2 Preoperative Evaluation

Preoperative evaluation is a key step in the workout of a revision surgery. Clinical and radiological information should be merged to obtain a precise diagnosis and an exhaustive surgical planning.

During clinical evaluation, a careful assessment of the scar of the previous surgery is important, to detect eventual wound dehiscence, drainage or reddening that could be suggestive of infection. ROM measurements should be taken both actively and passively, to assess stiffness and detect abnormal movements. A thorough evaluation of rotator cuff muscles is of utmost importance. When infection is suspected, it must be ruled out with blood testing and radiological evaluation.

Plain X-rays are the first step of radiological evaluation. They provide information regarding humeral stem placement and signs of loosening, of humeral subluxation, implant migration, and glenoid erosion.

Glenoid erosion is the first cause of HA revision and primary concern during glenoid component implantation.

Risk factors for the development of glenoid erosion after HA are gender, with women more prone to development of erosion; presence of glenoid cysts, that are markers of glenoid bone low quality; rheumatoid arthritis; and fatty infiltration of rotator cuff muscles. HA implantation for fracture demonstrated protection from glenoid erosion, probably because of good preoperative glenoid quality [17]. Interestingly, preoperative glenoid version, prosthetic humeral head size and inclination, and critical shoulder angle were not correlated with glenoid erosion [17, 18]. Implant design was updated throughout the years with the aim to reduce glenoid erosion with the adoption of pyrocarbon head HA; its tribological qualities and elastic properties resembling cortical bone were extremely promising, and good short-term clinical and radiographic results were obtained [19, 20]. Unfortunately, it did not prove to be a real game changer.

Typically, glenoid erosion can show two kinetic patterns: a continuous erosion over time and severe erosion rapidly after implantation [17].

Radiographic methods to evaluate glenoid erosion were proposed by Sperling [21] and Mercer [22].

Sperling proposed a four-grade qualitative classification of glenoid erosion: none; mild (erosion into the subchondral bone); moderate (medialization of the glenoid subchondral bone with hemispheric conforming deformation of the glenoid); or severe (complete hemispheric deformation of the glenoid with superior bone loss to the base of the coracoid base) [21].

Mercer and coworkers [22] proposed a quantitative method to determine medial translation of center of rotation in 2 planes plotted over time. Measurement was performed with the aid of templates that should be superimposed to shoulder radiographs to measure translation in millimeters. It proved to be complex to reproduce and demonstrated only fair interobserver agreement [17].

Deeper evaluation of glenoid erosion and bone stock deficit requires a CT scan evaluation. In order to correctly visualize the glenoid, appropriate window should be chosen and metal artifact suppression must be used [23]. There are no dedicated CT classifications of glenoid bone deficiencies for HA. Sperling classification has been adapted to CT evaluation with good results [17]. Furthermore, classifications described for different clinical scenarios were successfully adapted to HA glenoid erosion.

A classification of glenoid bone deficiencies was proposed by Antuna and coworkers [24]. It classified glenoid bone loss in 3 types: central, peripheral, or combined; each type was subsequently graded as mild, moderate, or severe. Gupta et al. [25] later updated the classification, dividing the defects as centric or eccentric; every type was subclassified in 4 grades depending on the percentage of glenoid bone stock erosion, ranging from none to >60% of glenoid bone stock.

Ideally, these classifications, through accurate definition of severity and location of the glenoid defect, should guide the surgeon in the choice of operative technique.

12.3 Surgical Technique

Revision of a failed HA is a complex procedure that should be approached with extreme care and extensive planning. In spite of the fact that the glenoid was not involved in the previous surgery, difficult steps can be required both in the management of the humeral side and of the glenoid. Humeral component loosening, tuberosities deficiencies, glenoid bone loss, and soft tissues deficiencies, that can be a consequence of previous surgery or of implant failure, are problems that should be assessed and solved to perform a successful surgery [26].

Implant choice is another key point in surgery planning, with options ranging from an RSA, to an aTSA to a new HA, with various procedures to be added to correct glenoid bone loss. Nowadays, the most common choice is an RSA, whose adoption is increasing over the years [27].

We routinely perform a deltopectoral approach in both primary and revision cases. Anterosuperior approach should not be advised in revision surgery as it is not extensile and may threaten the axillary nerve [26]. The first challenge a surgeon has to face in a revision setting is the correct identification of deltopectoral interval, as scar tissue and adherences will be present and cephalic vein will often be missing, having been closed during or as a consequence of the previous surgery. After separation of deltoid and pectoralis major, careful release of subdeltoid and subacromial space should be performed. Extensive soft tissue releases might be necessary to mobilize the humerus and expose the HA (Fig. 12.1). Failure

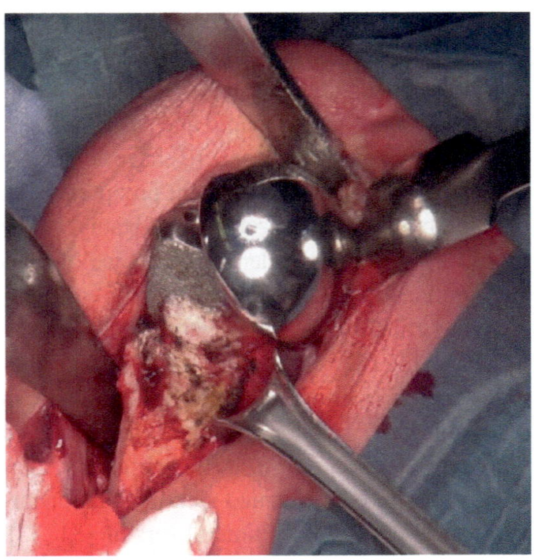

Fig. 12.1 Hemiarthroplasty exposure

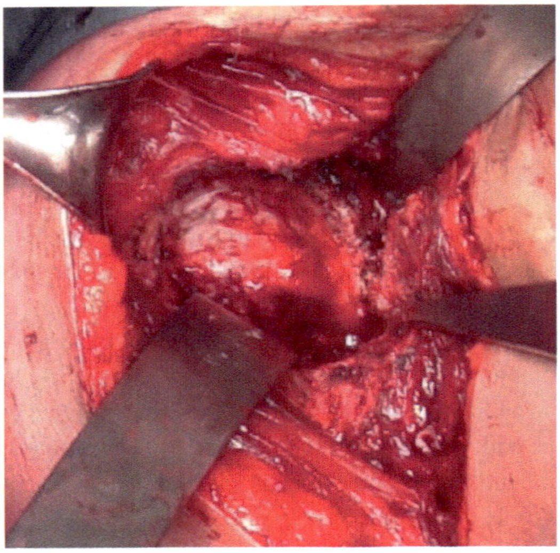

Fig. 12.2 Glenoid exposure after soft tissues release

in completing the release may lead to component malpositioning, thus posing a risk on the final outcome of the revision.

Once exposed, HA should be tested for loosening. If the prosthesis is loose, a revision is mandatory. If the HA is well-fixed, the surgeon has to choose whether to remove it or to convert it, if technically feasible. If a stable modular stem is present, its conversion, compared to its revision, allows shorter surgical times, reduced blood loss and decreased complications [28].

Adequate glenoid exposure is a mandatory step in revision surgery. Removal of scar tissue and capsule is necessary until complete visualization of glenoid edge is possible (Fig. 12.2).

Once the glenoid has been exposed, subsequent steps depend on glenoid and patients' characteristics. It is important to have correctly planned the glenoid management preoperatively. Glenoid bone stock and rotator cuff status are the main variables to consider in the choice of revision implant.

When rotator cuff is present and functionally reliable, an aTSA can be implanted. When glenoid erosion is minimal, a primary implant can be used [29, 30]. Minor erosion can be corrected with eccentric reaming or with the use of augmented glenoid. Augmented glenoid components allow recovery of glenohumeral version [31, 32].

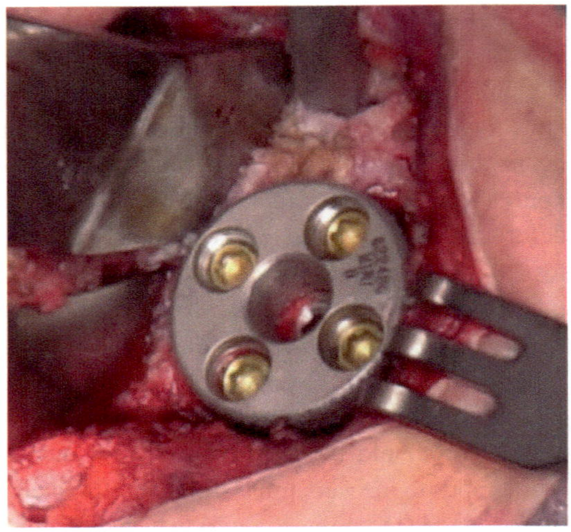

Fig. 12.3 Augmented glenoid implant

Good clinical results can be obtained with these implants [33, 34], but radiographic results are worse in patients with more preoperative retroversion, who needed thicker augments [34] and with incomplete retroversion correction [33], so care should be taken in revision settings.

When rotator cuff is insufficient or glenoid bone loss is too severe to allow for implantation of an aTSA, a RSA should be considered [35, 36]. To address glenoid erosion, eccentric glenoid reaming, augmented glenoid components (Fig. 12.3), and bone grafting techniques may be required. Sixty percentage of patients typically present with a mild erosion [35], that can be easily treated as a primary glenoid with eccentric reaming, standard, or augmented glenoid components (Fig. 12.4).

Severe bone loss with the need for bone grafting is detected in 17-25% of patients [35, 36]. In the setting of severe bone loss, various techniques are possible:

- No bone grafting and no implantation of glenoid component, revision to an HA.
- Bone grafting without glenoid implantation, revision to an HA.
- Single-stage bone grafting with reverse glenoid implantation.
- Dual-stage bone grafting with reverse glenoid implantation.

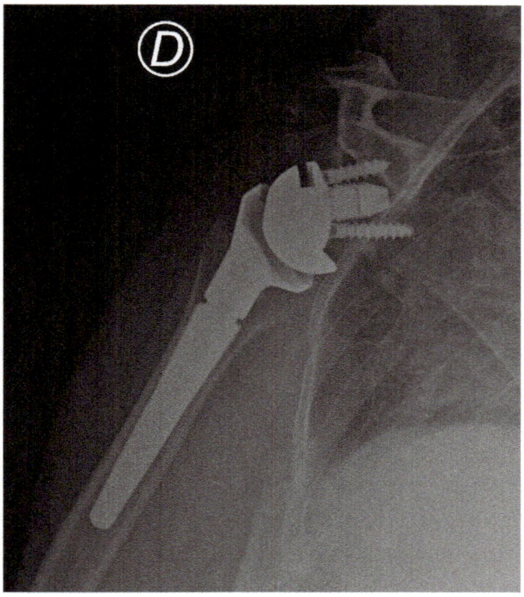

Fig. 12.4 Postoperative X-ray of an RSA for revision of a failed HA

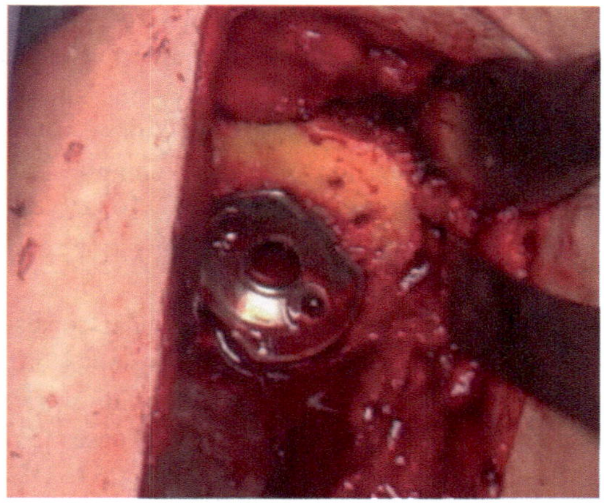

Fig. 12.5 Femoral head grafting and standard glenoid implant

As no autologous humeral head is available in a revision setting, need for a graft should be planned in advance: autologous iliac bone graft should be harvested, or an allograft femoral head, femoral neck, or humeral head should be available in the operating theatre. In extreme cases, a patient-specific implant may be necessary. In selected cases, placement of a medialized and inferiorly tilted glenoid, with peg stability found in the scapular pillar, is possible. Good clinical results have been demonstrated, comparable to that of bone grafting, but with higher rates of revision [37].

When no bone grafting is performed and no glenoid component is implanted, a CTA HA may be a viable surgical option. It can be extremely useful in cases with acromial fragmentation or axillary nerve palsy [38].

Bone grafting without glenoid implantation is another option: bicortical iliac crest bone grafting can be used to fill the glenoid bone deficit when placing a glenoid component is deemed impossible. Once harvested, the graft can be impacted into the glenoid, if the defect is centrally located, or, if a peripheral defect is present, the graft should be secured with screws. In both cases, the graft should be placed so that the cortical part of the graft opposes the humeral head, providing structural integrity and opposing medialization [39].

Dual-stage bone grafting with reverse glenoid implantation is an uncommon but possible option: a CTA HA can be implanted with a glenoid bone grafting aimed to restore a valid bone stock [38]. After graft healing, CTA HA can be converted to a definitive reverse prosthesis [40].

Single-stage bone grafting with reverse glenoid implantation is the most common option; grafting can range from filling with cancellous chips to femoral head allograft (Fig. 12.5) [35, 36, 41].

12.4 Outcomes

Outcomes of HA revision are poorly analyzed in literature. Few studies have been produced on the topic, and their evidence level is generally low, being mostly case series and cohort studies including a low number of patients [12, 13].

Revision of HA to aTSA is described in a small number of studies [29, 30, 42–46]. Reported results are generally good, yet results are inconsistent among patients and ample variability has been reported by different authors [30, 45]. After revision, significant improvement in range of motion and pain is reported [30, 42–44, 47–50], with good patient satisfaction after surgery, ranging from 45% to 81% [29, 30, 44]. Improvements in Constant scores were reported by some authors [42], but not confirmed by other authors [46]. Unfortunately, revision yields high complication rates, ranging from 12.5% to 50% [29, 42, 44, 47–50], with up to 21.4% requiring further surgery [29].

Use of an RSA to revise HA provides consistent results, with improvement in Constant score, pain, and ROM [13, 35, 51–54] and with overall good patient satisfaction in 79-83% of cases [51, 53]. Complications were registered in 26.6-32% of cases [51, 53], but only 6.6-7% required reoperations [35, 51]. Outcomes could even improve when revision is performed through stem retention and conversion of a modular implant [55–57].

Results obtained are not different from those of a primary RSA implanted for osteoarthritis, while revising an HA to another HA or an aTSA yields significantly worse results compared to those of a primary implant [14], appealing surgeons to the choice of an RSA.

Despite this generally encouraging results, a variability exists depending on the preoperative diagnosis: HA revision for fractures provide the worse postoperative range of motion compared to cuff tear arthropathy and osteonecrosis, with a trend toward worse results in PROMs exists [58]. Fracture as initial diagnosis carries a higher risk of re-revision, as well [58]. Complications occurred in 13.6-32% of patients [13, 47, 49, 50], with the majority of complications occurring in patients who underwent more than one previous surgery [47]. This does not imply that outcomes are intrinsically bad, as statistically significant improvement in pain scores, PROMs, and ROM can be obtained even in the setting of a revision of a HA implanted for fracture [47–50], but that the obtained results are significantly inferior to those of a primary RSA for an acute fracture [59, 60].

This variability can be explained by the fact that each diagnosis is associated with different typical amounts of bone loss, soft-tissue contracture, and muscle-tendon loss, that are somehow carried on from primary HA to revision RSA, providing the different results [58].

Hartel et al. [61] compared the outcomes of HA revision in aTSA and RSA. Shoulder function significantly increased with both procedures; yet patients revised to aTSA demonstrated better Constant and OSS score results than those revised to RSA. Interestingly, patients revised for implant failure performed better than patients revised for soft tissue failure, and those different causes distributed unevenly between patients revised to aTSA and RSA. This should remind us that despite RSA being the most reliable option for glenoid deformity, bone loss, and rotator cuff insufficiency, aTSA can provide extremely satisfactory results when used with appropriate indications. The expert surgeon should be able to select the most appropriate implant in each particular case, with results from the available literature being just a guide and not a cage.

12.5 Conclusion

Revision of a failed HA is a challenging procedure that should be carefully planned and evaluated. Key points in the choice of implant are glenoid erosion and rotator cuff tendon integrity. In the setting of a severe glenoid bone loss, glenoid management can be challenging, requiring the use of bone grafts or dedicated implants. Anyways, when correctly planned and performed, HA revision can provide acceptable results, both for the surgeon and the patients, with satisfactory functional recovery.

References

1. New Zealand Orthopaedic Association. The New Zealand Joint registry. 22 year report. NZJR; 2021. Available from: www.nzoa.org.nz/nzoa-joint-registry.
2. Farley KX, Wilson JM, Kumar A, Gottschalk MB, Daly C, Sanchez-Sotelo J, et al. Prevalence of shoulder arthroplasty in the United States and the increasing Burden of revision shoulder arthroplasty. JB JS Open Access. 2021;6:e20.00156.
3. Australian Orthopaedic Association National Joint Replacement Registry (AOANJRR). Hip, knee and shoulder arthroplasty: 2022 annual report. Adelaide:

AOA. p. 2022. Available from: https://aoanjrr.sahmri.com/annual-reports-2022
4. National Joint Registry. 19th Annual Report 2022. NJR; 2022. Available from: reports.njrcentre.org.uk.
5. Padegimas EM, Maltenfort M, Lazarus MD, Ramsey ML, Williams GR, Namdari S. Future patient demand for shoulder arthroplasty by younger patients: national projections. Clin Orthop Relat Res. 2015;473:1860–7.
6. Torre M, Ceccarelli S, Biondi A, Carrani E, Masciocchi M, Cornacchia A. Registro Italiano ArtroProtesi. In: Report Annuale 2020. Roma: Il Pensiero Scientifico Editore; 2021.
7. Registro Implantologia Protesica Ortopedica. Rendiconto Attività Registro Regionale di Implantologia Protesica Ortopedica. Dati complessivi interventi di protesi d'anca, di ginocchio e di spalla in Emilia Romagna 2000–2018. Regione Emilia Romagna; 2020.
8. Fevang B-TS, Lie SA, Havelin LI, Skredderstuen A, Furnes O. Risk factors for revision after shoulder arthroplasty: 1825 shoulder arthroplasties from the Norwegian Arthroplasty Register. Acta Orthop. 2009;80:83–91.
9. Unbehaun D, Rasmussen S, Hole R, Fenstad AM, Salomonsson B, Demir Y, et al. Low arthroplasty survival after treatment for proximal humerus fracture sequelae: 3245 shoulder replacements from the Nordic Arthroplasty Register Association. Acta Orthop. 2020;91(6):776–81.
10. Singh JA, Sperling JW, Cofield RH. Risk factors for revision surgery after humeral head replacement: 1431 shoulders over 3 decades. J Shoulder Elb Surg. 2012;21:1039–44.
11. Gauci M-O, Cavalier M, Gonzalez J-F, Holzer N, Baring T, Walch G, et al. Revision of failed shoulder arthroplasty: epidemiology, etiology, and surgical options. J Shoulder Elb Surg. 2020;29:541–9.
12. Davies A, Selmi H, Sabharwal S, Vella-Baldacchino M, Liddle AD, Reilly P. Revision shoulder hemiarthroplasty and total shoulder arthroplasty a systematic review and meta-analysis. J Shoulder Elb Arthroplast. 2022;6:24715492221095990.
13. Bois AJ, Knight P, Alhojailan K, Bohsali KI. Clinical outcomes and complications of reverse shoulder arthroplasty used for failed prior shoulder surgery: a systematic review and meta-analysis. JSES Int. 2020;4:156–68.
14. Rasmussen JV, Olsen BS, Al-Hamdani A, Brorson S. Outcome of revision shoulder arthroplasty after resurfacing hemiarthroplasty in patients with glenohumeral osteoarthritis. J Bone Joint Surg Am. 2016;98:1631–7.
15. Ödquist M, Hallberg K, Rahme H, Salomonsson B, Rosso A. Lower age increases the risk of revision for stemmed and resurfacing shoulder hemi arthroplasty. Acta Orthop. 2018;89:3–9.
16. Werner BC, Burrus MT, Begho I, Gwathmey FW, Brockmeier SF. Early revision within 1 year after shoulder arthroplasty: patient factors and etiology. J Shoulder Elb Surg. 2015;24:e323–30.
17. Herschel R, Wieser K, Morrey ME, Ramos CH, Gerber C, Meyer DC. Risk factors for glenoid erosion in patients with shoulder hemiarthroplasty: an analysis of 118 cases. J Shoulder Elb Surg. 2017;26:246–52.
18. Cerciello S, Morris BJ, Visonà E, Corona K, Edwards TB, Maffulli N, et al. No relationship between critical shoulder angle and glenoid erosion after shoulder hemiarthroplasty: a comparative radiographic study. Arch Orthop Trauma Surg. 2017;137:919–23.
19. Garret J, Harly E, Le Huec J-C, Brunner U, Rotini R, Godenèche A. Pyrolytic carbon humeral head in hemi-shoulder arthroplasty: preliminary results at 2-year follow-up. JSES Open Access. 2019;3:37–42.
20. Cointat C, Raynier JL, Vasseur H, Lareyre F, Raffort J, Gauci MO, et al. Short-term outcomes and survival of pyrocarbon hemiarthroplasty in the young arthritic shoulder. J Shoulder Elb Surg. 2022;31:113–22.
21. Sperling JW, Cofield RH, Schleck CD, Harmsen WS. Total shoulder arthroplasty versus hemiarthroplasty for rheumatoid arthritis of the shoulder: results of 303 consecutive cases. J Shoulder Elb Surg. 2007;16:683–90.
22. Mercer DM, Gilmer BB, Saltzman MD, Bertelsen A, Warme WJ, Matsen FA. A quantitative method for determining medial migration of the humeral head after shoulder arthroplasty: preliminary results in assessing glenoid wear at a minimum of two years after hemiarthroplasty with concentric glenoid reaming. J Shoulder Elb Surg. 2011;20:301–7.
23. Merolla G, Campi F, Paladini P, Cavagna E, Porcellini G. Multichannel computed tomography (MCCT) analysis of glenoid erosion in shoulder hemiarthroplasty: preliminary clinical applications. Musculoskelet Surg. 2010;94(Suppl. 1):S71–7.
24. Antuna SA, Sperling JW, Cofield RH, Rowland CM. Glenoid revision surgery after total shoulder arthroplasty. J Shoulder Elb Surg. 2001;10:217–24.
25. Gupta A, Thussbas C, Koch M, Seebauer L. Management of glenoid bone defects with reverse shoulder arthroplasty-surgical technique and clinical outcomes. J Shoulder Elb Surg. 2018;27:853–62.
26. Harrison AK, Knudsen ML, Braman JP. Hemiarthroplasty and total shoulder arthroplasty conversion to reverse total shoulder arthroplasty. Curr Rev Musculoskelet Med. 2020;13:501–8.
27. Wagner ER, Chang MJ, Welp KM, Solberg MJ, Hunt TJ, Woodmass JM, et al. The impact of the reverse prosthesis on revision shoulder arthroplasty: analysis of a high-volume shoulder practice. J Shoulder Elb Surg. 2019;28:e49–56.
28. Wieser K, Borbas P, Ek ET, Meyer DC, Gerber C. Conversion of stemmed hemi- or total to reverse total shoulder arthroplasty: advantages of a modular stem design. Clin Orthop Relat Res. 2015;473:651–60.
29. Sheth MM, Sholder D, Abboud J, Lazarus MD, Ramsey ML, Williams GR, et al. Revision of failed hemiarthroplasty for painful glenoid arthrosis to anatomic total shoulder arthroplasty. J Shoulder Elb Surg. 2018;27:1884–90.

30. Carroll RM, Izquierdo R, Vazquez M, Blaine TA, Levine WN, Bigliani LU. Conversion of painful hemiarthroplasty to total shoulder arthroplasty: long-term results. J Shoulder Elb Surg. 2004;13:599–603.
31. Das AK, Wright AC, Singh J, Monga P. Does posterior half-wedge augmented glenoid restore version and alignment in total shoulder arthroplasty for the B2 glenoid? J Clin Orthop Trauma. 2020;11:S275–9.
32. Grey SG, Wright TW, Flurin P-H, Zuckerman JD, Roche CP, Friedman RJ. Clinical and radiographic outcomes with a posteriorly augmented glenoid for Walch B glenoids in anatomic total shoulder arthroplasty. J Shoulder Elb Surg. 2020;29:e185–95.
33. Ho JC, Amini MH, Entezari V, Jun BJ, Alolabi B, Ricchetti ET, et al. Clinical and radiographic outcomes of a posteriorly augmented glenoid component in anatomic total shoulder arthroplasty for primary osteoarthritis with posterior glenoid bone loss. J Bone Joint Surg Am. 2018;100:1934–48.
34. Priddy M, Zarezadeh A, Farmer KW, Struk AM, King JJ, Wright TW, et al. Early results of augmented anatomic glenoid components. J Shoulder Elb Surg. 2019;28:S138–45.
35. Merolla G, Wagner E, Sperling JW, Paladini P, Fabbri E, Porcellini G. Revision of failed shoulder hemiarthroplasty to reverse total arthroplasty: analysis of 157 revision implants. J Shoulder Elb Surg. 2018;27:75–81.
36. Sheth MM, Sholder D, Getz CL, Williams GR, Namdari S. Revision of failed hemiarthroplasty and anatomic total shoulder arthroplasty to reverse total shoulder arthroplasty. J Shoulder Elb Surg. 2019;28:1074–81.
37. Verstuyft L, Vergison L, Van Tongel A, De Wilde L. Is bone grafting always necessary in revision reverse total shoulder arthroplasty with uncontained glenoid bone defects? J Shoulder Elb Surg. 2021;30:1891–8.
38. Smith TJ, Shah SS, Peterson JW, Ross G. The modern use of the extended humeral head (cuff tear arthropathy) hemiarthroplasty. JSES Int. 2021;5:142–8.
39. Neyton L, Walch G, Nové-Josserand L, Edwards TB. Glenoid corticocancellous bone grafting after glenoid component removal in the treatment of glenoid loosening. J Shoulder Elb Surg. 2006;15:173–9.
40. Hoffelner T, Moroder P, Auffarth A, Tauber M, Resch H. Outcomes after shoulder arthroplasty revision with glenoid reconstruction and bone grafting. Int Orthop. 2014;38:775–82.
41. Boileau P, Moineau G, Roussanne Y, O'Shea K. Bony increased offset-reversed shoulder arthroplasty (BIO-RSA). JBJS Essent Surg Tech. 2017;7:e37.
42. Postacchini R, Castagna A, Borroni M, Cinotti G, Postacchini F, Gumina S. Total shoulder arthroplasty for the treatment of failed hemiarthroplasty in patients with fracture of the proximal humerus. J Shoulder Elb Surg. 2012;21:1542–9.
43. Sperling JW, Cofield RH. Revision total shoulder arthroplasty for the treatment of glenoid arthrosis. J Bone Joint Surg Am. 1998;80:860–7.
44. Sassoon AA, Rhee PC, Schleck CD, Harmsen WS, Sperling JW, Cofield RH. Revision total shoulder arthroplasty for painful glenoid arthrosis after humeral head replacement: the nontraumatic shoulder. J Shoulder Elb Surg. 2012;21:1484–91.
45. Groh GI, Wirth MA. Results of revision from hemiarthroplasty to total shoulder arthroplasty utilizing modular component systems. J Shoulder Elb Surg. 2011;20:778–82.
46. Ravenscroft M, Charalambous CP, Haines JF, Trail IA. Outcome of stemmed shoulder hemi-arthroplasty revision. Arch Orthop Trauma Surg. 2009;129:797–9.
47. Uri O, Beckles V, Higgs D, Falworth M, Middleton C, Lambert S. Increased-offset reverse shoulder arthroplasty for the treatment of failed post-traumatic humeral head replacement. J Shoulder Elb Surg. 2014;23:401–8.
48. Castagna A, Delcogliano M, de Caro F, Ziveri G, Borroni M, Gumina S, et al. Conversion of shoulder arthroplasty to reverse implants: clinical and radiological results using a modular system. Int Orthop. 2013;37:1297–305.
49. Holschen M, Siemes M-K, Witt K-A, Steinbeck J. Five-year outcome after conversion of a hemiarthroplasty when used for the treatment of a proximal humeral fracture to a reverse total shoulder arthroplasty. Bone Joint J. 2018;100-B:761–6.
50. Merolla G, Tartarone A, Sperling JW, Paladini P, Fabbri E, Porcellini G. Early clinical and radiological outcomes of reverse shoulder arthroplasty with an eccentric all-polyethylene glenosphere to treat failed hemiarthroplasty and the sequelae of proximal humeral fractures. Int Orthop. 2017;41:141–8.
51. Valenti P, Kilinc AS, Sauzières P, Katz D. Results of 30 reverse shoulder prostheses for revision of failed hemi- or total shoulder arthroplasty. Eur J Orthop Surg Traumatol. 2014;24:1375–82.
52. Patel DN, Young B, Onyekwelu I, Zuckerman JD, Kwon YW. Reverse total shoulder arthroplasty for failed shoulder arthroplasty. J Shoulder Elb Surg. 2012;21:1478–83.
53. Levy J, Frankle M, Mighell M, Pupello D. The use of the reverse shoulder prosthesis for the treatment of failed hemiarthroplasty for proximal humeral fracture. J Bone Joint Surg Am. 2007;89:292–300.
54. Paladini P, Collu A, Campi E, Porcellini G. The inverse prosthesis as a revision prosthesis in failures of shoulder hemiarthroplasty. Chir Organi Mov. 2005;90:11–21.
55. Werner BS, Boehm D, Gohlke F. Revision to reverse shoulder arthroplasty with retention of the humeral component. Acta Orthop. 2013;84:473–8.
56. Williams PN, Trehan SK, Tsouris N, Dines JS, Dines DM, Craig EV, et al. Functional outcomes of modular conversion of hemiarthroplasty or total to reverse total shoulder arthroplasty. HSS J. 2017;13:102–7.
57. Reuther F, Irlenbusch U, Kääb MJ, Kohut G. Conversion of hemiarthroplasty to reverse shoulder arthroplasty with humeral stem retention. J Clin Med. 2022;11:834.

58. Franke KJ, Christmas KN, Downes KL, Mighell MA, Frankle MA. Does the etiology of a failed hemiarthroplasty affect outcomes when revised to a reverse shoulder arthroplasty? J Shoulder Elb Surg. 2020;29:S149–56.
59. Dezfuli B, King JJ, Farmer KW, Struk AM, Wright TW. Outcomes of reverse total shoulder arthroplasty as primary versus revision procedure for proximal humerus fractures. J Shoulder Elb Surg. 2016;25:1133–7.
60. Lollino N, Paladini P, Campi F, Merolla G, Rossi P, Porcellini G. Reverse shoulder prosthesis as revision surgery after fractures of the proximal humerus, treated initially by internal fixation or hemiarthroplasty. Chir Organi Mov. 2009;93(Suppl. 1):S35–9.
61. Hartel BP, Alta TD, Sewnath ME, Willems WJ. Difference in clinical outcome between total shoulder arthroplasty and reverse shoulder arthroplasty used in hemiarthroplasty revision surgery. Int J Shoulder Surg. 2015;9:69–73.

13 Revising the Failed Glenoid in TSA

Gianluca Ciolli, Edoardo Giovannetti de Sanctis, and Lionel Neyton

Abbreviations

HA	Hemiarthroplasty
RSA	Reverse total shoulder arthroplasty
TSA	Anatomic total shoulder arthroplasty

13.1 Introduction

Over the past decade, the incidence of total shoulder arthroplasty has increased exponentially. From 2012 to 2017, in the USA, the incidence of anatomic total shoulder arthroplasty (TSA) increased from 9.5 to 12.5 cases per 100,000 [1].

These figures are explained by the favorable results of shoulder replacement and by the excellent survival of implants (mean survival of 90% at 10 years) [2–4].

G. Ciolli
Ramsay Santé, Hôpital Privé Jean Mermoz, Centre Orthopédique Santy, Lyon, France

Fondazione Policlinico Universitario A. Gemelli, Rome, Italy

E. Giovannetti de Sanctis
Ramsay Santé, Hôpital Privé Jean Mermoz, Centre Orthopédique Santy, Lyon, France

IULS-Institut Universitaire Locomoteur et Sports, Pasteur 2 Hospital, CHU, Nice, France

L. Neyton (✉)
Ramsay Santé, Hôpital Privé Jean Mermoz, Centre Orthopédique Santy, Lyon, France

Subsequently, the increased number of total shoulder arthroplasties has led to a corresponding growth of prosthetic revisions [5].

The Australian Orthopaedic Association National Joint Replacement Registry Report of 2020 reported a 10-year cumulative revision rate of 12.3% for TSA.

Causes of revisions include aseptic loosening, infection, instability, secondary cuff rupture, joint stiffness, and neurological complications.

The glenoid component appears to be the weakest link in TSA because of component loosening, implant material failure, malposition, or wear. Glenoid component loosening occurs in 0% to 20% of cases of total shoulder arthroplasty and results in revision surgery in 0% to 6% of cases [6].

Radiographic evidence of glenoid loosening without pain and/or functional impairment is often treated nonoperatively. Glenoid loosening is often silent and well-tolerated by the patient, and it is not uncommon for pain to be absent before the bone stock is severely altered. In elderly patients and/or poor health conditions, conservative treatment should be preferred. In a younger, motivated patient, the revision surgery should be considered before progressing to more extensive bone damage.

Revision of a loose glenoid component in TSA is always a complex procedure, requiring a thorough analysis to validate the treatment strategy. It is not uncommon for several complica-

F. Franceschi et al. (eds.), *Revision Shoulder Arthroplasty*,
https://doi.org/10.1007/978-3-031-45944-3_13

tions to coexist, even if the revision of the glenoid component is the main problem [2, 7].

In these difficult revision cases, Wierks et al. [8] determined that the learning curve required seven revision cases. Accordingly, unexperienced surgeons should preferably seek the advice of a more experienced surgeon.

13.2 Preparing for Revision Shoulder Arthroplasty

The patient must be appropriately informed of the risks and possible adjustments during surgery. The patient must be informed of the increased risk of complications compared with primary surgery. The preoperative evaluation focuses on assessing the patient's operability and evaluating the bone stock.

13.3 Preoperative Examinations (Fig. 13.1)

Radiographic evaluation with AP views in neutral, internal, and external rotation and a profile view is systematic. Multiple classifications have been proposed to evaluate the glenoid radiographic status.

13.3.1 Classification According to Sperling [9]

Components are divided into radiographic zones for measurements of periprosthetic lucency; the glenoid has five zones. The lines are evaluated according to their presence or absence, location, and thickness. The maximum thickness of the line is measured within 0.5 mm. A glenoid component is "at risk" when a complete lucent line is present, some part of it being 1.5 mm or greater in width, or when at least 2 of 3 independent observers identify migration or tilt of the component.

13.3.2 Classification According to Molé [10]

The position of the radiolucent lines is established using six zones from the upper to the periphery of the keel and the middle part of the tray. Their thickness is measured in three grades: grade 1 (<1 mm), grade 2 (between 1 and 2 mm), and grade 3 (>2 mm).

The authors also calculate the radiolucent line score (RLL score). RLL score is the sum of each zone involved multiplied by its grade, giving a maximum of 18. The glenoid component is arbi-

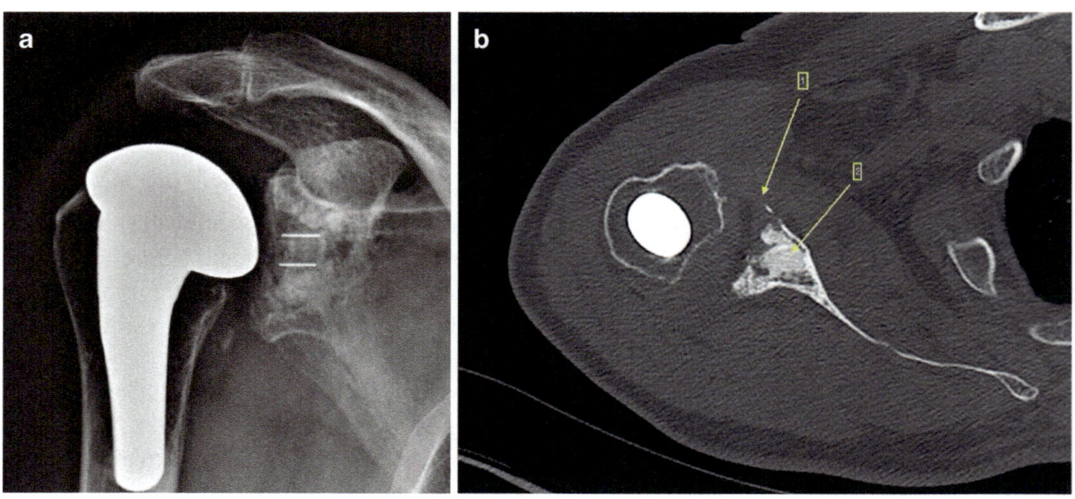

Fig. 13.1 Failure of total shoulder arthroplasty. AP X-Ray view with areas of osteolysis around the prosthetic stem (**a**). CT scan axial view (**b**) with articular bone loss (1) and glenoid bone resorption (2)

trarily considered as being loose if the score is greater than 12.

13.3.3 Classification According to Lazarus [11]

Grade 0: No radiolucency.
Grade 1: Incomplete radiolucency around 1 or 2 pegs.
Grade 2: Complete radiolucency (<2 mm wide) around 1 peg only, with or without incomplete radiolucency around one other peg.
Grade 3: Complete radiolucency (<2 mm wide) around 2 or more pegs.
Grade 4: Complete radiolucency (>2 mm wide) around 2 or more pegs.
Grade 5: Gross loosening.

Grade A: Complete component seating.
Grade B: <25% incomplete contact, single radiograph.
Grade C: 25–50% incomplete contact, single radiograph.
Grade D: <50% incomplete contact, both radiographs.
Grade E: >50% incomplete contact, single radiograph.

All these classifications attempt at establishing the degree of severity of the loosening.

It is generally admitted that a glenoid component is "at risk" for loosening when there is an incomplete lucent line surrounding the component.

Loosening of the glenoid component can be defined as follows [12, 13]:

- radiolucent line greater than 2 mm and complete;
- progression of radiolucent lines on several consecutive radiographs;
- fragmentation of cement; fracture of fixation screws;
- obvious migration/mobilization of the component.

A CT scan (ideally with the use of metal artifact reduction software) allows a more precise analysis of loosening and loss of bone stock. The use of 3D reconstructions, without or with subtraction of the humerus, also provides additional information and a better spatial representation of bone loss.

The causes of revision of a loose glenoid component are often multifactorial. Therefore, the options for revision of a glenoid implant, while influenced by the state of the glenoid bone stock, must also take into account possible associated problems such as prosthetic instability, cuff tear, acute or low-grade sepsis, or loosening of the humeral implant.

CT arthrography is indicated if doubts remain about the competence of the rotator cuff.

Lastly, a low-grade infection should often be suspected during surgical revision even in the absence of clinical evidence. Lucas et al. reported up to 54% positive cultures (at least 1 positive culture) for Cutibacterium acnes and/or staphylococcus in patients with glenoid loosening without clear evidence of infection [14].

13.4 How to Revise an Anatomic Glenoid Component?

It is important to know precisely the type of prosthesis that is to be revised and to ask the following questions:

- Is it a cemented implant?
- What is the model of the prosthesis?
- Is the implant convertible?
- Is it still available on the market?

Therefore, it is necessary to retrieve the operative report of the initial surgery (and any previous revisions), which usually contains all the necessary information.

In most cases, it is possible to order implant-specific instrumentation which allows the prosthesis to be removed in the best condition possible. Sometimes, the presence of the implant representative in the room can also be helpful for "tips and tricks."

The deltopectoral approach is the approach of choice for prosthetic revision. It allows both proximal and distal widening toward the humerus. The existence of a previous superior-external approach is not a contraindication to performing another adjacent incision.

13.4.1 Intraoperative Analysis (Fig. 13.2)

An intraoperative analysis is only performed after the implant has been removed.

Antuna classification is helpful to evaluate glenoid bone deficiencies after glenoid component removal [15].

Glenoid bone loss is categorized intraoperatively on the basis of location and severity.

The defects are categorized as central, peripheral, or combined. Based on the severity, deficiencies are categorized as mild (less than one-third of the glenoid rim or surface), moderate (between one-third and two-thirds), or severe (more than two-thirds).

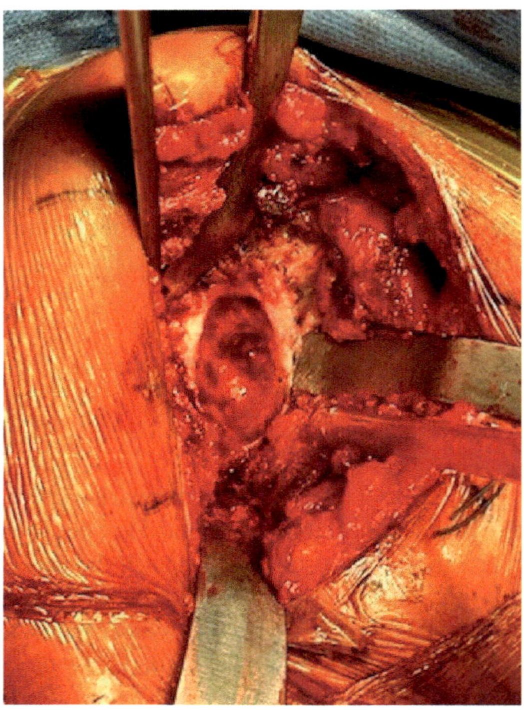

Fig. 13.2 Intraoperative evaluation of glenoid bone loss after removal of a previous implant

Williams and Iannotti made modifications in 2007 to Antuna's classification by adding the notions of contained or uncontained central deficit (depending on whether the glenoid arch is respected or not) and the notions of symmetrical or asymmetrical peripheral/combined deficits [16].

The surgical implications of Antuna's classification have been clarified in a "new" similar classification described by Gupta et al. in 2018 [17].

13.4.2 Revision of the Glenoid Component

Removal of the glenoid implant should be as conservative as possible to preserve the remaining bone stock. Fractures during glenoid implant removal are rare, as removal is often facilitated by the loosening of the bone [18].

For the removal of a cemented polyethylene (PE), the base of the keel can be cut by sliding an osteotome behind the plate or using an oscillating saw (preferably angled at 90°). The remaining piece of the keel and the cement are then removed with a rotating bur.

Once the implant is removed, several samples are taken. The various cavities are cleaned (false membranes/cement) using a curette and/or a small rotating bur. Debridement must be done carefully so as not to aggravate the bone defect. Optimal debridement is achieved with pulsed washing.

There are several surgical options:

- Bone grafting without reimplantation.
- Conversion to hemiarthroplasty:
  - simple removal of the loosened implant open or arthroscopic [19, 20],
  - implant removal and bone graft (impacted ± screw fixation) [6, 21, 22];
- Anatomic glenoid revision: cemented PE [7] or anatomic metal-back glenoid component [23];

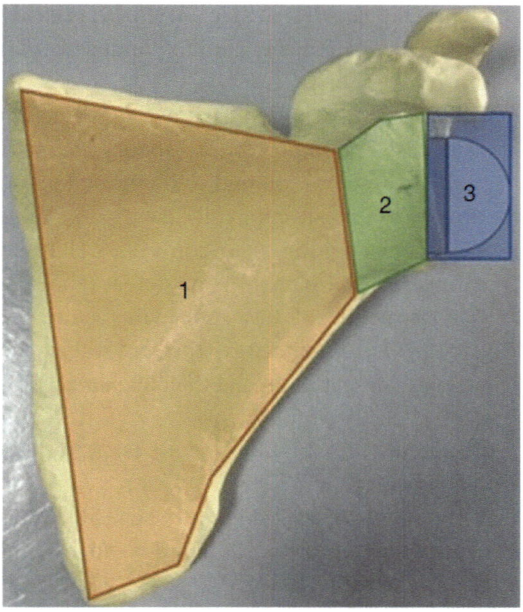

Fig. 13.3 Schematic representation of basic principles by zone

- Reverse glenoid revision: standard implant [24–27], augmented [28], custom-made [29, 30];
- two-stage surgical reconstruction [24],
- conversion to reverse hemiarthroplasty [31].

To clarify the treatment options, we define the following three zones (Fig. 13.3):

- Zone 1 corresponds to the scapula;
- Zone 2 corresponds to the native glenoid;
- Zone 3 corresponds to the glenoid implant.

13.4.3 Simple Removal of the Loosened Implant

When the patient is fragile and is not a candidate for major revision surgery, simple removal of the loosened implant is possible. This intervention, effective on pain, gives only mediocre results on function and mobility [32].

The implant is removed openly or under arthroscopy, and the joint is cleaned at the same time as the cement is removed. The loss of function observed in the aftermath is related to the reduction of the lever arm of the cuff and deltoid by medialization of the humeral head and wear of the remaining glenoid.

Hawkins et al. [33] consider simple ablation as an acceptable alternative to other technical solutions. Cofield and Edgerton [34] reported the results of 9 cases, and only one patient had no pain relief.

In addition, this wear of the bone stock compromises the subsequent possibility of reimplantation of a glenoid [32].

13.4.4 Bone Grafting Without Reimplantation

This option is chosen in case of a major defect to reconstruct the glenoid bone stock. Bone graft impaction is the treatment of choice when the patient is still young, the humeral implant is not loosened, and the rotator cuff can stabilize and center the humeral head. This option may be the first step before reimplantation once the graft is integrated. Although bone grafting is known to be effective in filling in the loss of substance, the type of graft remains a matter of debate. Several options are possible: fragmented or structural graft, allograft, autograft (iliac crest), and synthetic bone (demineralized bone matrix [DBM]).

Antuna et al. [15] report on their experience with impacted cancellous grafts (allograft) and note a significant average medialization (7.5 mm) of the humeral head on the glenoid. Despite this medialization, reimplantation in a second stage was possible in 3 cases. Nevertheless, the reconstructed bone stock available at the time of reimplantation was not equivalent to the initially impacted graft.

Frankle and Long [35] report the results of 14 massive allograft reconstructions during revision surgery. Eleven patients were followed up radiographically, in whom allograft resorption and medialization of the humeral head were found 4 times.

Norris et al. [24, 36, 37] recommend mixing the allograft with DBM. Many commercial forms can be used: Allomatrix custom® (Wright Medical Technology Inc., Memphis, Tennessee),

Dynagraft® (IsoTis OrthoBiologics US, Irvine, California), Grafton® (Osteotech, Eatontown, New Jersey), or Opteform® (Exactech, Gainsville, Florida). The reported results are satisfactory in terms of pain relief, but with progressive graft failure in a high number of cases. Thirteen percent of patients underwent repeated surgery within 3 years for persistent pain with reimplantation of a glenoid.

Our experience [6] with allograft use is similar, with compression and/or resorption of the graft, medialization of the humeral head, and loss of anterior elevation within one year of revision. These results prompted us to use a structural self-graft of iliac origin with the cortical surface facing the humeral head to provide mechanical resistance to medialization.

Young et al. [21] described a glenoid reconstruction technique using tricortical iliac crest graft supplemented with resorbable bone cement and showed that the addition of the resorbable bone cement improved the mechanical stability of the iliac crest tricortical graft used for glenoid reconstruction.

13.4.5 Conversion to Hemiarthroplasty

An intact and functional rotator cuff is the prerequisite for conversion to a HA.

HA remains a viable salvage option for truly unreconstructable glenoid bone loss in complex revision settings and intractable instability in a reverse shoulder replacement [38].

- The first option is to bypass the bone defect and proceed with the simple removal of the loosened implant.
- The removal can be performed open or under arthroscopy. The second solution is often preferred. The aim is to remove the implant minimally invasively through the rotator interval while respecting the subscapularis. This surgical technique was described by O'Driscoll et al. in 2005 [19].
- Under arthroscopy, the PE is fragmented using an osteotome. The PE fragments are extracted through the arthroscopic portals. Only the central block is left in place. If the PE is easily mobilized, it can be entirely removed with grasping forceps.
- Brochin et al. reported satisfactory results on pain at 55 months' follow-up despite poor mobility in elevation and two conversions to RSA (17%, persistent pain) [20].
- The second option is to convert to HA and reconstruct the glenoid bone defect (zone 2). Reconstruction of this zone will restore the lateral offset (reduced by the removal of the glenoid compartment and the bone defect).

Reconstruction of the glenoid is performed with a bone graft.

It is possible to use allograft bone [15], a femoral head allograft block [22], or a bi–/tricortical bone autograft [6, 21, 32].

There are different treatment options depending on whether the glenoid walls are intact (central bone defect) or deficient (combined bone defect).

13.4.6 Central Cavitary Bone Loss

When the walls are intact, our preference goes for an iliac tricortical bone graft. The size of the graft is adapted to the bone loss. The usual indication for this surgical option is the presence of a severe central bone defect. The graft measures approximately 2 cm long, 1 cm wide, and 1 cm thick. The cortical bone graft is contoured and then press-fit into the bone defect (Fig. 13.4).

If the stability of the bone graft is insufficient or when the defect is combined, the graft is secured with screws (absorbable or not) [6]. Note the risk of secondary wear of the bone graft with potential secondary contact with the humeral head.

13.4.7 Combined Bone Loss (Central and Peripheral)

A massive tricortical graft and cancellous bone chips are required. The graft is shaped to fill the defect, temporarily fixed with Kirschner wires,

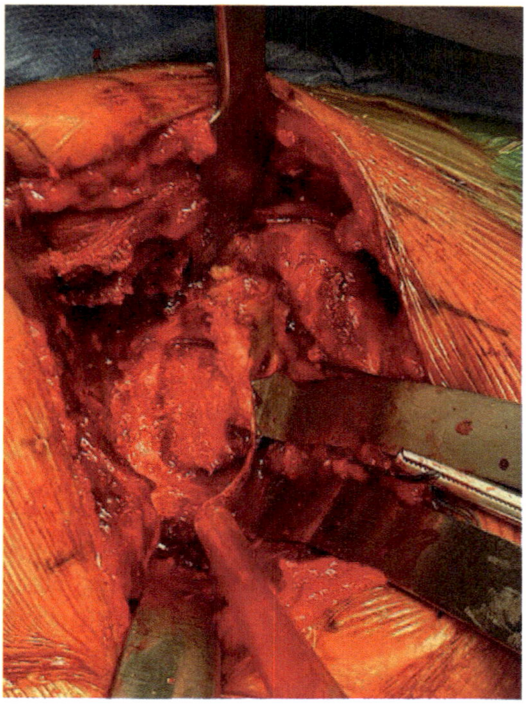

Fig. 13.4 Intraoperative evaluation of massive glenoid bone loss

and then screwed into the native glenoid with 3.5 mm screws. The screwing can be done from lateral to medial, provided that the screw heads are buried to avoid contact with the prosthetic head. Resorbable screws can also be used. Screwing can also be done from the front to the back in case of anterior substance loss. In the case of a posterior defect, exposure may be difficult. Screwing from posterior to anterior can be performed percutaneously through the posterior deltoid and facilitated by using an arthroscopic cannula.

13.4.8 Anatomic Glenoid Revision

Reimplantation of an anatomic glenoid component mostly relies on the status of the glenoid bone stock, the presence of glenohumeral instability, rotator cuff tears, and/or malunion of the greater tuberosity [39].

It is possible if the following criteria are met:

- The bone stock is sufficient in zones 1 and 2, and there is no damage to the walls, therefore, limited central bone loss;
- The rotator cuff is intact and functional;
- There is no associated instability component.

A central guide pin is inserted to restore a satisfactory inclination and a version to prevent eccentric glenoid loading. Minimal reaming is then performed to bring the native glenoid into accordance with the posterior implant design. A cemented PE or a metal base can be implanted.

When a cemented PE is chosen, a keeled implant should be preferred to allow anchorage in zone 2.

Although total shoulder arthroplasty provides better results than HA, glenoid loosening remains a major concern [6].

Also, reimplantation of a glenoid component does not solve the problem of loosening.

Bonnevialle et al. reported iterative loosening in 67% of cases, with a reoperation rate of 21% at a mean follow-up of 6 years [7].

According to the authors, the importance of iterative loosening is related to the preoperative underestimation of prosthetic instability and soft tissue incompetence.

Revision of the glenoid compartment with a metal-back component with anatomical PE is another option. However, this surgical strategy has not been proven to be effective in the long term. Moreover, a revision rate of 37% has been reported at a mean follow-up of 8.5 years in primary TSA, with 80% of revisions showing signs of wear of the PE [23].

13.4.9 Reimplantation of a Cemented Glenoid and Cementoplasty

This option is possible when the bone defect is weak or moderate. The bone loss is filled with cement before cementing the implant. The reported results are better than the simple removal of the loosened implant, but the risk of iterative loosening is high [15, 32, 33, 40].

When the bone defect is more significant, reconstruction is necessary.

13.4.10 Reimplantation of a Cemented Glenoid with a Graft

It is possible to consider an impacted or screw-fixed graft with concomitant cemented glenoid implantation, but this option is at high risk of iterative glenoid loosening with failure of graft fixation.

13.4.11 Reimplantation of an Uncemented Metal-back Glenoid with or without Graft

The use of metal-back implants in revision surgery provides advantages over cemented implants (fixation of a graft, primary stability) [32].

This option is only valid in cases of an intact cuff. In addition, the use of a metal-back implant with an unconstrained prosthesis is at risk of specific complications (PE dissociation, wear) [41, 42].

Antuna et al. [15] reported 8 cases of revision with an unconstrained uncemented glenoid implant. Three did not require grafting (no loss of bone stock or insignificant loss of central substance), and 5 were implanted with cancellous grafting. Although the efficacy on pain was satisfactory, a periprosthetic lucent line was found in 42% of cases in the medium term.

13.4.12 Conversion to Reverse Shoulder Arthroplasty

RSA is nowadays considered the primary option in case of glenoid loosening or failure occurring in association with other major complications such as severe glenoid bone loss, rotator cuff tears, subscapularis insufficiency, and/or prosthetic instability [32, 39, 43].

The two main advantages of an RSA conversion are:

- Reconstruction of the glenoid bone stock by fixing the bone graft with the help of metal back and screws;
- Concomitant management of associated complications by the semi-constrained design of the implant: prosthetic instability, rotator cuff tear, and subscapularis insufficiency.

Restoration of humeral length and glenoid offset (diameter of the glenosphere, lateralization, and inferiorization) of the implant are options to prevent prosthetic instability. The short- and medium-term clinical results are satisfactory. However, the reoperation rate is not negligible (20–21%, of which 64–85% is an arthroplasty revision), as is the glenoid loosening rate (8–17%) [39, 44].

Several treatment options exist:

- One-stage reconstruction;
- Two-stage reconstruction [24].

Revision must comply with a few basic principles:

- Anchoring the implant in zone 1 (scapula);
- Reconstruction of zone 2;
- Restoration of the lateral and inferior offset in zone 3.

The implant anchorage should ideally bridge zone 2 and reach the native scapula in zone 1. This is achieved with the metal-back baseplate with a long post or long central screw. Additional fixation is provided by the peripheral screws.

Different fixation areas are required to ensure the proper fit of the baseplate. In a cadaveric study, Humphrey et al. proposed three fixation areas in the scapula to optimize the fixation of the glenoid component (3-column concept area) [24]. These three columns, which have the highest bone density, are the base of the coracoid, the spine, and the lateral pillar (Fig. 13.5).

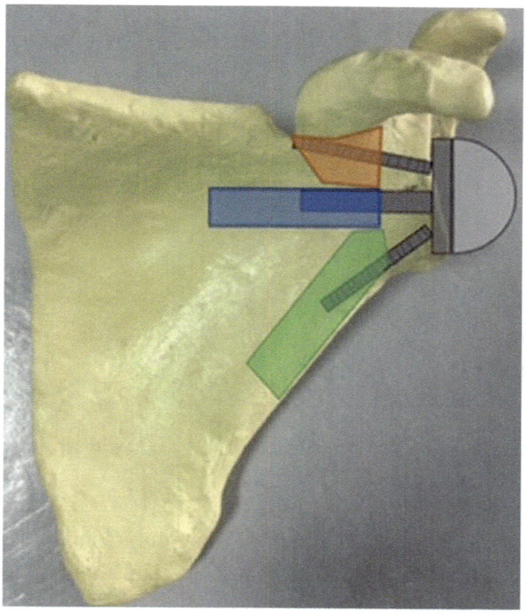

Fig. 13.5 Representation of the three-column concept, with the base of the coracoid in orange, the spine in blue and the lateral pillar in green

13.4.13 Reconstruction in One-Stage

13.4.13.1 Without Associated Grafting

The residual bone stock does not require reconstruction, and the remaining glenoid can be prepared as a native glenoid (placement of the guide pin, reaming, drilling).

Ideally, the baseplate is fully seated on the glenoid. Formaini et al. demonstrated in a biomechanical study that the use of a compensated graft or implant should be considered if the baseplate coverage is less than 50%.

13.4.13.2 With Associated Graft

Bone reconstruction or compensations (zones 1 and 2) should allow zone 3 to be managed by standard glenosphere in conditions as close as possible to those of the primary setting (lateralization, inferiorization, and diameter).

In case of significant loss of central substance or involvement of the walls, it is recommended to reconstruct the bone stock using a massive bone grafting technique. This reconstruction can be performed in one or two stages [9, 31].

If there is more central or combined bone loss and/or less than 50% base coverage, zone 2 reconstruction is required. If the walls are intact, a simple bone graft may be sufficient. If the walls are affected, the native glenoid structure must be restored.

The technique described by Norris is the gold standard [24].

This technique uses an iliac crest graft with a long-peg baseplate (25 or 30 mm) and locked screws. The graft is prepared in situ. To allow immediate solid fixation of the tricortical bone graft, the baseplate is implanted directly on the iliac crest. After exposure of the internal and external tables of the iliac crest, a guide pin is inserted at the top of the crest, targeting between the two bone tables. The base of the metal baseplate is then prepared with a burr, and the hole for the long post is made. The baseplate is attached to the ridge, and an oscillating saw is used to remove the entire iliac bone in one piece.

The bone graft is then trimmed to the volume of the bone defect. A new guide pin is placed in the native glenoid. Norris et al. recommended an entry point of 12 mm above the inferior border of the glenoid. The remaining native glenoid is prepared with a burr, and the center post hole is made. Finally, the basement/bone graft assembly is implanted and secured with locked screws in the areas described above.

To prevent donor site morbidity, the use of a femoral head allograft block has been proposed [25, 26]. The operative technique is similar to the use of an autologous graft. Tashjian et al. recommended perforating the allograft 10 to 15 times with a pin to facilitate integration and bone healing [26].

The allograft is either:

- Fixed temporarily with pins before the metal base is placed [26];
- The baseplate is pre-fixed to the allograft before implantation on the remaining glenoid [25, 45].

Augmented baseplates (half-wedge/full-wedge) have recently been introduced, making it possible to compensate for part of the deficit. Their use in revision surgery with or without

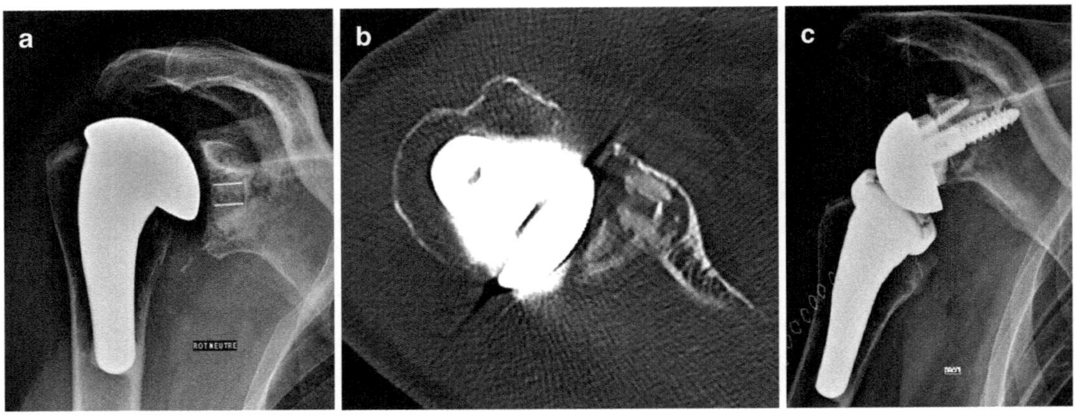

Fig. 13.6 Failure of total shoulder arthroplasty: AP X-Ray view (**a**) and CT scan axial view (**b**). Revision with a reverse shoulder arthroplasty (c)

an associated graft remains to be evaluated (Fig. 13.6).

13.4.14 Customized Augmented Metal Base

This therapeutic option requires specific planning (use of a CT scan and dedicated software) allowing a detailed analysis of the bone stock for precise positioning of the custom-made implant in the native bone. Several authors have reported the use of these augmented implants for first-line arthroplasty [29, 30].

Only Bodendorfer et al. reported short-term clinical results of their use in a mixed cohort (primary and revision setting) for a major glenoid bone defect (30 months follow-up, no loosening) [44].

13.4.15 Two-Stage Revision

Revision of a metal base is almost always possible. The stability of the construct is assessed after the reconstruction of zone 2 and anchoring in zone 1. In some cases, the reduction of the humeral implant may compromise the glenoid reconstruction due to excessive mechanical stress.

A two-stage revision of the glenoid should be considered. The treatment plan may then be as follows:

- The first stage of glenoid reconstruction with bone grafting and fixation of the baseplate with a sphere. The baseplate ensures the primary fixation of the graft.
- Spherical reaming of the humeral head to adapt to the sphere and trans osseous reinsertion of the subscapularis. The humeral component is not implanted to reduce glenoid stress.
- In the second surgical step (3–6 months), after control of the bone integration of the glenoid graft, the reimplantation of the humeral stem is performed.

13.5 Conversion to Reverse Hemiarthroplasty

In some cases, the second stage of surgery is not performed (poor general condition and refusal of general anesthesia, patient refusal). The patient may then be left in reverse HA. Kilian and Edwards, in three cases, reported a significant improvement in pain and function with the remodeling of the greater tuberosity [31]. Therefore, conversion to reverse HA is a viable option in selected patients.

13.6 Conclusion

Revision of a loose glenoid component TSA is a difficult surgery that requires a precise analysis:

- Reason for failure and loosening pattern.
- Implant type and brand.
- Associated complication.
- State of the bone stock and soft tissues.
- Operability of the patient.

Based on these parameters, the optimal operative strategy is defined. Many treatment options are possible, and conversion to RSA is today the preferred option.

References

1. Best MJ, Aziz KT, Wilckens JH, McFarland EG, Srikumaran U. Increasing incidence of primary reverse and anatomic total shoulder arthroplasty in the United States. J Shoulder Elb Surg. 2021;30(5):1159–66. https://doi.org/10.1016/j.jse.2020.08.010.
2. Neyton L, Kirsch JM, Collotte P, Collin P, Gossing L, Chelli M, et al. Mid- to long-term follow-up of shoulder arthroplasty for primary glenohumeral osteoarthritis in patients aged 60 or under. J Shoulder Elb Surg. 2019;28(9):1666–73. https://doi.org/10.1016/j.jse.2019.03.006.
3. Ernstbrunner L, Andronic O, Grubhofer F, Camenzind RS, Wieser K, Gerber C. Long-term results of reverse total shoulder arthroplasty for rotator cuff dysfunction: a systematic review of longitudinal outcomes. J Shoulder Elb Surg. 2019;28(4):774–81. https://doi.org/10.1016/j.jse.2018.10.005.
4. Bacle G, Nové-Josserand L, Garaud P, Walch G. Long-term outcomes of reverse total shoulder arthroplasty. J Bone Joint Surg Am. 2017;99(6):454–61. https://doi.org/10.2106/JBJS.16.00223.
5. Favard L. Revision of total shoulder arthroplasty. Orthop Traumatol Surg Res. 2013;99(Suppl. 1):S12–21. https://doi.org/10.1016/j.otsr.2012.11.010.
6. Neyton L, Walch G, Nové-Josserand L, Edwards TB. Glenoid corticocancellous bone grafting after glenoid component removal in the treatment of glenoid loosening. J Shoulder Elb Surg. 2006;15(2):173–9. https://doi.org/10.1016/j.jse.2005.07.010.
7. Bonnevialle N, Melis B, Neyton L, Favard L, Molé D, Walch G, et al. Aseptic glenoid loosening or failure in total shoulder arthroplasty: revision with glenoid reimplantation. J Shoulder Elb Surg. 2013;22(6):745–51. https://doi.org/10.1016/j.jse.2012.08.009.
8. Wierks C, Skolasky RL, Ji JH, McFarland EG. Reverse total shoulder replacement: intraoperative and early postoperative complications. Clin Orthop Relat Res. 2009;467(1):225–34. https://doi.org/10.1007/s11999-008-0406-1.
9. Sperling JW, Cofield RH, O'Driscoll SW, Torchia ME, Rowland CM. Radiographic assessment of ingrowth total shoulder arthroplasty. J Shoulder Elb Surg. 2000;9(6):507–13. https://doi.org/10.1067/mse.2000.109384.
10. Molé D, Roche O, Riand N, Lévigne C, Walch G. Cemented glenoid component: results in osteoarthritis and rheumatoid arthritis. In: Walch G, Boileau P, editors. Shoulder arthroplasty. Springer Science & Business Media; 2012. p. 163–71.
11. Lazarus MD, Jensen KL, Southworth C, Matsen FA. The radiographic evaluation of keeled and pegged glenoid component insertion. J Bone Joint Surg Am. 2002;84(7):1174–82. https://doi.org/10.2106/00004623-200207000-00013.
12. Deutsch A, Abboud JA, Kelly J, Mody M, Norris T, Ramsey ML, et al. Clinical results of revision shoulder arthroplasty for glenoid component loosening. J Shoulder Elb Surg. 2007;16(6):706–16. https://doi.org/10.1016/j.jse.2007.01.007.
13. Cheung EV, Sperling JW, Cofield RH. Revision shoulder arthroplasty for glenoid component loosening. J Shoulder Elb Surg. 2008;17(3):371–5. https://doi.org/10.1016/j.jse.2007.09.003.
14. Lucas RM, Hsu JE, Whitney IJ, Wasserburger J, Matsen FA. Loose glenoid components in revision shoulder arthroplasty: is there an association with positive cultures? J Shoulder Elb Surg. 2016;25(8):1371–5. https://doi.org/10.1016/j.jse.2015.12.026.
15. Antuna SA, Sperling JW, Cofield RH, Rowland CM. Glenoid revision surgery after total shoulder arthroplasty. J Shoulder Elb Surg. 2001;10(3):217–24. https://doi.org/10.1067/mse.2001.113961.
16. Wallace AL, Phillips RL, MacDougal GA, Walsh WR, Sonnabend DH. Resurfacing of the glenoid in total shoulder arthroplasty. A comparison, at a mean of five years, of prostheses inserted with and without cement. J Bone Joint Surg Am. 1999;81(4):510–8. https://doi.org/10.2106/00004623-199904000-00008.
17. Gupta A, Thussbas C, Koch M, Seebauer L. Management of glenoid bone defects with reverse shoulder arthroplasty—surgical technique and clinical outcomes. J Shoulder Elb Surg. 2018 May;27(5):853–62. https://doi.org/10.1016/j.jse.2017.10.004.
18. Barco R, Savvidou OD, Sperling JW, Sanchez-Sotelo J, Cofield RH. Complications in reverse shoulder arthroplasty. EFORT Open Rev. 2017;1(3):72–80. https://doi.org/10.1302/2058-5241.1.160003.
19. O'Driscoll SW, Petrie RS, Torchia ME. Arthroscopic removal of the glenoid component for failed total shoulder arthroplasty. A report of five cases. J Bone Joint Surg Am. 2005;87(4):858–63. https://doi.org/10.2106/JBJS.C.01732.
20. Brochin RL, Zastrow RK, Patel AV, Parsons BO, Flatow EL, Cagle PJ. Arthroscopic glenoid removal for aseptic loosening in total shoulder arthroplasty.

Semin Arthroplasty: JSES. 2021;31(2):197–201. https://doi.org/10.1053/j.sart.2020.11.012.
21. Young AA, Neyton L, Molony DC, Boileau P, Walch G. Glenoid tricortical iliac crest structural bone graft enhanced with resorbable cement for the treatment of aseptic glenoid loosening. Tech Shoulder Elbow Surg. 2011;12(1):12–7. https://doi.org/10.1097/BTE.0b013e31820b3517.
22. Scalise JJ, Iannotti JP. Bone grafting severe glenoid defects in revision shoulder arthroplasty. Clin Orthop Relat Res. 2008;466(1):139–45. https://doi.org/10.1007/s11999-007-0065-7.
23. Boileau P, Moineau G, Morin-Salvo N, Avidor C, Godenèche A, Lévigne C, et al. Metal-backed glenoid implant with polyethylene insert is not a viable long-term therapeutic option. J Shoulder Elb Surg. 2015;24(10):1534–43. https://doi.org/10.1016/j.jse.2015.02.012.
24. Norris TR, Ii JDK, Humphrey CS. Management of glenoid bone defects in revision shoulder arthroplasty: a new application of the reverse total shoulder prosthesis. Tech Should Elb Surg. 2007;8:37–46. https://doi.org/10.1097/BTE.0B013E318030D3B7.
25. Ozgur SE, Sadeghpour R, Norris TR. Revision shoulder arthroplasty with a reverse shoulder prosthesis. Orthopade. 2017;46(12):1055–62. https://doi.org/10.1007/s00132-017-3494-3.
26. Tashjian RZ, Broschinsky K, Stertz I, Chalmers PN. Structural glenoid allograft reconstruction during reverse total shoulder arthroplasty. J Shoulder Elb Surg. 2020;29(3):534–40. https://doi.org/10.1016/j.jse.2019.07.011.
27. Taylor JR, Schrumpf MA, Shea KE, Kelly JD. Distal clavicle autograft augmentation for glenoid bone loss in revision shoulder arthroplasty: results and technique. J Shoulder Elb Surg. 2020;29(10):e386–93. https://doi.org/10.1016/j.jse.2020.05.009.
28. Jones RB, Wright TW, Roche CP. Bone grafting the glenoid versus use of augmented glenoid baseplates with reverse shoulder arthroplasty. Bull Hosp Jt Dis (2013). 2015;73(Suppl. 1):S129–35.
29. Berger NM, Craig EV, Petrigliano FA. The use of a custom glenoid component for the treatment of severe glenoid bone loss in reverse total shoulder arthroplasty. Tech Should Elbow Surg. 2014;15(2):51–4. https://doi.org/10.1097/BTE.0000000000000008.
30. Stoffelen DVC, Eraly K, Debeer P. The use of 3D printing technology in reconstruction of a severe glenoid defect: a case report with 2.5 years of follow-up. J Shoulder Elb Surg. 2015;24(8):e218–22. https://doi.org/10.1016/j.jse.2015.04.006.
31. Kilian CM, Edwards TB. Reverse hemiarthroplasty? What happens when a patient forgoes the second stage of a 2-stage glenoid bone graft reconstruction in revision shoulder arthroplasty: a report of 3 cases. JSES Open Access. 2017;1(2):79–84. https://doi.org/10.1016/j.jses.2017.06.005.
32. Neyton L, Sirveaux F, Roche O, Molé D, Boileau P, Walch G. Résultats des reprises pour descellement glénoïdien. Rev Chir Orthop Reparatrice Appar Mot. 2004;90(2):111–21. https://doi.org/10.1016/s0035-1040(04)70032-x.
33. Hawkins RJ, Greis PE, Bonutti PM. Treatment of symptomatic glenoid loosening following unconstrained shoulder arthroplasty. Orthopedics. 1999;22(2):229–34. https://doi.org/10.3928/0147-7447-19990201-13.
34. Cofield RH, Edgerton BC. Total shoulder arthroplasty: complications and revision surgery. Instr Course Lect. 1990;39:449–62. PMID: 2186136
35. Frankle MA, Long RA. Glenoid component failure treated with a bulk allograft for revision total surgery. In: Presented at the 18th Annual Meeting of the American Shoulder and Elbow Surgeons ; Napa, Calif October 24–27, 2001; 2001.
36. Hill JM, Norris TR. Long-term results of total shoulder arthroplasty following bone-grafting of the glenoid. J Bone Joint Surg Am. 2001;83(6):877–83.
37. Neer CS II, editor. Shoulder reconstruction. Philadelphie: Saunders; 1990.
38. Malhas A, Rashid A, Copas D, Bale S, Trail I. Glenoid bone loss in primary and revision shoulder arthroplasty. Should Elbow. 2016;8(4):229–40. https://doi.org/10.1177/1758573216648601.
39. Melis B, Bonnevialle N, Neyton L, Lévigne C, Favard L, Walch G, et al. Glenoid loosening and failure in anatomical total shoulder arthroplasty: is revision with a reverse shoulder arthroplasty a reliable option? J Shoulder Elb Surg. 2012;21(3):342–9. https://doi.org/10.1016/j.jse.2011.05.021.
40. Bohsali KI, Wirth MA, Rockwood CA. Complications of total shoulder arthroplasty. Current concepts review. J Bone Joint Surg Am. 2006;88(10):2279–92. https://doi.org/10.2106/JBJS.F.0012.
41. Boileau P, Avidor C, Walch G. Prothèse totale d'épaule avec un implant glénoïdien métallique non scellé: étude prospective de 354 implants suivis à plus de deux ans. In: Boileau P, Walch G, Molé D, editors. 2000 shoulder prostheses: two-to-ten-year follow-up. Montpellier: Sauramps Médical; 2001. p. 489–507.
42. Cofield RH, Daly PJ. Total shoulder arthroplasty with a tissue-ingrowth glenoid component. J Shoulder Elb Surg. 1992;1(2):77–85. https://doi.org/10.1016/S1058-2746(09)80124-9.
43. Neyton L, Boileau P, Nové-Josserand L, Edwards TB, Walch G. Glenoid bone grafting with a reverse design prosthesis. J Shoulder Elb Surg. 2007;16(Suppl. 3):S71–8. https://doi.org/10.1016/j.jse.2006.02.002.
44. Bodendorfer BM, Loughran GJ, Looney AM, Velott AT, Stein JA, Lutton DM, et al. Short-term outcomes of reverse shoulder arthroplasty using a custom baseplate for severe glenoid deficiency. J Shoulder Elb Surg. 2021;30(5):1060–7. https://doi.org/10.1016/j.jse.2020.08.002.
45. Jones RB, Wright TW, Zuckerman JD. Reverse total shoulder arthroplasty with structural bone grafting of large glenoid defects. J Shoulder Elb Surg. 2016;25(9):1425–32. https://doi.org/10.1016/j.jse.2016.01.016.

14 Revising a Failed Glenoid in Reverse Total Shoulder Arthroplasty

Akshay V. Daji and Howard Routman

14.1 Incidence of Glenoid Revision in rTSA

With an increasing number of patients undergoing total shoulder arthroplasty and expanding indications for reverse total shoulder arthroplasty (RSA), there has been an increase in the incidence of RSA failures [1, 2]. Component survival for primary RSA is high at 93% [3]; however, functional outcomes at 10 years range from 58% to 76% [4, 5]. Revision rates and outcomes following revision RSA are poor compared to outcomes following primary RSA [4, 5]. Zumstein et al. found revision rates following primary and revision RSA to be 6% and 16%, respectively [6]. Complication rates range from 10% for primary RSA versus 40% for revision RSA [7]. Although relatively rare, glenoid-sided complications often lead to failure of the construct as a whole, with significant challenges presented to revise the component [8]. Reasons for failure of the glenoid component can be due to patient-related factors such as trauma, poor bone quality or ingrowth failure, or surgical factors like component malpositioning, postoperative infection, suprascapular neuropathy from errant screw placement, central screw fatigue and failure, and high-grade scapular notching with resultant destabilization of a well-fixed glenoid component. Superior placement or inclination of the glenosphere can result in excessive shear forces that compromise bone-implant fixation. If at the time of the index procedure, a bone graft was used behind the glenoid component, poor initial fixation or subsequent graft resorption can also result in glenoid component loosening.

With improvements in design, fixation, and surgical technique, glenoid components in reverse shoulder arthroplasty have been shown to be fairly durable in the absence of infection or high-grade scapular notching which results in polyethylene liner wear and osteolysis. Glenoid-sided complications include baseplate loosening, mechanical failure, acromial or scapular fracture with secondary decoupling of the scapula, high grade notching, and glenosphere dissociation [9]. Other infrequent reasons for the need to revise a glenoid like peri-prosthetic fractures occur but are rare. An early design of the Grammont prosthesis included a threaded glenosphere which screwed onto the baseplate. Cases of the glenosphere unscrewing itself have been reported, but this design was ultimately

A. V. Daji
HCA Florida JFK Hospital/University of Miami Miller School of Medicine Orthopaedic Surgery Residency Program, Palm Beach, FL, USA
e-mail: axd2048@miami.edu

H. Routman (✉)
HCA Florida JFK Hospital/University of Miami Miller School of Medicine Orthopaedic Surgery Residency Program, Palm Beach, FL, USA

Palm Beach Shoulder Service at Atlantis Orthopaedics, Palm Beach Gardens, FL, USA
e-mail: hdr@floridashoulder.com

F. Franceschi et al. (eds.), *Revision Shoulder Arthroplasty*,
https://doi.org/10.1007/978-3-031-45944-3_14

abandoned. The overall rate of glenoid-sided complications in the literature ranges from 0 to 60% [10]. The reported mechanical glenosphere failure rate differs based on RSA design with a range of 0–6.3% failure rate for the Grammont design [11–13] versus 0–11.7% for the DJO design [14, 15].

Options following glenoid-sided failure of RSA are revision RSA or in the setting of salvage operations, conversion to hemiarthroplasty, placement of an antibiotic spacer in the setting of infection, or glenohumeral arthrodesis [16, 17].

14.2 Imaging and Physical Exam Findings

Evaluation of failed RSA should begin with a careful history and physical exam. Determining whether a patients' chief complaint is pain, loss of function, or a combination of both can be helpful in delineating an etiology. Mechanical failure of the baseplate often results in both pain and loss of function. Particular attention should be paid to the postoperative course, chronicity of symptoms, as well as any history of trauma to the shoulder. Specific patient complaints that may be indicative of glenoid failure are mechanical symptoms such as crunching, catching, clicking, or metallic squeaking that can be audible.

Physical exam should begin with inspection assessing the previous incision, noting the approach, quality of the tissue, and for any signs of deformity or muscle atrophy. Particular attention should be paid to assessing for signs of infection including erythema, cellulitis, swelling, or drainage. Additionally, patients should be asked about any risk factors conferring susceptibility to infection including prior history of infection, diabetes with poor glycemic control, immunosuppression, and recent surgery or dental procedures. Neurovascular status should also be assessed with particular attention toward axillary nerve function.

Radiographic evaluation of glenoid failure begins with obtaining anteroposterior (AP), Grashey, axillary, and scapular Y views of the shoulder. Standard radiographs will allow the surgeon to evaluate for periprosthetic fracture, implant dislocation, and component malpositioning or loosening. Specifically, AP views establish implant position and may inform on inadequate soft tissue tension if inferior subluxation is present. Additionally, AP views may demonstrate malpositioned screws violating the suprascapular or spinoglenoid notch causing shoulder pain and weakness of the external rotators. This is uncommon with only a few case reports describing this occurrence in the literature however is treatable with the removal of the offending hardware or transection of the screw as it enters the notch [18, 19]. Confirmation of malpositioned screws can be achieved with an EMG study, advanced imaging, or a diagnostic injection of the notch [20]. Axillary views will demonstrate frank dislocation as well as allow for determination of glenosphere version. Common radiographic findings associated with glenoid loosening are proximal migration and superior inclination of the component. Migration may be a subtle process or acute in the setting of trauma. If possible, prior radiographs from the index operation and follow-up visits should be obtained. CT scans with metal artifact subtraction are helpful for evaluation of glenoid morphology, medialization, implant orientation, available bone stock, as well as potential impingement. Additionally, CT scans may demonstrate acromion or scapula fractures not appreciable on standard radiographs. Traditionally, the ability to use CT scans to preoperatively plan in 3D revision glenoid surgery has been limited because of the metallic artifact on the images, but recent developments have improved our ability to use traditional 3D planning software to plan revision reconstructions.

14.3 Published Results of Reverse-to-Reverse Revision Shoulder Arthroplasty

Although outcomes are not as good compared to primary RSA for rotator cuff arthropathy, massive rotator cuff tear, and osteoarthritis, revision RSA for failed primary RSA can be a reasonable salvage procedure. A retrospective review found an overall complication rate of 25% after primary RTSA and a 69% after revision RTSA [21]. A single institution, retrospective review of 27 patients with who underwent revision RSA found that the 5 year survival free of further revision was 85% with a 4% risk of further revision each postoperative year. Although the revision rate is higher than primary RSA, patients experienced significant pain relief and improvements in ROM and function [16]. Periprosthetic dislocation was found to be the most common complication and is the most common indication for further revision following revision RSA. Attenuation of soft tissues and difficult intraoperative assessment of tensioning are thought to contribute to the high instability and dislocation rate. This poses unique challenges given the diminished glenoid bone stock associated with revision RSA from glenoid-sided failure and that the second most frequent complication is glenoid loosening. During revision rTSA, a balance has to be struck between lateralizing the glenoid to improve prosthesis stability while reducing shear forces on the glenoid to ensure adequate glenoid fixation and decreased glenoid loosening. Additionally, surgeons must keep in mind the high rate of traction injury to the axillary nerve in revision RSA. When testing stability intraoperatively, surgeons should also keep in mind that scarring will tighten attenuated soft tissues in the postoperative period.

Future studies analyzing the complication and revision rate following revision RSA for failed RSA due to glenoid-sided complications are required given the unique challenges associated with this failure type.

14.4 Special Considerations: Surgical Exposure for Revising a Reverse Glenoid

Exposure of the glenoid in the revision setting is more difficult due to scarring, adhesion formation, and loss of normal surgical planes. Adequate exposure is crucial for the evaluation of glenoid bone stock as well as proper positioning of revision components. Superficial dissection can be more complicated in that even the deltopectoral interval can be hard to identify which can lead to denervation of a part of the deltoid during dissection. The layer between the pectoralis, the deltoid, and the conjoined tendon is frequently completely scarred together and at times the conjoined tendon, which is an important landmark to avoid medial dissection and surgical misadventure, can be very difficult to find. It is critical to remain patient during revision dissections and re-establish these planes as best as possible, with particular attention toward identifying the coracoid process and working lateral to the conjoined tendon to avoid inadvertent medial dissection into the plexus or vascular structures. The subscapularis can also be difficult to mobilize in revision arthroplasty and the area around the subscapularis for mobilization is prone to bleeding. Placement of a Fukuda or double pronged Bankart retractor on the posterior rim of the glenoid will aid in exposure of the inferior glenoid by displacing the proximal humerus posterolaterally and placing the postero-inferior capsule under tension. Particular care and attention should be paid to addressing the inferior rind of tissue that is frequently identified at revision reverse arthroplasty surgery; however, care must be taken because of its close proximity to neurovascular structures. A blunt Hohman can be placed between inferior capsule and the axillary nerve to protect it. With the nerve protected, capsule can be split or excised, depending on surgeon preference, to complete the inferior release of the glenoid. Frequently, this thickened inferior capsule is present in revision reverse patients that can block the insertion of spheres and limit visibility of the glenoid. Release and/or resection of this inferior rind will also improve postoperative arm abduction range of motion; however, the axillary nerve is directly underneath this structure, and resection needs to be done carefully. Following release of the anterior capsule, a double pronged Bankart retractor can be placed on the scapular neck to further expose the glenoid. Abduction and external rotation can aid in glenoid visualization but should be utilized with caution as these maneuvers can put excessive traction on the brachial plexus. Finally, the risk of intraoperative vascular injury is higher in revision shoulder arthroplasty and having a plan in place with vascular surgery support and supplies should be a part of the preoperative plan, especially in cases of bone deformity resulting in medialization of the humerus.

14.5 Special Considerations: What to Do If the Glenoid Component Is Stuck

With improvements in prosthesis design and porous trabecular metals, removing glenoid components while preserving bone stock has become an increasingly challenging problem. Preoperative preparation is critical to success. Instruments to consider having in the operating room include implant extraction tools, rigid and flexible osteotomes, microsagittal saws, and pencil tip high-speed burrs. Additionally well-fixed titanium screws are easy to strip so it may behoove surgeons to have screw removal kits ready. Specific technique to remove baseplates are dependent on implant type but generally require undercutting the baseplate with a high-speed burr. If this is unsuccessful in removing the baseplate, the center holes can be connected with a drill and explanted with a slap hammer (Fig. 14.1). If the baseplate remains well fixed, then the centerpost can be undercut, leaving the central design feature in the glenoid (Figs. 14.2 and 14.3). This technique produces large amounts of titanium dust which can be captured by putting sterile ultrasound gel in the wound prior to burring. Following glenoid retrieval, the gel and captured titanium shavings can be suctioned out.

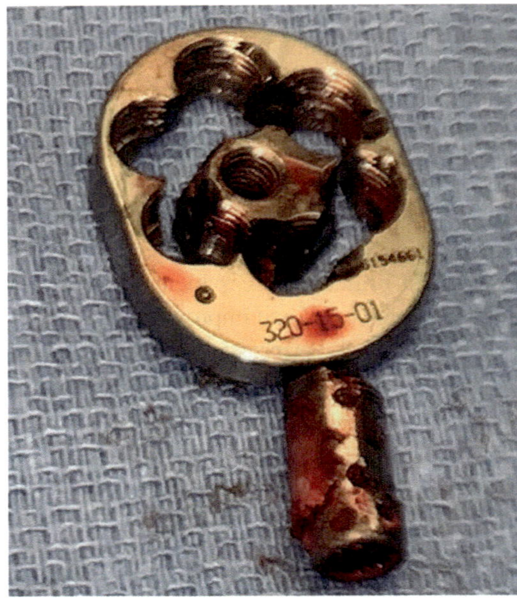

Fig. 14.1 Baseplate removed by connecting the center holes with a drill and explanting with a slap hammer. Photo courtesy of Howard Routman, DO

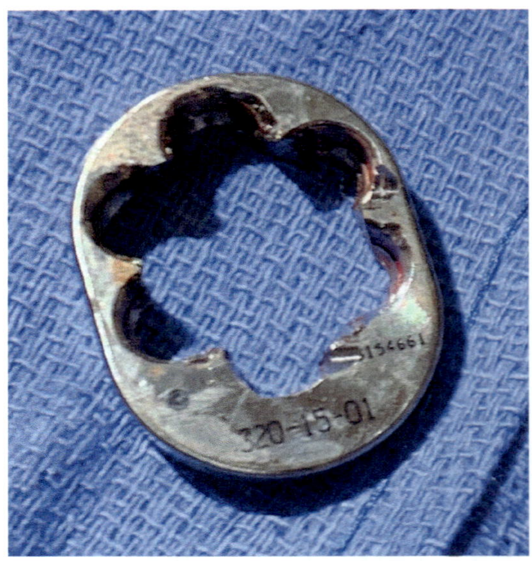

Fig. 14.2 Explanted baseplate with central design feature left in the glenoid. Photo courtesy of Howard Routman, DO

14.6 Special Considerations: Anticipate There Will Be Bone Loss

The implant used during the primary surgery can impact how much bone stock is available following the removing of the glenoid component in revision RSA for failed glenoids. Bone loss is variable and highly dependent on primary implant used, mode of failure, and the technique used to remove implant. Implants with a central screw only (Figs. 14.4a and 14.5a) with no in-vault on-growth design feature obtain long-term fixation onto the back of the baseplate only, whereas implants with in-growth material that resides in the vault (Figs. 14.4b and 14.5b) achieve on-growth inside the vault as well as onto the back side of the baseplate. Implants that have intra-osseous cages or long posts can obtain on-growth or through-growth inside the scapula. The unique features of each of these designs are critical to understand in order to remove the implant with minimal trauma and maximal bone stock preservation.

The Walch classification system is of little utility in the revision setting as patterns of bone loss are highly variable. Unaddressed superior erosion as classified by Sirveaux can be helpful as it can help the surgeon avoid glenoid malposition at the time of revision. Characterizing glenoid bone loss as either contained or uncontained (Fig. 14.6) or centric or eccentric (Figs. 14.7 and 14.8) will assist in determining how to best address the deficiencies [22, 23]. Options for addressing glenoid bone loss include augmented or patient-specific glenoids [24], alternative base plate positioning, and bone grafting.

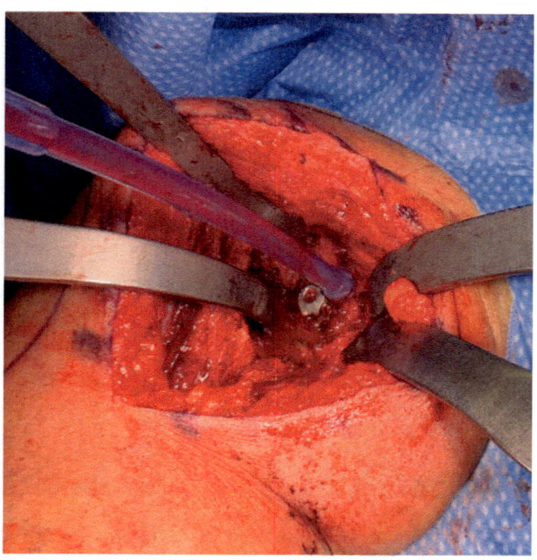

Fig. 14.3 Central design feature left in the glenoid by undercutting the centerpost. Photo courtesy of Howard Routman, DO

The amount of back-side baseplate coverage acceptable to proceed without graft varies from surgeon to surgeon and from implant to implant. Smaller baseplates with less opportunity for on-growth should have greater percentage contact, whereas larger baseplates with a large surface area and implants that have extensions for on-growth into the vault and scapula can tolerate less percentage contact with the glenoid face while remaining stable. If there is greater than 60–80% of bony coverage, then baseplate implantation can be achieved without the use of bone graft [25].

In cases of glenoid bone loss, Klein et al. has described an alternative technique whereby a post is placed within the scapular spine (the alternate center line) as opposed to the standard glenoid centerline referenced to the inferior rim [26]. This technique allows for robust initial fixation with a center screw despite glenoid bone loss and demonstrated no significant difference in ASES postoperative scores. Disadvantages of this technique include the risk of scapular body and spine fractures and possible impingement given the superior position of the baseplate. As such, this technique necessitates the use of a lateralized baseplate or glenosphere to limit impingement with adduction.

In cases of more significant glenoid bone loss, grafting is warranted. Debate exists regarding the indications for one- or two-stage procedures. Seidl et al. argues that two-stage procedures are rarely indicated unless infection is present or there is inadequate or excessive tension on the construct [25].

Defects can be characterized as contained or uncontained depending on if there is glenoid rim deficiency. With contained, central bone loss,

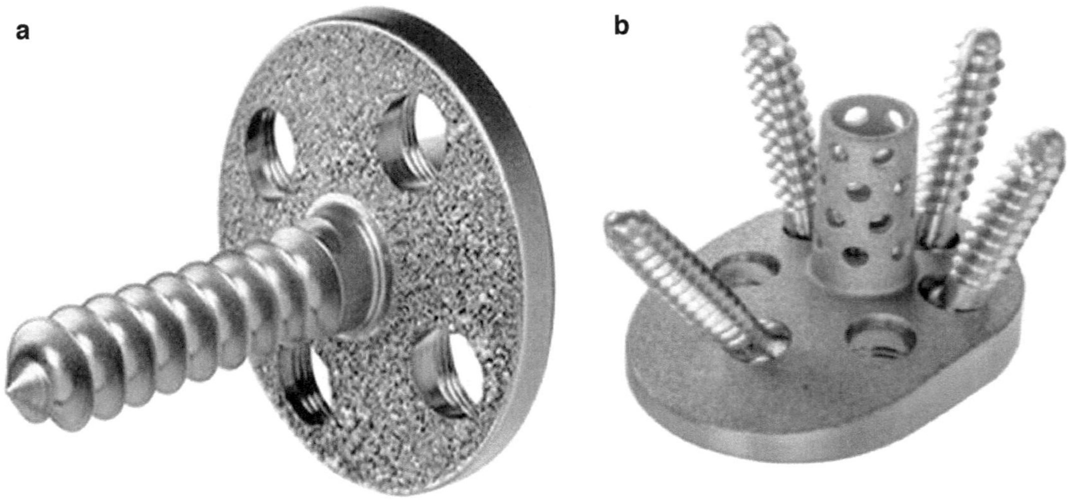

Fig. 14.4 (**a** and **b**) No in-vault osteointegration (left) versus in-vault osteointegration (right). (Figure **a** reproduced with permission from Walker, Matthew, Derek Pupello, and Mark Frankle. "Rationale, technique, and results of the DJO surgical reverse total shoulder arthroplasty." Operative Techniques in Orthopaedics 2011;21(1): 60–68. Figure **b** reproduced with permission from Jones, Richard B., et al. Accuracy and precision of placement of the glenoid baseplate in reverse total shoulder arthroplasty using a novel computer assisted navigation system combined with preoperative planning: a controlled cadaveric study. Seminars in Arthroplasty: JSES. 2020;30(1). WB Saunders)

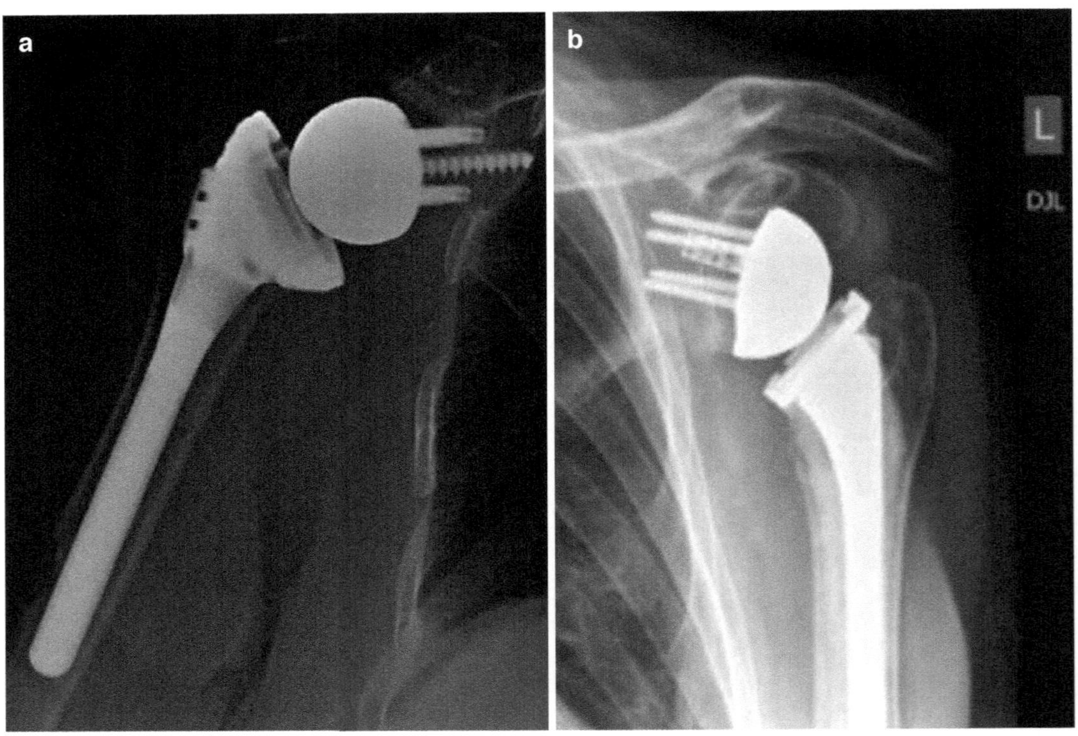

Fig. 14.5 (**a** and **b**) Radiographs of DJO central screw glenoid (left) versus in-vault osteointegration (right). (Figure **a** reproduced with permission from Ho, Jason C., et al. "Early radiographic failure of reverse total shoulder arthroplasty with structural bone graft for glenoid bone loss." Journal of Shoulder and Elbow Surgery 2020;29(3): 550–560. Figure **b** reproduced with permission from Jones, Richard B., Thomas W. Wright, and Joseph D. Zuckerman. "Reverse total shoulder arthroplasty with structural bone grafting of large glenoid defects." Journal of Shoulder and Elbow Surgery 2016;25(9):1425–1432)

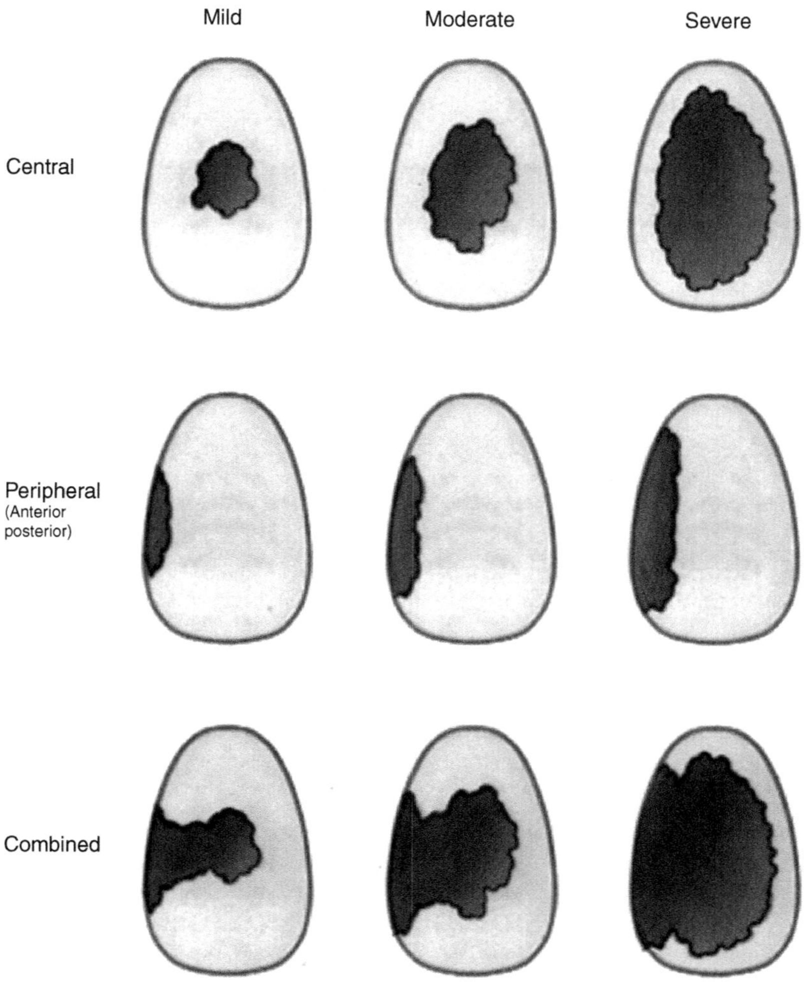

Fig. 14.6 Top row demonstrates contained glenoid defects, while bottom two rows demonstrate uncontained defects. (Reproduced with permission from Antuna, Samuel A., et al. "Glenoid revision surgery after total shoulder arthroplasty." *Journal of Shoulder and Elbow Surgery* 2001;10(3):217–224)

cancellous bone graft can be used to fill the void (Fig. 14.9). When cortical bone loss compromises the glenoid rim, corticocancellous bone graft can be utilized with the cortical surface facing laterally. This will prevent subsidence and medialization of the glenoid component [12].

Tricortical iliac crest autograft is commonly used to supplement glenoid bone deficits. A technique described by Norris et al. consists of implanting the long peg baseplate directly into the iliac crest prior to graft harvest [27]. Autograft is then harvested using osteotomes or an oscillating saw. Rongeurs or osteotomes can be used to then contour the graft to fill the glenoid defect. The graft is then impacted into the defect and secured with compression screws. A key benefit of this technique is the robust fixation of the baseplate to the autograft. A case series of 12 patients found ASES scores improved significantly with this technique with 80% of patients reporting that they were either satisfied or very satisfied [28]. Iliac crest autograft can also be used to fill the glenoid defect freely prior to implantation of the baseplate. Although this technique confers the advantage of being able to place a central wire in the glenoid without obstruction of anatomic landmarks, this is a more technically difficult and time-consuming process. Although humeral head is not an available option for autograft in revision settings, distal clavicle can be used as a local source of autograft bone.

Allograft can be used in combination or as a substitute for iliac crest autograft. An advantage of allograft usage is the lack of donor site mor-

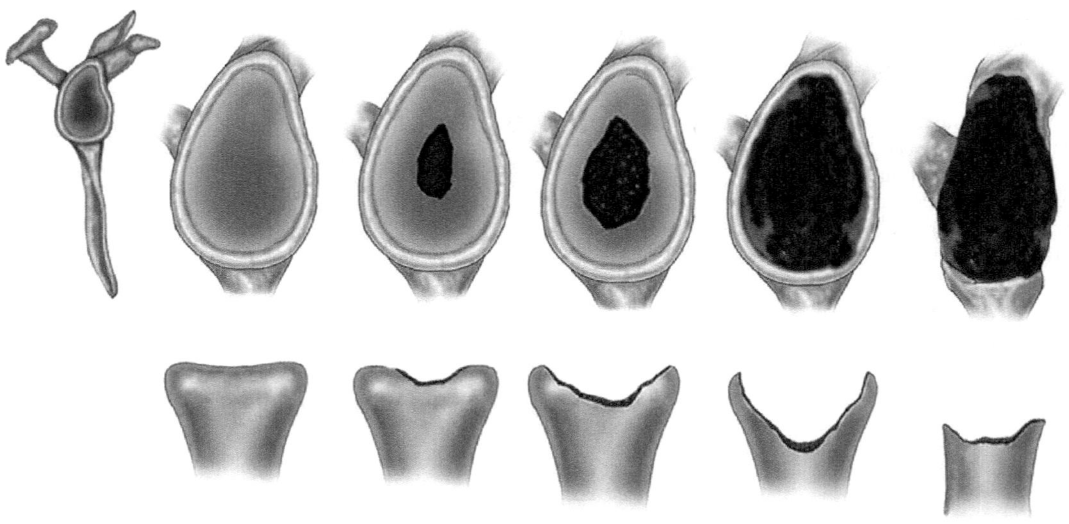

Fig. 14.7 Centric glenoid defects. (Reproduced with permission from Gupta A, Thussbas C, Koch M, Seebauer L. Management of glenoid bone defects with reverse shoulder arthroplasty—surgical technique and clinical outcomes. Journal of Shoulder and Elbow Surgery. 2018 May 1;27(5):853–62)

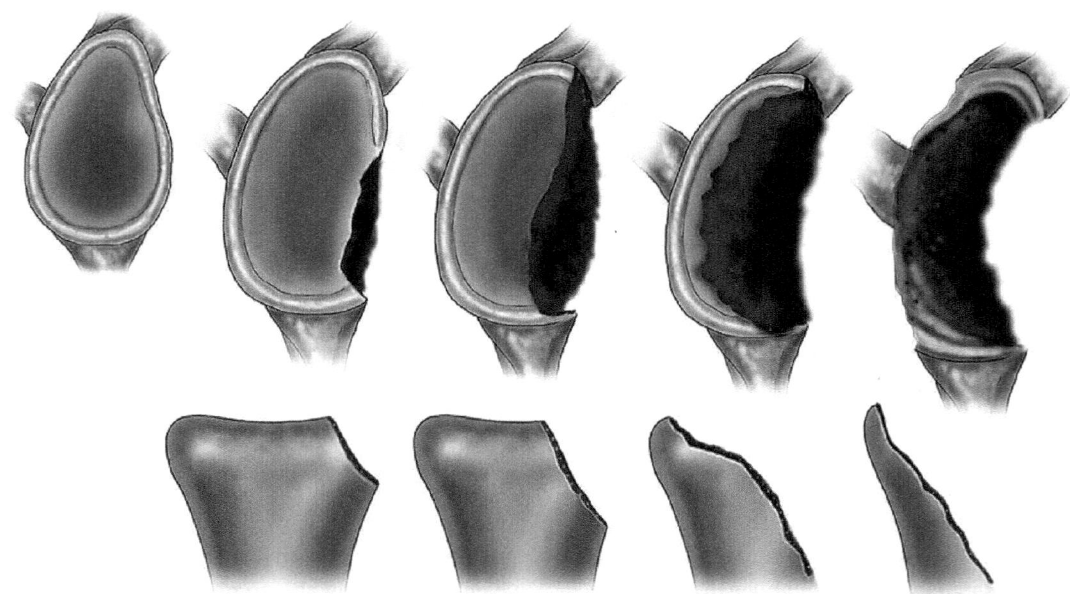

Fig. 14.8 Eccentric glenoid defects. (Reproduced with permission from Gupta A, Thussbas C, Koch M, Seebauer L. Management of glenoid bone defects with reverse shoulder arthroplasty—surgical technique and clinical outcomes. Journal of Shoulder and Elbow Surgery. 2018 May 1;27(5):853–62)

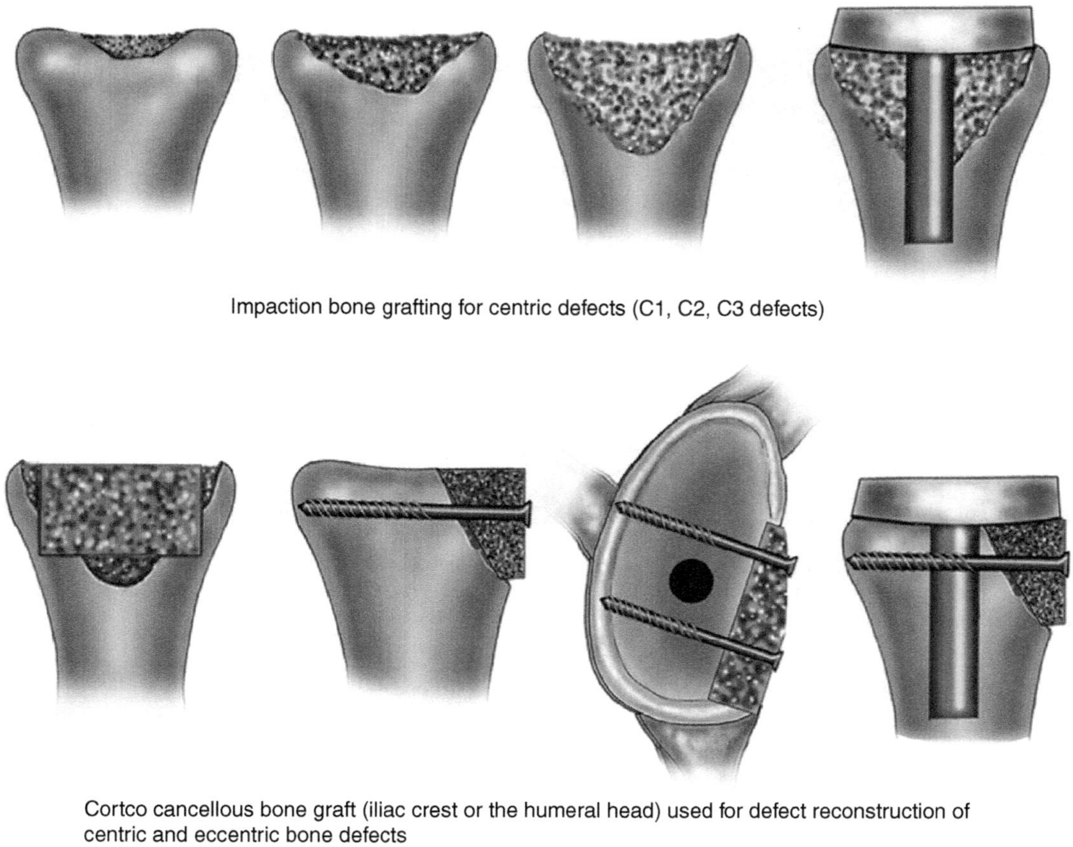

Fig. 14.9 Defect reconstruction technique differs based on centricity of defect. (Reproduced with permission from Gupta A, Thussbas C, Koch M, Seebauer L. Management of glenoid bone defects with reverse shoulder arthroplasty—surgical technique and clinical outcomes. Journal of Shoulder and Elbow Surgery. 2018 May 1;27(5):853–62)

bidity. Femoral neck allograft is a good choice given its dimensions mimic that of the glenoids and a study of 5 patients who underwent single-stage hybrid autograft and allografting of a glenoid defect demonstrated CT-confirmed graft incorporation for all 5 patients with no evidence of baseplate loosening [29]. A larger retrospective review comparing 44 patients who underwent either femoral head allografting, humeral head, or iliac crest autografting behind the baseplate found no difference in functional outcomes [24].

Augmented glenoid components have emerged as a popular alternative to bone grafting in the setting of glenoid bone loss. Studies are limited in the revision setting; however, Virk et al. found the use of augmented baseplates in primary RSA in patients with posterior glenoid wear to have good clinical and radiographic outcomes [30]. Advantages of augmented components over bone grafting primarily relate to donor site morbidity as well as the increased operative time and complications associated with graft retrieval, shaping, and fixation. An additional benefit is the baseplate rests against native bone potentially providing greater initial stability. Although bone grafting under a glenoid baseplate may compromise initial stability, if graft incorporation is achieved, the lever arm from the center of rotation is shorter reducing torque forces acting on the glenoid. In additional to a more favorable biomechanical profile, bone grafting has the

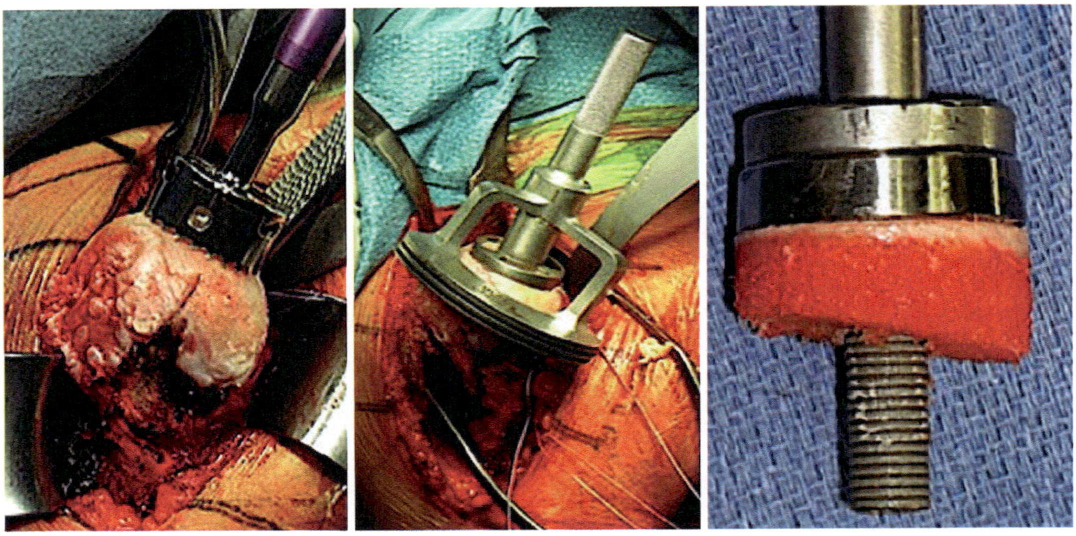

Fig. 14.10 Instrumentation for autograft harvesting. (Reproduced with permission from Beuckelaers, Ellen, et al. "Three-dimensional computed tomography scan evaluation of the pattern of erosion in type B glenoids." Journal of Shoulder and Elbow Surgery. 2014;23(1):109–116)

potential to add to native bone stock and restore or even lateralize the joint line. This may be critical given the high risk of reoperation following revision RSA. Lastly, bone graft has the advantage of being able to be shaped to fill the defect in the glenoid, whereas there is limited variability in augment shape and size and native glenoid has to be removed to ensure the augment fits. Instrumentation for allograft harvest can be the same as used for the bony-increased offset (BIO) RSA technique used to correct glenoid deficiency with humeral head autograft in primary RSA (Fig. 14.10).

Computer-aided manufacturing technology and 3D printing have garnered increased attention in orthopedics over the past few years as a solution for severe bone loss. Due to the early success of custom acetabular implants in THA [31], Zimmer Biomet developed the Comprehensive Vault Reconstruction System (VRS) patient-specific implant as a solution for severe glenoid bone loss in TSA. Proposed benefits include the ability to match the surface of the deformed glenoid and provide an adequately oriented and lateralized surface for the glenosphere. Potential benefits have to be balanced with the increased radiation exposure and time required for preoperative planning and manufacturing. Additionally, the VRS baseplate is significantly more expensive [32]. Given the recency of these implants availability on the market, long-term studies evaluating outcomes and longevity are lacking; however, small preliminary studies have been promising demonstrating satisfactory results [33–35]. When used specifically in the revision setting for 21 patients, postoperative ASES was improved at 3 year follow-up; however, the complication rate was 43% [36]. Given glenoid failure is often a slowly progressive process, studies with longer follow-up period are required before definitive conclusions can be made regarding the utility of patient-specific glenoid components. Given the early success surgeons are having with these 3D custom-printed components, multiple companies are now marketing this option which may drive the cost down.

14.7 Conclusion

In conclusion, revision of a failed glenoid in RSA is a challenging problem that requires careful preoperative and contingency planning. Potential difficulties faced intraoperatively are numerous including obtaining adequate exposure, removing well-fixed glenoids, and poor glenoid bone stock. Patterns of glenoid bone loss are highly variable and require careful consideration of the advantages and disadvantages of various surgical techniques including alternative base plate locations, bone grafting, metal baseplate augmentation, and custom 3D-printed glenoid components. The frequency of revision RSA is only expected to increase over the years to come and will likely be an area of significant innovation with newer implants and techniques to assist surgeons with this difficult procedure.

Conflict of Interest The authors received no funding for this chapter.

Financial Disclaimer None.

References

1. Palsis JA, Simpson KN, Matthews JH, Traven S, Eichinger JK, Friedman RJ. Current trends in the use of shoulder arthroplasty in the United States. Orthopedics. 2018;41(3):e416–23. https://doi.org/10.3928/01477447-20180409-05.
2. Farley KX, Wilson JM, Kumar A, Gottschalk MB, Daly C, Sanchez-Sotelo J, et al. Prevalence of shoulder arthroplasty in the United States and the increasing burden of revision shoulder arthroplasty. JB JS Open Access. 2021;6(3):e20.00156. https://doi.org/10.2106/JBJS.OA.20.00156.
3. Bacle G, Nové-Josserand L, Garaud P, Walch G. Long-term outcomes of reverse total shoulder arthroplasty: a follow-up of a previous study. J Bone Jt Surg. 2017;99(6):454–61.
4. Favard L, Levigne C, Nerot C, Gerber C, De Wilde L, Mole D. Reverse prostheses in arthropathies with cuff tear: are survivorship and function maintained over time? Clin Orthop. 2011;469(9):2469–75.
5. Morrey BF. Reverse total shoulder arthroplasty: survivorship analysis of eighty replacements followed for five to ten Years. Yearb Orthop. 2007;2007:233–5.
6. Zumstein MA, Pinedo M, Old J, Boileau P. Problems, complications, reoperations, and revisions in reverse total shoulder arthroplasty: a systematic review. J Shoulder Elb Surg. 2011;20(1):146–57.
7. Barco R, Savvidou OD, Sperling JW, Sanchez-Sotelo J, Cofield RH. Complications in reverse shoulder arthroplasty. EFORT Open Rev. 2016;1(3):72–80.
8. Boileau P, Melis B, Duperron D, Moineau G, Rumian AP, Han Y. Revision surgery of reverse shoulder arthroplasty. J Shoulder Elb Surg. 2013;22(10):1359–70.
9. Levy JC, Anderson C, Samson A. Classification of postoperative acromial fractures following reverse shoulder arthroplasty. J Bone Jt Surg-Am Vol. 2013;95(15):e104. -1–7
10. Holcomb JO, Cuff D, Petersen SA, Pupello DR, Frankle MA. Revision reverse shoulder arthroplasty for glenoid baseplate failure after primary reverse shoulder arthroplasty. J Shoulder Elb Surg. 2009;18(5):717–23.
11. Familiari F, Rojas J, Nedim Doral M, Huri G, McFarland EG. Reverse total shoulder arthroplasty. EFORT Open Rev. 2018;3(2):58–69.
12. Neyton L, Walch G, Nové-Josserand L, Edwards TB. Glenoid corticocancellous bone grafting after glenoid component removal in the treatment of glenoid loosening. J Shoulder Elb Surg. 2006;15(2):173–9.
13. Ivaldo N, Mangano T, Caione G, Rossoni M, Ligas A. Customized tantalum-augmented reverse shoulder arthroplasty for glenoid bone defect and excessive medialization: description of the technique. Musculoskelet Surg. 2016;100(S1):13–8.
14. Frankle M, Siegal S, Pupello D, Saleem A, Mighell M, Vasey M. The reverse shoulder prosthesis for glenohumeral arthritis associated with severe rotator cuff deficiency. A minimum two-year follow-up study of sixty patients. J Bone Joint Surg Am. 2005;87(8):1697–705. https://doi.org/10.2106/JBJS.D.02813.
15. Cuff DJ, Pupello DR, Santoni BG, Clark RE, Frankle MA. Reverse shoulder arthroplasty for the treatment of rotator cuff deficiency: a concise follow-up, at a minimum of 10 years, of previous reports*. J Bone Jt Surg. 2017;99(22):1895–9.
16. Casier S, Middernacht B, Van Tongel A, De Wilde L. Revision of reversed shoulder arthroplasty: is a reoperation possible? Obere Extrem. 2017;12(1):16–24.
17. Wagner ER, Farley KX, Higgins I, Wilson JM, Daly CA, Gottschalk MB. The incidence of shoulder arthroplasty: rise and future projections compared with hip and knee arthroplasty. J Shoulder Elb Surg. 2020;29(12):2601–9.
18. Jang YH, Oh SY, Kim SH. Three-dimensional analysis of baseplate screw penetration in reverse total shoulder arthroplasty: risk of iatrogenic suprascapular neuropathy by screw violation. J Shoulder Elb Surg. 2022;31(5):940–7.
19. Wang J, Singh A, Higgins L, Warner J. Suprascapular neuropathy secondary to reverse shoulder arthroplasty: a case report. J Shoulder Elb Surg. 2010;19(3):e5–8.
20. Kahan JB, Iannotti J, Donohue K. Suprascapular neuropathy from malpositioned baseplate screws in primary reverse shoulder arthroplasty: two case reports. JBJS Case Connect. 2020;10(4):e20.00096.
21. Saltzman BM, Chalmers PN, Gupta AK, Romeo AA, Nicholson GP. Complication rates comparing primary with revision reverse total shoulder arthroplasty. J Shoulder Elb Surg. 2014;23(11):1647–54.
22. Antuna SA, Sperling JW, Cofield RH, Rowland CM. Glenoid revision surgery after total shoulder arthroplasty. J Shoulder Elb Surg. 2001 May;10(3):217–24.
23. Gupta A, Thussbas C, Koch M, Seebauer L. Management of glenoid bone defects with reverse

shoulder arthroplasty—surgical technique and clinical outcomes. J Shoulder Elb Surg. 2018;27(5):853–62.
24. Jones RB. Bone grafting the glenoid versus use of augmented glenoid baseplates with reverse shoulder arthroplasty. Bull Hosp Jt Dis (2013). 2015;73(Suppl. 1):S129–35.
25. Seidl AJ, Williams GR, Boileau P. Challenges in reverse shoulder arthroplasty: addressing glenoid bone loss. Orthopedics. 2016;39(1):14–23.
26. Klein SM, Dunning P, Mulieri P, Pupello D, Downes K, Frankle MA. Effects of acquired glenoid bone defects on surgical technique and clinical outcomes in reverse shoulder arthroplasty. J Bone Jt Surg-Am. 2010;92(5):1144–54.
27. Norris TR, Ii JDK, Humphrey CS. Management of glenoid bone defects in revision shoulder arthroplasty: a new application of the reverse total shoulder prosthesis. Tech Shoulder Elb Surg. 2007;8(1):10.
28. Kelly JD, Zhao JX, Hobgood ER, Norris TR. Clinical results of revision shoulder arthroplasty using the reverse prosthesis. J Shoulder Elb Surg. 2012;21(11):1516–25.
29. Bateman E, Donald SM. Reconstruction of massive uncontained glenoid defects using a combined autograft-allograft construct with reverse shoulder arthroplasty: preliminary results. J Shoulder Elb Surg. 2012;21(7):925–34.
30. Virk M, Yip M, Liuzza L, Abdelshahed M, Paoli A, Grey S, et al. Clinical and radiographic outcomes with a posteriorly augmented glenoid for Walch B2, B3, and C glenoids in reverse total shoulder arthroplasty. J Shoulder Elb Surg. 2020;29(5):e196–204.
31. Berend ME, Berend KR, Lombardi AV, Cates H, Faris P. The patient-specific Triflange acetabular implant for revision total hip arthroplasty in patients with severe acetabular defects: planning, implantation, and results. Bone Jt J. 2018;100-B(Suppl. A):50–4.
32. Bodendorfer BM, Loughran GJ, Looney AM, Velott AT, Stein JA, Lutton DM, et al. Short-term outcomes of reverse shoulder arthroplasty using a custom baseplate for severe glenoid deficiency. J Shoulder Elb Surg. 2021;30(5):1060–7.
33. Rangarajan R, Blout CK, Patel VV, Bastian SA, Lee BK, Itamura JM. Early results of reverse total shoulder arthroplasty using a patient-matched glenoid implant for severe glenoid bone deficiency. J Shoulder Elb Surg. 2020;29(7):S139–48.
34. Chammaa R, Uri O, Lambert S. Primary shoulder arthroplasty using a custom-made hip-inspired implant for the treatment of advanced glenohumeral arthritis in the presence of severe glenoid bone loss. J Shoulder Elb Surg. 2017;26(1):101–7.
35. Uri O, Bayley I, Lambert S. Hip-inspired implant for revision of failed reverse shoulder arthroplasty with severe glenoid bone loss: improved clinical outcome in 11 patients at 3-year follow-up. Acta Orthop. 2014;85(2):171–6.
36. Uri O, Beckles V, Falworth M, Higgs D, Lambert S. Revision arthroplasty with a hip-inspired computer-assisted design/computer-assisted manufacturing implant for glenoid-deficient shoulders. J Shoulder Elb Surg. 2014;23(2):205–13.

Options for Glenoid Reconstruction: Graft vs. Metal vs. Combined

15

Marko Nabergoj, Patrick J. Denard, Philippe Collin, Tiago Martinho, Arash Amiri, Jeanni Zbinden, and Alexandre Lädermann

15.1 Introduction

Glenoid bone loss is technically challenging to manage given the inherently limited bone stock. Glenoid bone loss is frequently encountered in the revision setting but can also be present in the primary setting including cuff tear arthropathy, glenohumeral arthritis, rheumatoid arthritis, chronic instability, trauma, neoplasms, and congenital malformations [1]. Baseplate fixation and position are critical for osseous integration (Fig. 15.1) [2], optimal range of motion, as well as avoidance of complications including instability [3, 4] and scapular notching [5]. Acquired glenoid bone deformities thus often require modifying standard surgical techniques to achieve successful glenoid reconstruction.

Reverse shoulder arthroplasty (RSA) has increasingly become the primary method of addressing glenoid bone loss because of the improved fixation obtainable with a baseplate, ability to achieve to appropriate soft-tissue tension with lateralization on the glenoid or humerus [6], and constrained nature which compensates for associated rotator cuff deficiency. Technical options to address glenoid bone loss with RSA range from acceptance of incomplete baseplate seating, reaming of the glenoid to achieve partial or complete correction [7], bone grafting [8], the use of metallic augments, or a combination of the above [9]. Currently, there are no clear guidelines on how to address these deformities. Thus, the optimal method of treatment often depends on defect size and patient characteristics such as bone quality and surgeon preference.

The present chapter reviews the biomechanics, surgical technique, and clinical outcomes of RSA in the setting of severe glenoid bone loss. Preoperative planning, navigation, and classification are reviewed in Chaps. 5, 6 and 9, respectively, and will not be addressed in the present chapter.

M. Nabergoj (✉)
Valdotra Orthopaedic Hospital, Ankaran, Slovenia

Faculty of Medicine, University of Ljubljana, Ljubljana, Slovenia

P. J. Denard
Oregon Shoulder Institute, Medford, OR, USA

P. Collin
American Hospital of Paris, Neuilly-sur-Seine, France

T. Martinho · A. Amiri · J. Zbinden
Division of Orthopaedics and Trauma Surgery, La Tour Hospital, Meyrin, Switzerland
e-mail: tiago.martinho@latour.ch

A. Lädermann
Division of Orthopaedics and Trauma Surgery, La Tour Hospital, Meyrin, Switzerland

Faculty of Medicine, University of Geneva, Geneva, Switzerland

Division of Orthopaedics and Trauma Surgery, Department of Surgery, Geneva University Hospitals, Geneva, Switzerland

F. Franceschi et al. (eds.), *Revision Shoulder Arthroplasty*,
https://doi.org/10.1007/978-3-031-45944-3_15

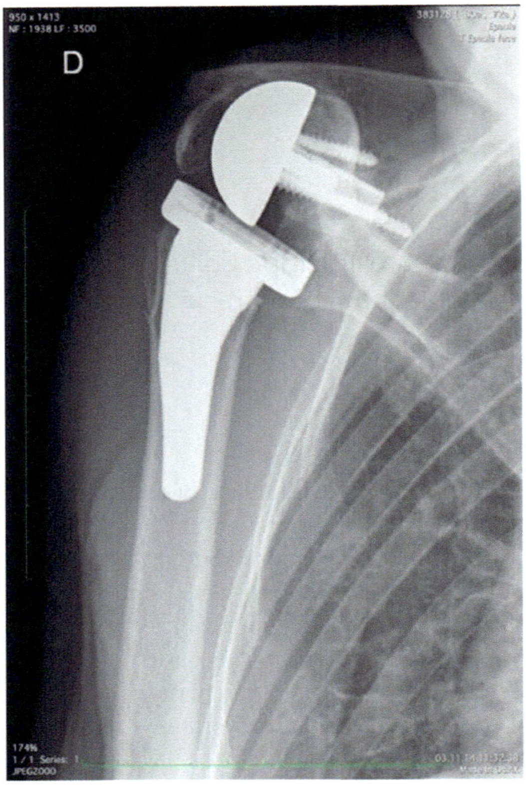

Fig. 15.1 X-ray of the right shoulder, anteroposterior view. Acute superior glenoid implant migration is seen

15.2 Biomechanics

Specific anatomic and morphological parameters are subject to interperson variability, with different bone morphology and different muscle volume. Although each patient has different glenohumeral offset and muscle moment arm lengths, much of planning for bone loss currently relies upon population averages. Based on three-dimensional (3D) computed tomography (CT) measurements, mean glenoid retroversion is approximately 6° ± 4° and mean inclination is 7 ± 5 degrees of superior tilt [10].

Interestingly, most studies have focused on correction of glenoid version and inclination but have not specifically evaluate restoration of glenoid joint line. Nonetheless, glenoid medialization implies altered deltoid and rotator cuff moment arms, reduced deltoid wrapping around the greater tuberosity [11], modified capsular tension [12], as well as implant malpositioning, all having potential undesirable effects on the outcomes. Restoration of the joint line is thus critical to tension the deltoid [3, 13], improve deltoid wrapping and bone stock, maximize function [14], and limit friction- and abutment-type impingements [15], as well as instability. Norris et al. [16] demonstrated that with significant medial glenoid wear, the deltoid can actually generate a laterally directed distraction force that could result in prosthetic instability. Additionally, through a biomechanical study, Codsi et al. demonstrated that the presence of large central cavitary defect, potentially seen in revision settings, resulted in greater initial micromotion of the glenoid implant, affecting the initial fixation and stability of the construct [17]. The reference normal glenohumeral joint line is at a mean of 9 mm lateral to the lateral aspect of the coracoid process' base (Fig. 15.2)

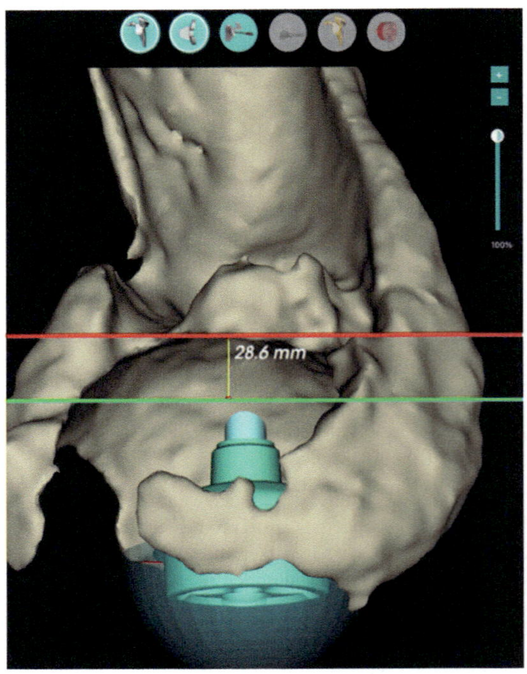

Fig. 15.2 3D CT scan reconstruction of a left shoulder with a planification software (Imascap Glenosys, Imascap SAS, 29280 Plouzané, France), superior view. Two reference points are identified and marked on the scapula; 1) the lateral aspect of the base of the coracoid (green line), and 2) the point of the glenoid at the site of its deepest erosion (red line). In the present case, a massive medialization (28 mm + 9 mm) of the joint line is observed

[18, 19]. The glenoid vault model has also been proposed as a method of assessing the premorbid glenoid vault anatomy and joint line [20] but is not widely available for use.

The aim of glenoid reconstruction from a mechanical standpoint is to achieve adequate contact between the native glenoid bone and the baseplate or the graft for osseous integration. It commonly felt that to allow for bone ingrowth, baseplate micromotion must be under 150 um [21]. Werner et al. have observed that in order to achieve a satisfying fixation between the native glenoid and the baseplate, the adequate contact should be at least 50% [22]. Additionally, Formaini et al. have shown that the fixation of the baseplate does not differ if a contact is at 100%, 75%, or 50% [23]. However, they noticed a significantly greater micromotion above 150 μm threshold when the coverage of the baseplate was at 25%. Consequently, as general guidelines if at least 50% baseplate contact with a central screw or 75% baseplate contact with a central post are not attainable, other techniques such as reaming, bone grafting, or augments should be used [23]. However, individual patient characteristics such bone quality and the amount of glenoid lateralization are also necessary to consider on an individual basis.

The optimal screw configuration to enhance initial stability is long (>17 mm inside the glenoid) and large (diameter > 3.5 mm), and divergent (around 30 degrees) screws [24]. A locking inferior screw may have an advantage inferiorly as tensile forces are the highest at the inferior border secondary to humeral loading [25]. However, from a technical perspective, inferior compression screws may be considered in the setting of a central post so as to promote inferior tilt. Superior tilt leads to a decrease of stabilizing compressive forces and an increase in destabilizing shear forces directed toward glenoid baseplate during contraction of the deltoid, which could result in early loosening [26, 27]. Superior tilt should thus always be avoided as stress at the bone interface increases.

15.3 Prevalence

By some reports, glenoid bone loss is present in approximately 40% of patients undergoing RSA [28, 29]. The prevalence of glenoid defects in patients undergoing RSA procedure has likely increased due to improved preoperative recognition with CT evaluation [30]. Among them, around half required bone grafting in one series [29], although augmented designs were not available in that series. Erosions can develop in any part of the glenoid, but they usually occur either on the posterior part (18%), superior part (9%), anterior part (4%), or as a global erosion (6%) in patients undergoing RSA [28, 29]. Lévigne et al., in their multicenter study, retrospectively observed glenoid deformity in 47% of cases (E1 glenoid in 17%, E2 glenoid in 12%, E3 glenoid in 15%, and E4 in 3%) [31].

15.4 Treatment Options

The goals of glenoid reconstruction are: 1) stable baseplate fixation to achieve osseous integration and 2) re-approximation of the native glenoid joint line to achieve appropriate soft-tissue tension. Meeting these goals in the bone loss scenario often requires modification of standard surgical techniques. Current treatment options in RSA that address severe glenoid bone loss range from implantation of both autograft and allograft, the use of metallic augments and custom prosthesis, or a combination of the above [9, 32]. Initial evaluation includes plain radiographs of the affected shoulder. The axillary view is particularly helpful in assessing glenoid morphology. A 3-dimensional (3D) CT scan allows for further assessment of glenoid bone stock, preoperative planning [33], and even placement [34–36] assisted or not by augmented reality [37] but may be limited by metal artifacts in the setting of revision.

It is well established that the superior tilt of the baseplate should be avoided to limit the risk of loosening. On the other hand, there appears to be more tolerance regarding postoperative version [38]. Some remaining retroversion might be beneficial for soft tissue balance and postoperative range of motion [39]. Increased retroversion may facilitate complex posterior glenoid reconstruction and prevent anterior impingement [40]. Conversely, an alternate center line with increased anteversion has been demonstrated to be clinically acceptable and not substantially limit postoperative range of motion.

It has been previously stated that at least 10 mm of a central post length should be inserted in the native glenoid during primary RSA to obtain initial stability and ingrowth potential. Although central post design theoretically provides increased ingrowth potential, initial stability is higher with a central screw. Furthermore, in the setting of bone loss, the amount of native bone around the post may be compromised (Fig. 15.3). Consequently, the use of central screw with cortical fixation offering a tremendous initial compression is often a viable option [9, 41]. Some designs in fact have a "screw post" with ingrowth the proximal portion of the screw or a short post with an independent central screw that provides the advantages of both a post and central screw.

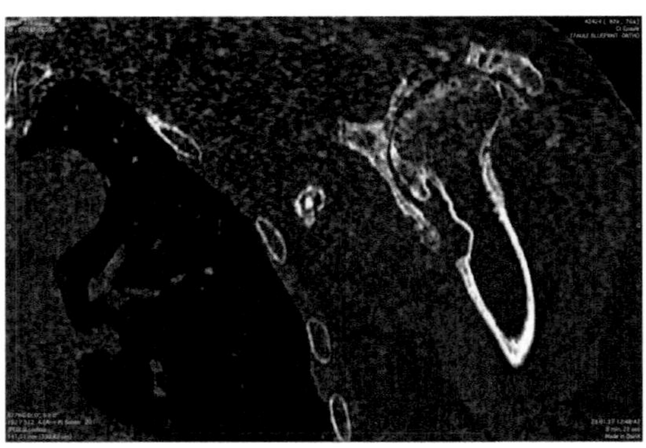

Fig. 15.3 Coronal view of a left shoulder CT scan. Observed the thin glenoid vault allowing only millimetric bone ingrowth around a central peg

Depending on the reconstruction, hybrid peripheral screw fixation using combinations of locked and nonlocked screws seems to offer more security [42]. Even if the number of screws do not seems to play a significant role without bony defect [43], the use of four screws seems necessary in case of complex glenoid reconstruction, without counting any independent screws used to stabilize a bone graft (Fig. 15.4).

15.4.1 Local Autograft

15.4.1.1 Humeral Head

Most series reporting outcomes of correction of glenoid deformity have used autograft. Two techniques are currently used. In the first, the whole humeral head autograft is harvested and prepared to match the size and location of the glenoid defect. When the glenoid is sufficiently exposed, the eroded part of the glenoid is predrilled in order to improve vascularization and bone healing between the native glenoid and the autograft (Fig. 15.5). The graft is temporarily fixed to the native glenoid or held by the post during impaction or screw insertion [44]. Advantages of this technique are the reconstruction of potentially massive erosion and preservation of the hard subchondral bone that often matches the glenoid defect.

Boileau et al. introduced the bony increased-offset (BIO)-RSA technique wherein a cylinder of humeral head is placed around the post of a baseplate [44]. Initially described as a cylinder for the purposes of symmetric lateralization, the graft may also be shaped to accommodate asymmetric defects. After dislocation of the humeral head, a slight pre-cut is done to remove the remaining cartilage. A Kirschner-wire is inserted in the center of humeral head perpendicular to the bone surface. Then, a bell saw, guided along the guidewire, is used to create a cylinder of cancellous bone. While BIO-RSA has been associated with high rates of integration and low rate of scapular notching [44], this technique is limited by the fact that it is cancellous only, it is not available in the revision setting, and complete graft

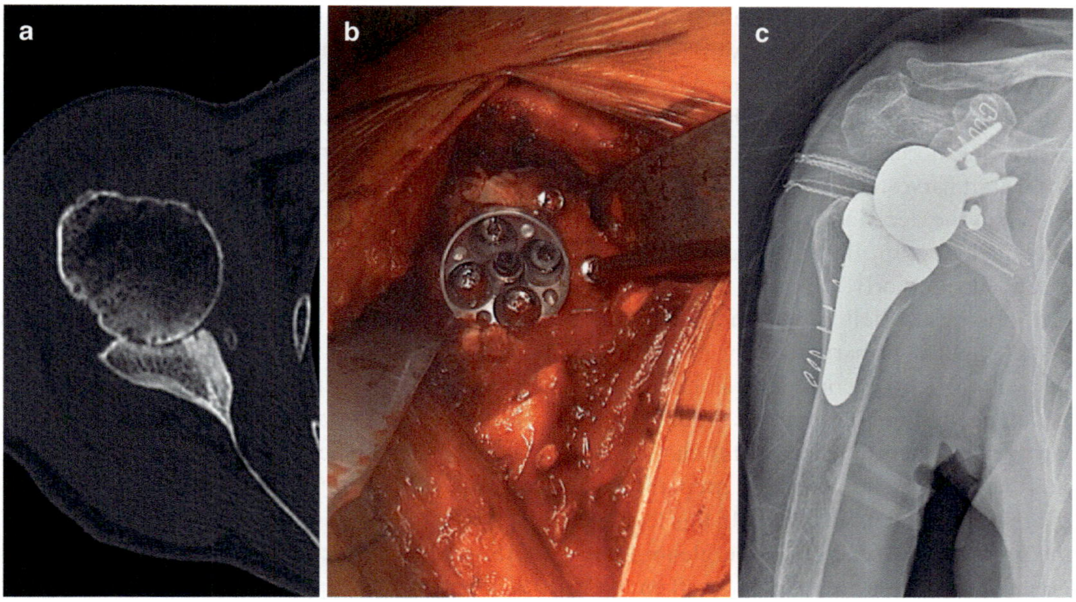

Fig. 15.4 Independent screws for right anterior glenoid reconstruction. (**a**) Anterior locked dislocation with D-type Walch glenoid. (**b**) Intraoperative view. Two independent 4.5 cortical screws replace Kirscher-wire. (**c**) Postoperative X-ray

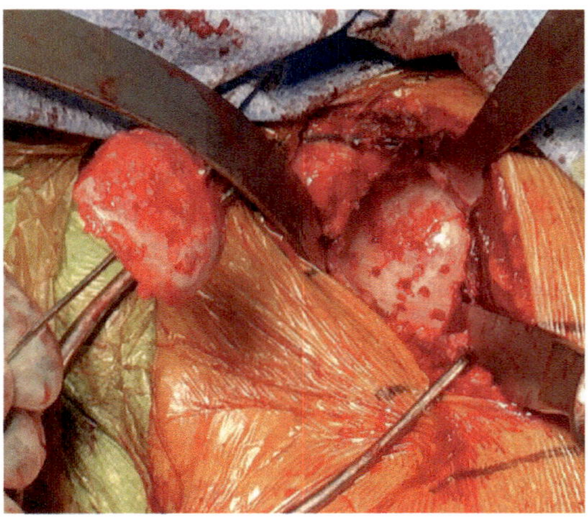

Fig. 15.5 A whole left humeral head autograft has been harvested and the glenoid predrilled to improve vascularization. From Nabergoj et al. with permission [9]

resorptions are occasionally observed in the long term (Fig. 15.6).

15.4.1.2 Distal Clavicle

The distal clavicle autograft can be used to reconstruct central or peripheral defects. In the former, the graft can be compressed during baseplate placement. In the latter, the cortical structure can

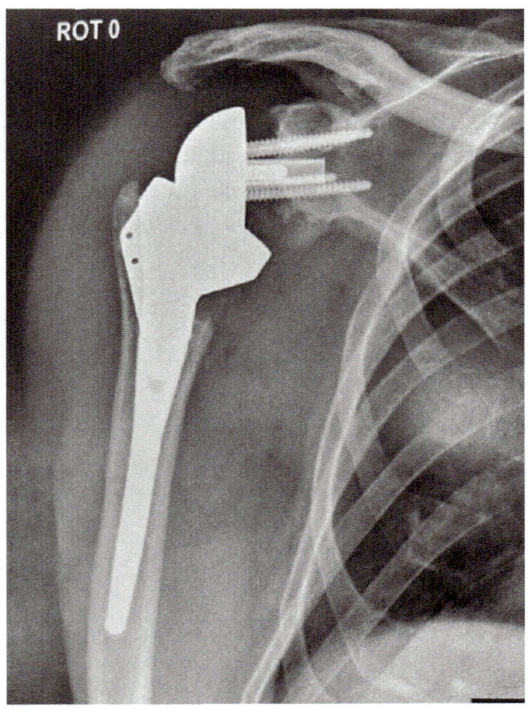

Fig. 15.6 Right RSA with 5 years follow-up. Observed on the glenoid side the complete disappearance of the graft and the bony scapular spur, and humeral stress shielding [5]

be left untouched, allowing the use of the distal clavicle to reconstruct glenoid wall defects. This technique has not only similar advantages to other bone grafting techniques but also limits the donor site morbidity associated with iliac crest bone graft harvesting.

When the decision is made to use the distal clavicle autograft, the deltopectoral incision is extended superiorly, exposing the lateral clavicle between the deltoid and the trapezius. The distal clavicle is harvested by a sagittal saw just lateral to the coracoclavicular ligaments which need to be preserved in order to prevent iatrogenic instability. The distal clavicle autograft needs to be meticulously prepared to specifically fit the glenoid defect. In this technique, the graft can be secured to the glenoid with a guide Kirschner-wire, which is then drilled with a cannulated drill or reamer for the baseplate placement. It is again critical that the baseplate post is fixed in the native scapula as inability to do so greatly increases the chance of failure. An alternative technique involves placing the baseplate on the distal clavicle before harvesting with the sagittal saw. This technique is recommended in orthogonal central glenoid defects or those with wall defects. After the guide pin is placed, the top part of the clavicle is decorticated using the reamer for the baseplate. Then, the guide pin is overdrilled with a cannulated reamer or a drill, and a baseplate with a long post is placed on the clavicle. Afterward, the clavicle is osteotomized medial to the baseplate avoiding injury to the coracoclavicular ligaments. Then, a glenoid guide pin is placed and overdrilled, and the composite implant and clavicle graft can be implanted into the prepared hole in the glenoid [45].

The advantage of the distal clavicle graft is that it is local and inexpensive. The disadvantage to this technique is cosmetic effect due to an extended deltopectoral approach and the possibility of causing iatrogenic instability in case of injuring the coracoclavicular ligaments during harvesting.

15.4.1.3 Coracoid Process

The technique is potentially applicable to mild or moderate central, peripheral anterior, and combined anterior types [46] as well as superior bone loss (E3) [47]. A 90° angled saw blade or a curved osteotome is used to perform a coracoid process osteotomy at its base. The coracoid undersurface and length are conformed to the later prepared glenoid defect. In case of a central defect, the underside of the coracoid graft is impacted directly into the central defect with the conjoined tendon positioned at the inferior glenoid (Fig. 15.7a, b). When the defect is anterior or combined anterior and central, the graft can

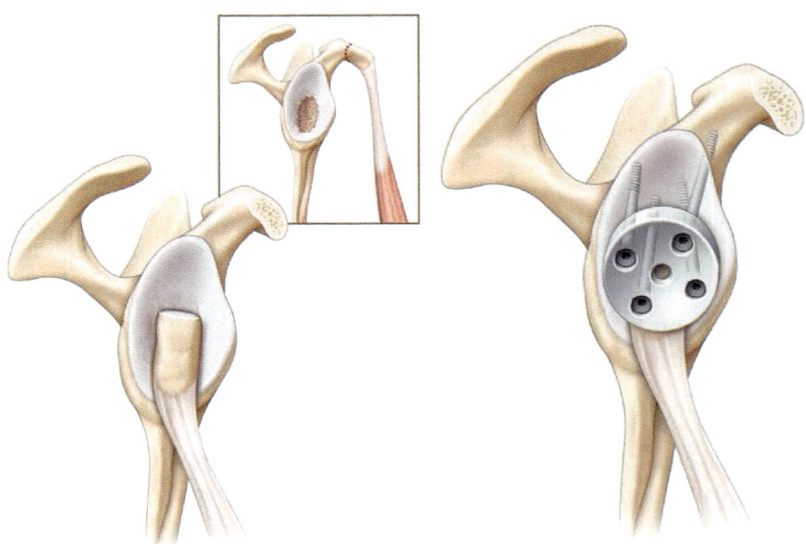

Fig. 15.7 (**a**) Illustration of a right shoulder with a central defect. The coracoid graft is impacted directly into the central defect with the conjoined tendon positioned at the inferior glenoid. (**b**) Illustration after fixation of the baseplate. Reproduced from Lädermann et al., with permission [8]

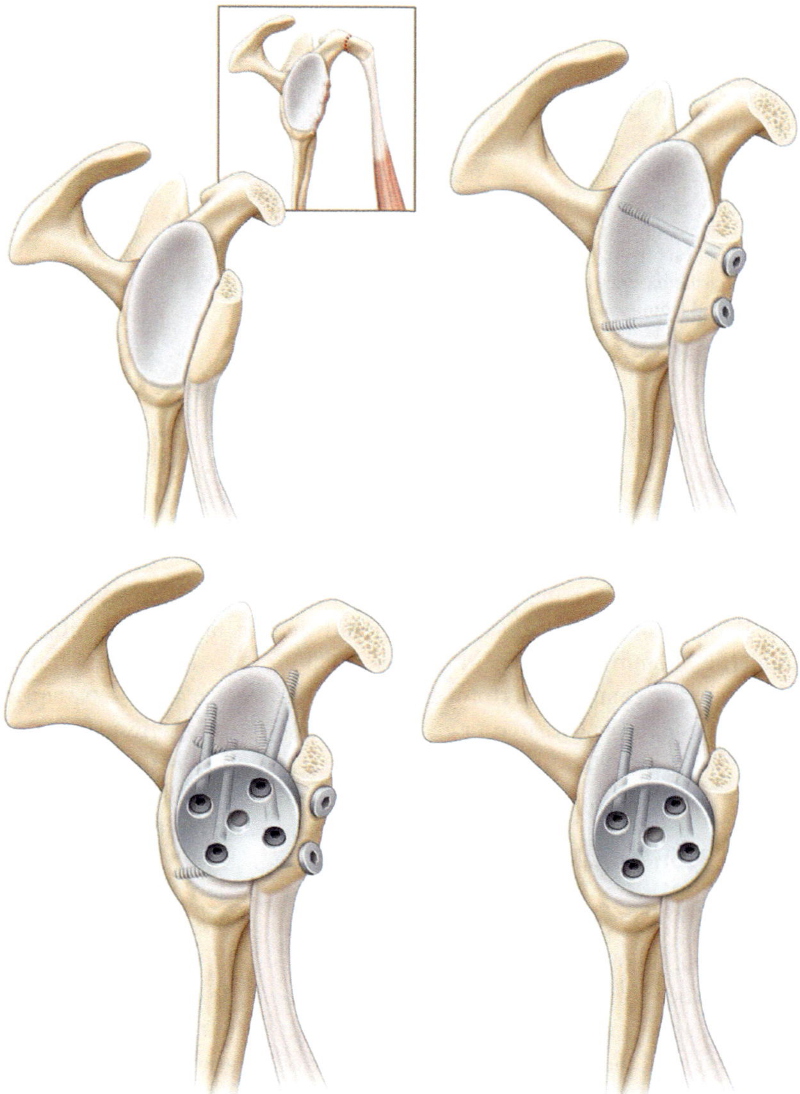

Fig. 15.8 (a) Illustration of a right shoulder with an anterior defect. (**b**, **c**) Illustration with (**b** and **c**) or without (**d**) additional anteroposterior screw fixation of the graft. Reproduced from Lädermann et al., with permission [8]

be placed anteriorly [48], as in the Latarjet procedure [49] (Fig. 15.8a–d), with the conjoined tendon exiting from the glenoid anteroinferiorly. Finally, superior defects could be reconstructed by fixing the coracoid process horizontally with the conjoined tendon exiting the glenoid anterosuperiorly (Fig. 15.9a, b), provided that the subscapularis tendon would be absent or left unrepaired. Like for humeral head autografts, the coracoid can be temporarily fixed on glenoid with wires before placement of the baseplate or mounted on the baseplate and directly impacted [8].

The coracoid graft technique has the benefit of being local, unexpensive, and vascularized which may lower the risk of resorption or nonunion, commonly seen with other grafts [50]. Coracoid graft has, however, many limitations. The experience and the follow-up are limited. Moreover, the graft size is limited by the size of the coracoid

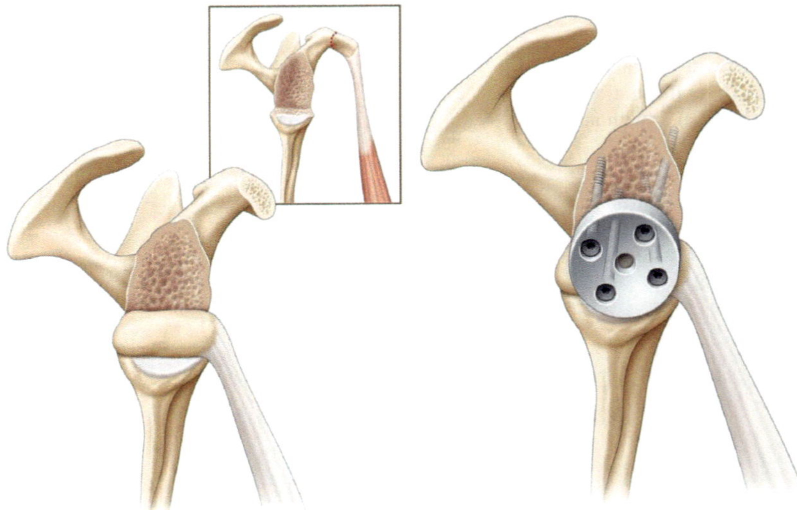

Fig. 15.9 (**a**) Illustration of a right shoulder with a superior defect reconstructed by fixing the coracoid process horizontally with the conjoined tendon exiting the glenoid anterosuperiorly. (**b**) Illustration after fixation of the baseplate. Reproduced from Lädermann et al., with permission [8]

process. Furthermore, the central peg or screw of the glenoid component must thus be relatively small (i.e., 10 mm) to avoid graft fracture. Finally, this procedure cannot be performed in the setting of previous Latarjet, Bristow, or certain acromioclavicular stabilizations.

15.4.2 Non-Local Autograft

15.4.2.1 Iliac Crest

Another option of an autograft represents the use of a tricortical iliac crest graft. Its use is recommended in revision cases, when a large autograft is desired, and the humeral head is absent or of poor quality. This technique has been reported for cavitary defects of the glenoid and in absence of either the anterior or posterior wall [51]. The iliac crest graft is harvested from the lateral ilium wall as the superior bone bridge is preserved to avoid any stress riser and also to keep the iliac contour intact. The inner and outer ileum cortex are exposed, and a guidewire is inserted from outside to inside via a template, while the superior bone bridge is left untouched. The outer surface is reamed to match the baseplate concavity, and a central peg hole is drilled. Then, the chosen peg and baseplate are implanted. The bone graft-implant composite is then removed from the ilium. The graft can then be reshaped using rongeurs before implantation in the glenoid [52].

An iliac crest graft is an inexpensive autograft; however, a separate incision is needed for harvesting. Besides that, donor site morbidity, postoperative hematoma, seroma, pain, and fracture of the ilium have been previously described in the literature [52, 53].

15.4.3 Allograft

The use of an allograft is commonly utilized in the revision setting but has been associated with variable healing rates. The source of the allograft has most commonly been the proximal femur, femoral shaft, plateau of the tibia, or proximal humerus [54, 55]. As with humeral head autograft, the graft may either be placed independently or around the post of the baseplate by prepping the graft to accept the baseplate [56].

The advantage of the allograft compared to an autograft is that in terms of volume of bone graft, they are larger and consequently can be used to reconstruct greater glenoid defects. However, allografts must often be ordered in advance and are not readily available in every operating room. Benninger et al. reported that the cost of commercially available allografts ranges from €1672 to €2149 [57]. Such expense is not affordable in every setting and must be considered as the burden of revision arthroplasty increases.

However, long-term results of massive allografts need to be scrutinized as follow-ups in other joint has been associated with catastrophic failures [58]. Around the hip, allografts are failing causing acetabular cup instability in 25% after only 2 years, 50% after 5 years, and 85% after 10 years [58].

15.4.4 Metallic Augments and Custom Glenoids

Metallic build-up is increasingly used to reconstruct glenoid deformity via either augmented glenoid components or patient-specific (custom) glenoids. As with the use of bone graft, preoperative planning is ideal to determine the ability of a specific augment to match the specific deformity. Initially augments were designed with predetermined angles (half or full wedge) with specific posterior build-ups (typically 4 to 8 mm). More recently, the computer-aided design and 3D printing enable surgeons to reconstruct the damaged glenoid vault with a metallic, patient-specific glenoid component which can range from simply matching a deformity to large reconstructions of 15 mm or more (Fig. 15.10).

Advantages of metallic augmentations are (1) permanent availability for revision surgery, (2) non-reliance on quality of bone graft, (3) increase prosthesis surface contact area with cortical bone, (4) the need to only achieve healing on one side as opposed to the dual-sided healing required for bone graft, (5) improved mechanics compared to bone graft, and (6) the ability to reconstruct larger defects than achievable with bone graft (i.e., >10 to 15 mm of bone loss) [59–61]. Positive clinical results have been reported with augmented baseplates in a variety of eroded glenoids [62, 63].

Regarding patient-specific implants, they are usually designed to treat more severely eroded glenoids. Limitations in the latter group are the scarcity of clinical results and high costs which are two to three times higher than that of a standard baseplate [64]. Bodendorfer et al. reported eleven patients with a mean age of 68 years and a mean follow-up time of 30 months. They found that a median improvement in pain score was 7 points, a SANE score at 43%, and ASES

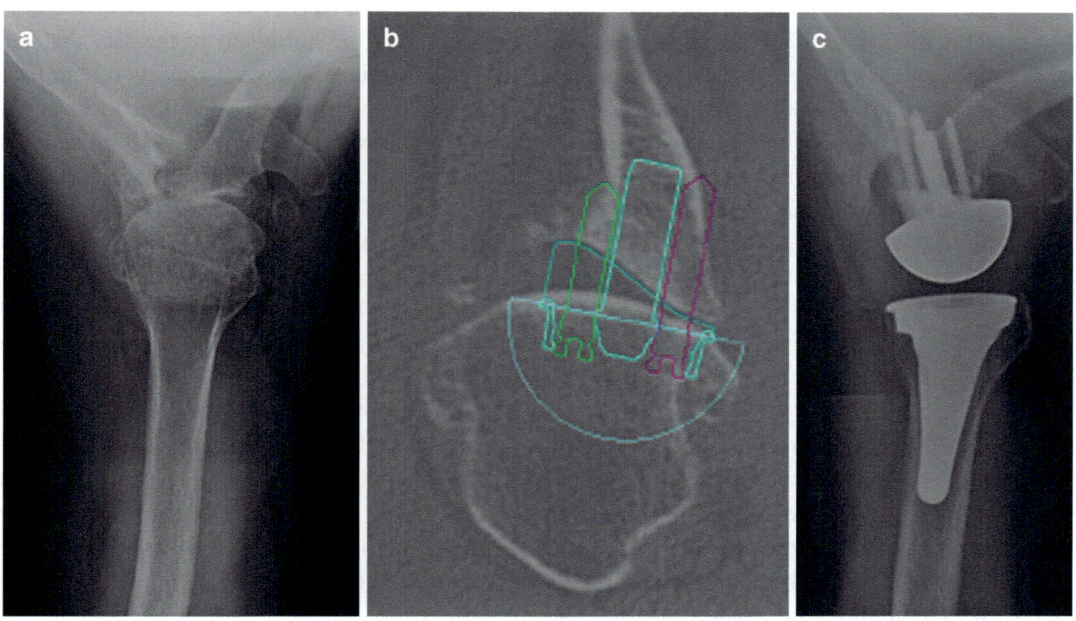

Fig. 15.10 (**a**) Axial CT scan of an 81-year-old woman with a left B2 deformity according to Walch. (**b**) A patient-specific glenoid component has been planned and implanted (**c**). Courtesy of Robert Tashjian

score at 45 points, and a Penn Shoulder Score 49 points. All implants were radiographically stable at follow-up, and no complications were reported [64]. Rangarajan et al. published the results of 19 patient-matched glenoid implants. Complications including greater tuberosity fracture, humeral cortical perforation, and recurrent instability were observed in approximately 20% of cases. However, all measured scores (Disabilities of the Arm, Shoulder and Hand (DASH), Constant, ASES, Simple Shoulder Test, SANE, and pain scores) improved significantly, and no radiographic complication was observed [65].

15.4.5 Combined Bony and Metallic Augmentation

An alternative to patient-specific glenoids is to use a combination of bone graft and an augment to reconstruct very large defects (Figs. 15.11 and 15.12).

Bone autograft (humeral head or iliac crest) is first meticulously shaped to precisely fill the void in the glenoid. Then, Kirschner-wires or 4.5 mm cortical screw(s) are placed to fix the bone graft so that they do not interfere with later placement of the baseplate. The graft surface is flattened out with a reamer that is placed over a central guidewire. Next, the drill-hole for placement of the baseplate central screw or long central peg is prepared, followed by fixation of the baseplate with metal augmentation (half- or full wedge baseplates for B2, B3, C, D, E3, or E4 glenoids) (Fig. 15.13).

15.4.6 Graft Healing

Literature shows mixed results regarding graft healing or incorporation with the results generally favoring autograft over allograft. The use of an autograft and an allograft to reconstruct the glenoid during RSA has been analyzed in three studies with a minimum two-year follow-up [54, 56, 66].

Mahylis et al. analyzed 15 patients who received structural iliac crest bone autograft and 15 patients who received nonstructural bone allograft. They observed no significant differences between the two groups in terms of bone graft integration [66]. Lopiz et al. analyzed 13 patients who underwent structural allografting and 7 patients who underwent autografting for severe glenoid deformity with RSA. Tibial plateau (11 cases) and proximal femur (2 cases) allografts were used. They analyzed radiographic allograft incorporation with computed tomography scans and found that 8% of allografts (1 out of 13) did not incorporate compared to 0% of patients with autograft [54]. Jones et al. analyzed 44 patients (29 received humeral head autograft, one received iliac crest autograft, and 14 received femoral head allograft) who underwent bone grafting for glenoid defects in the setting of RSA. The autograft group showed a higher rate of graft incorporation (86% complete or partial incorporation vs. 66.6% for allografts) [56]. Ozgur et al. analyzed 20 patients undergoing RSA with structural allograft with a minimum follow-up of 1 year. Compared to the Jones et al. study, they reported an even worse healing rate as only 45% (9 of 20 grafts) were still in place at 1 year postoperatively. The difference in the healing rate could be attributed to the fact that the cohort of Ozgur et al. was much more complex compared to the group of patients of Jones et al., as they underwent an average of 3.9 procedures prior to allografting. Additionally, Ozgur et al. used a mix of femoral shaft and femoral neck allografts, and they showed that femoral shaft allografts did very poorly as only 12.5% (1 out of 8) survived [67]. Iannotti et al. analyzed the use of structural allograft in the management of large glenoid defects. They noted >50% graft resorption in 6 out of 19 patients [68]. Ho et al. retrospectively analyzed 44 patients who underwent RSA with structural bone grafting of glenoid defects (allo- and autograft) and showed that 25% had radiographic baseplate loosening associated with resorption [69].

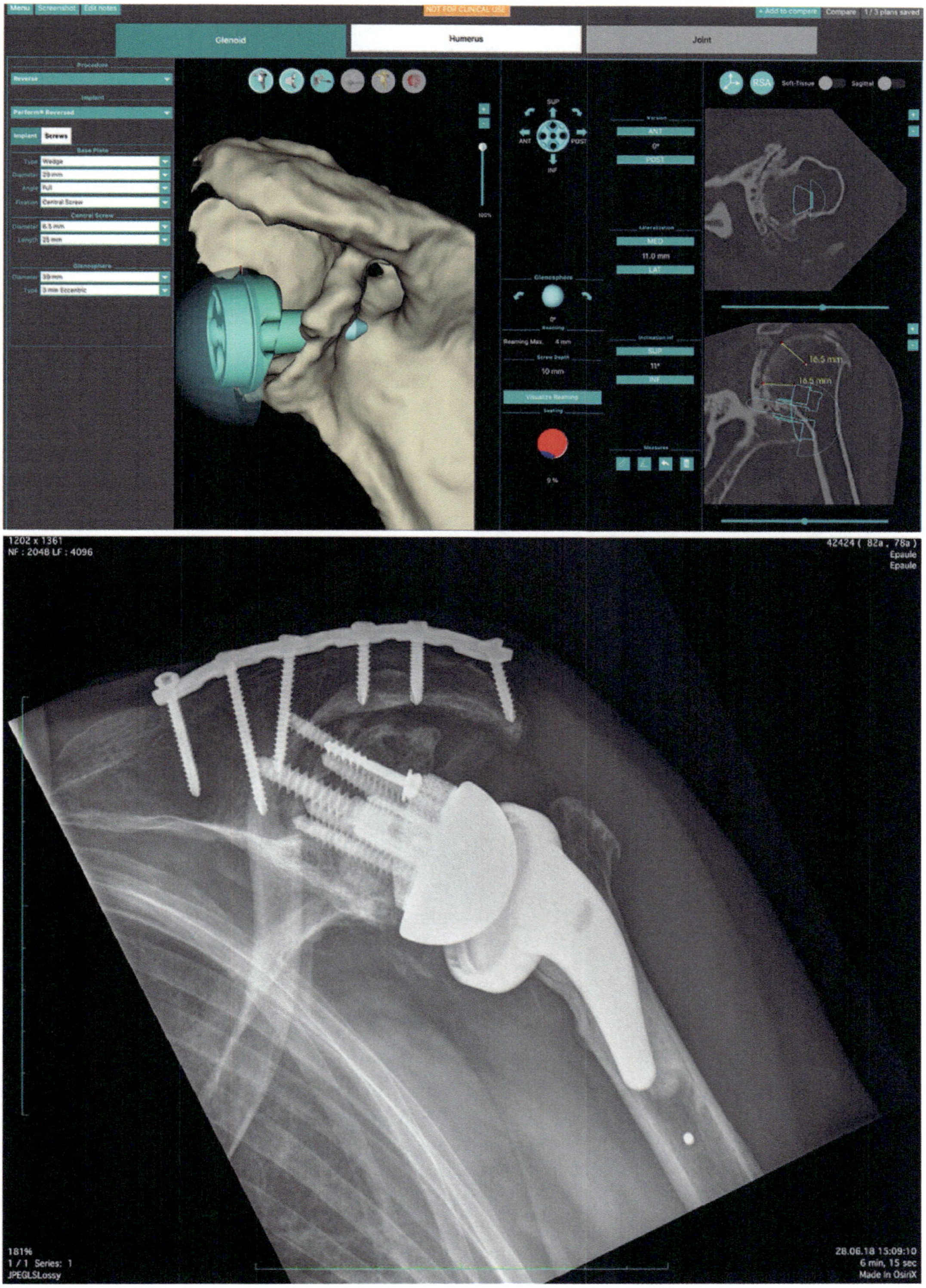

Fig. 15.11 (**a**) Coronal and axial views of a 3-dimensional (3D) reconstruction of a left massive glenoid erosion. Preoperative planning reveals that metallic augmentation alone would not achieve optimal joint line restoration. A full wedge baseplate is required to obtain inferior tilt that will transform shear into compression forces. (**b**) A preoperative spine fracture that has been fixed at the same time. Four-year radiographic follow-up that demonstrates restoration of the joint line and good incorporation of the graft and healing of the spine

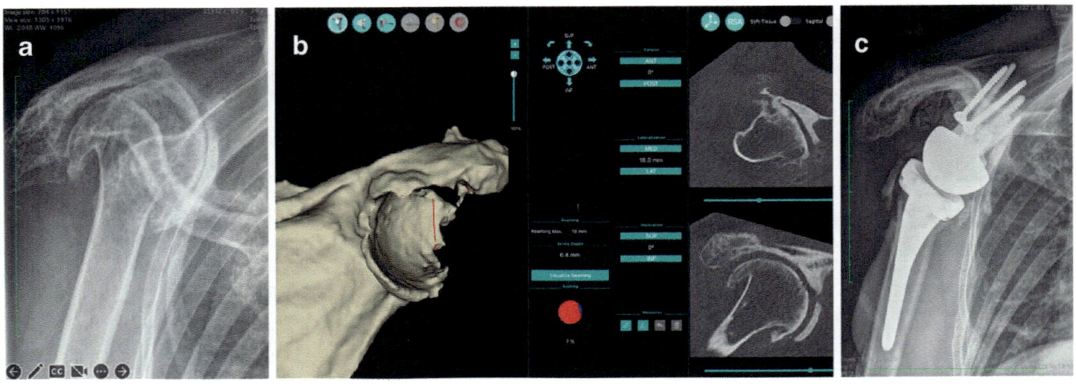

Fig. 15.12 (**a**) Preoperative anteroposterior X-ray and (**b**) 3D reconstruction of a right massive glenoid erosion. (**c**) Three-year radiographic follow-up demonstrating incorporation of the graft and satisfactory inferior tilt with combined bony and metallic reconstruction

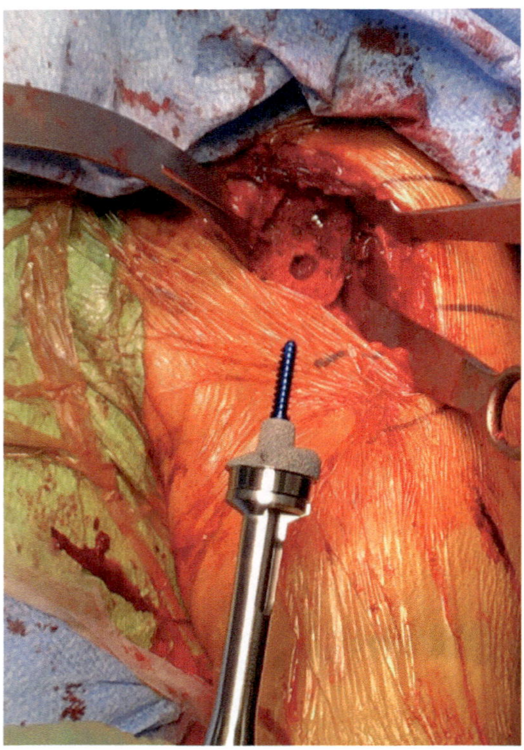

Fig. 15.13 Intraoperative view of a left glenoid reconstruction after humeral bone autograft. According to planification, the entire humeral head is not sufficient to compensate for the bony erosion. A full wedge baseplate is therefore screwed

15.4.7 Bony vs. Metallic Augmentation

In comparison to bone grafts, the advantages of metallic augments are its easier technique and absence of complications otherwise observed with the use of bone grafts, like nonunion or graft resorption. Although, the disadvantages are significantly higher costs, especially if the humeral head is used as an autograft [70], and less flexibility with the implant as the degree of correction that the augmented baseplate can provide is limited to the manufacturers augment dimensions [32, 71]. Colasanti et al. compared the outcomes of primary RSA utilizing bone grafting to primary RSA utilizing metal augments with a minimum of two-year follow-up. They compared the results of 520 patients treated with bone grafting compared to 47 patients who received a metal augment for correction of the glenoid defect. The average follow-up was 37 and 53 months, respectively. They demonstrated that the use of metal augments for insufficient glenoid bone stock is superior according to multiple patient-reported outcome measures, range of motion metrics, minimum clinically important difference, and substantial clinical benefit when compared to bone graft augmentation. The use of metal augments also outperformed bone grafting in complication and revision rates [72]. Jones et al. also compared the postoperative results of metal augments and bone grafting of the glenoid defects during RSA. They reviewed 80 patients (39 in the metal augment group and 41 in the bone grafting group) and reported a lower complication rate and scapular notching rate with the use of metal augments [62]. On the Contrary, in a recent review comparing outcomes

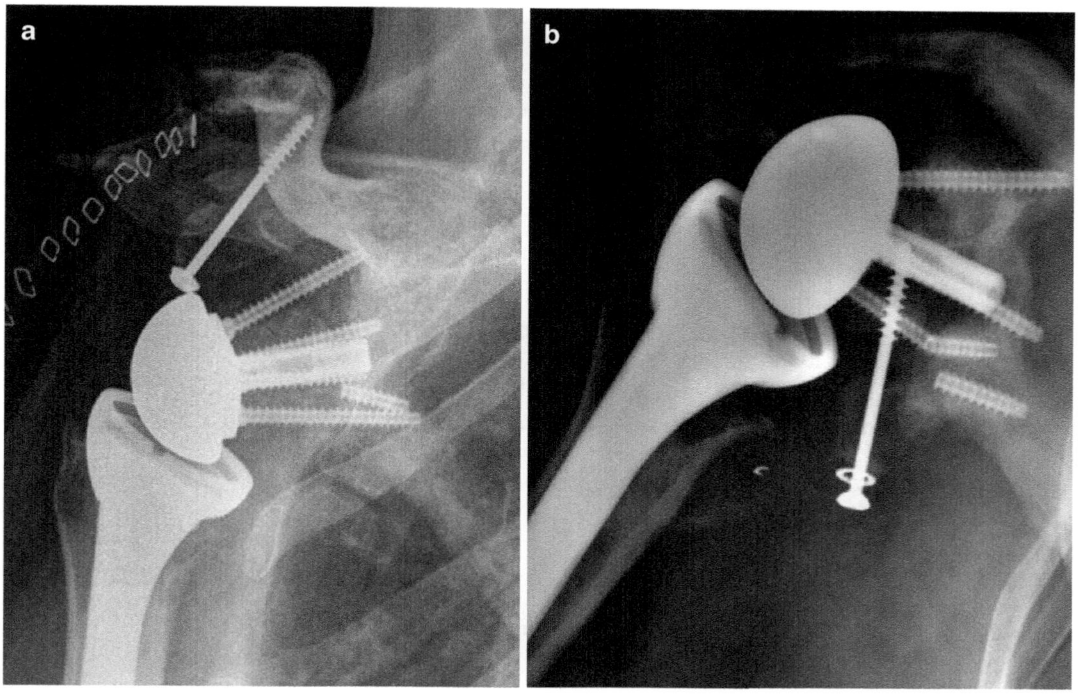

Fig. 15.14 Postoperative X-rays of right massive glenoid bone loss reconstruction and implantation of a straight stem. On the left, less than 10 mm of the central post has been impacted in the native glenoid despite long peg. Humeral lateralization could have been useful to compensate for medialization. Reproduced from Lädermann et al. [74], with permission

of RSA using either bone graft or augmented baseplates for the management of glenoid bone loss and deformity, Lanham et al. did not find difference between the two options [73].

15.4.8 Humeral Lateralization

Interestingly, the literature focuses only on glenoid reconstruction in case of glenoid bone loss. However, complete restoration of the joint line is not always required (Fig. 15.11), and other types of compensation such as humeral lateralization may be used to obtain satisfactory global lateralization (Fig. 15.14). However, one limitation of such an approach is the ability to achieve joint reduction. In the setting of chronic bone loss, soft tissue contracture may be difficult to obtain humeral lateralization once the glenoid joint line is restored. Thus, our recommendation is to restore the glenoid as much as possible, then determine whether or not humeral lateralization is possible or required based on intraoperative stability testing.

15.4.9 One- or Two-stages

The advantage of a one-stage procedure is avoiding the surgical morbidity of a second surgery. Nevertheless, conversion to a two-stage approach is recommended when intraoperative stability of the baseplate is suboptimal [2].

15.4.10 Rehabilitation Protocol

Rehabilitation protocol as used by the authors is described. Postoperatively, the arm is placed in an abduction pillow sling for 6 weeks for complex glenoid reconstruction to promote compression instead of shear forces. After

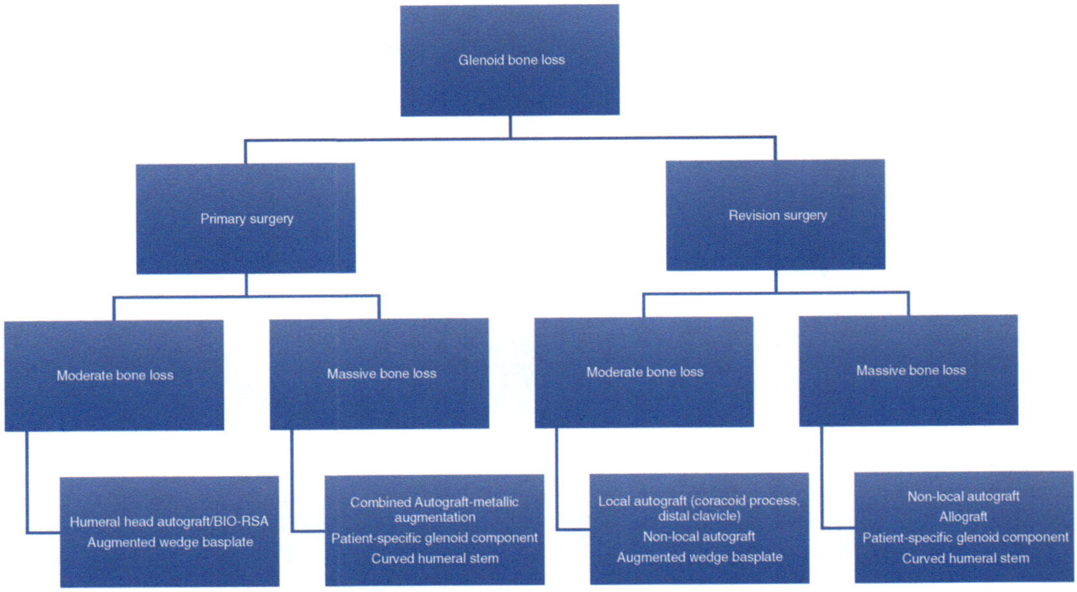

Fig. 15.15 Treatment paradigm proposed by the authors for patients with glenoid bone loss

6 weeks, the immobilization is discontinued and active-assisted range of motion can be then initiated. Activities of daily living are progressed, but strengthening is not specifically recommended [75].

15.5 Author's Preferred Treatment

Treatment is based on patient factors and associated pathology as previously discussed (Fig. 15.15).

15.6 Conclusion

In this chapter, we described our preferred surgical techniques for management of severe glenoid deformity. Varying amounts of bone loss produce distinctly different types of deformity which require different surgical approaches. Adequate preoperative planning is crucial to make the best decisions regarding the appropriate approach. This procedure is technically demanding independently of the chosen approach to address the bone defect. Autograft should be preferred to allografts, whenever possible. Longer-term clinical and radiographic follow-up studies for the use of bone grafting and metallic augments in RSA are necessary to find the best management protocol for this challenging pathology.

Conflict of Interest Disclosure Statement Marko Nabergoj is a consultant for Smith & Nephew.

Patrick J Denard P.J.D. has received consulting fees from Arthrex, royalties from Arthrex, and research grants from Arthrex.

Tiago Martinho has nothing to declare.

Philippe Collin P.C. has received personal fees from Advanced Medical Applications, ConMed, Smith & Nephew, Stortz, and Stryker.

Alexandre Lädermann is a paid consultant for Arthrex, Stryker, and Medacta. He received royalties from Stryker. He is the founder of FORE, Med4Cast, and BeeMed.

Source of Funding FORE (Foundation for Research and Teaching in Orthopaedics, Sports Medicine, Trauma, and Imaging in the Musculoskeletal System). Grant id FORE 2022-40.

References

1. Kozak T, Bauer S, Walch G, Al-Karawi S, Blakeney W. An update on reverse total shoulder arthroplasty: current indications, new designs, same old problems. EFORT Open Rev. 2021;6(3):189–201. https://doi.org/10.1302/2058-5241.6.200085.

2. Lädermann A, Schwitzguebel AJ, Edwards TB, Godeneche A, Favard L, Walch G, et al. Glenoid loosening and migration in reverse shoulder arthroplasty. Bone Joint J. 2019;101-B(4):461–9. https://doi.org/10.1302/0301-620X.101B4.BJJ-2018-1275.R1.
3. Lädermann A, Williams MD, Mélis B, Hoffmeyer P, Walch G. Objective evaluation of lengthening in reverse shoulder arthroplasty. J Shoulder Elb Surg. 2009;18(4):588–95. https://doi.org/10.1016/j.jse.2009.03.012.
4. Tashjian RZ, Martin BI, Ricketts CA, Henninger HB, Granger EK, Chalmers PN. Superior baseplate inclination is associated with instability after reverse total shoulder arthroplasty. Clin Orthop Relat Res. 2018;476(8):1622–9. https://doi.org/10.1097/CORR.0000000000000340.
5. Mélis B, DeFranco M, Lädermann A, Mole D, Favard L, Nerot C, et al. An evaluation of the radiological changes around the Grammont reverse geometry shoulder arthroplasty after eight to 12 years. J Bone Joint Surg Br. 2011;93(9):1240–6. https://doi.org/10.1302/0301-620X.93B9.25926.
6. Lädermann A, Denard PJ, Boileau P, Farron A, Deransart P, Terrier A, et al. Effect of humeral stem design on humeral position and range of motion in reverse shoulder arthroplasty. Int Orthop. 2015;39(11):2205–13. https://doi.org/10.1007/s00264-015-2984-3.
7. Walch G, Moraga C, Young A, Castellanos-Rosas J. Results of anatomic nonconstrained prosthesis in primary osteoarthritis with biconcave glenoid. J Shoulder Elb Surg. 2012;21(11):1526–33. https://doi.org/10.1016/j.jse.2011.11.030.
8. Lädermann A, AlAmer N, Denard PJ, Martinho T, Hurtado JA, Collin P. Glenoid reconstruction bone loss with a pediculated coracoid autograft during shoulder arthroplasty. A technical note. Orthop Traumatol Surg Res. 2023;109(4):103542. https://doi.org/10.1016/j.otsr.2022.103542.
9. Nabergoj M, Neyton L, Bothorel H, Ho SWL, Wang S, Chong XL, et al. Reverse shoulder arthroplasty with bony and metallic versus standard bony reconstruction for severe glenoid bone loss. A retrospective comparative cohort study. J Clin Med. 2021;10(22) https://doi.org/10.3390/jcm10225274.
10. Gauci MO, Deransart P, Chaoui J, Urvoy M, Athwal GS, Sanchez-Sotelo J, et al. Three-dimensional geometry of the normal shoulder: a software analysis. J Shoulder Elb Surg. 2020;29(12):e468–e77. https://doi.org/10.1016/j.jse.2020.03.042.
11. Roche CP. Reverse shoulder arthroplasty biomechanics. J Funct Morphol Kinesiol. 2022;7(1) https://doi.org/10.3390/jfmk7010013.
12. Boileau P, Walch G. The three-dimensional geometry of the proximal humerus. Implications for surgical technique and prosthetic design. J Bone Joint Surg Br. 1997;79(5):857–65.
13. Lädermann A, Edwards TB, Walch G. Arm lengthening after reverse shoulder arthroplasty: a review. Int Orthop. 2014;38(5):991–1000. https://doi.org/10.1007/s00264-013-2175-z.
14. Lädermann A, Denard PJ, Boileau P, Farron A, Deransart P, Walch G. What is the best glenoid configuration in onlay reverse shoulder arthroplasty? Int Orthop. 2018;42(6):1339–46. https://doi.org/10.1007/s00264-018-3850-x.
15. Lädermann A, Gueorguiev B, Charbonnier C, Stimec BV, Fasel JH, Zderic I, et al. Scapular notching on kinematic simulated range of motion after reverse shoulder arthroplasty is not the result of impingement in adduction. Medicine (Baltimore). 2015;94(38):e1615. https://doi.org/10.1097/MD.0000000000001615.
16. Norris T, Kelly J, Humphrey CS. Management of glenoid bone defects in revision shoulder arthroplasty: a new application of the reverse total shoulder prosthesis. Tech Shoulder Elbow Surg. 2007;8:37–46.
17. Codsi MJ, Iannotti JP. The effect of screw position on the initial fixation of a reverse total shoulder prosthesis in a glenoid with a cavitary bone defect. J Shoulder Elb Surg. 2008;17(3):479–86. https://doi.org/10.1016/j.jse.2007.09.002.
18. Bhatia DN, de Beer JF, du Toit DF. Coracoid process anatomy: implications in radiographic imaging and surgery. Clin Anat. 2007;20(7):774–84. https://doi.org/10.1002/ca.20525.
19. Italia KR, Green N, Maharaj J, Launay M, Gupta A. Computed tomographic evaluation of glenoid joint line restoration with glenoid bone grafting and reverse shoulder arthroplasty in patients with significant glenoid bone loss. J Shoulder Elb Surg. 2021;30(3):599–608. https://doi.org/10.1016/j.jse.2020.09.031.
20. Ricchetti ET, Hendel MD, Collins DN, Iannotti JP. Is premorbid glenoid anatomy altered in patients with glenohumeral osteoarthritis? Clin Orthop Relat Res. 2013;471(9):2932–9. https://doi.org/10.1007/s11999-013-3069-5.
21. Jasty M, Bragdon C, Burke D, O'Connor D, Lowenstein J, Harris WH. In vivo skeletal responses to porous-surfaced implants subjected to small induced motions. J Bone Joint Surg Am. 1997;79(5):707–14. https://doi.org/10.2106/00004623-199705000-00010.
22. Werner BS, Bohm D, Abdelkawi A, Gohlke F. Glenoid bone grafting in reverse shoulder arthroplasty for long-standing anterior shoulder dislocation. J Shoulder Elb Surg. 2014;23(11):1655–61. https://doi.org/10.1016/j.jse.2014.02.017.
23. Formaini NT, Everding NG, Levy JC, Santoni BG, Nayak AN, Wilson C, et al. The effect of glenoid bone loss on reverse shoulder arthroplasty baseplate fixation. J Shoulder Elb Surg. 2015;24(11):e312–9. https://doi.org/10.1016/j.jse.2015.05.045.
24. Goetti P, Denard PJ, Collin P, Ibrahim M, Mazzolari A, Lädermann A. Biomechanics of anatomic and reverse shoulder arthroplasty. EFORT Open Rev. 2021;6(10):918–31. https://doi.org/10.1302/2058-5241.6.210014.
25. Chebli C, Huber P, Watling J, Bertelsen A, Bicknell RT, Matsen F 3rd. Factors affecting fixation of the glenoid component of a reverse total shoulder prothesis.

J Shoulder Elb Surg. 2008;17(2):323–7. https://doi.org/10.1016/j.jse.2007.07.015.
26. Gutierrez S, Greiwe RM, Frankle MA, Siegal S, Lee WE 3rd. Biomechanical comparison of component position and hardware failure in the reverse shoulder prosthesis. J Shoulder Elb Surg. 2007;16(Suppl. 3):S9–S12. https://doi.org/10.1016/j.jse.2005.11.008.
27. Gutierrez S, Walker M, Willis M, Pupello DR, Frankle MA. Effects of tilt and glenosphere eccentricity on baseplate/bone interface forces in a computational model, validated by a mechanical model, of reverse shoulder arthroplasty. J Shoulder Elb Surg. 2011;20(5):732–9. https://doi.org/10.1016/j.jse.2010.10.035.
28. Frankle MA, Teramoto A, Luo ZP, Levy JC, Pupello D. Glenoid morphology in reverse shoulder arthroplasty: classification and surgical implications. J Shoulder Elb Surg. 2009;18(6):874–85. https://doi.org/10.1016/j.jse.2009.02.013.
29. Klein SM, Dunning P, Mulieri P, Pupello D, Downes K, Frankle MA. Effects of acquired glenoid bone defects on surgical technique and clinical outcomes in reverse shoulder arthroplasty. J Bone Joint Surg Am. 2010;92(5):1144–54. https://doi.org/10.2106/JBJS.I.00778.
30. Budge MD, Lewis GS, Schaefer E, Coquia S, Flemming DJ, Armstrong AD. Comparison of standard two-dimensional and three-dimensional corrected glenoid version measurements. J Shoulder Elb Surg. 2011;20(4):577–83. https://doi.org/10.1016/j.jse.2010.11.003.
31. Levigne C, Boileau P, Favard L, Garaud P, Mole D, Sirveaux F, et al. Scapular notching in reverse shoulder arthroplasty. J Shoulder Elb Surg. 2008;17(6):925–35. https://doi.org/10.1016/j.jse.2008.02.010.
32. Ascione F, Routman HD. Severe glenoid erosion (B2, B3, C, E2, E3) treated with RSA. In: Tashjian R, editor. Complex and revision shoulder arthroplasty. Cham: Springer; 2019. p. 59–73.
33. Berhouet J, Jacquot A, Walch G, Deransart P, Favard L, Gauci MO. Preoperative planning of baseplate position in reverse shoulder arthroplasty: still no consensus on lateralization, version and inclination. Orthop Traumatol Surg Res. 2022;108(3):103115. https://doi.org/10.1016/j.otsr.2021.103115.
34. Berhouet J, Slimane M, Facomprez M, Jiang M, Favard L. Views on a new surgical assistance method for implanting the glenoid component during total shoulder arthroplasty. Part 2: From three-dimensional reconstruction to augmented reality: feasibility study. Orthop Traumatol Surg Res. 2019;105(2):211–8. https://doi.org/10.1016/j.otsr.2018.08.021.
35. Theopold J, Pieroh P, Scharge ML, Marquass B, Hohmann T, Josten C, et al. Improved accuracy of K-wire positioning into the glenoid vault by intraoperative 3D image intensifier-based navigation for the glenoid component in shoulder arthroplasty. Orthop Traumatol Surg Res. 2016;102(5):575–81. https://doi.org/10.1016/j.otsr.2016.03.013.
36. Verborgt O, Hachem AI, Eid K, Vuylsteke K, Ferrand M, Hardy P. Accuracy of patient-specific guided implantation of the glenoid component in reversed shoulder arthroplasty. Orthop Traumatol Surg Res. 2018;104(6):767–72. https://doi.org/10.1016/j.otsr.2018.01.010.
37. Rojas JT, Lädermann A, Ho SWL, Rashid MS, Zumstein MA. Glenoid component placement assisted by augmented reality through a head-mounted display during reverse shoulder arthroplasty. Arthrosc Tech. 2022;11(5):e863–e74. https://doi.org/10.1016/j.eats.2021.12.046.
38. Elmallah R, Swanson D, Le K, Kirsch J, Jawa A. Baseplate retroversion does not affect postoperative outcomes after reverse shoulder arthroplasty. J Shoulder Elb Surg. 2022;31(10):2082–8. https://doi.org/10.1016/j.jse.2022.02.043.
39. Keener JD, Patterson BM, Orvets N, Aleem AW, Chamberlain AM. Optimizing reverse shoulder arthroplasty component position in the setting of advanced arthritis with posterior glenoid erosion: a computer-enhanced range of motion analysis. J Shoulder Elb Surg. 2018;27(2):339–49. https://doi.org/10.1016/j.jse.2017.09.011.
40. Cunningham G, Lädermann A. Redefining anterior shoulder impingement: a literature review. Int Orthop. 2017; https://doi.org/10.1007/s00264-017-3515-1.
41. Achors K, Diaz MA, Simon P, Hill B, Christmas KN, Cronin KJ, et al. Avoiding glenoid baseplate fixation failure by altering surgical technique for varying bone densities. JBJS Open Access. 2022;7(3) https://doi.org/10.2106/JBJS.OA.22.00003.
42. Formaini NT, Everding NG, Levy JC, Santoni BG, Nayak AN, Wilson C. Glenoid baseplate fixation using hybrid configurations of locked and unlocked peripheral screws. J Orthop Traumatol. 2017;18(3):221–8. https://doi.org/10.1007/s10195-016-0438-3.
43. Lung TS, Cruickshank D, Grant HJ, Rainbow MJ, Bryant TJ, Bicknell RT. Factors contributing to glenoid baseplate micromotion in reverse shoulder arthroplasty: a biomechanical study. J Shoulder Elb Surg. 2019;28(4):648–53. https://doi.org/10.1016/j.jse.2018.09.012.
44. Boileau P, Moineau G, Roussanne Y, O'Shea K. Bony increased-offset reversed shoulder arthroplasty: minimizing scapular impingement while maximizing glenoid fixation. Clin Orthop Relat Res. 2011;469(9):2558–67. https://doi.org/10.1007/s11999-011-1775-4.
45. Taylor JR, Schrumpf MA, Shea KE, Kelly JD 2nd. Distal clavicle autograft augmentation for glenoid bone loss in revision shoulder arthroplasty: results and technique. J Shoulder Elb Surg. 2020;29(10):e386–e93. https://doi.org/10.1016/j.jse.2020.05.009.
46. Antuna SA, Sperling JW, Cofield RH, Rowland CM. Glenoid revision surgery after total shoulder arthroplasty. J Shoulder Elb Surg. 2001;10(3):217–24. https://doi.org/10.1067/mse.2001.113961.
47. Favard L, Lautmann S, Sirveaux F, Oudet D, Kerjean Y, Huguet D. Hemiarthroplasty versus reverse arthro-

plasty in the treatment of osteoarthritis with massive rotator cuff tear. In: Walch G, Boileau P, Mole D, editors. 2000 Shoulder prostheses two to ten years follow-up. Paris: Sauramps Medical; 2001. p. 261–8.
48. Garofalo R, Brody F, Castagna A, Ceccarelli E, Krishnan SG. Reverse shoulder arthroplasty with glenoid bone grafting for anterior glenoid rim fracture associated with glenohumeral dislocation and proximal humerus fracture. Orthop Traumatol Surg Res. 2016;102(8):989–94. https://doi.org/10.1016/j.otsr.2016.09.009.
49. Lädermann A, Lubbeke A, Stern R, Cunningham G, Bellotti V, Gazielly DF. Risk factors for dislocation arthropathy after Latarjet procedure: a long-term study. Int Orthop. 2013;37(6):1093–8. https://doi.org/10.1007/s00264-013-1848-y.
50. Hussain ZB, Godin JA, Sanchez G, Kennedy NI, Cinque ME, Ferrari MB, et al. Reverse total shoulder arthroplasty with humeral head autograft fixed onto glenoid for treatment of severe glenoid retroversion. Arthrosc Tech. 2017;6(5):e1691–e5. https://doi.org/10.1016/j.eats.2017.06.025.
51. Norris TR. Glenoid bone loss in reverse shoulder arthroplasty treated with bone graft techniques. Am J Orthop. 2018;47(3) https://doi.org/10.12788/ajo.2018.0016.
52. Singh J, Odak S, Neelakandan K, Walton MJ, Monga P, Bale S, et al. Survivorship of autologous structural bone graft at a minimum of 2 years when used to address significant glenoid bone loss in primary and revision shoulder arthroplasty: a computed tomographic and clinical review. J Shoulder Elb Surg. 2021;30(3):668–78. https://doi.org/10.1016/j.jse.2020.06.015.
53. Almaiman M, Al-Bargi HH, Manson P. Complication of anterior iliac bone graft harvesting in 372 adult patients from May 2006 to May 2011 and a literature review. Craniomaxillofac Trauma Reconstr. 2013;6(4):257–66. https://doi.org/10.1055/s-0033-1357510.
54. Lopiz Y, Garcia-Fernandez C, Arriaza A, Rizo B, Marcelo H, Marco F. Midterm outcomes of bone grafting in glenoid defects treated with reverse shoulder arthroplasty. J Shoulder Elb Surg. 2017;26(9):1581–8. https://doi.org/10.1016/j.jse.2017.01.017.
55. Malahias MA, Chytas D, Kostretzis L, Brilakis E, Fandridis E, Hantes M, et al. Bone grafting in primary and revision reverse total shoulder arthroplasty for the management of glenoid bone loss: a systematic review. J Orthop. 2020;20:78–86. https://doi.org/10.1016/j.jor.2019.12.005.
56. Jones RB, Wright TW, Zuckerman JD. Reverse total shoulder arthroplasty with structural bone grafting of large glenoid defects. J Shoulder Elb Surg. 2016;25(9):1425–32. https://doi.org/10.1016/j.jse.2016.01.016.
57. Benninger E, Zingg PO, Kamath AF, Dora C. Cost analysis of fresh-frozen femoral head allografts: is it worthwhile to run a bone bank? Bone Joint J. 2014;96-B(10):1307–11. https://doi.org/10.1302/0301-620X.96B10.33486.
58. Delimar D, Aljinovic A, Bicanic G. Failure of bulk bone grafts after total hip arthroplasty for hip dysplasia. Arch Orthop Trauma Surg. 2014;134(8):1167–73. https://doi.org/10.1007/s00402-014-2006-8.
59. Friedman R, Stroud N, Glattke K, Flurin PH, Wright TW, Zuckerman JD, et al. The impact of posterior wear on reverse shoulder glenoid fixation. Bullet Hosp Joint Dis. 2015;73(1):15–20.
60. Roche CP, Stroud NJ, Martin BL, Steiler CA, Flurin PH, Wright TW, et al. Achieving fixation in glenoids with superior wear using reverse shoulder arthroplasty. J Shoulder Elb Surg. 2013; https://doi.org/10.1016/j.jse.2013.03.008.
61. Roche CP, Stroud NJ, Palomino P, Flurin PH, Wright TW, Zuckerman JD, et al. The impact of anterior glenoid defects on reverse shoulder glenoid fixation in a composite scapula model. Bullet Hosp Joint Dis. 2018;76(2):116–22.
62. Jones RB, Wright TW, Roche CP. Bone grafting the glenoid versus use of augmented glenoid baseplates with reverse shoulder arthroplasty. Bullet Hosp Joint Dis. 2015;73(1):129–35.
63. Virk M, Yip M, Liuzza L, Abdelshahed M, Paoli A, Grey S, et al. Clinical and radiographic outcomes with a posteriorly augmented glenoid for Walch B2, B3, and C glenoids in reverse total shoulder arthroplasty. J Shoulder Elb Surg. 2020;29(5):e196–204. https://doi.org/10.1016/j.jse.2019.09.031.
64. Bodendorfer BM, Loughran GJ, Looney AM, Velott AT, Stein JA, Lutton DM, et al. Short-term outcomes of reverse shoulder arthroplasty using a custom baseplate for severe glenoid deficiency. J Shoulder Elb Surg. 2021;30(5):1060–7. https://doi.org/10.1016/j.jse.2020.08.002.
65. Rangarajan R, Blout CK, Patel VV, Bastian SA, Lee BK, Itamura JM. Early results of reverse total shoulder arthroplasty using a patient-matched glenoid implant for severe glenoid bone deficiency. J Shoulder Elb Surg. 2020;29(7S):S139–S48. https://doi.org/10.1016/j.jse.2020.04.024.
66. Mahylis JM, Puzzitiello RN, Ho JC, Amini MH, Iannotti JP, Ricchetti ET. Comparison of radiographic and clinical outcomes of revision reverse total shoulder arthroplasty with structural versus nonstructural bone graft. J Shoulder Elb Surg. 2019;28(1):e1–9. https://doi.org/10.1016/j.jse.2018.06.026.
67. Ozgur SE, Sadeghpour R, Norris TR. Revision shoulder arthroplasty with a reverse shoulder prosthesis : Use of structural allograft for glenoid bone loss. Der Orthop. 2017;46(12):1055–62. https://doi.org/10.1007/s00132-017-3494-3.
68. Iannotti JP, Frangiamore SJ. Fate of large structural allograft for treatment of severe uncontained glenoid bone deficiency. J Shoulder Elb Surg. 2012;21(6):765–71. https://doi.org/10.1016/j.jse.2011.08.069.
69. Ho JC, Thakar O, Chan WW, Nicholson T, Williams GR, Namdari S. Early radiographic failure of reverse total shoulder arthroplasty with structural

bone graft for glenoid bone loss. J Shoulder Elb Surg. 2020;29(3):550–60. https://doi.org/10.1016/j.jse.2019.07.035.
70. Liuzza L, Mai DH, Grey S, Wright TW, Flurin PH, Roche CP, et al. Reverse total shoulder arthroplasty with a superior augmented glenoid component for Favard type-E1, E2, and E3 glenoids. J Bone Joint Surg Am. 2020;102(21):1865–73. https://doi.org/10.2106/JBJS.19.00946.
71. Collin P, Liu X, Denard PJ, Gain S, Nowak A, Lädermann A. Standard versus bony increased-offset reverse shoulder arthroplasty: a retrospective comparative cohort study. J Shoulder Elb Surg. 2018;27(1):59–64. https://doi.org/10.1016/j.jse.2017.07.020.
72. Colasanti CA, Lin CC, Ross K, Luthringer T, Elwell JA, Roche C, et al. Augmented baseplates yield optimum outcomes when compared to bone graft augmentation for managing glenoid deformity during reverse total shoulder arthroplasty-a retrospective comparative study. J Shoulder Elb Surg. 2022; https://doi.org/10.1016/j.jse.2022.10.015.
73. Lanham NS, Peterson JR, Ahmed R, Pearsall C, Jobin CM, Levine WN. Comparison of glenoid bone grafting versus augmented glenoid baseplates in reverse shoulder arthroplasty: a systematic review. J Shoulder Elb Surg. 2022; https://doi.org/10.1016/j.jse.2022.11.017.
74. Lädermann A, Collin P, Denard P. Range of motion after RSA: which combinations of humeral stem and glenosphere work the best? Obere Extremität. 2020;15:172–8. https://doi.org/10.1007/s11678-020-00599-5.
75. Collin P, Matsukawa T, Denard PJ, Gain S, Lädermann A. Pre-operative factors influence the recovery of range of motion following reverse shoulder arthroplasty. Int Orthop. 2017;41(10):2135–42. https://doi.org/10.1007/s00264-017-3573-4.

16 Single-stage vs. Two-stage Reconstruction of Glenoid Defects in Revision Shoulder Arthroplasty

Ashish Gupta, Kristine Italia, Roberto Pareyon, Mohammad Jomaa, Marine Launay, Jashint Maharaj, Luke Gilliland, James Nielsen, and Ludwig Seebauer

16.1 Introduction

Glenoid pathologies are one of the main indications for revision surgery in both anatomical and reverse shoulder replacements [1–10]. Significant glenoid defects are often seen during revision, usually requiring extensive bony reconstruction [11–21].

Moreover, one of the main problems of the anatomical hemi-arthroplasty is early glenoid erosion, with an incidence of up to 30% in the individual studies [22, 23]. Revision to an anatomic total shoulder arthroplasty (TSA) in these cases is only promising when the bony erosion is not too advanced, the rotator cuff is intact, and the shoulder joint is well centered [24, 25]. Otherwise, revision to anatomic TSA with bony glenoid reconstruction in these cases has unsatisfactory results due to resorption of the bony augmentation and early loosening of the glenoid component [17, 26].

In primary anatomic TSA, the loosening of the glenoid components, which occurs rather later, is usually accompanied by massive glenoid defects. It is also often associated with rotator cuff insufficiencies or ruptures [1, 7]. Similarly, revision to another anatomic TSA with glenoid bone grafting shows unsatisfactory results due to premature resorption of the bone graft with subsequent recurrent loosening [15, 24, 27]. The biomechanics of anatomic TSA is characterized by eccentric glenoid loading [28]. Additional rotator cuff insufficiency significantly increases this eccentric loading, which then may lead to early component loosening due to the so-called "rocking horse" phenomenon [29]. As a result of the moderate success in attempts to revise these cases to anatomic TSA with a bony structure while retaining the anatomical principle, revision to reverse shoulder arthroplasty (RSA) is now generally practiced in the case of extensive glenoid defects. Exceptions may be young patients with well-preserved rotator cuffs [30]. In these cases of extensive glenoid defects, the revision is always performed with RSA with bony or metallic glenoid augments due to the accompanying rotator cuff insufficiency. Depending on the size of the

A. Gupta (✉)
Queensland Unit for Advanced Shoulder Research (QUASR), Brisbane, Australia

Greenslopes Private Hospital, Brisbane, Australia
e-mail: research@qoc.com.au

K. Italia · R. Pareyon · M. Jomaa
M. Launay · J. Maharaj · L. Gilliland · J. Nielsen
Queensland Unit for Advanced Shoulder Research (QUASR), Brisbane, Australia
e-mail: kristine@akunah.com; ropareyon@gmail.com; dr.mohammadnedaljomaa@gmail.com; marine@akunah.com; jashint@qoc.com.au; luke@akunah.com; james@akunah.com

L. Seebauer
Center for Orthopaedics, Trauma Surgery and Sports Medicine—München-Klinik Bogenhausen, Munich, Germany
e-mail: ludwig.seebauer@extern.lrz-muenchen.de; seebauer@schulterorthopaedie.de

F. Franceschi et al. (eds.), *Revision Shoulder Arthroplasty*,
https://doi.org/10.1007/978-3-031-45944-3_16

defect and concomitant pathology (e.g. low-grade infection), the procedure is performed in one or two stages. In rare cases, definitive revision to a humeral hemiprosthesis or resection arthroplasty is indicated [3, 6, 9].

16.2 Classification of Glenoid Defects in Revision Surgery

16.2.1 Antuna Classification

Antuna et al. [14] presented a classification system for glenoid defects in the revision of anatomical TSA in 2001. The main characteristic is that it distinguishes between centric and peripheral, or a combination of both, in three different degrees of severity (mild, moderate, and severe).

16.2.2 Seebauer-Gupta Classification

One of the senior authors (LS) further developed this classification system for the management of glenoid bone defects in RSA [11] and presented it for the first time in 2005 [31]. In this classification system, we differentiate between 4 centric and 4 eccentric degrees of severity (Table 16.1). In the case of eccentric defects, the main direction of the defect is also specified.

The detailed classification system should serve as a decision-making tool regarding the one- or two-stage procedure, as well as surgical tactics and techniques. This will be discussed in more detail in the following sections. This classification system is independent of the underlying etiology and is defined purely by the morphology of the defect. Therefore, it can be applied for both primary and revision shoulder arthroplasties.

16.2.2.1 Characterization of the Types According to the Seebauer-Gupta Classification [11]

Basically, a distinction is made between centric-contained defects (C defects) and eccentric-uncontained defects (E defects) (Fig. 16.1a–d). In centric defects, the central depth and medial erosion of the defect are the important reference points, as well as the lateral and medial attachment point of the coracoid (Fig. 16.1a). The peripheral bony ring of the glenoid wall and the glenoid cavity ("glenoid vault") are fully preserved [10].

In eccentric defects, the bony substance of the glenoid is eroded in at least one or more directions. The volume loss of the glenoid bone substance and the extent of the maximum medial erosion are used to subdivide the defect size (Fig. 16.1b).

Combined defects are not uncommon (Fig. 16.1c). It is important to include the main direction of eccentricity in the classification (Fig. 16.1d), since the difficulty and type of defect reconstruction in predominantly anterior or posterior eccentric defects is technically far more demanding than in superior or inferior orientation.

A special form is the C4 defect, in which the entire glenoid bone base has eroded medially up to the exit of the scapular spine and only the scapula bone is left with or without contact of the coracoid with the scapula (see Fig. 16.1c).

Table 16.1 Characterization of the glenoid defects according to our classification [11]

	Centric defects		Eccentric defects
C1	Shallow (Depth < 50% of AP glenoid diameter)	E1	Small or shallow
C2	Deep (Depth > 50% of AP glenoid diameter + stable vault)	E2	Medium (<30% of the glenoid bone stock)
C3	Cavitary (C2 + unstable vault)	E3	Large (30–60% of the glenoid bone stock)
C4	Destructive (significant destruction of the glenoid vault)	E4	Massive (>60% of the glenoid bone stock)

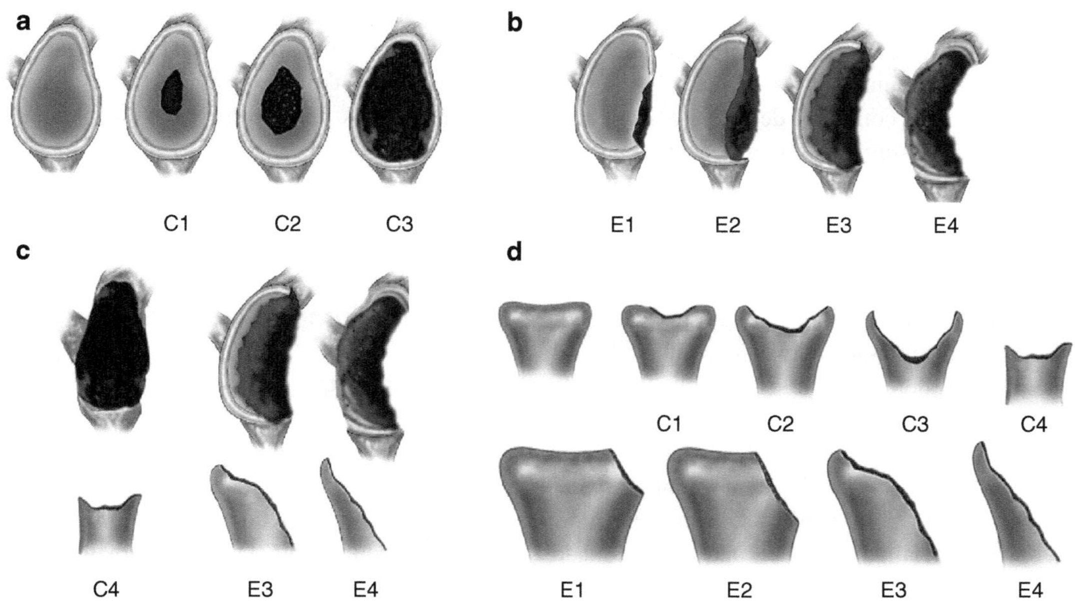

Fig. 16.1 (**a**–**d**) Schematic representation of the glenoid defects: (**a**) centric-contained, (**b**) eccentric-noncontained, (**c**) combined, (**d**) main direction of the defect in the sagittal plane. (Images reprinted from J Shoulder Elbow Surg Vol 27, Gupta et al., "Management of glenoid bone defects with reverse shoulder arthroplasty – surgical technique and clinical outcomes," 853–862, ©2018 [11])

16.2.3 Gohlke and Werner Classification

A similar classification system was presented by Gohlke in 2017 [32] for glenoid defects, whereby only 5 types are differentiated. Based on this classification, the author [33] gives recommendations for the surgical technique of a revision arthroplasty. Type 2 corresponds to the Seebauer-Gupta type C2, type 3 to the Seebauer-Gupta type E2 to E3, type 4 to the Seebauer-Gupta type C3, and type 5 to the Seebauer-Gupta type E4.

16.2.4 Other Classifications

In the meantime, other classification systems have been published in connection with the reconstruction of bony defects during revisions with RSA [34–36], which assess the glenoid defect to varying degrees. Malhas et al. [34] combined the "Antuna" concept with that of Williams et al. [10] 2007 and Page et al. [25] "Glenoid Vault" concept presented in 2009. Kocsis et al. [35] focused mainly on the degree of medialization of the glenoid erosion. However, a more detailed analysis of the 3D configuration and orientation of the defect is not performed. Mahylis et al. [36] used the extended "glenoid vault" model presented by Williams and Iannotti in 2007 [10] for classifying bony glenoid defects.

To date, there is no uniform classification system for assessing glenoid defects in revision shoulder arthroplasty similar to the defect classification of the acetabulum according to Paprosky [37] in revision hip arthroplasty.

16.3 Assessment of Glenoid Defects

This review will focus exclusively on the treatment of extensive bone defects in revision shoulder arthroplasty, which are the defects E3 and E4, as well as C3 and C4, or a combination of these defect sizes according to our classification (Seebauer-Gupta). These correspond to defect sizes 3 to 5 according to Gohlke, types 2 and 3 according to Kocsis, and the severe defect types according to Antuna.

Since centric contained defects are much easier to address surgically than eccentric uncontained defects, it is important to differentiate the defects regarding these morphological criteria and not only according to the defect depth.

For an exact assessment of the reconstructability and for the planning of the surgical technique, a distinction between contained and uncontained defects is essential. On the other hand, it is certainly critical to have an exact description of the extent and the degree of medialization to determine the appropriate surgical technique (i.e., bony construct, composite graft technique, metallic construct, and custom-made implant "PSI") and the decision to perform a one or two stage procedure. This is achieved by using the revision indications of our classification, Gohlke's classification, or the extended Vault model by Williams and Iannotti [10].

In the assessment of the bony defect and the planning of surgical technique, the following factors should be considered:

- Glenoid wall ring present (contained or centric defect) or absent (eccentric defect).
- Volume of the bony defect.
- Degree of maximum medial extent of the defect (degree of medialization of the glenoid joint line "Zero Line").
- Main direction of eccentric glenoid erosion.

Frankle et al. [38] presented in 2009 a purely 3D morphological descriptive classification of glenoid defects in primary reverse prosthesis indications (osteoarthritis and rotator cuff arthropathy), and Klein et al. [39] in 2010 presented their implications for the surgical technique. The latter showed for the first time that in the case of extensive eccentric defects (anterior–inferior–posterior), the fixation of the glenoid baseplate should be performed alternatively in the scapular spine center line (alternative center line).

All classifications presented so far do not consider the bone quality of the residual scapular-glenoid bone. The influence on the surgical strategy (bony vs metallic reconstruction) and the short- and long-term loosening of the glenoid component has not yet been sufficiently investigated.

16.4 Preoperative Imaging Diagnostics and Computerized Planning

16.4.1 Imaging

In addition to X-rays in 3 planes (anteroposterior (AP), Y view, and axial), a computed tomography (CT) scan is always recommended. Nowadays, there is no doubt that 3D imaging of the bone defect, preferably by means of a 3D CT, provides the best visualization of the extent of the defect and the basis for planning the surgery [40] (Fig. 16.2). The 3D imaging provides a much more accurate information regarding the extent of the bony defect to help the surgeon plan the necessary size and shape of the bone graft to fill the defect and the ideal type of revision glenoid baseplate implant. Furthermore, it provides a better visualization and understanding of the remaining bony structures for stable anchorage of the central implant anchoring peg and/or screw or the peripheral screws to achieve optimal primary and long-term stability.

16.4.2 Computerized Planning

Computerized planning is absolutely necessary in cases of revision surgeries associated with bony defects. The process involves uploading CT images of the patient's glenoid and scapula to create a virtual 3D model. Reflect COMPLEX planning by Akunah (Brisbane, Australia) enables an accurate assessment of the glenoid morphology with the measurement of inclination, version after the removal of the metal artifacts, extent of bone loss, estimates of the Zero Line or normal glenoid joint line, and dimensions of the graft required. This aids the surgeon in planning for the 3D position of the baseplate on the physiolog-

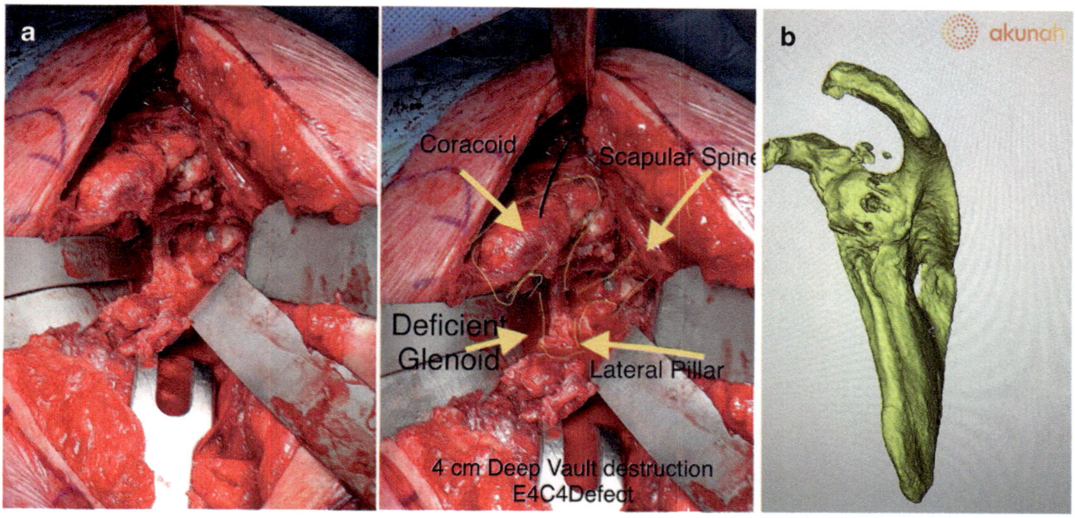

Fig. 16.2 (**a**, **b**) Eccentric E4 defect. (**a**) Intraoperative view of E4 defect after the removal of implants and (**b**) preoperative 3D imaging (image from Reflect COMPLEX (Akunah, Brisbane, Australia))

ical joint line with correct inclination and version.

16.4.2.1 Patient-Specific Instruments (PSI)

The use of preoperative 3D planning software and PSI for shoulder arthroplasty is now clinically established [41]. Manufacturer-specific algorithms applied to the 3D model allow the creation of guidewire implantation templates for the planned positioning of the central peg/screw(s) and determining the correct baseplate position. The creation of an individual bone model of the pathological glenoid facilitates the intraoperative presentation of the pathology. The patient-specific drill guide is used intraoperatively on the pathological glenoid as planned and, if necessary, for cross-checking again on the sterilized glenoid model to determine the optimal entry point and as a patient-specific drill guide for guide wire alignment.

16.4.2.2 Mixed Reality and Navigation

Preoperative planning coupled with mixed reality (MR) or other augmented reality techniques provide enhanced visualization with multiple plans intraoperatively for glenoid reconstruction. This has the advantage over PSI whereby the surgeon is not limited to a single plan as often glenoid baseplate removal can result in larger defects than planned. In the future, MR with navigation for intraoperative guidance of the instruments, especially of the guidewire and preparation of the glenoid surface by reaming or oblique or stepped sawing, will make execution very reliable and precise. However, these techniques also require CT data of the residual glenoid bone free of metal artifacts in order to enable reliable planning and virtual visualization or navigation control of the individual surgical steps [42–44].

16.4.3 Solutions to Metal Artifacts

In the case of revision surgeries, metallic implants in situ often impede visualization due to radiological interference artifacts [45]. These cannot be completely eliminated even with the most modern CT and software technology, which hinders an optimal 3D CT imaging and reliable acquisition of the bony image data. However, the latter are required for the recommended computerized, software-supported 3D planning of the surgical intervention.

If an implant is present and a single-stage procedure is planned, the use of specific CT examina-

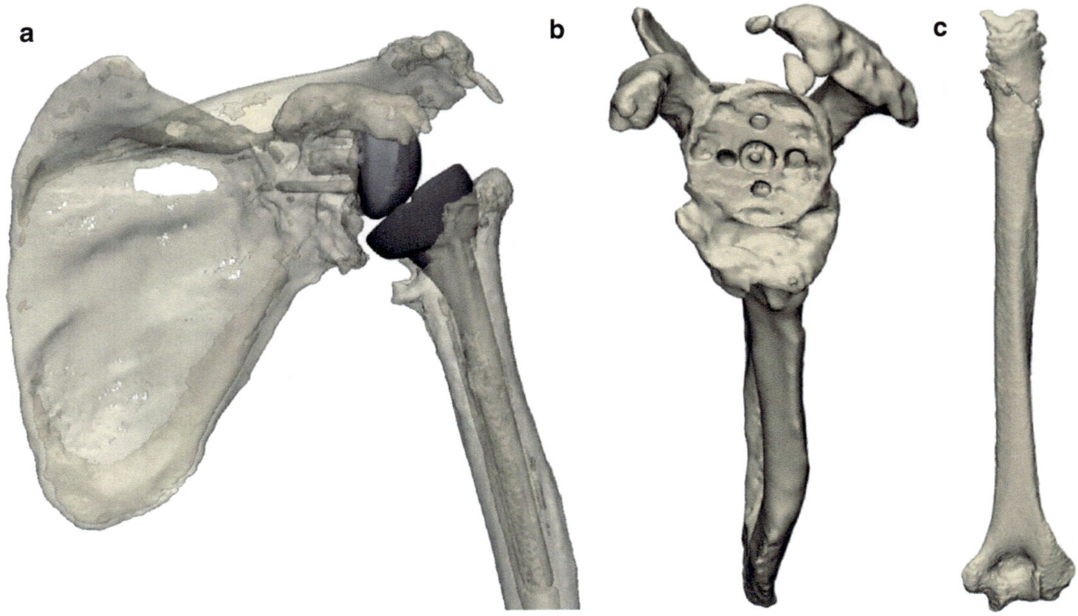

Fig. 16.3 (**a**–**c**) Planning with computer-assisted software with the implants in place (**a**). After subtraction of the primary implants in situ, 3D reconstructions of the scapula (**b**) and humerus (**c**) can be obtained (images from Reflect COMPLEX (Akunah, Brisbane, Australia)). (Images reprinted from J. Clin. Med. Vol 11(24), Italia et al. "Single-Stage Revision Reverse Shoulder Arthroplasty: Preoperative Planning, Surgical Technique, and Mixed Reality Execution", ©2022, https://doi.org/10.3390/jcm11247422 [48])

tion techniques and algorithms may be used to suppress metal artifacts (O-MAR™; https://www.philips.co.uk/healthcare/product/HCNOCTN192/omar-metal-artifact-reduction -for-orthopedic-implants) [45–47].

However, in case that 3D planning using the automated planning software from many suppliers is not possible due to disruptive metal artifacts, planning should at least be carried out on the 2D sectional images reformatted in the 3 spatial planes in all planes (iplan 3.0™, Brainlab AG, Munich or MediCad®-2D; mediCAD Hectec GmbH, D-84032 Altdorf/Landshut).

Recently, the Reflect COMPLEX planning by Akunah (Brisbane, Australia) has made it possible to segment CT images even with primary implants in situ (Fig. 16.3). This software has the ability to subtract implants in place and produce accurate 3D representation of the residual scapula and humerus, allowing precise evaluation of bony defects and manufacturer-independent planning of the surgical treatment.

16.5 Surgical Strategy and Technique

All planning and surgical considerations must have the goal to restore the 3D glenoid anatomy (restore the glenoid joint line to the Zero Line) and achieve reliable primary and long-term fixation of the glenoid component (baseplate) in the residual glenoid bone or scapula. A single-stage approach is preferred over a two-stage procedure to avoid repetitive surgery-related soft tissue trauma, risks of perioperative infections and fractures, and secondary arthrofibrosis.

The following should be given special consideration in the decision-making process:

- Fixation points and method (central peg, central screw, and central peg with screw).
- One-stage or two-stage reconstruction of extensive defects.
- Autologous vs allogeneic bone grafts.
- Composite graft (bone graft in combination with standard baseplate or metal-augmented baseplate).
- Metallic defect filling—patient-specific custom-made implants.

In addition to the residual bone quality, the type, extent, and location of the defect play a decisive role in these different surgical considerations:

- Centric-contained vs eccentric-uncontained.
- Localization of the eccentric defect.

With any technique chosen, the anteversion, retroversion, and inclination of the glenoid articular surface must be restored as best as possible [49, 50]. The medial displacement of the joint line due to the glenoid defect must also be taken into account. This can already be assessed based on a good AP X-ray image. However, the best way is to evaluate the joint line and plan using 3D CT and 3D planning software [40].

16.5.1 Restoration of the Joint Line

The restoration of the joint line (Fig. 16.4) in the coronal plane with the formation of a sufficiently long scapular neck is a critical factor in avoiding inferior glenoid notching, optimization of basic tension, lever arm and torque of all deltoid muscle components and the residual rotator cuff muscles and, above all, on intrinsic stability with the arm adducted. With a medialized joint line, the adduction capacity of the arm is reduced, early inferior mechanical impingement occurs with lat-

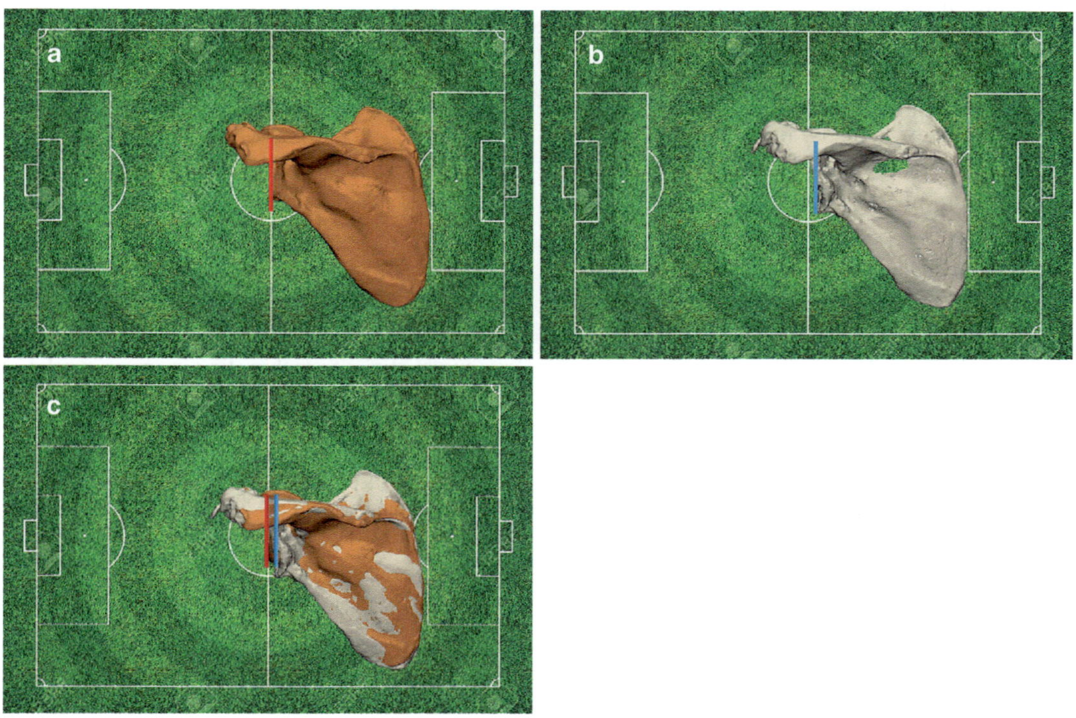

Fig. 16.4 Evaluation of the premorbid anatomy allows to locate the native joint line (red line) (**a**) and the subsequent amount of medialization in the pathological anatomy (blue line) (**b**), thus providing information on the reconstruction necessary to restore the native joint line (distance between the blue and red lines) (**c**). (Images reprinted from J. Clin. Med. Vol 11(24), Italia et al. "Single-Stage Revision Reverse Shoulder Arthroplasty: Preoperative Planning, Surgical Technique, and Mixed Reality Execution", ©2022, https://doi.org/10.3390/jcm11247422 [48])

eralizing joint-destabilizing pressure on the humeral component, and the risk of early inferior bony glenoid erosion (inferior notching) increases. Furthermore, medialization weakens the residual external rotators, generates a lateralizing, and thus destabilizes force vector in the start phase of the deltoid muscles from the adduction position (reduction of the compression effect of the deltoid muscles) [51–53].

In addition, knowledge of the premorbid glenohumeral joint line during reconstructive procedures allows for an adequate length-tensioning relationship of the rotator cuff, the conjoint tendon, the deltoid, as well as the periscapular muscles [40, 48].

16.5.1.1 Centric—Contained Defects

In these defects, the glenoid ring is completely or sufficiently preserved, and the medialization has not yet reached the so-called red line (perpendicular to the medial coracoid attachment). Techniques on restoring the joint line depend on the depth of the defect and mechanical strength of the residual glenoid bone stock.

1. *Impaction bone grafting (*Fig. 16.5*).*

   In smaller defects, filling with cancellous bone or corticocancellous chips and impaction grafting are sufficient.
2. *Corticocancelous bone grafting.*

   In advanced C3 defects with partial smaller wall defects or poor anterior or posterior bony glenoid rim quality, the additional insertion of a corticocancellous chip is recommended. This usually does not have to be fixed with additional screws. It can be fixed directly with primary stability via the central peg and the peripheral screws. The central peg of the baseplate must be of sufficiently long to allow at least 50% of its length to sit in the native scapular bone. A temporary fixation with Kirschner wire (K wire) during the preparation of the glenoid and the graft to receive the implant is recommended.
3. *Composite graft technique.*

   Alternatively, larger defects can also be addressed using the so-called composite graft technique. This is the preferred approach, especially in the case of advanced or combined C3 defects and C4 defects (Fig. 16.6). This technique is further discussed later.

16.5.1.2 Eccentric-Uncontained Defects

Structural corticocancellous bone grafts are fundamentally necessary to reconstruct these defects. In the case of revision, the humeral head is not available. Hence, only the autologous iliac crest graft or allograft can be considered.

There are different tactics for reconstructing these defects.

1. *Preparation of the glenoid defect.*

   The first step is to adapt the shape and contact surface of the corticocancellous bone graft to the defect as well as possible in three dimensions. In the case of difficult defect geometry and bone graft modeling, it is sometimes helpful to make a bone cement model of the defect. It is also helpful to orient yourself

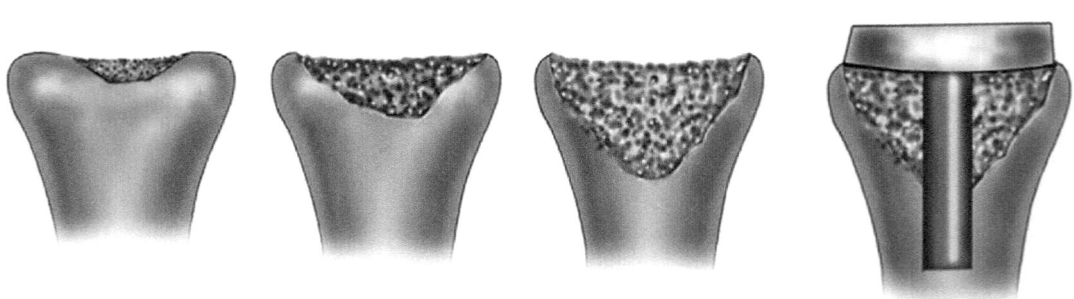

Fig. 16.5 Treatment of a contained C3 defect with an impaction graft and metaglene with a long peg. (Images reprinted from J Shoulder Elbow Surg Vol 27, Gupta et al., "Management of glenoid bone defects with reverse shoulder arthroplasty – surgical technique and clinical outcomes," 853–862, ©2018 [11])

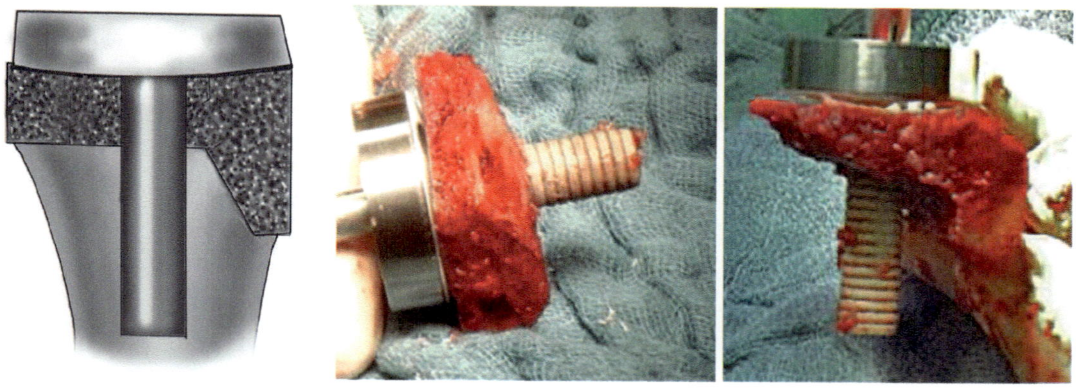

Fig. 16.6 "Composite-Graft": corticocancellous graft is applied directly to the central peg of the metaglene and then inserted together into the central anchoring hole in the scapula. (Images reprinted from J Shoulder Elbow Surg Vol 27, Gupta et al., "Management of glenoid bone defects with reverse shoulder arthroplasty – surgical technique and clinical outcomes," 853–862, ©2018 [11])

on the existing non-eroded parts of the glenoid. Moreover, formation of a good bearing surface for the corticocancellous bone graft with a stepped configuration is optimal here. During osteotomy of the bearing surface, care must be taken to preserve as much native glenoid/scapular bone as possible.

2. *Impaction bone grafting of smaller, central defects.*

   After thorough debridement and freshening up, the central cystic or lacunar parts of the defect are filled by impacting cancellous or corticocancellous bone. Any minor unevenness on the glenoid contact surface should also be evened out with milled corticocancellous bone graft. Firm impaction of bone graft is necessary to get a stable base for baseplate fixation.

3. *Reconstruction of the defect.*

   The main defect can now be reconstructed in three ways:

   (a) Definitive defect filling.

   The corticocancellous graft is directly inserted into the defect (cortical surface peripherally on the glenoid edge and centrally in the contact area of the glenoid baseplate) (Fig. 16.7). The graft is temporarily fixed using two to three 1.2 mm K wires and can later be fixed with a cannulated 4.0 mm cancellous screw if the fixation with the peripheral screws of the baseplate is not sufficient. Then, the guidewire of the glenoid reamer with the guide template is inserted into the desired scapula position (standard or alternative scapular spine center line). Care must be taken not to create a superior tilt and to achieve sufficient fixation depth in the native scapula. We aim for at least 50% of the central glenoid peg or screw length in the native bone. If anything is unclear, an intraoperative fluoroscopy should be performed in the correct anterior–posterior projection. This is followed by the careful and economical reaming of the remaining peripheral glenoid bone or the surface of the chip, followed by drilling of the central hole. The metal baseplate (standard or metallic augmented form) is then inserted and fixed with at least two peripheral locking screws. Protruding bone that obstructs the placement of the glenosphere is carefully reamed off.

   (b) Extracorporeal graft preparation.

   Alternatively, the central guidewire can be inserted into the previously planned scapular position before the definitive defect filling with the corticocancellous graft using a guide template or a patient-specific defect-adapted setting

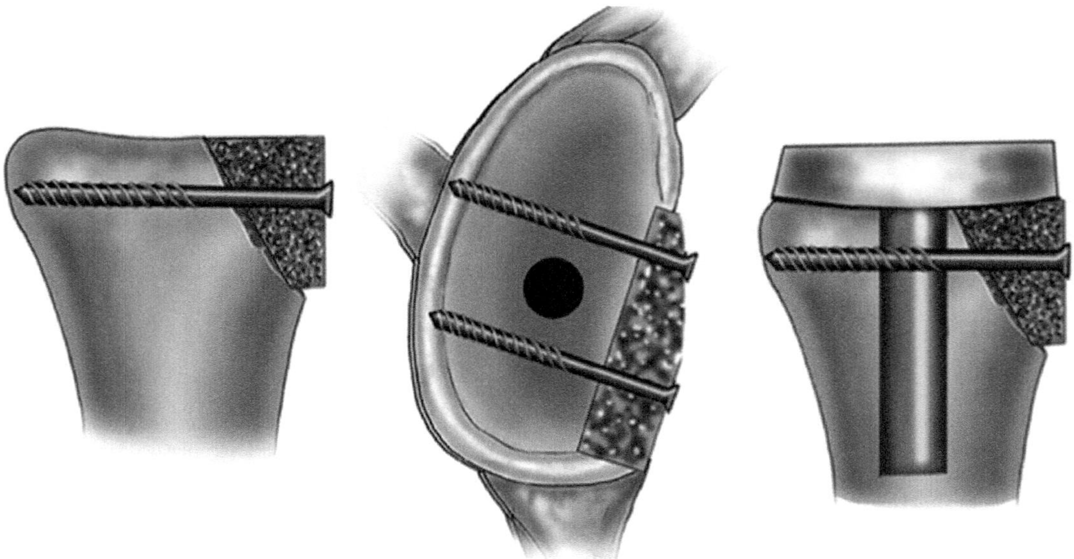

Fig. 16.7 Corticocancellous bone graft of anterior glenoid defect with an oblique (or stepped osteotomy) and fixed with screws from anterior to posterior. (Images reprinted from J Shoulder Elbow Surg Vol 27, Gupta et al., "Management of glenoid bone defects with reverse shoulder arthroplasty – surgical technique and clinical outcomes," 853–862, ©2018 [11])

instrument (PSI) or holograms. In this case, the exact position of the guidewire must be marked on the prepared graft and the hole for the central peg or screw of the baseplate must be prepared extracorporeally with the graft. After the graft has been inserted, the subsequent procedure is as described above. (Temporary graft fixation with K wires, surface reaming, drilling of the central fixation, and insertion of the definitive implant).

(c) Composite graft technique.

As described above, a precisely fitting corticocancellous graft is prepared. This is then applied directly to the metallic baseplate (Fig. 16.7). Prior to inserting the composite graft, the surface of the native glenoid is reamed and the hole for central fixation of the baseplate is drilled. Central cystic-lacunar defects are filled with mulched cancellous bone, and the bearing surface on the glenoid is covered with soft cancellous bone. The baseplate and the graft are then introduced together into the prepared central hole of the glenoid. Finally, the construct is fixed definitely with at least two peripheral angle-stable screws in a compressive and angle-stable manner.

The two last-mentioned methods allow better visualization, as well as 3D orientation and guidance, when inserting the central guidewire into the planned scapula position (standard or scapula spine center line). This is particularly useful, especially in cases with very extensive defects.

Whether additional screw fixation is necessary depends essentially on the main direction of the eccentricity and less on the extent of the defect (E3 < 60% or E4 > 60% glenoid). Anterior or posterior extensive defects are usually more technically challenging and usually require additional screw fixation. Bone grafts of superior or inferior defects can usually be sufficiently fixed with the superior or inferior screw of the baseplate.

16.5.2 Surgical Technique Basic Principles for Revision Shoulder Arthroplasty

16.5.2.1 Debridement—Freshening—Jet Lavage

After explantation of existing implants, every defect must be thoroughly debrided of all foreign materials from the previous operation (cement and metallosis). Scar and granulation tissue, as well as necrotic bone material, must also be meticulously removed. All nonviable tissues must be excised. However, as much native glenoid/scapular bone as possible should also be preserved. At least three tissue samples from the glenoid and bone–soft–tissue interface should be sent for microbiological and histopathological examination, having a total of five samples from the entire joint area.

16.5.2.2 Positioning and Implantation Depth of the Central Anchorage in Native Glenoid/Scapular Bone

To achieve adequate primary and long-term stability, we recommend that at least 50% of the length of the central peg and/or screw lies in the native bone of the glenoid or scapula. Koenigshausen [54] et al. have described an anchorage depth of 30% of the central peg length as sufficient in biomechanical studies. Gohlke [33] suggested an anchorage depth of at least 1 cm in the native bone.

In the case of extensive anterior or posterior–inferior defects (E3 or E4 according to the Seebauer-Gupta classification), it is not possible to achieve sufficient bony purchase of the central peg or screw for primary stability when implanting the baseplate centered on the so-called standard glenoid line. In such cases, we recommend using the so-called alternative scapula spine center line for central fixation [39]. It must be taken into account that this leads to an anteversion and inferior inclination of the baseplate of 10° each.

16.5.2.3 Screw Fixation of the Baseplate

In order to achieve a permanent firm fixation and bony osteointegration of the baseplate as well as stable healing of the bone graft, it is important that the fixing screws apply sufficient compression pressure of the glenoid baseplate against the residual glenoid surface and the implanted bone graft. To achieve adequate primary stability, it is recommended to use at least 2 screws with stable angles. It is optimal if the screws used are primarily inserted compressively and can finally be fixed at a stable angle. The screws must be inserted with sufficient length in the native glenoid/scapular bone. We recommend a minimum of 40 mm for the inferior screw and a minimum of 30 mm for the superior screw.

Extensive glenoid defects limit the spatial options for screw placement. According to the "3-pillar" principle by Norris [17, 33], it is imperative that an inferior screw be placed in the lateral margin of the scapula and the superior screw in the coracoid base. Contrary to Humphrey and Norris [17], we consider a posterior screw in the scapular spine to be critical, as it could also be the cause of secondary spinal fractures [55]. Computerized planning software enables planning of the optimal orientation of the baseplate in the sagittal plane in order to be able to insert the longest possible screws in the desired anchorage zone (Fig. 16.8).

16.5.2.4 One- vs Two-Stage Reconstruction

1. One-stage reconstruction.

   In principle, one-stage reconstruction is generally possible for E3 and C3 defects.

   1a. *E3 defects.*

   With E3 defects, it is necessary to achieve the most stable contact surface possible. If the remaining glenoid bone stock allows, we convert the oblique defect into a stepped configuration, since the primary stability of the bone graft is greater this way [56, 57]. A bi- or even

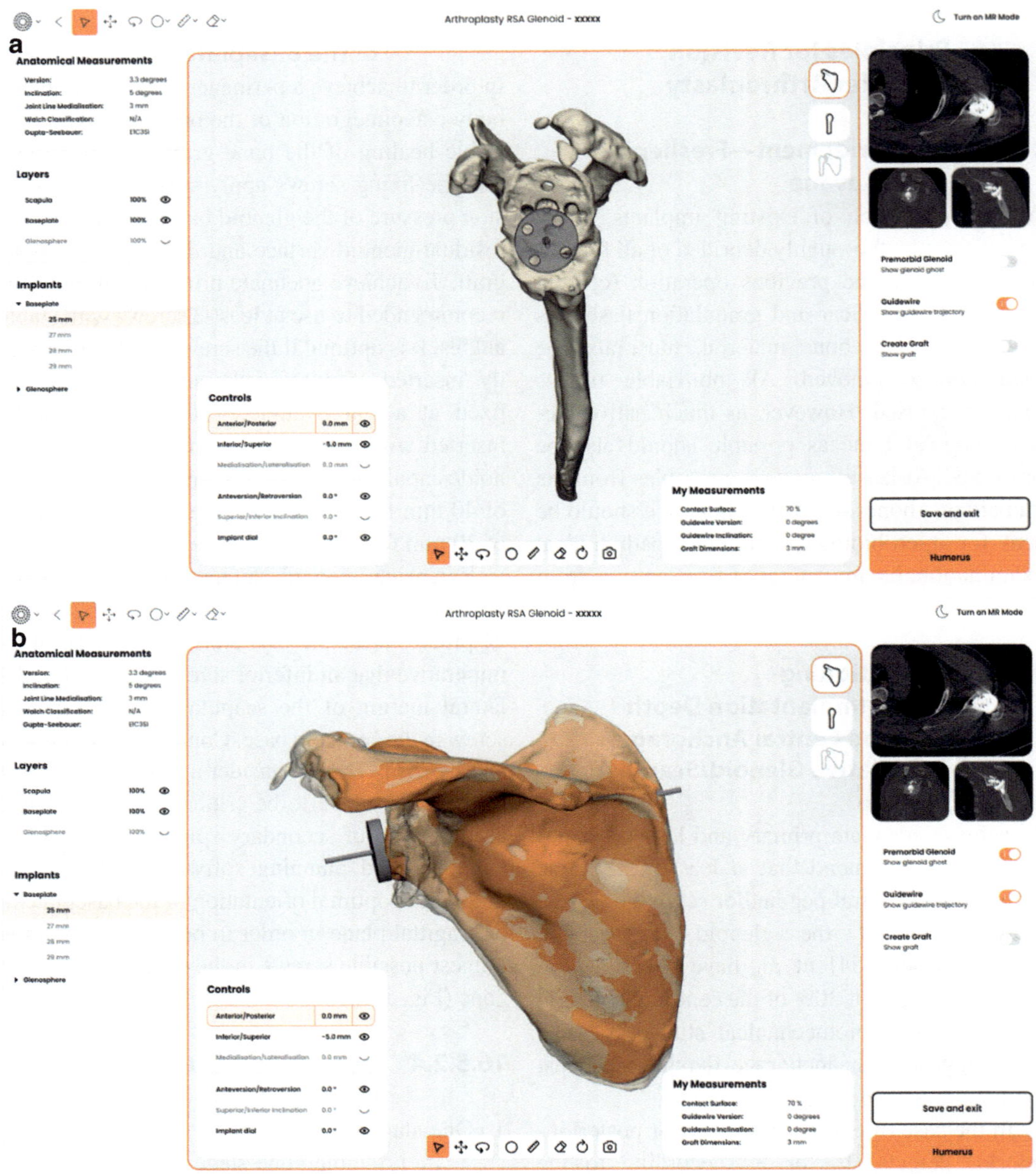

Fig. 16.8 3D planning of the baseplate position and orientation, as well as screw position and length with computerized planning software (images from Reflect™ (Akunah, Brisbane, Australia)). (Images reprinted from J. Clin. Med. Vol 11(24), Italia et al. "Single-Stage Revision Reverse Shoulder Arthroplasty: Preoperative Planning, Surgical Technique, and Mixed Reality Execution," ©2022, https://doi.org/10.3390/jcm11247422 [48])

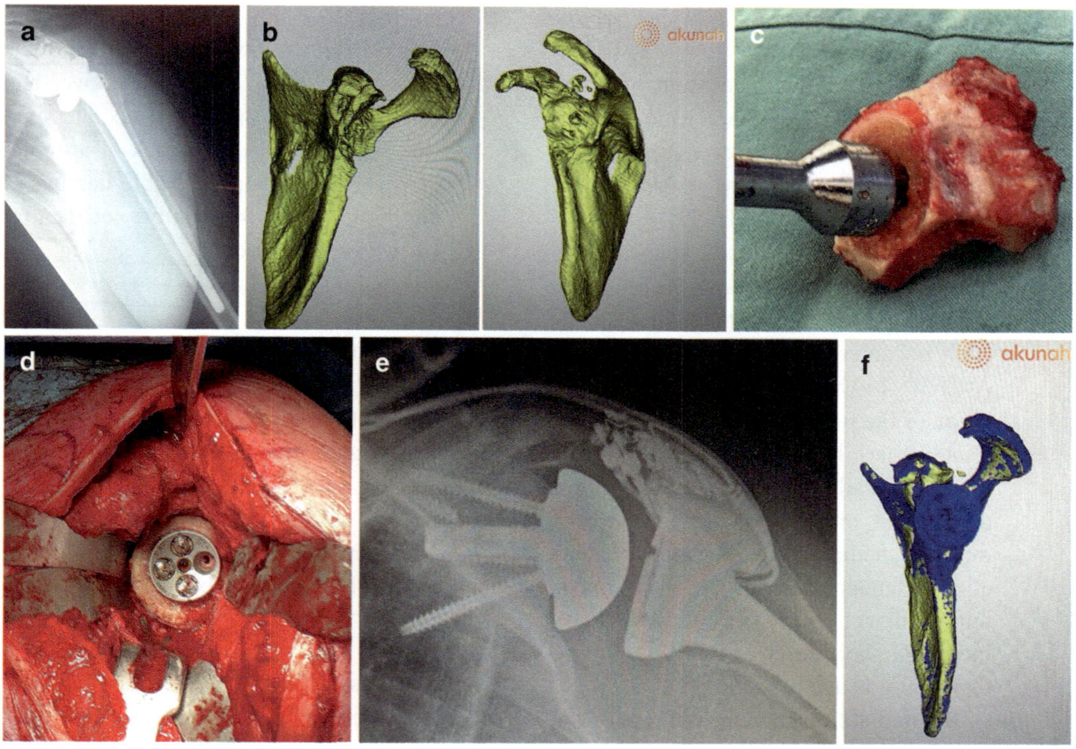

Fig. 16.9 (**a–f**) L-Span technique for reconstruction of advanced E4 and C4 defects. (**a**) Preoperative radiograph. (**b**) Preoperative 3D model with implant subtraction, (**c**) Figure 7 or L-shaped composite allograft, (**d**) Intraoperative view showing the construct performed using single-stage revision, (**e**) 2-year postoperative radiograph, and (**f**) 2-year postoperative 3D model with implant subtraction

tri-cortical iliac crest bone graft is always necessary for this.

1b. *C3 defects.*

In the case of C3 defects, we fill the central defect with cancellous or corticocancellous bone. The medialization of the joint line is then corrected with a corticocancellous bone graft made of monocortical iliac crest bone. We usually insert the bone graft as a composite graft directly with the baseplate.

1c. *E4 defects.*

In E4 defects, one-stage reconstruction is still possible if there is sufficient bone stock (i.e. approximately 30% of the native glenoid bone), if the defect no longer has a rudimentary posterior or anterior posterior glenoid wall, and if the central fixation part of the baseplate can be anchored with at least 50% of its length in the native scapula.

If possible, we use the composite graft technique with a corresponding L-shaped corticocancellous graft, especially for combined E3 and E4 defects with significant medialization (asymmetric C3 situation) (see Fig. 16.9). It is important to cover the defect surface with soft cancellous bone for optimal support and to compensate for minor irregularities.

2. Two-stage reconstruction.

A two-stage approach is necessary in cases where the central fixation of the baseplate does not gain sufficient depth and fixation in the native scapula, when there is only a paper-thin layer of the glenoid (E4 advanced) left on one side, or when the glenoid bone base is completely absent.

2a. *L-Span technique for two-stage reconstruction of the glenoid.*

As an alternative to custom implants [58], the reconstruction of the glenoid and the implantation of the reverse prosthesis can be carried out in two stages using a large L-shaped bone graft [59].

In the first stage, the L-shaped bone graft is fixed with screws to the posterior (in the case of anterior defects) scapular wall or anterior–inferior glenoid wall. After 10–12 weeks, the definitive implantation of the metaglene takes place. If the joint line is still medialized, it is advisable to use a metallic augmented baseplate for the second intervention. In the case of minimal medialization (−4 mm), a lateralized glenosphere may be used (maximum of 6 mm) since significantly increased shear forces occur when more than 8 mm is used [60].

In 2015 at the Annual Congress of the German Association for Shoulder and Elbow Surgery (DVSE) in Mannheim, we presented a case study of 7 patients who were reconstructed using this technique between June 2013 and June 2014. One-year follow-up showed that both the bone graft from the first stage and the prosthesis had healed stably. In two cases, osteoporosis caused scapular spine fracture or sagittal scapular fracture and one horizontal scapular dissociation 2 years postoperatively.

2b. *Humeral reconstruction.*

Based on our experience, we generally recommend leaving the humeral component in place or restoring it with a convex hemiprosthesis only in cases where a concentric joint without subluxation tendency is noted during revision. Only in these cases, the contact pressure of the hemiprosthetic articulation can help to accelerate the healing process of the bone graft. In the case of a preexisting subluxation or chronic persistent posterior or anterior dislocation of the prosthesis to be revised, we generally recommend removing the preexisting humerus component, glenoid defect reconstruction using the L-Span technique described above, and leaving the joint in an intermediate sine-sine situation. Despite a lack of articulation pressure, adequate stable healing of the bone graft is usually noted after 12 weeks, ready for the second stage of prosthetic implantation.

16.5.2.5 Autograft or Allograft

When deciding between an autologous and an allogeneic corticocancellous bone graft, the resected humeral head as an option for bone graft is already eliminated in the revision procedure. This is usually sufficient for primary RSA with the need for corticocancellous reconstruction of extensive glenoid bone defects.

1. Autograft.

   In the case of revision, only the iliac crest can be considered as a source for autologous bone graft. In older and osteoporotic patients, only moderate-quality bone is often found here. In addition, the harvest results in a considerable donor-site morbidity with corresponding possible complications, including secondary debilitating iliac wing fractures [61]. Therefore, when removing larger tricortical iliac crest bone graft, we always perform a prophylactic plating of the iliac crest that bridges the removal zone using a 1/3 tubular plate.

   Autologous corticocancellous bone graft reconstruction of bone defects in RSA shows good healing and no graft resorption in over 90% of all studies, even over the long term [11, 13, 16, 33, 54, 55, 62, 63].

2. Allograft.

   Results reported in the literature using corticocancellous allograft show a mixed picture (Table 16.2). This is probably due to the type of allograft material used with varying biological potency due to preparation, preservation, and storage. One of the senior authors (AG) routinely uses allograft reconstruction for all C3 C4/E3 E4 defects and has had successful clinical outcome with minimal resorp-

Table 16.2 Healing of allografts for the reconstruction of glenoid defects (primary and revision surgeries)

Author	n	Kind of graft	Preparation method	Failure rate
Bateman [19]	5	femoral neck	Hybrid: Autograft & Fresh frozen allograft	0%
Jones [20]	14	femoral head	–	33.3%
Lopiz [62]	13	Tibial plateau, femoral head	Fresh frozen	5%
Ozgur [64]	8	femoral stem	Thermodisinfected, deep frozen	87.5%
Ozgur [64]	9	femoral head	Thermodisinfected, deep frozen	33.3%
Tashjian [65]	22	femoral head	Fresh frozen	17.5%
Ho [66]	4	Hip, humeral head, fibula	Fresh frozen	50%

tion, whereas the other senior author (LS) due to mixed results with thermo-disinfected deep frozen structural allografts only use cortico-cancellous allograft chips for impaction grafting of centric defects. In eccentric defect with the need for a structural graft, he recommends the iliac crest autograft. Custom-made patient- or defect-specific allografts can now be made using the Reflect COMPLEX (Akunah, Brisbane, Australia). However, surgeons globally have had mixed results with allografts. Local factors and graft preparation techniques may play a significant role. In older patients, we use a metal-augmented glenoid baseplate in these cases. In contained centric C3 defects, central filling with allogeneic corticocancellous graft using the impaction technique is a reasonable alternative.

16.6 Discussion

In addition to the senior author's (LS) first series [31] of 9 patients with significant glenoid defects (> C3, > E3) reported at the European Society for Surgery of the Shoulder and the Elbow (SECEC) 2005 meeting in Rome, Neyton et al. in 2007 [67] were the next to report relevant numbers of patients with significant glenoid defects who underwent structural bone grafting with RSA in one or two stages. There were 3 primary RSAs for defect arthropathy, in which the defect was classified according to Favard [68] and the defect was filled with autologous humeral head. The other 6 patients underwent revision surgery using the autologous iliac crest as a graft. There was no precise description of the defect size and type. The mean postoperative Constant score was 53 (range 22–79), which was lower than for primary RSA without glenoid augmentation. Despite this, patients were subjectively satisfied with the outcome due to the significant reduction in pain. Radiographically, there was no glenoid loosening or graft resorption. Significant glenoid notching was observed in 66% (6 patients). A surgical treatment algorithm based on a defect classification could not be found in this work. It was more of a retrospective evaluation of individual intraoperative surgical decisions.

In contrast, in 2005 [31], one of the senior authors (LS) presented a treatment algorithm regarding the type of bone graft (cancellous, corticocancellous chips, or structural corticocancellous graft) and its fixation depending on our purely pathomorphological-based defect classification.

A defect-related analysis regarding the surgical procedure and fixation technique of the glenoid baseplate was shown for the first time by Klein et al. in 2010 [39] by positioning the central fixation of the glenoid baseplate not in the standard glenoid center line but alternatively in the scapula spine center line for certain extensive defects. In this study, defects are divided into anterior, posterior, inferior, superior, or global defects based on their main extent. There is no scaled quantitative defect classification, but the inclination, version, distance from the coracoid, and acromion were linearly measured for each defect. The scapular spine center line is chosen as the fixation for all eccentric, non-contained defects where fixation in the standard center line would not result in sufficient anchorage depth. A bone graft was also performed in 22 of 65 patients with anchorage in the scapular spine center line. The clinical results are not different for patients with or without bone grafting. The healing of the glenoid component is the same in both groups, with no relevant resorptions observed in the patients with bone augmentation. The defects were observed during primary implantations of the reverse prosthesis.

Bateman et al. [19] reported in 2012 on the use of a combination of long peg baseplate onto which a combined autologous-allograft bone graft was placed and then used as a composite graft for the single-stage treatment of extensive glenoid defects in reverse shoulder replacement. There were 5 patients with extensive, massive, uncontained glenoid defects, the extent of which was not further classified. A single-stage reconstruction was performed with a combined autologous and allograft bone graft applied directly onto the long peg glenoid baseplate and then incorporated as a "composite-graft baseplate" construct in a single-stage procedure. He reported no glenoid component loosening or relevant graft resorption after a minimum follow-up of at least 1 year. Postoperative CT scans showed a complete healing of the construct after 6 months at the latest.

Jones et al. [20] reported in 2016 on 44 patients who underwent single-stage primary or revision RSA with large structural bone grafting for an extensive bone defect. Twenty-nine humeral autografts, 1 iliac crest autograft, and 14 femoral head allografts were used. Eighty one percent of cases showed complete or adequate partial graft incorporation. Baseplate loosening occurred in 6 cases. The healing potential for autograft and allograft was reported to be equivalent. All patients who received a bone augmentation showed significantly better functional and clinical results postoperatively. There was no difference between autologous and allogeneic defect augmentation. However, the clinical results were poorer when compared with an age- and sex-matched comparison group without major bone defects treated with RSA. Overall, there were 6 (14%) complications requiring revision (1 dislocation, 1 humeral loosening, 2 aseptic glenoid loosening, and 2 infections).

Boileau et al. [13] described the use of a 3D corticocancellous autologous chip in combination with a long peg glenoid baseplate composite graft to restore neutral glenoid version and inclination in multiplanar eccentric defects. The defects were classified in the coronal plane according to Favard [68] and in the horizontal plane according to Bercik and Walch [69]. After 3D planning, patient-specific chips and guide templates were used. At a mean follow-up of 36 months in 54 patients, complete graft incorporation was observed in 91%. Baseplate loosening occurred in one case. Mild notching occurred in 25% of cases. The Constant score was 68 points, and the SSV was 83% at final follow-up.

Kelly and Norris [16, 17] gave recommendations regarding the surgical approach depending on the type of defect. They recommended using autologous humeral head or iliac crest for structural support of the baseplate and glenosphere. A distinction is made between 3 types of defects according to Kocsis [35]. For defect type 2 (1 wall and parts of the glenoid cavity still present), he recommends the use of the tricortical iliac crest and insertion as a composite graft threaded onto the central peg of the baseplate. Secure anchoring in the native scapula is necessary for a single-stage procedure. In the case of global type 3 defects (glenoid cavity completely missing), he recommends a two-stage procedure. It should be noted that bone substitutes, such as calcium orthophosphate, are not adequate substitute material.

Taylor et al. [63], using the same defect classification (according to Kocsis [35]) like Kelly and Norris, used the autologous lateral clavicle as graft instead of the autologous iliac crest. Glenoid component loosening and graft resorption occurred in only 1 of 20 cases, and secondary instability of the acromioclavicular joint occurred in only one case, which was not clinically significant in the follow-up examination. The reason given for the loosening was an intraoperative technical error (graft fracture) and the use of a non-osteointegrating central screw instead of using another baseplate with central compressive peg.

When using the humeral head as a structural autograft to fill glenoid defects, Tashjian et al. [70] reported loosening of the glenoid component in 1 case out of 26 primary reverse shoulder endoprostheses after an average of 2.6 years, but no chip resorption in any case. In our retrospective analysis of 94 patients treated with a structural autograft, with 83% having mainly eccentric defects, the bone augmentation could be carried out at the same time as the primary RSA in 93% of patients [11]. In one case, premature loosening of the glenoid component occurred because a sufficiently long central peg was not used. There was no radiological loosening during the follow-up period. Baseplate migration (1 superior and 1 medial) was observed in 2 cases. Resorption was noted in parts of the bone graft not covered by the baseplate, but never below the baseplate, with the exception of an inferior glenoid notching. Significant notching was observed in 3 cases. Clinical function improved significantly postoperatively with an increase in the Constant score of 61, as did the SST (increase of 5.8 points). The clinical outcome was independent of gender, age, defect size, and location. The overall complication rate was 13%. If the anchorage in the native scapula is not deep enough and the primary stability is insufficient, we recommend a two-stage procedure.

Gohlke et al. [33] reported on the treatment of large (58% type 2 and 3 of their classification [32]) and very large glenoid defects (42% type 4 and 5) in 145 patients. Autologous iliac crest was used as a structural graft in 56 patients and allograft in 5 cases. Twenty-five percent of the cases were carried out in two stages. The success rate (healing of the graft without loosening of the glenoid component) was over 90% for both the one- and two-stage procedures.

Mahylis et al. [36] compared the healing rates of structural autologous iliac crest grafts with nonstructural allografts in a retrospective study. Defects were significantly larger in cases with structural autografts. Radiologic follow-up at least 2 years postoperatively showed no difference between the two groups in terms of graft integration and resorption, glenosphere tilt and version, and notching rate. There was also no difference in clinical outcomes. Glenoid component loosening occurred in one patient with the iliac crest graft.

The retrospective study by Ho et al. [66] of 44 patients (37 primary and 7 revision indications) with structural bone grafting for glenoid defects with RSA showed graft resorption and glenoid component loosening in 25% after a median of 20 months. The resorption rate for the allografts was 50%. Correcting extensive version discrepancies appears to affect resorption and loosening rates. Important to note that primary RSAs were included in this study.

Tashjian et al. [65] came to a completely different conclusion who retrospectively analyzed 22 patients (12 indications for revision) with a femoral head allograft and a minimum follow-up of 2 years. Differentiated defect classification preoperatively was not used. The decision to reconstruct the defect was made intraoperatively based on the extent of superior inclination, version deviation, and medial erosion. A bone graft was used when the inclination and the version could not be restored to ±10°, and the joint line could not be restored physiologically by reaming. After 1 year postoperatively, complete graft incorporation was observed in 82% of the cases. Baseplate migration or radiographic loosening occurred in 2 patients without the need for surgical revision. Secondary acromion fractures with subsequent pseudoarthrosis occurred in 2 patients.

Nabergoj et al. [71] in a recently published study compared the clinical and radiographic results of defect reconstruction using bone augmentation and combined bony and metallic augmentation. The size and depth of the glenoid defect were significantly larger in the latter group. Despite the less favorable initial condition, postoperative flexion was better in the combined treatment. During a minimum 2-year follow-up, there was no relevant graft resorption or glenoid component loosening noted in any group. Partial inferior graft resorption was observed in 3 of 8 cases with bone augmentation alone.

Singh et al. [72] carried out the reconstruction of extensive glenoid defects in 43 patients with a structural autograft combined with a special glenoid baseplate made of trabecular titanium, inserted as a composite graft. RSA was performed in 25 patients, 19 of which were revision surgeries, in which the autologous iliac crest was used as the graft. CT scans at 2 years postoperatively showed satisfactory bone graft incorporation (at least 50%) in 90% of the cases. The average improvement in the Constant score was 36 points. The complication rate was relatively high: acromion/scapular spine fracture 2, infection 1, loosening 1, hematoma on iliac crest 1, brachial plexus damage 1, and notching 9 (1 with grade ≥ 3).

With the exception of one study, the few cohort studies show that with a precise understanding of the defect morphology and geometry of the residual glenoid bone, one- or two-stage reconstruction using structural bone grafting with RSA results in good success in more than 90% of cases of this extreme difficult pathology, even in extensive bone defects of the glenoid. The clinical results can be described as good but do not reach the results of RSA that do not require structural bone augmentation. In the short and medium term, no increased loosening of the glenoid component can be observed. At least a partial biomechanically sufficient healing of the bone structure is regularly observed.

16.7 Conclusion for Practice

- It is important to carry out a sufficiently differentiated and detailed imaging preoperatively. If possible, 3D CT analysis and software-supported computerized planning of the surgical procedure should be performed while avoiding disruptive metal artifacts.
- Determining the ideal entry point and depth of central peg and/or screw of the glenoid baseplate is critical. The defect must be filled with bone in such a way that the medio-lateral position and the inclination of the glenoid joint line in the coronal plane are physiologically restored. Version deviations in retroversion or anteversion can be tolerated at 10° from normal. 3D CT-based imaging and planning techniques also aid in volumetric and morphological analysis of the required bone graft.
- Anterior or posterior E4 defects or advanced C4 centric defects are the most difficult to treat, since sufficient purchase of the central peg and/or screw of the baseplate is often not possible to achieve with single-stage reconstruction. It is also often difficult to insert the angle-stable screws required according to the "3-pillar" principle with sufficient depth and strength into the coracoid base and lateral margin of the scapula in order to obtain sufficient primary stability.
- In the case of anterior or posterior extensive eccentric defects, direct screw fixation of the bone graft is recommended. An alternative is the so-called composite graft technique.
- If at least 50% of the central peg and/or screw of the baseplate and 2 locking screws in the coracoid and lateral margin of the scapula cannot be anchored well, we recommend a two-stage procedure.
- In principle, the use of special glenoid baseplates with a long central anchoring part (peg and/or screw) is necessary for the treatment of extensive defects due to the medialization of the pathological joint line.
- In younger and non-osteoporotic patients with an extensive eccentric defect, we recommend the autologous iliac crest if revision is indicated. When removing a large tricortical graft, a prophylactic bridge plating of the iliac crest is recommended.
- In the case of extensive eccentric reconstructions and/or nonoptimal primary stability with poor bone quality, we recommend a 45-degree abduction sling for 6 weeks, and passive or assistive exercise up to the horizontal plane, but no combination movements.

Conflict of Interest A Gupta is a consultant for Zimmer and Founder of Akunah.

K Italia, M Launay, L Gilliland, J Nielsen, and J Maharaj are employees of Akunah.

L. Seebauer is a consultant for Depuy Synthes Inc. Ltd. Leeds UK and receives royalties from this company.

Compliance with Ethical Guidelines For the studies listed, the ethical guidelines stated therein apply in each case.

References

1. Bohsali AI, Bois AJ, Wirth MA. Complications of shoulder arthroplasty. [Review]. J Bone Jt Surg Am. 2017;99:256–69.
2. Boileau P, Melis B, Duperron D, Moineau G, Rumian AP, Han Y. Revision surgery of reverse shoulder arthroplasty. J Shoulder Elb Surg. 2013;22(10):1359–70. https://doi.org/10.1016/j.jse.2013.02.004.
3. Boileau P. Complications and revision of reverse total shoulder arthroplasty. Orthop Traumatol Surg Res. 2016;102(1S):S33–43. https://doi.org/10.1016/j.otsr.2015.06.031.
4. Gonzalez JF, Alami GB, Baque F, Walch G, Boileau P. Complications of unconstrained shoulder prostheses. J Shoulder Elb Surg. 2011;20(4):666–82. https://doi.org/10.1016/j.jse.2010.11.017.
5. Boileau P, Moineau G, Morin-Salvo N, et al. Metal-backed glenoid implant with polyethylene insert is not a viable long-term therapeutic option. J Shoulder Elb Surg. 2015;24(10):1534–43. https://doi.org/10.1016/j.jse.2015.02.012.
6. Seidl AJ, Williams GR, Boileau P. Challenges in reverse shoulder arthroplasty: addressing glenoid bone loss. Orthopedics. 2016;39(1):14–23. https://doi.org/10.3928/01477447-20160111-01.
7. Gauci MO, Cavalier M, Gonzalez JF, et al. Revision of failed shoulder arthroplasty: epidemiology, etiology, and surgical options. J Shoulder Elb Surg. 2020;29(3):541–9. https://doi.org/10.1016/j.jse.2019.07.034.
8. Chalmers PN, Boileau P, Romeo AA, Tashjian RZ. Revision reverse shoulder arthroplasty. J Am Acad Orthop Surg. 2019;27(12):426–36. https://doi.org/10.5435/JAAOS-D-17-00535.
9. Koch M, Lifka J, Gupta A, Seebauer L. Revision of reverse shoulder arthroplasty. In: Abstr Pap 229 Present Annu Meet Am Acad Orthop Surg 2016, Orlando, USA; 2016.
10. Williams GR, Iannotti JP. Options for glenoid bone loss: Composites of prosthetics and biologics. J Shoulder Elbow Surg. 2007;19107:267–72. https://doi.org/10.1016/j.jse.2007.05.003.
11. Gupta A, Thussbas C, Koch M, Seebauer L. Management of glenoid bone defects with reverse shoulder arthroplasty—surgical technique and clinical outcomes. J Shoulder Elb Surg. 2018;27:853–62. https://doi.org/10.1016/j.jse.2017.10.004.
12. Werner BS, Böhm D, Abdelkawi A, et al. Glenoid bone grafting in reverse shoulder arthroplasty for long-standing anterior shoulder dislocation. J Shoulder Elb Surg. 2014;23(11):1655–61. https://doi.org/10.1016/j.jse.2014.02.017.
13. Boileau P, Morin-Salvo N, Gauci MO, et al. Angled BIO-RSA (bony-increased offset-reverse shoulder arthroplasty): a solution for the management glenoid bone loss and erosion. J Shoulder Elb Surg. 2017;26(12):1–10. https://doi.org/10.1016/j.jse.2017.05.024.
14. Antuna SA, Sperling JW, Cofield RH, Rowland CM. Glenoid revision surgery after total shoulder arthroplasty. J Shoulder Elbow Surg. 2001;10(3):217–24. https://doi.org/10.1067/mse.2001.113961.
15. Phipatanakul WP, Norris TR, Linda L, Francisco S. Treatment of glenoid loosening and bone loss due to osteolysis with glenoid bone grafting. J shoulder Elbow Surg. 2006;15:84–7. https://doi.org/10.1016/j.jse.2005.06.004.
16. Norris TR. Glenoid bone loss in reverse shoulder arthroplasty treated with bone graft techniques. Am J Orthop (Belle Mead NJ). 2018;47(3) https://doi.org/10.12788/ajo.2018.0016.
17. Norris TR, Kelly JD, Humphrey CS. Management of glenoid bone defects in revision shoulder arthroplasty: a new application of the reverse total shoulder prosthesis. Tech Shoulder Elb Surg. 2007;8(1):37–46. https://doi.org/10.1097/BTE.0b013e318030d3b7.
18. Kelly JD, Zhao JX, Hobgood ER, Norris TR. Clinical results of revision shoulder arthroplasty using the reverse prosthesis. J Shoulder Elb Surg. 2012;21(11):1516–25. https://doi.org/10.1016/j.jse.2011.11.021.
19. Bateman E, Ortho F, Donald SM. Reconstruction of massive uncontained glenoid defects using a combined autograft-allograft construct with reverse shoulder arthroplasty: preliminary results. J Shoulder Elb Surg. 2012;21(7):925–34. https://doi.org/10.1016/j.jse.2011.07.009.
20. Jones RB, Wright TW, Zuckerman JD. Reverse total shoulder arthroplasty with structural bone grafting of large glenoid defects. J Shoulder Elb Surg. 2016; https://doi.org/10.1016/j.jse.2016.01.016.
21. Scalise JJ, Iannotti JP. Bone grafting severe glenoid defects in revision shoulder arthroplasty. Clin Orthop Relat Res. 2008;466(1):139–45. https://doi.org/10.1007/s11999-007-0065-7.
22. Herschel R, Wieser K, Morrey ME, Ramos CH, Gerber C, Meyer DC. Risk factors for glenoid erosion in patients with shoulder hemiarthroplasty: an analysis of 118 cases. J Shoulder Elb Surg. 2017;26(2):246–52. https://doi.org/10.1016/j.jse.2016.06.004.
23. Levine WN, Fischer CR, Nguyen D, Flatow EL, Ahmad CS, Bigliani LU. Long-term follow-up of shoulder hemiarthroplasty for glenohumeral osteoarthritis. J Bone Jt Surg. 2012;94(22):1–7. https://doi.org/10.2106/JBJS.K.00603.
24. Elhassan B, Ozbaydar M, Higgins LD, Warner JJP. Glenoid reconstruction in revision shoulder arthroplasty. Clin Orthop Relat Res. 2008;466:599–607. https://doi.org/10.1007/s11999-007-0108-0.
25. Page RS, Haines JF, Trail I. Impaction bone grafting of the glenoid in revision shoulder arthroplasty:

classification, technical description and early results. Shoulder Elb. 2009;1(2):81–8. https://doi.org/10.1111/j.1758-5740.2009.00017.x.
26. Sheth MM, Sholder D, Abboud J, et al. Revision of failed hemiarthroplasty for painful glenoid arthrosis to anatomic total shoulder arthroplasty. J Shoulder Elb Surg. 2018;27(10):1884–90. https://doi.org/10.1016/j.jse.2018.03.018.
27. Deutsch A, Abboud JA, Kelly J, et al. Clinical results of revision shoulder arthroplasty for glenoid component loosening. J Shoulder Elb Surg. 2007;16(6):706–16. https://doi.org/10.1016/j.jse.2007.01.007.
28. Wang T, Abrams GD, Behn AW, Lindsey D, Giori N, Cheung EV. Posterior glenoid wear in total shoulder arthroplasty: eccentric anterior reaming is superior to posterior augment. Clin Orthop Relat Res. 2015;473(12):3928–36. https://doi.org/10.1007/s11999-015-4482-8.
29. Jackins SE, Barrett WP, Matsen FA. Glenoid loosening in total shoulder arthroplasty: association with rotator cuff deficiency. J Arthroplast. 1988;3(1):39–46. https://doi.org/10.1016/S0883-5403(88)80051-2.
30. Sheth MM, Sholder D, Getz CL, Williams GR, Namdari S. Revision of failed hemiarthroplasty and anatomic total shoulder arthroplasty to reverse total shoulder arthroplasty. J Shoulder Elb Surg. 2019;28(6):1074–81. https://doi.org/10.1016/j.jse.2018.10.026.
31. Seebauer L, Goebel M. Management of glenoid defects in reversed shoulder arthoplasty. In: Abstr Pap Present SECEC-congress 2005, Rome, Italy; 2005.
32. Gohlke F, Werner B. Humeral and glenoidal bone defects in shoulder arthroplasty: classification and treatment principles. Orthopedist. 2017;46(12):1008–14. https://doi.org/10.1007/s00132-017-3484-5.
33. Gohlke F, Werner B, Wiese I. Glenoid reconstruction in revision shoulder arthroplasty. Opera Orthop Traumatol. 2019;31(2):98–114. https://doi.org/10.1007/s00064-019-0594-8.
34. Malhas A, Rashid A, Copas D, Bale S, Trail I. Glenoid bone loss in primary and revision shoulder arthroplasty. Shoulder Elbow. 2016;8(4):229–40. https://doi.org/10.1177/1758573216648601.
35. Kocsis G, Thyagarajan DS, Fairbairn KJ, Wallace WA. A new classification of glenoid bone loss to help plan the implantation of a glenoid component before revision arthroplasty of the shoulder. Bone Jt J. 2016;98B(3):374–80. https://doi.org/10.1302/0301-620X.98B3.36664.
36. Mahylis JM, Puzzitiello RN, Ho JC, Amini MH, Iannotti JP, Ricchetti ET. Comparison of radiographic and clinical outcomes of revision reverse total shoulder arthroplasty with structural versus nonstructural bone graft. J Shoulder Elb Surg. 2019;28(1):e1–9. https://doi.org/10.1016/j.jse.2018.06.026.
37. Paprosky W, Magnus R. Principles of bone grafting in revision total hip arthroplasty. Clin Orthop Relat Res. 1994;(298):147–55.
38. Frankle MA, Teramoto A, Luo Z, Levy JC, Pupello D. Glenoid morphology in reverse shoulder arthroplasty: classification and surgical implications. J Shoulder Elb Surg. 2009;18(6):874–85. https://doi.org/10.1016/j.jse.2009.02.013.
39. Klein SM, Dunning P, Mulieri P, Pupello D, Downes K, Frankle MA. Effects of acquired glenoid bone defects on surgical technique and clinical outcomes in reverse shoulder arthroplasty. J Bone Joint Surg Am. 2010;92(5):1144–54. https://doi.org/10.2106/JBJS.I.00778.
40. Italia KR, Green N, Maharaj J, Launay M, Gupta A. Computed tomographic evaluation of glenoid joint line restoration with glenoid bone grafting and reverse shoulder arthroplasty in patients with significant glenoid bone loss. J Shoulder Elb Surg. 2021;30(3):599–608. https://doi.org/10.1016/j.jse.2020.09.031.
41. Raiss P, Walch G, Wittmann T, Athwal GS. Is preoperative planning effective for intraoperative glenoid implant size and type selection during anatomic and reverse shoulder arthroplasty? J Shoulder Elb Surg. 2020;29(10):2123–7. https://doi.org/10.1016/j.jse.2020.01.098.
42. Kriechling P, Loucas R, Loucas M, Casari F, Fürnstahl P, Wieser K. Augmented reality through head-mounted display for navigation of baseplate component placement in reverse total shoulder arthroplasty: a cadaveric study. Arch Orthop Trauma Surg. 2023;143(1):169–75. https://doi.org/10.1007/s00402-021-04025-5.
43. Schlueter-Brust K, Henckel J, Katinakis F, et al. Augmented-reality-assisted K-wire placement for glenoid component positioning in reversed shoulder arthroplasty: a proof-of-concept study. J Pers Med. 2021;11(8) https://doi.org/10.3390/jpm11080777.
44. Leafblad N, Asghar E, Tashjian RZ. Innovations in shoulder arthroplasty. J Clin Med. 2022;11(10) https://doi.org/10.3390/jcm11102799.
45. Shim E, Kang Y, Ahn JM, et al. Metal artifact reduction for orthopedic implants (O-MAR): usefulness in CT evaluation of reverse total shoulder arthroplasty. Am J Roentgenol. 2017;209(4):860–6. https://doi.org/10.2214/AJR.16.17684.
46. Mohammadinejad P, Baffour FI, Adkins MC, et al. Benefits of iterative metal artifact reduction and dual-energy CT towards mitigating artifact in the setting of total shoulder prostheses. Skelet Radiol. 2021;50(1):51–8. https://doi.org/10.1007/s00256-020-03528-3.
47. Zhang K, Han Q, Xu X, et al. Metal artifact reduction of orthopedics metal artifact reduction algorithm in total hip and knee arthroplasty. Medicine (Baltimore). 2020;99(11):e19268. https://doi.org/10.1097/MD.0000000000019268.
48. Italia K, Launay M, Gilliland L, Nielsen J, Pareyon R, Hollman F, Salhi A, Maharaj J, Jomaa M, Cutbush K, Gupta A. Single-stage revision reverse shoulder arthroplasty: preoperative planning, surgical technique, and mixed reality execution. J Clin Med. 2022;11:7422. https://doi.org/10.3390/jcm11247422.

49. Maurer A, Fucentese SF, Pfirrmann CWA, et al. Assessment of glenoid inclination on routine clinical radiographs and computed tomography examinations of the shoulder. J Shoulder Elb Surg. 2012;21(8):1096–103. https://doi.org/10.1016/j.jse.2011.07.010.
50. Boileau P, Gauci M, Wagner ER, Walch G, Clowez G, Chaoui J. The reverse shoulder arthroplasty angle: a new measurement of glenoid inclination for reverse shoulder arthroplasty. J Shoulder Elb Surg. 2019;28(7):1281–90. https://doi.org/10.1016/j.jse.2018.11.074.
51. Boileau P, Moineau G, Roussanne Y, O'Shea K. Bony increased-offset reversed shoulder arthroplasty minimizing scapular impingement while maximizing glenoid fixation. Clin Orthop Relat Res. 2011;469(9):2558–67. https://doi.org/10.1007/s11999-011-1775-4.
52. Walker DR, Struk AM, Matsuki K, Wright TW, Banks SA. How do deltoid muscle moment arms change after reverse total shoulder arthroplasty? J Shoulder Elb Surg. 2015;25(4):581–8. https://doi.org/10.1016/j.jse.2015.09.015.
53. Walker M, Brooks J, Willis M, Frankle M. How reverse shoulder arthroplasty works. Clin Orthop Relat Res. 2011;469(9):2440–51. https://doi.org/10.1007/s11999-011-1892-0.
54. Königshausen M, Jettkant B, Sverdlova N, et al. Influence of different peg length in glenoid bone loss: a biomechanical analysis regarding primary stability of the glenoid baseplate in reverse shoulder arthroplasty. Technol Heal Care. 2015;23(6):855–69. https://doi.org/10.3233/THC-151031.
55. Kennon JC, Lu C, Mcgee-lawrence ME, Crosby LA. Scapula fracture incidence in reverse total shoulder arthroplasty using screws above or below metaglene central cage: clinical and biomechanical outcomes. J Shoulder Elb Surg. 2017;26(6):1023–30. https://doi.org/10.1016/j.jse.2016.10.018.
56. Königshausen M, Sverdlova N, Ehlert C, et al. Bone grafting in oblique versus prepared rectangular uncontained glenoid defects in reversed shoulder arthroplasty. A biomechanical comparison. Clin Biomech. 2017;50:7–15. https://doi.org/10.1016/j.clinbiomech.2017.09.011.
57. Königshausen M, Sverdlova N, Mersmann C, et al. Biomechanical analysis of anterior bone graft augmentation with reversed shoulder arthroplasty in large combined glenoid defects compared with total bony joint line reconstruction (modified bony-increased-offset reversed shoulder arthroplasty). J Shoulder Elb Surg. 2017;26(10):1765–74. https://doi.org/10.1016/j.jse.2017.04.021.
58. Porcellini G, Micheloni GM, Tarallo L, Paladini P, Merolla G, Catani F. Custom-made reverse shoulder arthroplasty for severe glenoid bone loss: review of the literature and our preliminary results. J Orthop Traumatol. 2021;22(1) https://doi.org/10.1186/s10195-020-00564-6.
59. De Biase CF, Ziveri G, De Caro F, Roberts N, Delcogliano M. Reverse shoulder arthroplasty using a "L" shaped allograft for glenoid reconstruction in a patient with massive glenoid bone loss: case report. Eur Rev Med Pharmacol Sci. 2014;18(1 Suppl):44–9. http://www.ncbi.nlm.nih.gov/pubmed/24825041
60. Parry S, Stachler S, Mahylis J. Lateralization in reverse shoulder arthroplasty: a review. J Orthop. 2020;22(February):64–7. https://doi.org/10.1016/j.jor.2020.03.027.
61. Shin SR, Tornetta P. Donor site morbidity after anterior iliac bone graft harvesting. J Orthop Trauma. 2016;30(6):340–3. https://doi.org/10.1097/BOT.0000000000000551.
62. Lopiz Y, García-Fernández C, Arriaza A, Rizo B, Marcelo H, Marco F. Midterm outcomes of bone grafting in glenoid defects treated with reverse shoulder arthroplasty. J Shoulder Elb Surg. 2017;26(9):1581–8. https://doi.org/10.1016/j.jse.2017.01.017.
63. Taylor JR, Schrumpf MA, Shea KE, Kelly JD. Distal clavicle autograft augmentation for glenoid bone loss in revision shoulder arthroplasty: results and technique. J Shoulder Elb Surg. 2020;29(10):e386–93. https://doi.org/10.1016/j.jse.2020.05.009.
64. Ozgur SE, Sadeghpour R, Norris TR. Revision shoulder arthroplasty with reverse shoulder prosthesis: use of a structured allograft to treat glenoid bone loss. Orthopedist. 2017;46(12):1055–62. https://doi.org/10.1007/s00132-017-3494-3.
65. Tashjian RZ, Broschinsky K, Stertz I, Chalmers PN. Structural glenoid allograft reconstruction during reverse total shoulder arthroplasty. J Shoulder Elb Surg. 2020;29(3):534–40. https://doi.org/10.1016/j.jse.2019.07.011.
66. Ho JC, Thakar O, Chan WW, Nicholson T, Williams GR, Namdari S. Early radiographic failure of reverse total shoulder arthroplasty with structural bone graft for glenoid bone loss. J Shoulder Elb Surg. 2020;29(3):550–60. https://doi.org/10.1016/j.jse.2019.07.035.
67. Neyton L, Boileau P, Nové-josserand L, Edwards TB. Glenoid bone grafting with a reverse design prosthesis. J Shoulder Elb Surg. 2007;16(Suppl. 3):71–8. https://doi.org/10.1016/j.jse.2006.02.002.
68. Favard L, Berhouet J, Walch G, Chaoui J, Lévigne C. Superior glenoid inclination and glenoid bone loss. Orthopade. 2017:1015–21. https://doi.org/10.1007/s00132-017-3496-1.
69. Bercik MJ, Ii KK, Yalizis M, Gauci M, Chaoui J, Walch G. A modification to the Walch classification of the glenoid in primary glenohumeral osteoarthritis using three-dimensional imaging. J Shoulder Elb Surg. 2016;25(10):1601–6. https://doi.org/10.1016/j.jse.2016.03.010.
70. Tashjian RZ, Granger E, Chalmers PN. Structural glenoid grafting during primary reverse total shoulder arthroplasty using humeral head autograft. J Shoulder Elb Surg. 2018;27(1):e1–8. https://doi.org/10.1016/j.jse.2017.07.010.

71. Nabergoj M, Neyton L, Bothorel H, et al. Reverse shoulder arthroplasty with bony and metallic versus standard bony reconstruction for severe glenoid bone loss. A retrospective comparative cohort study. J Clin Med. 2021;10(22):5274. https://doi.org/10.3390/jcm10225274.
72. Singh J, Odak S, Neelakandan K, et al. Survivorship of autologous structural bone graft at a minimum of 2 years when used to address significant glenoid bone loss in primary and revision shoulder arthroplasty: a computed tomographic and clinical review. J Shoulder Elb Surg. 2021;30(3):668–78. https://doi.org/10.1016/j.jse.2020.06.015.

17 Surgical Management of Periprosthetic Scapular Spine and Acromion Fractures

Ludwig Seebauer, Kristine Italia, Roberto Pareyon, Mohammad Jomaa, and Ashish Gupta

17.1 Introduction

Fractures of the acromion and the scapular spine are uncommon in anatomic total shoulder arthroplasty but are significant in patients with reverse shoulder arthroplasty (RSA). Over the last 25 years, RSA has gained great popularity. The indications have expanded, and the number of procedures has increased exponentially. Periprosthetic fractures of the acromion and scapular spine have been reported increasingly as a complication of RSA with an associated decline in clinical outcome [1–7]. The fracture rate after RSA averages in recent meta-analyses and reviews [8–10] between 4 and 5% but reached up to 25% in a single report [11]. The literature from the first decade of year 2000s reported very small numbers with heterogeneous data on the incidence, etiology, and treatment options. In a review of the literature in 2013, Rouleau et al. [12] found 56 reported cases in 6 studies. Bohsali et al. [2] reported in 2017 an incidence of 1.0% (40 cases in 4124 RSAs). In a systematic review of 90 articles (9048 RTAs) in 2019, King et al. [4] found the incidence of acromial and/or scapular spine fracture to be 2.8%. Despite this increasing incidence of acromial and/or scapular spine fractures after RSA, there is still no consensus on the management of these fractures.

L. Seebauer (✉)
Center for Orthopaedics, Trauma Surgery and Sports Medicine—München-KlinikBogenhausen, Munich, Germany
e-mail: ludwig.seebauer@muenchen-klinik.de

K. Italia · R. Pareyon · M. Jomaa
Queensland Unit for Advanced Shoulder Research (QUASR), Brisbane, Australia
e-mail: kristine@akunah.com

A. Gupta
Queensland Unit for Advanced Shoulder Research (QUASR), Brisbane, Australia

Greenslopes Private Hospital, Brisbane, Australia
e-mail: research@qoc.com.au

17.2 Incidence

RSA medializes the center of rotation and lengthens the moment arm for the deltoid muscle. This increases the load on the acromion and subsequently the risk for postoperative fatigue fractures. There are two different designs of reverse arthroplasty: the classic Grammont type design, where the center of rotation is at the bone–implant interface, and a design with a glenosphere with a lateral offset (more than a half sphere). These different designs result in different biomechanics and, therefore, may have different incidences of postoperative acromion and scapula spine fractures. Modification of the original Grammont design with a more lateralized glenosphere and changed humeral implant design (onlay design, less inclination) seems to increase the incidence of this difficult-to-treat complication [4, 7, 13–16].

F. Franceschi et al. (eds.), *Revision Shoulder Arthroplasty*,
https://doi.org/10.1007/978-3-031-45944-3_17

Over the last decade, nearly 50 different RSA designs have come into the market. Their biomechanical characteristics of the implants can be summarized as follows [17]:

- Medialized glenoid (MG) and medialized humerus (MH): MGMH
- Medialized glenoid (MG) and lateralized humerus (LH): MGLH
- Lateralized glenoid (LG)) and medialized humerus (LH): LGMH
- Lateralized glenoid (LG) and lateralized humerus (LH): LGLH

The reported incidence of acromial/scapula spine fractures after RSA varies between 1% and 12% (Table 17.1). In 2014, Teusink et al. [25] reported an incidence of 3.1% in a series of over 1000 RSA with a lateralized design. In our study [1] between 2008 and 2014 when 1483 RSA (Grammont type) were implanted as primary or revision arthroplasties, 20 patients had to be treated because of an acromion or scapular spine fracture (incidence 1.35%). Surprisingly, the incidence of fractures in the reverse-for-revision group in several studies is significantly lower (0-0.6%) than for primary indications [4, 34–36].

The most comprehensive analysis of 90 studies on 9083 RSA by King et al. [4] disclosed the highest incidences of periprosthetic acromion/scapular spine fractures in primary RSA for inflammatory arthritis (10.9%), massive cuff tear (3.8%) and cuff tear arthropathy (3.5%). Interestingly, the incidence in the acute trauma subgroup is 0%.

Werthel et al. [26] reported 1082 primary RSA with an incidence of acromial fractures of 1.11% in their series in a 2-year follow-up, reporting osteoporosis as the main cause of this complication.

Furthermore, in one of the newest systemic reviews, Shah et al. [37] reported an overall incidence of 2.6% (371 of 14,235 RSAs) of acromial stress fractures, similar to King et al. [4], in a mean overall follow-up of 4.3 years with no statistical difference between component designs.

Otto et al. [11] showed that blinded reviewers identified only 79% of the fractures with plain radiographs. Therefore, generally, the reported incidences are probably an underestimate of the true incidence, since this complication is often missed and underreported.

Table 17.1 Summary of literature on acromial and scapular spine fractures after reverse shoulder arthroplasty

Author	Year	Lateralized design (n)	Incidence acromion/ scapular spine fracture	Standard design (n)	Incidence acromion/ scapular spine fracture	Comment
Frankle [18]	2005	60	5%			Reverse shoulder Encore Medical
Werner [19]	2005			58	4 (6.9%)	Delta 3 (MGMH)
Walch [20]	2009			457	4 (0.9%)	9% of all cases had preoperative acromial pathology
Hattrup [21]	2010			125	9 (7.2%)	Delta 3 (MGMH), Zimmer Trabecular metal (MGMH)
Goebel [22]	2010			259	9 (3.5%)	
Hamid [23]	2011			162	8 (4.9%)	
Crosby [24]	2011	400	22 (5.5%)	400	22 (5.5%)	Mixed: MGMH and MGLH+
Teusink [25]	2014	1018	32 (3.1%)			Reverse shoulder DJO (DJO Surgical, Austin, TX, USA).
Koch [1]	2016			1483	20 (1.4%)	Grammont-type
Werthel [26]	2018	756	5 (0.66%)	326	7 (2.14%)	Lateralized design: Comprehensive + DJO Grammont style: Delta xtend, Aequalis, Delta III
King [4]	2019	1698 LG/MH 1936 MG/LH	65 (3.8%) 28 (1.5%)	2352 MGMH	58 (2.5%)	Mixed implants, but classified
Neyton [27]	2019			1953	26 (1.3%)	Grammont-type
Haidamous [15]	2020	Onlay (84)	10 (11.9%)	Inlay* (342) **But DJO is LGMH > mixed*	16 (4.7%)	-Arthrex Universe Revers™ (MGMH) -DJO Altivate Revers™ (LGMH) - Ascend flex Tornier™ (MGLH)
Marigi [28]	2020	2172	36 (1.6%)	2172	36 (1.6%)	Mixed
Nyffeler [16]	2020	189	12 (5.8%)			Duocentric ™ (Aston Medical, Saint-Etienne, France) (LGLH)
Routman [29]	2020	4125	61 (1.5%)			Equinoxe, Exactech (MGLH)

(continued)

Table 17.1 (continued)

Author	Year	Lateralized design (n)	Incidence acromion/ scapular spine fracture	Standard design (n)	Incidence acromion/ scapular spine fracture	Comment
Schenk [30]	2020	924 MGLH+	18 (1.9%)	222 MGMH	3 (1.4%)	– Delta 3 (MGMH) – Inverse/reverse (Zimmer Biomet) (MGLH+)
Zmistovski [31]	2020	LH 106 LG 430	5 (4.7%) 32 (7.4%)	MH 793 MG 469	51 (6.4%) 24 (5.1%)	Mixed but categorized
Moverman [32]	2021	1479	54 (3.7%)			DJO prosthesis (DJO Surgical, Austin, TX, USA) LGMH
Mahendrajai [5]	2021	6755	264 (3.9%)	6755	264 (3.9%)	Mixed: No breakdown for categories
Meshram [33]	2022	71 onlay	0%	79 inlay	2 (2.8%)	

17.3 Diagnosis

17.3.1 History and Clinical Examination

A careful patient history gives a high suspicion of an acromial/scapular spine fracture. The typical patient has an unremarkable postoperative period with significant improvement in range of motion and excellent pain relief. Suddenly, the patient experiences severe pain over the shoulder and inability to lift the arm. In most instances, these are atraumatic events where the fracture is caused by daily tasks (insufficiency fracture). Most cases occur during the first year, but fractures after many years have been reported. The three most common complications during the first year are periprosthetic infection, dislocation, or acromial/scapular spine fractures. These complications have different clinical characteristics that can help differentiate among them (Table 17.2). Physical examination reveals tenderness over the posterior part of acromion or scapular spine. Sudden loss of active elevation with posterior shoulder pain is often a typical presenting complaint.

17.3.2 X-Ray and CT Scan

A plain radiograph can be diagnostic, but a fracture may often be missed. Therefore, a computed tomography (CT) scan should be performed if patient history or clinical examination results in suspicion of a fracture. The "tilted acromion sign" is mainly seen on plain radiographs (Fig. 17.1a) in type 1 or anterior type 2 fractures (type 2a) but rarely in the acute situation in type

Table 17.2 Clinical characteristics for periprosthetic infection, dislocation, and postoperative fractures of acromion or scapular spine after a reverse total shoulder arthroplasty

Pain	Range of motion	Diagnosis
Gradual increase of pain at rest	Increasing stiffness	Periprosthetic infection
No or limited pain	Sudden loss of active elevation	Dislocation
Sudden severe pain	Sudden loss of active elevation	Fracture of scapular spine

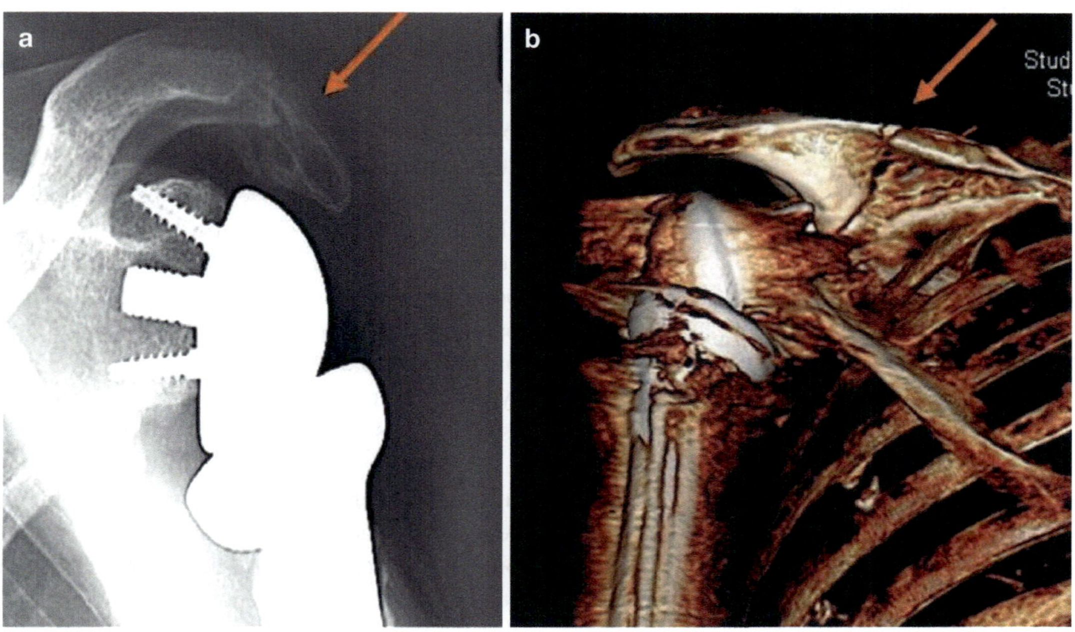

Fig. 17.1 (**a**) "Tilted Acromion Sign" in a type 1 acromial fracture. (**b**) 3D-CT of a type 3 scapular spine fracture

2 posterior (2b) or type 3 fractures. Therefore frequently, only a CT scan can confirm the fracture and its location (Fig. 17.1b). It is essential to ask the radiologist to specifically look for a fracture of the acromion and scapular spine in all painful RSA.

Otto et al. [11] found that 17 of 53 patients (32%) had a delayed diagnosis. Therefore, whenever there is clinical suspicion of a periprosthetic acromion fracture after RSA, a CT scan, preferably with 3D image formatting, should be performed to confirm the diagnosis and plan therapy.

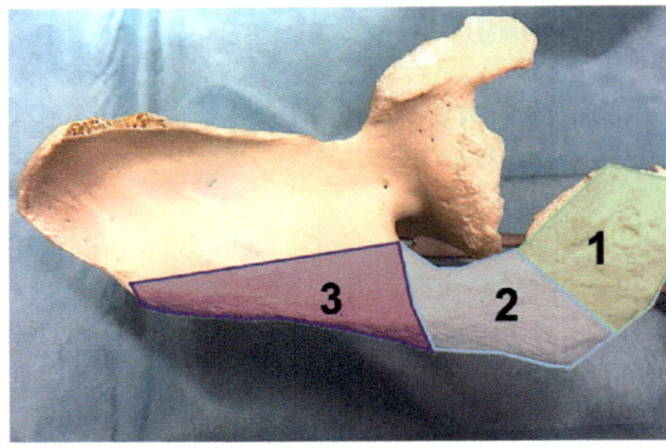

Fig. 17.2 Classification of acromion and scapular spine fracture after reverse shoulder arthroplasty based on location according to Levy et al. [38]

17.3.3 SPECT-CT

A single-photon emission computed tomography (SPECT)-CT may be requested if the clinical suspicion is high. Undisplaced fractures will be picked up with a SPECT-CT, which may not be evident on a standard CT metal subtraction sequence.

Zmitowski et al. [31] reported an incidence of acromial stress fractures (4.2%) and acromial stress reactions (6.4%) in a series of 1170 RSA cases. Acromial stress reaction was defined as pain or tenderness on the acromion with a decrease in shoulder function but without changes of the bone in the imaging studies. The result of this analysis brings to the conclusion that sometimes SPECT-CT could be necessary for the correct diagnosis.

17.4 Classification

In our first series [22] of 9 cases presented in 2010 at the Annual German Shoulder and Elbow Society meeting, we distinguished three types. Type 1 is a fatigue fracture of chronically eroded acromion. Type 2 is an acromial edge fracture (metacromial fracture). Type 3 is scapular spine fracture.

In 2011, Crosby et al. [24] proposed a classification system of postoperative acromial fractures based on a retrospective analysis of 22 cases. Type 1 is an avulsion fracture of the anterior acromion, type 2 is a fracture of the acromion posterior of the acromioclavicular joint, and type 3 is a fracture of the spine of the scapula.

Levy et al. [38] classified 18 patients with postoperative fractures of the acromion and scapular spine into three types according to the anatomical position (Fig. 17.2). Type 1 is fracture of mid-acromion involving the anterior and portion of middle deltoid origin, type 2 involves the entire middle and part of the posterior deltoid origin (posterior part of acromion), and type 3 involves the entire middle and posterior deltoid origin (scapula spine). The interobserver reliability was found to be excellent.

These classification systems are only based on the location of the fracture. No studies on subtypes of fractures and outcomes are available that can be used for therapeutic guidance.

Within the last years, we expanded Levy's classification type 2 into type 2a (posterolateral acromion edge = transition type from middle to posterior deltoid insertion) and type 2b (acromial base = acromial-spine isthmus = transition type of acromion into scapular spine), and type 3 into type 3a (scapular spine fracture) and type 3b (sagittal transscapular fracture) (Fig. 17.3).

With longer follow-up in our series, we identify some patients with very poor bone quality in which the scapular spine fractures extend not only in the scapular spine but penetrate from the scapular spine to the glenoid–scapular junction through the entire scapula (type 3b) (Fig. 17.3).

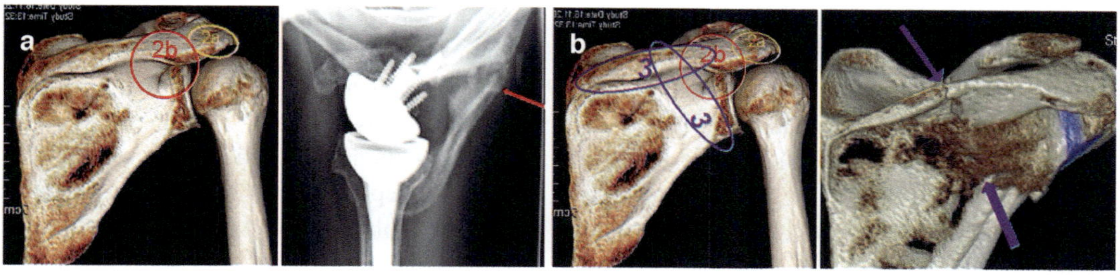

Fig. 17.3 Critical subtypes of acromial base ("Isthmus") fractures (type 2b), scapular spine fractures (type 3a), and sagittal transscapular fracture (type 3b)

17.5 Etiology

RSA increases the load on acromion due to the medialization of the center of rotation and the lengthening of the deltoid muscle. Many authors believe these fractures result from arm lengthening and increased tension in the deltoid muscle [13, 21, 39, 40]. However, finite element studies [41], biomechanical experiments [42, 43], and several clinical studies [31, 44] cannot approve this hypothesis.

Some authors [11, 24, 45, 46] found that many fractures of the scapula spine occurred at the superior fixation screw of the glenoid base plate. However, in other studies, an increased relative risk due to surgical technique or screw placement could not be found [11]. In our revision of RSA and retrospective analysis [1] of management of periprosthetic acromion or scapular spine fractures, we could not find in the 17 cases a superior or posterior screw as a stress riser for a fatigue fracture. Otherwise, there was no case in which, following Norris's [47] "three-column" fixation recommendation, a third screw reached the base of the scapular spine. Within our implantation technique, we put the superior screw into the coracoid base and aim not to penetrate the medial cortex of the coracoid base. In addition, we avoid reaching the scapular spine with the posterior screw.

Another theory [13, 27] has been that the greater tuberosity in onlay designs impinges on acromion in abduction resulting in a fatigue fracture.

Taylor et al. [48] postulated homogenous strain distribution by an intact coracoacromial ligament and identified higher strain to the scapular spine by dissecting this ligament during the surgical approach. In the superolateral approach wherein this ligament is routinely dissected, a higher incidence of scapular spine fractures would be expected. Cho et al. [8] showed that the opposite is the case.

Nyfeller et al. [16] ascribed the majority of fractures to a traumatic fall. He associated this with the more exposed and less soft tissue-covered acromion with the reverse prosthesis design, which makes it more vulnerable to direct trauma.

Without any doubt, major trauma can cause a periprosthetic fracture of the acromion and/or the scapular spine after RSA. However, in the majority of the studies [4, 5, 9], local poor bone quality or generalized osteoporosis is consistently seen as the main factor. Osteoporosis has been shown to increase the risk for postoperative acromial or scapula spine fractures [4, 11, 30, 40, 49].

Besides King's [4] extensive meta-analysis of 90 reports, the most recent publication of the ASES Complications of RSA Multicenter Research Group by Mahendraraj et al. [5] is the most comprehensive analysis with a retrospective study of 6755 primary and revision reverse arthroplasty of 15 institutes across the USA identified 3.0% (n = 200) symptomatic acromial stress fractures and 0.9% (n = 64) scapular spine stress fractures. This means an overall fracture rate of 3.9% with 21.2% (n = 56) following a trauma. Predictive factors for acromial fracture were chronic dislocation, massive rotator cuff tear without arthritis, rotator cuff arthropathy, self-reported osteoporosis, inflammatory arthritis, female sex, and older age. Factors independently associated with the development of scapular spine fractures included osteoporosis, female sex, rotator cuff arthropathy, and inflammatory arthritis. The impact of prosthetic factors, as well as other peri- and postoperative factors, could be deducted by this multicenter retrospective study.

Moreover, Werthel [26] proposed the theory that lateralized designs that do not excessively verticalize the deltoid line of pull on the acromion may decrease the risk of postoperative acromial fractures, whereas osteoporosis, greater arm lengthening, and thinner acromion were risk factors. On the other hand, the systemic review reported by Zmistowski [31] showed no relationship between different implants and the risk of acromial stress fractures.

However, not quite explainable is the fact that in anatomic total shoulder arthroplasty with a similar at-risk cohort for osteoporosis, the occurrence of acromion and/or scapular spine fractures is nearly unknown. Therefore, further studies are needed to clarify the specific causing mechanisms and risk factors in RSA for periprosthetic acromial and scapula spine fractures.

17.6 Treatment

The systematic comprehensive review of King et al. [4] reports the frequency of acromial fracture to be 2.5 times higher (2%) than that of scapular spine fractures (0.8%), which is very close to the distribution by the American Shoulder and Elbow Surgeons (ASES) Complications of RSA Multicenter Research Group [5]. Acromial fractures, especially of the anterior third of the acromion, are clinically and biomechanically less significant than of the posterior third of the acromion or through the scapular spine. This could explain the heterogeneous recommendations for conservative versus operative treatment and the variable results for both treatment options. In most of these small number studies, no clear distinction is made between the fracture locations and subtypes. In addition, no consistent treatment algorithm based on a biomechanical-pathomorphological classification is available.

The overrepresentation of acromial fractures could be explained by two reasons. First, in advanced massive cuff tears or cuff tear arthropathy, the static superior subluxation of the humeral head causes secondary acromion bone erosion. Second, preexisting os acromiale, in combination with rotator cuff tears, which have a prevalence of up to 6% [50], could get symptomatic postoperatively and confirmed by the radiologic "inferior acromial tilt" sign.

17.6.1 Conservative Treatment

The fractures of the anterior acromion (Crosby type 1, Levy type 1) can be treated nonoperatively in a sling or abduction brace or by open reduction and internal fixation (ORIF).

Asymptomatic acromial fractures (especially type 1), which are detected incidentally by follow-up routine radiographs, do not need a specific treatment. Asymptomatic acromial fractures have no significant adverse effects on patient outcomes or range of motion, but close observation is warranted [51]. Often, they represent preoperatively overseen os acromiale. In our series, we have one patient becoming symptomatic after 2-year follow-up, even though the acromion-tilt sign was visible at the immediate postoperative X-ray. The other patients with an obvious postoperative acromion-tilt sign stayed asymptomatic with the acromial fracture but developed a scapular spine fracture (type 3) 4 years postoperatively.

Most reported acromial fractures (type 1 and 2) could be treated successfully nonoperatively [20, 21]. The conservative treatment means immobilization for at least 6 weeks in an abduction brace or sling. The abduction position takes some tension out of the deltoid, reducing the downward pull on the acromion. Teusink et al. [25] compared 25 patients who were treated nonoperatively with a minimum of 2-year follow-up with a cohort of matched patients without this complication as controls. The fracture patients had inferior outcomes but improved compared to the preoperative function.

Symptomatic nonunion, with the need for secondary surgical intervention, occur frequently. Neyton et al. [27] reported a nonunion rate of 66% in a series of 10 acromial base and 9 scapular spine fractures. The primary treatment strategy for all acute nondisplaced fractures was conservative treatment with immobilization.

Patterson et al. [9], in their systematic review of outcomes of acromial spine fractures following RSA, found a variable union rate between 50% and 60% with nonoperative treatment. In cases with conservative fracture healing, pain and shoulder function improved significantly better.

17.6.2 Operative Treatment

Crosby et al. [24] performed ORIF of four fractures of the spine of the scapula (type 3). One fixation failed and had to be revised. No detailed outcome was reported. The authors recommended ORIF for type 3 fractures. Wahlqvist et al. [52] reported on five postoperative acromial base fractures. One was acutely treated with ORIF, and two cases were later treated surgically due to a nonunion of the base of the acromion. Limited pain but poor functional outcome was reported at follow-up, and no recommendations for treatment could be given. Different surgical techniques have been used for these fractures, such as plating, double-plating, or tension-band wiring. In one of Ekelund's series [53] of 1000 RSAs, 15 postoperative fractures were identified. There were 13 women and 2 men with a mean age of 75 years (range 57–89). Six patients had a significant trauma causing the fracture, while the remaining 9 had a sudden onset of pain during normal activities. The nontraumatic fractures occurred at a mean of 4 months postoperatively (range 2–6 months), while the traumatic fractures occurred at a mean of 16 months postoperatively (range 1–36 months). Five patients underwent open reduction and plate fixation. Two of these healed. Nonunion of the spine of the scapula (type 3 fractures) increases the risk for dislocation of the RSA due to poor deltoid tensioning. In 2021, Kriechling [54] et al., in a series of 854 primary RSAs, reported an incidence of 5.4% (46 cases) acromial stress fractures and 5.2% (44 cases) acromial stress reactions. They reported that the healing rate was much higher with surgical management. Nevertheless, fracture consolidation does not result in better clinical outcomes than nonunion.

It is crucial to distinguish preexisting thinned eroded acromion, acromion and scapular fatigue fractures, and os acromiale from postoperative fractures. Walch et al. [20] found a significant prevalence of weakened acromion/scapular spine (41/457 = 9%) in patients with RSA for cuff tear arthropathy and revision of failed arthroplasties. He also found similar good clinical results in preexisting acromion pathologies (os acromiale, fatigue fracture, eroded acromion, and severe acetabularization). Preoperative acromial pathology, surgical approach, and amount of inferior acromial tilt did not diminish the postoperative range of motion, Constant score, or subjective results when compared to patients without acromial pathology. On the other hand, he found 4 postoperative fractures (0.8%) with significantly worse functional and subjective outcomes. In addition, Walch [20] et al. reported that both acquired and congenital preoperative lesions of the acromion are not a contraindication of RSA. Moreover, the results obtained are not different from patients with normal acromia.

17.6.3 Based on Fracture Type

As already recommended by Crosby et al. [24] in 2011, a consensus of nonoperative treatment of type 1 fractures (anterior and lateral acromion fractures) in the publications of the last ten years [12, 23, 27, 40] could be found. This fracture presents as a harmless complication after RSA, which is sometimes even asymptomatic. The results of conservative treatment are generally good.

The treatment recommendations for type 2 fractures are variable. The tendency is for conservative treatment of acute nondisplaced fractures. Operative treatment is only recommended in symptomatic delayed unions or nonunions.

For type 3 fractures, the recommendations favor primary operative treatment, whereby the opinion regarding acute nondisplaced fractures with traumatic origin is also discussed controversially.

For the treatment decision, it is critical to distinguish in fractures occurring in type 2 and 3 between traumatic fractures on healthy bone from fatigue and stress fractures of osteoporotic bone. Also, it is essential to subclassify type 2 into the more lateral type (type 2a) and the more medial fractures at the base of the acromion adjacent to the scapular spine (type 2b).

Undisplaced fractures in type 2a could be attempted by conservative treatment. Surgical intervention is only indicated if there is a symptomatic progressive dislocation or nonunion by conservative strategy. Type 2a fractures could sometimes be treated successfully by minimally invasive tension-band-wiring.

In type 2b, the chance of bone healing and regaining a satisfactory functional result by conservative treatment is minimal. We also tried different operative fixation techniques in this patient subgroup. We often could not achieve adequate bone healing by single-plating, tension-band-wiring, and even by double-plate osteosynthesis. We consider this fatigue fractures in type 3 and medial type 2 (type 2b subtype at the acromial base junction to the scapular spine) as a symptom of a bone that is too weak for the nonphysiologic load applied by the reverse prosthesis design.

17.6.4 Double-Plate Osteosynthesis in Combination with Structural Bone Graft

Because the current treatment recommendations for this insufficiency fracture in the area of the base of the acromion and spine of the scapula after RSA are very controversial and the reported results are often disappointing, we retrospectively analyzed our results on single- and double-plate osteosynthesis from 2009 to 2016. We observed a high rate of hardware failure and nonunion in the atraumatic patient group with poor bone quality.

The rate of nonunion is high and is always associated with a deterioration in function. In order to bring about a safe bony consolidation after ORIF, structural iliac crest autograft was attached to the fracture and fixed with 2 cortical screws or an additional small plate. This technique was later extended to double-plate osteosynthesis combined with an iliac crest autograft to increase stability (Figs. 17.4c, d and 17.5c, d).

In detail, the double-plating technique consists of a 3.5 locking compression palte (LCP) or Reconstruction plate along the scapular spine's posterior aspect and the acromion's postero-lateral aspect, and a superior small plate placed superior to the bone graft in the supraspinatus fossa (Fig. 17.5). The screws in the acromial end of the strong 3.5-posterior locking plate should be placed bicortical in a transverse direction in the acromial bone to gain an intraosseous length as long as possible. At least 3 screws with adequate fixation strength should be placed at each fracture site.

From a total of 19 cases between 2016 and 2020, 4 plate osteosynthesis and 5 double-plate osteosynthesis were reviewed with a follow-up period of at least 1 year. The radiological images at 12 months postoperatively were examined for bony consolidation and radiological abnormalities. In addition, an evaluation of the clinical function of the shoulder joint was carried out at the same time and osteosynthesis-associated complications in the postoperative course were noted. In the case of insufficiency fractures treated with single-plate osteosynthesis and autologous cancellous bone graft, 2 out of 4 (50%) showed bony consolidation after 1 year, compared to double-plate osteosynthesis with iliac crest autograft with 4 out of 5 (80%) fracture healing. There were no cases of loosening of the osteosynthesis material. Interestingly, there was no correlation between clinical function and the consolidation rate. One patient with simple plate fixation suffered a spontaneous refracture medial to the fixation. The results indicate a radiologically and functionally better outcome of double-plate osteosynthesis with iliac crest autograft compared to single-plate osteosynthesis with cancellous bone autograft after 1 year. Therefore,

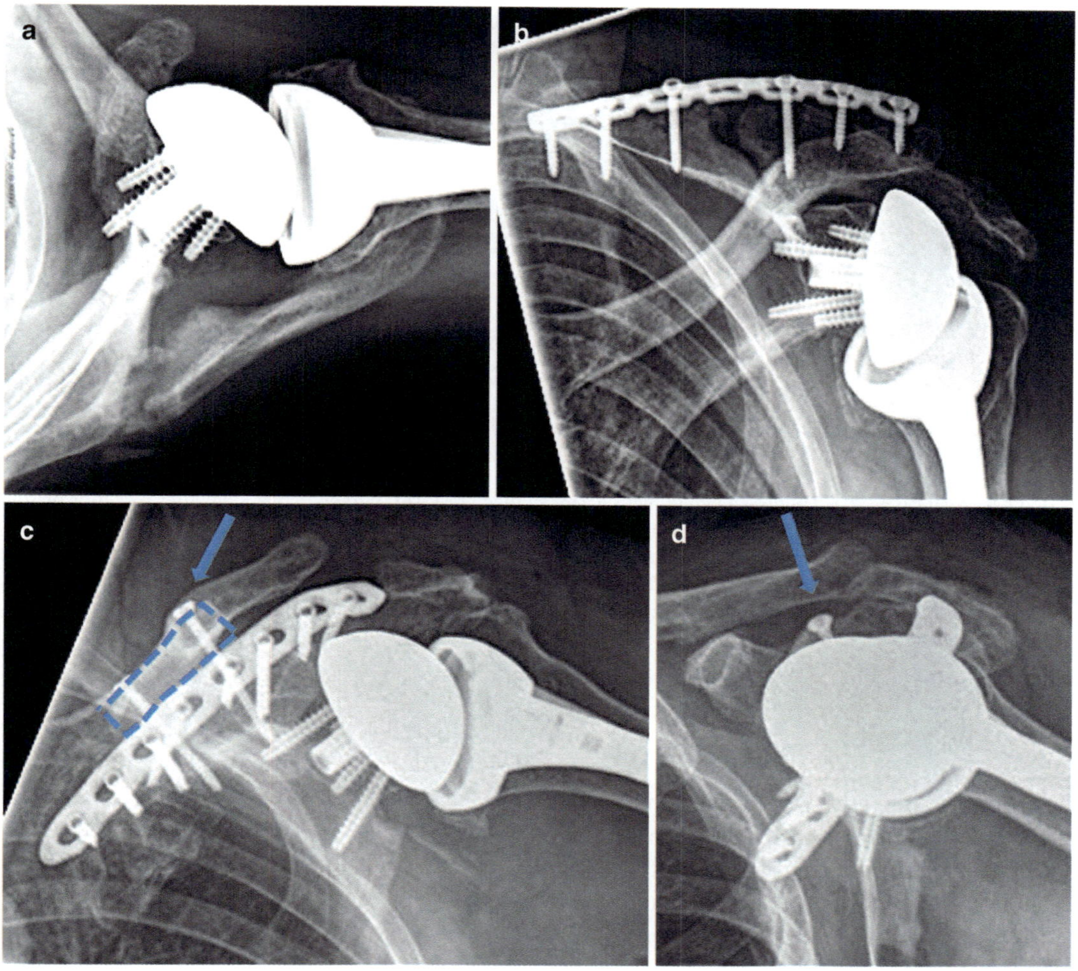

Fig. 17.4 (**a**) Type 2b fatigue fracture at the base of the coracoid. (**b**) Nonunion of single plating by LCP-Reco plate of a type 3 fracture. (**c** and **d**) Salvage by "indirect double-plating" by posterior 3,5-LCP plate and structural iliac crest graft in the supraspinatus fossa with strong crest cortex fixed by perpendicular screws to the posterior plate

we emphasize fixing the insufficiency fracture of the base of the acromion (Levy type 2) and scapular spine (Levy type 3) by a right angular positioned double-plating combined with augmentation with structural osseous autograft (Fig. 17.5).

In addition, a case report on a double-plating technique of a scapular spine fracture by Bauer et al. [55] also reported a good clinical outcome despite secondary fracture of the acromion adjacent to the end of the plate. Also, Toft and Moro [56], in a small case series of 4 patients (2 acute and 2 delayed union), reported good functional results and pain relief by double-plating technique. Further studies are needed to support the results of these case series.

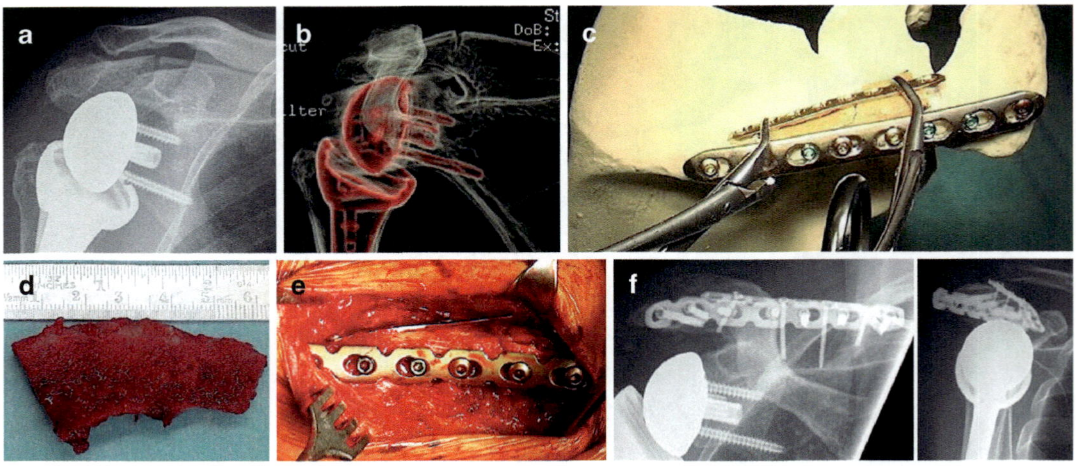

Fig. 17.5 Acute type 2 b fracture: Double-plate osteosynthesis combined with structural iliac crest graft. (**a**, **b**). X-ray and CT scan. (**c**). Illustration of the double-plating technique and additional structural bone graft for bridging and enforcing the acromial base—scapular spine junction. (**d**). Corticocancellous autograft of the inner wall of the iliac crest. (**e**). Intraoperative view after posterior plating of the scapular spine and acromion with 3.5 locking compression plate (LCP) Reconstruction plate and additional bone graft and 2.4 LCP on the supraspinatus fossa. (**f**). Postoperative x-ray AP and Y views

17.7 Discussion

Postoperative fractures of the acromion or scapula spine are, together with periprosthetic joint infection and instability, one of the most common early complications after RSA. Careful history and physical examination can give a strong suspicion for postoperative acromion/scapular spine fracture, but plain radiographs are often negative. Therefore, a CT scan should be performed in painful reverse arthroplasties. Furthermore, it is critical to assess the preoperative osseous condition of the acromion and spine of the scapulae. Specifically, in long-standing cuff tear arthropathy with excessive superior migration, a severely eroded glenoid or even acromion fractures are preexisting. Also, in patients with poor bone quality (e.g., rheumatoid arthritis), preexisting stress fractures of the base of the acromion and/or scapular spine are often overseen. There are no good treatment recommendations for preexisting fatigue fractures in type 2 and 3. We neglect acromion erosions or fatigue fractures in type 1 but avoid further weakening of the deltoid suspension structures on the antero-lateral acromion and delto-trapezIal fascia by an anterior-superior (McKenzie) approach. In these cases, we always use an anterior deltopectoral approach, avoid over-tensioning of the deltoid or mechanical stress to fornix humeri by too aggressive sizing or excessive inferior overlap and/or lateralization of the glenosphere or lateralized humeral epiphysis design (onlay design, 135° or 145° inclination).

The existing classification systems [24, 38] are descriptive and cannot be used generally as guidance for the treatment of postoperative fractures, as they do not consider the etiology (traumatic vs. fatigue fracture), bone quality, and timing (undisplaced acute fractures vs. nonunions). Levy type 3 fractures are more probably candidates for ORIF. Even though these fracture patients improve compared to preoperative function, the results are inferior compared to patients without this complication. In younger patients with displaced fractures in the posterior part of the acromion or spine of the scapula (type 3), the authors perform ORIF. However, there is limited evidence in the literature supporting surgical management for these fractures. Further studies are needed to define the best treatment for these fractures.

17.8 Conclusion

Postoperative fractures of the base of the acromion or the spine of the scapula are a common complication after reverse shoulder arthroplasty. It has a negative impact on functional outcomes and is challenging to treat. The recommendations for treatment are variable, but based on the published literature, no recommendation can be given regarding treatment. Further studies are needed to define the best treatment for these fractures.

Conflict of Interest L Seebauer is a consultant for Depuy Synthes Inc. Ltd. Leeds UK and receives royalties from this company.

A Gupta is a Consultant for Zimmer and Founder of Akunah Ltd., Brisbane, Queensland, Australia.

K Italia is employee of Akunah.

Compliance with Ethical Guidelines For the studies listed, the ethical guidelines stated therein apply in each case.

References

1. Koch M, Lifka J, Gupta A, Seebauer L. Revision of reverse shoulder arthroplasty. In: Abstr Pap 229 Present Annu Meet Am AcadOrthop Surg 2016, Orlando, USA; 2016.
2. Bohsali KI, Bois AJ, Wirth MA. Complications of shoulder arthroplasty. [Review]. J Bone Jt Surg Am. 2017;99:256–69.
3. Gauci MO, Cavalier M, Gonzalez JF, et al. Revision of failed shoulder arthroplasty: epidemiology, etiology, and surgical options. J Shoulder Elb Surg. 2020;29(3):541–9. https://doi.org/10.1016/j.jse.2019.07.034.
4. King JJ, Dalton SS, Gulotta LV, Wright TW, Schoch BS. How common are acromial and scapular spine fractures after reverse shoulder arthroplasty? Bone Jt J. 2019;101 B(6):627–34. https://doi.org/10.1302/0301-620X.101B6.BJJ-2018-1187.R1.
5. Mahendraraj KA, Abboud J, Armstrong A, et al. Predictors of acromial and scapular stress fracture after reverse shoulder arthroplasty: a study by the ASES Complications of RSA Multicenter Research Group. J Shoulder Elb Surg. 2021;30(10):2296–305. https://doi.org/10.1016/j.jse.2021.02.008.
6. Colliton EM, Jawa A, Kirsch JM. Acromion and scapular spine fractures following reverse total shoulder arthroplasty. Orthop Clin North Am. 2021;52(3):257–68. https://doi.org/10.1016/j.ocl.2021.03.006.
7. Kozak T, Bauer S, Walch G, Al-karawi S, Blakeney W. An update on reverse total shoulder arthroplasty: current indications, new designs, same old problems. EFORT Open Rev. 2021;6(3):189–201. https://doi.org/10.1302/2058-5241.6.200085.
8. Cho CH, Jung JW, Na SS, Bae KC, Lee KJ, Kim DH. Is acromial fracture after reverse total shoulder arthroplasty a negligible complication? A systematic review. Clin Orthop Surg. 2019;11(4):427–35. https://doi.org/10.4055/cios.2019.11.4.427.
9. Patterson DC, Chi D, Parsons BO, Cagle PJ. Acromial spine fracture after reverse total shoulder arthroplasty: a systematic review. J Shoulder Elb Surg. 2019;28(4):792–801. https://doi.org/10.1016/j.jse.2018.08.033.
10. Lau SC, Large R. Acromial fracture after reverse total shoulder arthroplasty: a systematic review. Shoulder Elb. 2020;12(6):375–89. https://doi.org/10.1177/1758573219876486.
11. Otto RJ, Virani NA, Levy JC, Nigro PT, Cuff DJ, Frankle MA. Scapular fractures after reverse shoulder arthroplasty: Evaluation of risk factors and the reliability of a proposed classification. J Shoulder Elb Surg. 2013;22(11):1514–21. https://doi.org/10.1016/j.jse.2013.02.007.
12. Rouleau DM, Gaudelli C. Successful treatment of fractures of the base of the acromion after reverse shoulder arthroplasty: case report and review of the literature. Int J Shoulder Surg. 2013;7(4):149–52. https://doi.org/10.4103/0973-6042.123531.
13. Ascione F, Kilian CM, Laughlin MS, et al. Increased scapular spine fractures after reverse shoulder arthroplasty with a humeral onlay short stem: an analysis of 485 consecutive cases. J Shoulder Elb Surg. 2018;27(12):2183–90. https://doi.org/10.1016/j.jse.2018.06.007.
14. Shah SS, Gentile J, Chen X, et al. Influence of implant design and parasagittal acromial morphology on acromial and scapular spine strain after reverse total shoulder arthroplasty: a cadaveric and computer-based biomechanical analysis. J Shoulder Elb Surg. 2020;29(11):2395–405. https://doi.org/10.1016/j.jse.2020.04.004.
15. Haidamous G, Lädermann A, Frankle MA, Gorman RA, Denard PJ. The risk of postoperative scapular spine fracture following reverse shoulder arthroplasty is increased with an onlay humeral stem. J Shoulder Elb Surg. 2020;29(12):2556–63. https://doi.org/10.1016/j.jse.2020.03.036.
16. Nyffeler RW, Altioklar B, Bissig P. Causes of acromion and scapular spine fractures following reverse shoulder arthroplasty: a retrospective analysis and literature review. Int Orthop. 2020;44(12):2673–81. https://doi.org/10.1007/s00264-020-04813-5.
17. Werthel JD, Walch G, Vegehan E, Deransart P, Sanchez-Sotelo J, Valenti P. Lateralization in reverse shoulder arthroplasty: a descriptive analysis of different implants in current practice. Int Orthop. 2019;43(10):2349–60. https://doi.org/10.1007/s00264-019-04365-3.
18. Klatte TO, Junghans K, Al-Khateeb H, et al. Single-stage revision for peri-prosthetic shoulder infection.

J Shoulder Elb Surg. 2015;24(4):1–8. https://doi.org/10.1016/j.jse.2015.09.027.
19. Werner CML, Steinmann PA, Gilbart M, Gerber C. Treatment of painful pseudoparesis due to irreparable rotator cuff dysfunction with the Delta 3 reverse-ball-and-socket total shoulder prosthesis. J Bone Jt Surg. 2005;87(7):1476–86. https://doi.org/10.2106/JBJS.D.02342.
20. Walch G, Mottier F, Wall B, Boileau P, Molé D, Favard L. Acromial insufficiency in reverse shoulder arthroplasties. J Shoulder Elb Surg. 2009;18(3):495–502. https://doi.org/10.1016/j.jse.2008.12.002.
21. Hattrup SJ. The influence of postoperative acromial and scapular spine fractures on the results of reverse shoulder arthroplasty. Orthopedics. 2010;33(5) https://doi.org/10.3928/01477447-20100329-04.
22. Goebel M, Klinc P, Seebauer L. Stressfrakturen der Scapula nachinversemSchultergelenksersatz – Inzidenz und Behandlungstratgie. In: Abstr V4 DVSE-Jahreskongress 2010, Rosenheim, Ger; 2010.
23. Hamid N, Connor PM, Fleischli JF, D'Alessandro DF. Acromial fracture after reverse shoulder arthroplasty. Am J Orthop (Belle Mead NJ). 2011;40(7):125–9.
24. Crosby LA, Hamilton A, Twiss T. Scapula fractures after reverse total shoulder arthroplasty: classification and treatment. Clin Orthop Relat Res. 2011;469(9):2544–9. https://doi.org/10.1007/s11999-011-1881-3.
25. Teusink MJ, Otto RJ, Cottrell BJ, Frankle MA. What is the effect of postoperative scapular fracture on outcomes of reverse shoulder arthroplasty? J Shoulder Elb Surg. 2014;23(6):782–90. https://doi.org/10.1016/j.jse.2013.09.010.
26. Werthel J-D, Schoch BS, van Veen SC, et al. Acromial fractures in reverse shoulder arthroplasty: a clinical and radiographic analysis. J Shoulder Elbow Arthroplasty. 2018:2. https://doi.org/10.1177/2471549218777628.
27. Neyton L, Erickson J, Ascione F, et al. Grammont Award 2018: scapular fractures in reverse shoulder arthroplasty (Grammont style): prevalence, functional, and radiographic results with minimum 5-year follow-up. J Shoulder Elb Surg. 2019;28(2):260–7. https://doi.org/10.1016/j.jse.2018.07.004.
28. Marigi E, Bartels D, Tangtiphaiboontana J, Ivanov D, Nguyen NT, Sanchez-Sotelo J. Acromial and spine fractures after reverse arthroplasty: prevalence and risk factors. Semin Arthroplast: JSES. 2020;30(3):237–41. https://doi.org/10.1053/j.sart.2020.07.006.
29. Routman HD, Simovitch RW, Wright T, Flurin P, Zuckerman JD, Roche CP. Acromial and scapular fractures after reverse total shoulder arthroplasty with a medialized glenoid and lateralized humeral implant. J Bone Jt Surg Am. 2020;102:1724–33.
30. Schenk P, Aichmair A, Beeler S, Ernstbrunner L, Meyer DC, Gerber C. Acromial fractures following reverse total shoulder arthroplasty: a cohort controlled analysis. Orthopedics. 2020;43(1):15–22. https://doi.org/10.3928/01477447-20191031-03.
31. Zmistowski B, Gutman M, Horvath Y, Abboud JA, Williams GR, Namdari S. Acromial stress fracture following reverse total shoulder arthroplasty: incidence and predictors. J Shoulder Elb Surg. 2020;29(4):799–806. https://doi.org/10.1016/j.jse.2019.08.004.
32. Moverman MA, Menendez ME, Mahendraraj KA, Polisetty T, Jawa A, Levy JC. Patient risk factors for acromial stress fractures after reverse shoulder arthroplasty: a multicenter study. J Shoulder Elb Surg. 2021;30(7):1619–25. https://doi.org/10.1016/j.jse.2020.09.012.
33. Meshram P, Joseph J, Zhou Y, Srikumaran U, McFarland EG. Lateralized glenosphere reverse shoulder arthroplasty: inlay and onlay designs have similar clinical outcomes in patients with glenohumeral osteoarthritis. J Shoulder Elb Surg. 2022;31(4):747–54. https://doi.org/10.1016/j.jse.2021.08.016.
34. Saltzman BM, Chalmers PN, Gupta AK, Romeo A, a, Nicholson GP. Complication rates comparing primary with revision reverse total shoulder arthroplasty. J Shoulder Elb Surg. 2014;23(11):1647–54. https://doi.org/10.1016/j.jse.2014.04.015.
35. Groh GI, Groh GM. Complications rates, reoperation rates, and the learning curve in reverse shoulder arthroplasty. J Shoulder Elb Surg. 2014;23(3):388–94. https://doi.org/10.1016/j.jse.2013.06.002.
36. Merolla G, Wagner E, Sperling JW, Paladini P, Fabbri E, Porcellini G. Revision of failed shoulder hemiarthroplasty to reverse total arthroplasty: analysis of 157 revision implants. J Shoulder Elb Surg. 2018;27(1) https://doi.org/10.1016/j.jse.2017.06.038.
37. Shah SS, Roche AM, Sullivan SW, Gaal BT, Dalton S, Sharma A, King JJ, Grawe BM, Namdari S, Lawler M, Helmkamp J, Garrigues GE, Wright TW, Schoch BS, Flik K, Otto RJ, Jones R, Jawa A, McCann P, Abboud J, Horneff G, Ross G, Friedman R, Ricchetti ET, Boardman D, Tashjian RZ, Gulotta LV. The modern reverse shoulder arthroplasty and an updated systematic review for each complication: Part II. JSES Int. 2020;5(1):121–37. https://doi.org/10.1016/j.jseint.2020.07.018.
38. Levy JC, Anderson C, Samson A. Classification of postoperative acromial fractures. JBJS. 2013;104:1–7.
39. Lopiz Y, Garcia-coiradas J, Garcia-fernandez C, Marco F. Proximal humerus nailing: a randomized clinical trial between curvilinear and straight nails. J Shoulder Elb Surg. 2014;23(3):369–76. https://doi.org/10.1016/j.jse.2013.08.023.
40. Mayne IP, Bell SN, Wright W, Coghlan JA. Acromial and scapular spine fractures after reverse total shoulder arthroplasty. Shoulder Elb. 2016;8(2):90–100. https://doi.org/10.1177/1758573216628783.
41. Terrier A, Merlini F, Farron A. Simulated joint and muscle forces in reversed and anatomic shoulder prostheses. J Bone Joint Surg Br. 2008;90(6):751–6. https://doi.org/10.1302/0301-620X.90B6.19708.
42. Henninger HB, Barg A, Anderson AE, Bachus KN, Burks RT, Tashjian RZ. Effect of lateral offset center of rotation in reverse total shoulder arthro-

plasty: a biomechanical study. J Shoulder Elb Surg. 2012;21(9):1128–35. https://doi.org/10.1016/j.jse.2011.07.034.
43. Ackland DC, Roshan-zamir S, Richardson M, Pandy MG. Muscle and joint-contact loading at the glenohumeral joint after reverse total shoulder arthroplasty. J Orthop Res. 2011;29(12):1850–8. https://doi.org/10.1002/jor.21437.
44. Dubrow S, Streit JJ, Muh S, Shishani Y, Gobezie R. Acromial stress fractures: correlation with acromioclavicular osteoarthritis and acromiohumeral distance. Orthopedics. 2014;37(12):e1074–9. https://doi.org/10.3928/01477447-20141124-54.
45. Kennon JC, Lu C, Mcgee-lawrence ME, Crosby LA. Scapula fracture incidence in reverse total shoulder arthroplasty using screws above or below metaglene central cage: clinical and biomechanical outcomes. J Shoulder Elb Surg. 2017;26(6):1023–30. https://doi.org/10.1016/j.jse.2016.10.018.
46. Eroğlu ON, Hüsemoğlu B, Başçı O, Özkan M, Havıtçıoğlu H, Hapa O. Scapular spine base fracture with long outside-in superior or posterior screws with reverse shoulder arthroplasty. Clin Shoulder Elb. 2021;24(3):141–6. https://doi.org/10.5397/cise.2021.00213.
47. Norris TR, Kelly JD, Humphrey CS. Management of glenoid bone defects in revision shoulder arthroplasty: a new application of the reverse total shoulder prosthesis. Tech Shoulder Elb Surg. 2007;8(1):37–46. https://doi.org/10.1097/BTE.0b013e318030d3b7.
48. Taylor SA, Shah SS, Chen X, et al. Scapular ring preservation. J Bone Jt Surg. 2020;102(15):1358–64. https://doi.org/10.2106/jbjs.19.01118.
49. Casp AJ, Montgomery SR, Cancienne JM, Brockmeier SF, Werner BC. Osteoporosis and implant-related complications after anatomic and reverse total shoulder arthroplasty. J Am AcadOrthop Surg. 2020;28(3):121–7. https://doi.org/10.5435/JAAOS-D-18-00537.
50. Boehm TD, Rolf O, Martetschlaeger F, Kenn W, Gohlke F. Rotator cuff tears associated with osacromiale. Acta Orthop. 2005;76(2):241–4. https://doi.org/10.1080/00016470510030643.
51. Burkholz KJ, Roberts CC, Hattrup SJ. Scapular spine stress fracture as a complication of reverse shoulder arthroplasty. Radiol Case Rep. 2007;2(2):78–82. https://doi.org/10.2484/rcr.v2i2.105.
52. Wahlquist TC, Hunt AF, Braman JP. Acromial base fractures after reverse total shoulder arthroplasty: report of five cases. J Shoulder Elb Surg. 2011;20(7):1178–83. https://doi.org/10.1016/j.jse.2011.01.029.
53. Ekelund A, Seebauer L. Acromial and scapular spine fractures after reverse shoulder arthroplasty. Obere Extrem. 2017;12:32–7.
54. Kriechling P, Hodel S, Paszicsnyek A, Schwihla I, Borbas P, Wieser K. Incidence, radiographic predictors, and clinical outcome of acromial stress reaction and acromial fractures in reverse total shoulder arthroplasty. J Shoulder Elb Surg. 2022;31(6):1143–53. https://doi.org/10.1016/j.jse.2021.11.012.
55. Bauer S, Traverso A, Walch G. Locked 90°-double plating of scapular spine fracture after reverse shoulder arthroplasty with union and good outcome despite plate adjacent acromion fracture. BMJ Case Rep. 2020;13(9):1–4. https://doi.org/10.1136/bcr-2020-234727.
56. Toft F, Moro F. Does ORIF of rare scapular spine fractures sustained after reverse shoulder arthroplasty benefit elderly patients? A case-series appraisal. Orthop Traumatol Surg Res. 2019;105(8):1521–8. https://doi.org/10.1016/j.otsr.2019.07.023.

Part IV

Humerus

18 Humeral Stress Shielding and Bony Adaptations in Shoulder Arthroplasty

E. Fumina Kobayashi and William R. Aibinder

18.1 Introduction

Primary anatomic total shoulder arthroplasty (aTSA) and reverse total shoulder arthroplasty (rTSA) have become more common recently. As a result, the estimated rate of revisions is 10% at 10 years, rising to between 20% and 30% within 20 years of an index arthroplasty [1]. Historically, traditional length cemented humeral stems were utilized in shoulder arthroplasty with low rates of loosening [2]. These stems were problematic as the use of cement increased operative time, could hypothetically lead to risk of fat embolism, and increased the complexity of revision procedures. Consequently, uncemented traditional length stems gained popularity. As fixation and integration improved with third and fourth generation cementless stems, these shoulders demonstrated high rates of bony resorption up to 82% at long-term follow-up [2–10]. Progressive humeral bone loss raises concern for associated bone atrophy and weakness which may lead to decreased function and contribute to the difficulty of obtaining stable fixation during revision arthroplasty. In an attempt to decrease this bony resorption, several modifications of the humeral implant have been implemented with the shift of design to shorter stems, and even stemless implants [11–16].

Shorter humeral implants obtain fixation in the metaphysis of the proximal humerus which has been shown to decrease the rate of proximal bone resorption in nonclinical studies [17, 18]. Further advantages of shorter implants include ease of removal at revision procedures, avoidance of mid-diaphyseal stress risers which lead to challenging periprosthetic fractures, easier implantation when faced with substantial proximal humerus deformity, and decreased surgical time [17]. While studies have demonstrated a low rate of aseptic implant loosening, proximal bone resorption is still seen in radiographic follow-up [6, 10, 11, 13–16, 19]. Despite the known prevalence of stress shielding and bony adaptions, the clinical significance and risk factors are not well borne out in the literature. This chapter will focus on defining various forms of bone resorption, including stress shielding, and review the nonclinical, clinical, and radiographic data.

18.2 Causes of Bone Loss

Terminology in the literature is oftentimes misleading in studies regarding stress shielding and other bone adaptations. Commonly, osteolysis is used interchangeably in several studies. Consistent with Wolff's law, *stress shielding* is

E. F. Kobayashi · W. R. Aibinder (✉)
Orthopaedic Surgery, University of Michigan, Ann Arbor, MI, USA
e-mail: evangelk@med.umich.edu; waibinde@med.umich.edu

F. Franceschi et al. (eds.), *Revision Shoulder Arthroplasty*,
https://doi.org/10.1007/978-3-031-45944-3_18

defined as bony adaptations due to altered distributions of stress on the bone [20]. There are two mechanisms of stress shielding that have been proposed. With arthroplasty, increase in axial bending stiffness from the native bone to the implant will cause bone adaptations due to the stem rigidity [21, 22]. Secondly, when fixation is distal in the diaphysis, there is decreased load or stress proximal to this area leading to bone resorption [21]. Resulting changes in the bone are seen through external remodeling with cortical thinning or internal remodeling with the bone becoming more porous and osteopenic, ultimately resulting in resorption of the greater tuberosity or calcar [22]. The clinical consequence of stress shielding is not entirely elucidated. The reports on outcomes range from loosening and subsidence occurring secondary to stress shielding [23] to no clinical difference in function or radiographic evidence of at risk stems [7, 11, 24–26]. A humeral implant is classified as "at risk" for loosening if a radiolucent lines of 2 mm or greater are present in three or more zones [27]. Radiolucent lines under the humeral tray are more concerning for osteolysis as this region of bone should see increased stresses due to the loading of the reverse articulation [26].

In contrast to stress shielding, *osteolysis* is commonly used to refer to bone loss that is a bone response to wear particulate debris formation of various materials, such as polyethylene, ceramics, cement, and metals. This leads to macrophage response with the activation of osteoclasts [28, 29]. Further osteoclast activation leads to osteolysis around the prosthesis leading to micromotion which can further increase particle wear and further bone resorption, eventually resulting in loosening of the implant and potential catastrophic failure. Osteolysis is described as endosteal scalloping, cortical thinning, or cystic changes within the metaphyseal bone of the humerus [30].

It can be challenging to differentiate bone resorption from osteolysis. Stress shielding should be suspected in cases with no glenoid component wear or loosening in the case of aTSA, no scapular notching in the case of rTSA, and uncemented stem fixation in the case of aTSA, rTSA, or hemiarthroplasty. Regardless of the underlying cause, bone loss is concerning with an associated risk of implant failure, loosening, and periprosthetic fractures that may require revision procedures [8]. Furthermore, bone resorption at the time of revision surgery increases the difficulty of restoring native humeral length and obtaining stable fixation, particularly in the case of calcar resorption. Tuberosity resorption affects the ability to optimize rotation, joint stability, deltoid wrap, and ultimately function.

18.3 Radiographic Evaluation

A true glenohumeral anteroposterior (AP) view (Grashey view) and axillary radiographs are commonly obtained for evaluation for stress shielding. It is important to ensure the projection of the humerus is similar when comparing sequential radiographs whether the humerus be neutral, internally rotated, or externally rotated. Additionally, exposure technique at various time points can alter interpretations of the radiographs. If possible, radiographs should be obtained with the same protocol and at the same facility.

Classifications of radiographic changes were described by Nagels et al. [6] and applied to a shorter stem by Schnetzke et al. [19]. Bony adaptations, particularly stress shielding, are assessed by dividing the proximal humerus into zones, such as the greater and lesser tuberosities, proximal medial and lateral cortices, and around the distal end of the implant on serial postoperative radiographs at various follow-up time points [31]. This has also been adapted to stemless implants [24, 31].

External bony adaptations, such as cortical thinning, are easily evaluated and compared on sequential radiographs. External remodeling can be quantified by measuring the distance between the stem and outer lining of the cortex [6]. Other notable radiographic changes in the literature are spot welds or periprosthetic endosteal bone formation demonstrating osseointegration, condensation lines, or pedestal formation demonstrating new endosteal bone formation distal to the stem

[5]. These latter findings are more commonly found with hip arthroplasty.

Internal bony adaptations, including bone density, can be difficult to determine, given the contrast and brightness of radiographs must be similar to be able to evaluate these changes [6]. Some authors have attempted to quantify this in several studies [24, 32].

In the evaluation of stress shielding and bony adaptation, the canal fill index or relative stem size is an important factor to consider. It is defined as the ratio between the inner diameter of the humerus and the stem size [6, 19]. This can be measured proximally in the metaphysis and distally in the diaphysis depending on the length of the stem. A lower canal fill index is consistent with a smaller stem, while a higher canal fill index is associated with a larger diameter stem. Additionally, varus and valgus alignment of the stem should be evaluated as malalignment has been shown to be associated with bony adaptations [26]. When comparing the immediate postoperative radiograph, subsidence and tilt of the implant can be assessed with sequential imaging [2, 27].

18.4 Nonclinical Outcomes

18.4.1 Finite Element Analysis

Bone loss in the setting of total hip arthroplasty has been extensively studied through various computer-based finite element analyses. Although the stress on the glenohumeral joint is mostly due to muscle action rather than direct weight-bearing load like the hip, similar and significant differences in bone stresses have been noted in a study by Razfar et al. [18]. In the native humerus, the force is transmitted throughout the bone by the surrounding cortex. With stemmed implants, the load is carried through the implant and then contacting the distal cortex. Traditional length stems with fixation in the diaphysis demonstrated the greatest reduction in stress in the metaphyseal and epiphyseal cortical regions of the humerus. This was due to transfer of load over a longer distance to the point where the stem was in contact with the cortex [19]. Additional increases in stem length resulted in the load on the cortex to be more distal in the bone. Furthermore, larger stem diameters can also exacerbate stress shielding with fixation occurring more distal in the proximal humerus, decreasing load sharing through the remaining cancellous and metaphyseal bone, and lead to peripheral bone resorption [6, 19].

In short stem designs which are typically between 50–100 mm in length, proximal humeral cortical bone stresses were noted to be 78% of the native bone stress compared with only 58% with traditional length stems [19]. Like the longer standard stems, shorter and thinner implants that do not completely fill the canal were beneficial in decreasing stress shielding in a similar model [33]. This appears to result in better load sharing between the implant and the proximal humeral bone structure.

Native bone stress is most closely mimicked in stemless models as the joint reaction force is transferred across a shorter distance [19]. Stemless implants have varying designs and include a central peg, peripheral fins, or boundary-crossing (central and peripheral) fixation techniques [34]. The least bone changes were noted with central and thinner peripheral fixations, while the boundary-crossing implants had the highest changes in bone stress. The greatest changes in bone stress occur directly beneath the humeral resection and surrounding trabecular bone due to the fixation in the metaphysis [34]. Similar results were found using single-photon emission computed tomography integrated with multidetector computed tomography (SPECT/CT) imaging with the highest levels of metabolic activity in the most proximal segment of bone directly under the prosthesis within 3 months of implantation [35].

Conversely, Quental et al. noted stress shielding secondary to axial loading may not be a key factor for failure of humeral implants [36]. Models without muscle acting on the bone had significantly more bone resorption in three or more regions than in models with muscle acting on the bone. These authors also noted when the bone is considered healthy, no bone resorption was seen regardless of fixation technique. In contrast, bone resorption was seen in several regions in the humerus when the bone had initial poorer quality which may demonstrate preexisting bone quality to be another notable issue. SPECT/CT imaging, however, did not show a decreased metabolic response in osteopenic or osteoporotic patients after implantation of short stems [35].

While these studies provide a computational understanding of the effect of stem length and diameter on bone stress and ultimately stress shielding, it is important to value the clinical studies that address bone resorption. In the next sections, we will review the literature based on stem length, fixation technique, and highlight some comparative studies.

18.5 Radiographic Outcomes

18.5.1 Traditional Length Stem

Cemented traditional length stems demonstrate low rates of stress shielding, and loosening is exceptionally rare with rates reported as low as 0–2% in the long-term studies [37, 38]. While this data is positive, the use of cement in standard length stems did lead to challenges with revision procedures as previously discussed. Similarly, stress shielding with this type of fixation, even with longer stems, is rare since the stress from the stem is dissipated throughout the entire length of the stem by way of the cement [31].

The early generations of uncemented stems were straight, cylindrical, and uncoated stems. These stems relied on distal fixation. Up to 55.6% of these stems were noted to be at risk of radiographic loosening [2]. Despite this high rate, the authors noted a 19% rate of proximal humeral bone resorption as a surrogate for stress shielding. Verborgt et al. reported on a similar series of 37 patients with uncoated traditional length stems (Neer II or Modular Shoulder Prosthesis, 3 M, St. Paul, MN) [39]. At a mean follow-up of 9 years, the authors noted a similar rate of lucencies at 59% but only 5% of shoulders with evidence of resorption or stress shielding. This is counterintuitive to the finite element analysis findings that report that the proximal humeral bone stress is 58% of the native state with traditional length stems [18].

Despite these findings, several other studies have evaluated uncemented standard length stems. At mid-term follow-up of 5 years with a rectangular stem with diaphyseal fixation (Promos, Smith & Nephew, Memphis, TN), proximal bone resorption was reported 17% of aTSAs [7]. The larger the ratio of the stem diameter to the diameter of the canal, the increased risk of developing stress shielding was noted. Specifically, high canal filling ratios have been found to increase the risk of resorption 2.3 times higher if the canal filling index of 1.3–1.4 [7].

Metaphyseal tapered stems were suspected of increasing proximal fixation and thus decreasing diaphyseal fit along with the resultant stress shielding. Matsen et al. demonstrated that only 8.6% of shoulders had a radiolucent line greater than or equal to 1 mm, with 39% of shoulders having no radiolucencies [3]. Thus, optimizing proximal fixation may improve humeral implant survivability and decrease the rate of bony adaptations. One such technique that has been proposed is impaction grafting [40]. This can be particularly helpful in osteoporotic bone and allow for implantation of a prosthesis with a low canal filling ratio. In a comparison between a press-fit stem (Equinoxe, Exactech, Gainesville, FL) with metaphyseal taper placed with and without impaction grafting (low versus high filling ratio, respectively), they noted significantly decreased stress shielding at one-year postoperatively with the low filling ratio with impaction grafting [41]. Lucas et al. found that this technique even with the use of standard, smooth tapered humeral stems was with durable fixation with only 6.6% subsidence short- and mid-term follow-up [42].

Stress shielding, specifically in traditional length stems, is also associated with the amount of ingrowth surface. This can be adapted from the hip literature as well where high rates of stress shielding have also been seen in fully ingrown stems compared with proximally ingrown stems [43]. Uncoated press-fit stems (BioModular, Biomet, Warsaw, IN) are noted to have external stress shielding in 9% of shoulders at a follow-up of about 5 years [6]. In contrast, the previously discussed rectangular stem (Promos, Smith & Nephew, Memphis, TN) is grit blasted along the entirety of its length, and thus the rate of remodeling was noted to be 17% [7]. Similar studies have been noted with more novel stems with proximal ingrowth only, and the rate of stress shielding is reported at 6.5–7% [27, 30].

Raiss et al. performed a large multicenter study evaluating another specific metaphyseal taper designed stem (Aequalis, Stryker, Mahwah, NJ) [10]. Similar to the aforementioned studies, the stem is designed to minimize distal fixation and rely on proximal metaphyseal stability of the implant. In this study, the authors also compared fixation type (cement versus no cement) and hemiarthroplasty versus aTSA. In a comparison between similar hemiarthroplasties and TSA, 43% with osteolysis of the greater tuberosity and 39% of the medial calcar with osteolysis occurred only in the aTSA group [10, 42]. Within the aTSA group, 94.5% of the shoulders with glenoid loosening had humeral bone adaptations with multiple radiolucent lines and osteolysis around the implant at short- and mid-term follow-up [10, 44] This supports the finding that osteolysis is predominantly related to polyethylene wear.

Additionally, the authors reported a rate of stress shielding of 63% with uncemented stems, while there was no stress shielding with cement which dissipates the stress throughout the entirety of the humerus [10]. However, it should be noted that authors focused on stress shielding as internal remodeling with intact cortices which may affect the results. Some of the osteolysis noted in these stems not associated with glenoid loosening could be severe stress shielding with external remodeling. This may be also why the authors found no correlation with canal filling ratio and the level of stress shielding.

When comparing studies evaluating similar uncemented and cemented stems in the setting of rTSA, a significant number of stems at risk for loosening or subsided were those with evidence of scapular notching and subsequent polyethylene wear [5, 30, 45]. A notable concern with significant bone resorption at the greater tuberosity is the diminishing effect of deltoid wrapping causing instability after rTSA or decreased function [46]. Other risk factors of bone resorption in rTSA include female sex and the use of an onlay-type stem [46, 47] (Fig. 18.1). The proximal fixation of a stem with an inlay-type design decreases the reliance on distal stem fixation.

Stress shielding of the proximal humerus with traditional length stems has been reported as high as 63% [10, 19]; however, the definition in these studies is entirely variable with the use of internal or external remodeling, proximal bone resorption, or osteolysis as terms noted in the results sections of the aforementioned studies. Nonetheless, in the setting of traditional length stems, decreasing distal fixation through the use of cement, impaction grafting, or the use of a metaphyseal tapered stem may decrease the rate of stress shielding in. This trend toward more proximal fixation has led to the development of shorter stems.

18.5.2 Short Stems (SS)

Short stems were designed and intended to decrease bone-implant load sharing to a smaller region of the proximal humerus [17]. This would allow for more stress to be seen by the native proximal bone and thus potentially decrease bony adaptations [48]. In a comparison of a short stem and traditional length stem from a single vendor (Arthrex, Naples, FL), the short stem implants had a statistically significant decrease in the rate of cortical thinning and bone resorption rates [12]. However, short stems were still noted to have cortical thinning in 50% of shoulders, while 23% had evidence of calcar osteolysis [12]. These rates were not significantly improved compared to the aforementioned rates with other traditional length stems discussed in the previous section. It should also be noted that 86% of short stem cases had stems that were not placed in an anatomic position. In a study with a different short stemmed implant (Comprehensive Micro, Biomet, Warsaw, IN), Aibinder et al. noted that 95% of components were placed in anatomic alignment [32].

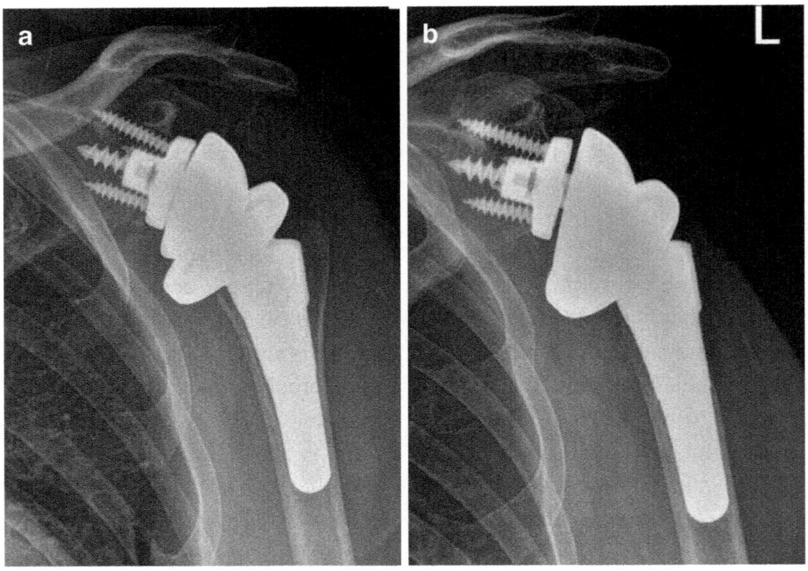

Fig. 18.1 Immediate postoperative (**a**) and 2-year postoperative (**b**) anteroposterior radiograph of a 55-year-old female who underwent a left reverse total shoulder arthroplasty for Hamada 4 cuff tear arthropathy with severe stress shielding of the greater tuberosity and medial calcar. At 2-year follow-up, the patient had a 30° decrease in forward elevation compared to her 1-year follow-up and developed an external rotation lag and evidence of a hornblower sign. This may be related to loss of her infraspinatus and teres minor insertion, as well as loss of the deltoid wrap effect. Review of the radiograph does demonstrate a large metaphyseal and diaphyseal fill ratio

Two studies evaluated the bony adaptations and stress shielding noted with a short stem metaphyseal tapered proximally coated implant (Ascend, Stryker, Mahwah, NJ) [14, 16, 19, 23, 25]. Schnetzke et al. reported medical calcar osteopenia or cortical thinning in 83% of cases [19]. In contrast, Casagrande et al. evaluated 73 shoulders and noted partial medial calcar osteolysis in 14.5% of cases and complete calcar osteolysis in 2.9% [14]. An earlier study by Schnetzke et al. evaluating the same stem reported a medial calcar stress shielding rate of 13.6% [23]. These studies highlight the importance of understanding the differences in terminology and the radiographic assessment in different studies. These studies focus on the stem prior to the addition of a proximal porous coating (Ascend Flex, Stryker, Mahwah, NJ). In a comparison of these 2 stems, Morwood et al. demonstrated a decreased rate of loosening risk and radiolucencies with the proximal coating, although the authors did not report on stress shielding, remodeling, osteolysis, or other bony adaptations [49]. Specifically, with an uncoated stem, the rate of "at risk" stems was 21% with radiolucencies reported up to 44%, while a coated stem of a similar design had an "at risk" loosening rate of 3% and radiolucencies in only 21% of shoulders [14, 49, 50]. Similar outcomes were seen with other proximally coated stems [16, 36].

Similar to the traditional length stems, short stems were noted to have a higher rate of bony adaptations, including stress shielding, internal and external remodeling, condensation lines, and spot welds with higher metaphyseal and diaphyseal filling ratios [19]. Thus, the larger the stem, the higher the rate of bony adaptations. In a cadaveric study, decreases in cortical and trabecular bone stress was most significant beneath the humeral cut plane with the most drastic decrease in shoulders with a large canal filling ratio [51]. Shoulders with a metaphyseal filling ratio of less than 68% had significantly fewer radiographic changes compared to those with filling ratio of 74% or greater [52]. Additionally, shoulders with a diaphyseal filling ratio of 85% had significantly more radiographic changes compared to those with lower filling ratio of 77%. It should also be noted that larger stems are often required in patients with poor bone quality in order to obtain initial stability with metaphyseal fixation as these stems do not rely on distal diaphyseal fit [19, 26]. Specifically with the curved oval stem design of the Ascend Flex, when stability is unable to be achieved with a small stem, consideration should be given toward impaction grafting to assist with stability or the use of a traditional length stem.

Stem shape and geometry may also play a significant role. For instance, in a study comparing a short stem (Revers Apex, Arthrex, Naples, FL) and a traditional length stem (Univers Revers, Arthrex, Naples, FL) in the setting of rTSA, the short stem had greater metaphyseal and diaphyseal canal fill ratio compared to traditional length stem group [53]. This is likely related to the rectangular and straight shape of the implant. The design in implant shape has also been assessed with finite element analysis comparing implant designs. An oval or semi-angular stem design closely reproduced native bone stresses, whereas angulated stems significantly increased surrounding bone stresses by 40% [54]. This increase is concerning as it can result in cracks in the cortex and eventual fracture [32]. With regard to torsional stability, angular and semi-angular stems were significantly more stable than oval stem designs [54]. In a clinical study, Denard et al. compared the rectangular-shaped short stem with a collar (Apex, Arthrex Inc., Naples, FL) to the metaphyseal tapered stem (Ascend, Stryker, Mahwah, NJ) and noted a decreased rate of medial calcar osteolysis (0% versus 7%), medial cortical thinning (63% versus 95%), and lateral cortical thinning (20% versus 79%) with the rectangular stem [11]. These authors noted the collared design might also be a significant design difference that is protective of the risk of bone adaptations.

Additionally, varus or valgus implant malalignment is associated with increased rates of medial or lateral metaphyseal cortical thinning, respectively [26]. In a finite element analysis, valgus alignment resulted in the largest changes in stress and increased bone resorption in the medial and lateral cortices [55].

Two studies also evaluated the outcome of a short stem proximally coated straight cylindrical stem that comes in 2 lengths [15, 32]. The short stem comes in two lengths: 83 mm (Biomet Comprehensive Mini, Warsaw, IN) and 55 mm (Biomet Comprehensive Micro, Warsaw, IN) with a proximal plasma spray [15, 32, 50]. Aibinder et al. evaluated the 55 mm stem and assessed both greater tuberosity stress shielding and medial calcar resorption [32]. The authors also graded these findings. Specifically, greater tuberosity stress shielding was graded as mild if there was only internal remodeling, moderate if there was cortical thinning, and severe if there was osteolysis. Medial calcar resorption was graded as mild if bone loss involved less than one-third of the coating of the implant, severe if it went beyond the implant coating, and moderate in between. In their study, the authors noted a greater tuberosity resorption rate of 14% with severe osteolysis in 3 cases, while medial calcar resorption was noted in 23% of cases. While these results are favorable compared to the oval metaphyseal tapered stem, the severe greater tuberosity resorption is concerning (Fig. 18.1).

While shorter stems should improve the rate of bony adaptations compared to traditional length stems, the current literature does not completely support this objective. It is likely that in patients with poor bone quality, larger diameter short stems seeking to achieve implant stability increase the filling ratio at the metaphysis and in the proximal diaphysis resulting in deleterious effects on stress distribution.

18.5.3 Stemless Implants

Stemless implants have been introduced with advantages of bone preservation and canal-sparing options for humeral fixation [56]. There is also the added benefit of decreased operative time by an average 25 min shorter compared to stemmed implants [57]. Stemless components can be fixed through impaction or through the use of a screw-in design (Eclipse, Arthrex Inc., Naples, FL). When compared to traditional length stems of the same vendor, a screw-in stemless component demonstrated a lower rate of internal remodeling, overall stress shielding, and humeral radiolucencies at short- and mid-term follow-up [57–59]. However, there continues to be reported decreases in proximal bone density with rates up to 41% at mid- to long-term follow-up, which is not insignificant [57–59]. Despite this, only 1% of shoulders demonstrates radiolucent lines at 5-year follow-up [58]. Longer-term studies on this implant demonstrated no stem loosening [60].

Early radiographic outcomes of impaction-type designs demonstrate no evidence of radiolucency, migration, subsidence, osteolysis, or stress shielding with two different designs (Simpliciti, Stryker, Mahwah, NJ; TESS, Zimmer Biomet, Warsaw, IN) [61, 62]. In one study, stemless implants were used in only 31% of aTSAs performed in the study period which may be a bias toward younger patients and those with good bone quality [62]. These impaction-type implants have a solid collar with an ingrowth surface that load shares across the cut surface. This is also present on the aforementioned screw-in design.

In a comparison between an impaction anchor fin design without a trunnion or collar (Sidus, Zimmer Biomet, Warsaw, IN) and a hollow screw-in fixation with a trunnion (Eclipse Arthrex, Inc., Naples, FL), the former had a significantly increased medial calcar resorption rate (33% versus 0%) at a minimum follow-up of 2 years [63]. The trunnion may distribute the axial load more evenly, decreasing the risk of calcar remodeling. This is consistent with the study by Aibinder et al. that reviewed 152 stemless aTSA using the anchor fin design and demonstrated an overall rate of stress shielding of 41% [24]. The authors also graded the stress shielding based on whether there was only decreased bone density, associated cortical thinning, or complete resorption. They found that severe stress shielding was noted to occur along the calcar in 7 shoulders compared to only 1 shoulder having the greater tuberosity affected. In contrast, Habermeyer et al. reviewed 78 patients who underwent aTSA with a hollow screw-in implant and noted decreased bone density in 46% of cases with the majority occurring along the greater tuberosity [58]. Thus, while the trunnion may be protective of the calcar in regard to stress shielding, it may be at the expense of loads at the greater tuberosity. In a systematic review, the screw-in fixation was noted to have significantly higher annual osteolysis rates than impaction-type fixations overall [64]. This was also demonstrated in a finite element analysis comparing different stemless fixation designs, in which the hollow screw design had significantly worse bone resorption and bone adaptation rates due to the preferential transfer of loads through the central screw [18, 65]. In this computational model, stemless designs with fixation in the periphery (SMR Stemless, LimaCorporate, San Daniele del Friuli, Italy) allow transfer of loads from the humeral component to the surrounding bone and may be protective of stress shielding like the trunnion [65].

Subscapularis management may also affect rates of stress shielding. There are decreased rates of stress shielding with lesser tuberosity osteotomy versus subscapularis peel [24]. This may be due to two factors. First, the peel technique detaches the entire subscapularis attachment along the lesser tuberosity and anteromedial calcar regions, often with incomplete healing of the inferior muscular portion of the subscapularis [24]. As seen in finite element analyses, the models without muscles acting on the bone had significantly more bone resorption, and thus with incomplete tendon healing the calcar region would experience less stress [36]. Secondly, the bone healing that occurs with an osteotomy and thus the resulting bone remodeling may be protective of stress shielding.

18.6 Clinical Outcomes

In the current literature, proximal humeral bone adaptations have not demonstrated a statistically significant influence of clinical outcomes at early follow-up regardless of stem length or design [7, 11, 12, 16, 19, 24–26, 32, 63]. Even in shoulders considered to be "at risk" for humeral loosening, outcomes were not associated with pain or decreased function [39]. All patients were noted to have significant improvements from preoperative to postoperative with regard to patient-reported outcome scores (PROs) and range of motion (ROM) at short- [14, 24, 57, 62], mid- [59], and long-term follow-ups [1, 66]. The majority of patients were satisfied or very satisfied with their shoulder [14, 57]. In a long-term follow-up of stemless aTSA, there was a 96.5% 10-year survivorship [66].

When comparing traditional length stems and short stems for aTSA (Univers II and Apex, Arthrex, Inc., Naples, FL), there were significant improvements in postoperative ROM and functional outcomes with no difference between groups despite a higher rate of cortical thinning in the traditional length group [12]. A similar study was performed for rTSA from the same vendor (Univers Revers and Revers Apex, Arthrex, Inc., Naples, FL) [53]. In this study, the short stem group had significantly better ASES scores, better forward elevation, and internal rotation postoperatively at the two-year follow-up [53]. Furthermore, several studies have compared the clinical outcomes of traditional length stems to stemless designs, and while both groups have significant improvements in PROs, ROM, and patient satisfaction, there is no significant clinical difference between the groups at short- and mid-term follow-ups [59, 67].

In contrast, patients with osteolysis associated with glenoid loosening and polyethylene wear had poorer clinical outcomes, significantly lower Constant scores, less elevation, and less external rotation at short- and long-term follow-up up to 9.5 years in both aTSA and rTSA [10, 68, 69].

18.7 Conclusion

While larger longer-term studies are needed, the current literature appears to support that stress shielding is not uncommon with shorter stemmed and stemless prostheses. There does not appear to be a significant effect on clinical outcomes. Few studies have systematically evaluated stress shielding based on severity, and there is no standard grading scale. Thus, future studies should evaluate internal and external bone remodeling of the proximal humerus in a standard way. Nonetheless, structural bone loss in severe cases may lead to implant failure and certainly increases the complexity of revision arthroplasty. Osteolysis related to polyethylene wear or infection, however, does lead to clinical deterioration and should be evaluated and addressed appropriately.

References

1. Raiss P, Bruckner T, Rickert M, Walch G. Longitudinal observational study of total shoulder replacements with cement: fifteen to twenty-year follow-up. J Bone Joint Surg Am. 2014;96:198–205. https://doi.org/10.2106/JBJS.M.00079.
2. Sanchez-Sotelo J, Wright TW, O'Driscoll SW, Cofield RH, Rowland CM. Radiographic assessment of uncemented humeral components in total shoulder arthroplasty. J Arthroplast. 2001;16:180–7. https://doi.org/10.1054/arth.2001.20905.
3. Matsen FA, Iannotti JP, Rockwood CA. Humeral fixation by press-fitting of a tapered metaphyseal stem: a prospective radiographic study. J Bone Joint Surg Am. 2003;85:304–8. https://doi.org/10.2106/00004623-200302000-00018.
4. Inoue K, Suenaga N, Oizumi N, Yamaguchi H, Miyoshi N, Taniguchi N, et al. Humeral bone resorption after anatomic shoulder arthroplasty using an uncemented stem. J Shoulder Elb Surg. 2017;26:1984–9. https://doi.org/10.1016/j.jse.2017.04.012.
5. Melis B, DeFranco M, Lädermann A, Molé D, Favard L, Nérot C, et al. An evaluation of the radiological changes around the Grammont reverse geometry shoulder arthroplasty after eight to 12 years. J Bone Joint Surg Br. 2011;93:1240–6. https://doi.org/10.1302/0301-620X.93B9.25926.
6. Nagels J, Stokdijk M, Rozing PM. Stress shielding and bone resorption in shoulder arthroplasty. J Shoulder Elb Surg. 2003;12:35–9. https://doi.org/10.1067/mse.2003.22.
7. Spormann C, Durchholz H, Audigé L, Flury M, Schwyzer H-K, Simmen BR, et al. Patterns of proximal humeral bone resorption after total shoulder arthroplasty with an uncemented rectangular stem. J Shoulder Elb Surg. 2014;23:1028–35. https://doi.org/10.1016/j.jse.2014.02.024.
8. Torchia ME, Cofield RH, Settergren CR. Total shoulder arthroplasty with the neer prosthesis: Long-term results. J Shoulder Elb Surg. 1997;6:495–505. https://doi.org/10.1016/S1058-2746(97)90081-1.
9. Throckmorton TW, Zarkadas PC, Sperling JW, Cofield RH. Radiographic stability of ingrowth humeral stems in total shoulder arthroplasty. Clin Orthop Relat Res. 2010;468:2122–8. https://doi.org/10.1007/s11999-010-1299-3.

10. Raiss P, Edwards TB, Deutsch A, Shah A, Bruckner T, Loew M, et al. Radiographic changes around humeral components in shoulder arthroplasty. J Bone Joint Surg Am. 2014;96:e54. https://doi.org/10.2106/JBJS.M.00378.
11. Denard PJ, Noyes MP, Walker JB, Shishani Y, Gobezie R, Romeo AA, et al. Radiographic changes differ between two different short press-fit humeral stem designs in total shoulder arthroplasty. J Shoulder Elb Surg. 2018;27:217–23. https://doi.org/10.1016/j.jse.2017.08.010.
12. Denard PJ, Noyes MP, Walker JB, Shishani Y, Gobezie R, Romeo AA, et al. Proximal stress shielding is decreased with a short stem compared with a traditional-length stem in total shoulder arthroplasty. J Shoulder Elb Surg. 2018;27:53–8. https://doi.org/10.1016/j.jse.2017.06.042.
13. Szerlip BW, Morris BJ, Laughlin MS, Kilian CM, Edwards TB. Clinical and radiographic outcomes after total shoulder arthroplasty with an anatomic press-fit short stem. J Shoulder Elb Surg. 2018;27:10–6. https://doi.org/10.1016/j.jse.2017.08.012.
14. Casagrande DJ, Parks DL, Torngren T, Schrumpf MA, Harmsen SM, Norris TR, et al. Radiographic evaluation of short-stem press-fit total shoulder arthroplasty: short-term follow-up. J Shoulder Elb Surg. 2016;25:1163–9. https://doi.org/10.1016/j.jse.2015.11.067.
15. Giuseffi SA, Streubel P, Sperling J, Sanchez-Sotelo J. Short-stem uncemented primary reverse shoulder arthroplasty: clinical and radiological outcomes. Bone Joint J. 2014;96-B:526–9. https://doi.org/10.1302/0301-620X.96B3.32702.
16. Schnetzke M, Preis A, Coda S, Raiss P, Loew M. Anatomical and reverse shoulder replacement with a convertible, uncemented short-stem shoulder prosthesis: first clinical and radiological results. Arch Orthop Trauma Surg. 2017;137:679–84. https://doi.org/10.1007/s00402-017-2673-3.
17. Harmer L, Throckmorton T, Sperling JW. Total shoulder arthroplasty: are the humeral components getting shorter? Curr Rev Musculoskelet Med. 2016;9:17–22. https://doi.org/10.1007/s12178-016-9313-3.
18. Razfar N, Reeves JM, Langohr DG, Willing R, Athwal GS, Johnson JA. Comparison of proximal humeral bone stresses between stemless, short stem, and standard stem length: a finite element analysis. J Shoulder Elb Surg. 2016;25:1076–83. https://doi.org/10.1016/j.jse.2015.11.011.
19. Schnetzke M, Coda S, Raiss P, Walch G, Loew M. Radiologic bone adaptations on a cementless short-stem shoulder prosthesis. J Shoulder Elb Surg. 2016;25:650–7. https://doi.org/10.1016/j.jse.2015.08.044.
20. Wolff J. The law of bone remodelling. Berlin, Heidelberg: Springer; 1986.
21. Engh CA, Bobyn JD. The influence of stem size and extent of porous coating on femoral bone resorption after primary cementless hip arthroplasty. Clin Orthop Relat Res. 1988;231:7–28.
22. Huiskes R, Weinans H, van Rietbergen B. The relationship between stress shielding and bone resorption around total hip stems and the effects of flexible materials. Clin Orthop Relat Res. 1992;274:124–34.
23. Schnetzke M, Coda S, Walch G, Loew M. Clinical and radiological results of a cementless short stem shoulder prosthesis at minimum follow-up of two years. Int Orthop. 2015;39:1351–7. https://doi.org/10.1007/s00264-015-2770-2.
24. Aibinder WR, Uddin F, Bicknell RT, Krupp R, Scheibel M, Athwal GS. Stress shielding following stemless anatomic total shoulder arthroplasty. Shoulder Elbow. 2023;15(1):54–60. https://doi.org/10.1177/17585732211058804.
25. Schnetzke M, Rick S, Raiss P, Walch G, Loew M. Mid-term results of anatomical total shoulder arthroplasty for primary osteoarthritis using a short-stemmed cementless humeral component. Bone Joint J. 2018;100-B:603–9. https://doi.org/10.1302/0301-620X.100B5.BJJ-2017-1102.R2.
26. Peduzzi L, Goetzmann T, Wein F, Roche O, Sirveaux F, Mole D, et al. Proximal humeral bony adaptations with a short uncemented stem for shoulder arthroplasty: a quantitative analysis. JSES Open Access. 2019;3:278–86. https://doi.org/10.1016/j.jses.2019.09.011.
27. Sperling JW, Cofield RH, O'Driscoll SW, Torchia ME, Rowland CM. Radiographic assessment of ingrowth total shoulder arthroplasty. J Shoulder Elb Surg. 2000;9:507–13. https://doi.org/10.1067/mse.2000.109384.
28. Dumbleton JH, Manley MT, Edidin AA. A literature review of the association between wear rate and osteolysis in total hip arthroplasty. J Arthroplast. 2002;17:649–61. https://doi.org/10.1054/arth.2002.33664.
29. Gupta SK, Chu A, Ranawat AS, Slamin J, Ranawat CS. Review article: osteolysis after total knee arthroplasty. J Arthroplast. 2007;22:787–99. https://doi.org/10.1016/j.arth.2007.05.041.
30. Brolin TJ, Cox RM, Horneff Iii JG, Namdari S, Abboud JA, Nicholson K, et al. Humeral-sided radiographic changes following reverse total shoulder arthroplasty. Arch Bone Jt Surg. 2020;8:50–7. https://doi.org/10.22038/abjs.2019.36065.1951.
31. Denard PJ, Raiss P, Gobezie R, Edwards TB, Lederman E. Stress shielding of the humerus in press-fit anatomic shoulder arthroplasty: review and recommendations for evaluation. J Shoulder Elb Surg. 2018;27:1139–47. https://doi.org/10.1016/j.jse.2017.12.020.
32. Aibinder WR, Bartels DW, Sperling JW, Sanchez-Sotelo J. Mid-term radiological results of a cementless short humeral component in anatomical and reverse shoulder arthroplasty. Bone Joint J. 2019;101-B:610–4. https://doi.org/10.1302/0301-620X.101B5.BJJ-2018-1374.R1.
33. Synnott S, Langohr GDG, Reeves JM, Johnson JA, Athwal GS. The effect of humeral implant thickness and canal fill on interface contact and bone stresses

in the proximal humerus. JSES Int. 2021;5:881–8. https://doi.org/10.1016/j.jseint.2021.05.006.
34. Reeves JM, Langohr GDG, Athwal GS, Johnson JA. The effect of stemless humeral component fixation feature design on bone stress and strain response: a finite element analysis. J Shoulder Elb Surg. 2018;27:2232–41. https://doi.org/10.1016/j.jse.2018.06.002.
35. Berth A, März V, Wissel H, Awiszus F, Amthauer H, Lohmann CH. SPECT/CT demonstrates the osseointegrative response of a stemless shoulder prosthesis. J Shoulder Elb Surg. 2016;25:e96–103. https://doi.org/10.1016/j.jse.2015.09.009.
36. Quental C, Folgado J, Fernandes PR, Monteiro J. Bone remodelling analysis of the humerus after a shoulder arthroplasty. Med Eng Phys. 2012;34:1132–8. https://doi.org/10.1016/j.medengphy.2011.12.001.
37. Raiss P, Schmitt M, Bruckner T, Kasten P, Pape G, Loew M, et al. Results of cemented total shoulder replacement with a minimum follow-up of ten years. J Bone Joint Surg Am. 2012;94:e1711–0. https://doi.org/10.2106/JBJS.K.00580.
38. Sanchez-Sotelo J, O'Driscoll SW, Torchia ME, Cofield RH, Rowland CM. Radiographic assessment of cemented humeral components in shoulder arthroplasty. J Shoulder Elb Surg. 2001;10:526–31. https://doi.org/10.1067/mse.2001.118482.
39. Verborgt O, El-Abiad R, Gazielly DF. Long-term results of uncemented humeral components in shoulder arthroplasty. J Shoulder Elb Surg. 2007;16:S13–8. https://doi.org/10.1016/j.jse.2006.02.003.
40. Hacker SA, Boorman RS, Lippitt SB, Matsen FA. Impaction grafting improves the fit of uncemented humeral arthroplasty. J Shoulder Elb Surg. 2003;12:431–5. https://doi.org/10.1016/S1058-2746(03)00053-3.
41. Kim SC, Park JH, Bukhary H, Yoo JC. Humeral stem with low filling ratio reduces stress shielding in primary reverse shoulder arthroplasty. Int Orthop. 2022;46:1341–9. https://doi.org/10.1007/s00264-022-05383-4.
42. Lucas RM, Hsu JE, Gee AO, Neradilek MB, Matsen FA. Impaction autografting: bone-preserving, secure fixation of a standard humeral component. J Shoulder Elb Surg. 2016;25:1787–94. https://doi.org/10.1016/j.jse.2016.03.008.
43. Huiskes R. The various stress patterns of press-fit, ingrown, and cemented femoral stems. Clin Orthop Relat Res. 1990;261:27–38.
44. DeVito P, Judd H, Malarkey A, Elson L, McNeely E, Berglund D, et al. Medial calcar bone resorption after anatomic total shoulder arthroplasty: does it affect outcomes? J Shoulder Elb Surg. 2019;28:2128–38. https://doi.org/10.1016/j.jse.2019.03.017.
45. Ascione F, Domos P, Guarrella V, Chelli M, Boileau P, Walch G. Long-term humeral complications after Grammont-style reverse shoulder arthroplasty. J Shoulder Elb Surg. 2018;27:1065–71. https://doi.org/10.1016/j.jse.2017.11.028.
46. Inoue K, Suenaga N, Oizumi N, Yamaguchi H, Miyoshi N, Taniguchi N, et al. Humeral bone resorption after reverse shoulder arthroplasty using uncemented stem. JSES Int. 2020;4:138–43. https://doi.org/10.1016/j.jses.2019.11.007.
47. Polisetty TS, Baessler AM, Levy JC, Badman BL. Onlay versus inlay reverse total shoulder arthroplasty: a retrospective comparison of radiographic and clinical outcomes. Semin Arthroplasty: JSES. 2021;31:202–8. https://doi.org/10.1053/j.sart.2020.11.013.
48. Huiskes R, Weinans H, Grootenboer HJ, Dalstra M, Fudala B, Slooff TJ. Adaptive bone-remodeling theory applied to prosthetic-design analysis. J Biomech. 1987;20:1135–50. https://doi.org/10.1016/0021-9290(87)90030-3.
49. Morwood MP, Johnston PS, Garrigues GE. Proximal ingrowth coating decreases risk of loosening following uncemented shoulder arthroplasty using mini-stem humeral components and lesser tuberosity osteotomy. J Shoulder Elb Surg. 2017;26:1246–52. https://doi.org/10.1016/j.jse.2016.11.041.
50. Jost PW, Dines JS, Griffith MH, Angel M, Altchek DW, Dines DM. Total shoulder arthroplasty utilizing mini-stem humeral components: technique and short-term results. HSS J. 2011;7:213–7. https://doi.org/10.1007/s11420-011-9221-4.
51. Langohr GDG, Reeves J, Roche CP, Faber KJ, Johnson JA. The effect of short-stem humeral component sizing on humeral bone stress. J Shoulder Elb Surg. 2020;29:761–7. https://doi.org/10.1016/j.jse.2019.08.018.
52. Raiss P, Schnetzke M, Wittmann T, Kilian CM, Edwards TB, Denard PJ, et al. Postoperative radiographic findings of an uncemented convertible short stem for anatomic and reverse shoulder arthroplasty. J Shoulder Elb Surg. 2019;28:715–23. https://doi.org/10.1016/j.jse.2018.08.037.
53. Erickson BJ, Denard PJ, Griffin JW, Wittman T, Raiss P, Gobezie R, et al. A 135° short inlay humeral stem leads to comparable radiographic and clinical outcomes compared with a standard-length stem for reverse shoulder arthroplasty. JSES Int. 2022;6:802–8. https://doi.org/10.1016/j.jseint.2022.05.003.
54. Barth J, Garret J, Geais L, Bothorel H, Saffarini M, Institute SF, et al. Influence of uncemented humeral stem proximal geometry on stress distributions and torsional stability following total shoulder arthroplasty. J Exp Orthop. 2019;6:8. https://doi.org/10.1186/s40634-019-0178-4.
55. Tavakoli A, Spangenberg G, Reeves JM, Faber KJ, Langohr GDG. Humeral short stem varus–valgus alignment affects bone stress. J Orthop Res. 2022;40:2169–78. https://doi.org/10.1002/jor.25239.
56. Churchill RS, Athwal GS. Stemless shoulder arthroplasty-current results and designs. Curr Rev Musculoskelet Med. 2016;9:10–6. https://doi.org/10.1007/s12178-016-9320-4.
57. Heuberer PR, Brandl G, Pauzenberger L, Laky B, Kriegleder B, Anderl W. Radiological changes do

not influence clinical mid-term outcome in stemless humeral head replacements with hollow screw fixation: a prospective radiological and clinical evaluation. BMC Musculoskelet Disord. 2018;19:28. https://doi.org/10.1186/s12891-018-1945-6.
58. Habermeyer P, Lichtenberg S, Tauber M, Magosch P. Midterm results of stemless shoulder arthroplasty: a prospective study. J Shoulder Elb Surg. 2015;24:1463–72. https://doi.org/10.1016/j.jse.2015.02.023.
59. Uschok S, Magosch P, Moe M, Lichtenberg S, Habermeyer P. Is the stemless humeral head replacement clinically and radiographically a secure equivalent to standard stem humeral head replacement in the long-term follow-up? A prospective randomized trial. J Shoulder Elb Surg. 2017;26:225–32. https://doi.org/10.1016/j.jse.2016.09.001.
60. Hawi N, Magosch P, Tauber M, Lichtenberg S, Habermeyer P. Nine-year outcome after anatomic stemless shoulder prosthesis: clinical and radiologic results. J Shoulder Elb Surg. 2017;26:1609–15. https://doi.org/10.1016/j.jse.2017.02.017.
61. Huguet D, DeClercq G, Rio B, Teissier J, Zipoli B, Group T. Results of a new stemless shoulder prosthesis: radiologic proof of maintained fixation and stability after a minimum of three years' follow-up. J Shoulder Elb Surg. 2010;19:847–52. https://doi.org/10.1016/j.jse.2009.12.009.
62. Churchill RS, Chuinard C, Wiater JM, Friedman R, Freehill M, Jacobson S, et al. Clinical and radiographic outcomes of the Simpliciti canal-sparing shoulder arthroplasty system: a prospective two-year multicenter study. J Bone Joint Surg Am. 2016;98:552–60. https://doi.org/10.2106/JBJS.15.00181.
63. Alikhah A, Imiolczyk J-P, Krukenberg A, Scheibel M. Screw fixation in stemless shoulder arthroplasty for the treatment of primary osteoarthritis leads to less osteolysis when compared to impaction fixation. BMC Musculoskelet Disord. 2020;21:295. https://doi.org/10.1186/s12891-020-03277-3.
64. Willems JIP, Hoffmann J, Sierevelt IN, van den Bekerom MPJ, Alta TDW, van Noort A. Results of stemless shoulder arthroplasty: a systematic review and meta-analysis. EFORT Open Rev. 2021;6:35–49. https://doi.org/10.1302/2058-5241.6.200067.
65. Comenda M, Quental C, Folgado J, Sarmento M, Monteiro J. Bone adaptation impact of stemless shoulder implants: a computational analysis. J Shoulder Elb Surg. 2019;28:1886–96. https://doi.org/10.1016/j.jse.2019.03.007.
66. Magosch P, Lichtenberg S, Habermeyer P. Survival of stemless humeral head replacement in anatomic shoulder arthroplasty: a prospective study. J Shoulder Elb Surg. 2021;30:e343–55. https://doi.org/10.1016/j.jse.2020.09.034.
67. Razmjou H, Holtby R, Christakis M, Axelrod T, Richards R. Impact of prosthetic design on clinical and radiologic outcomes of total shoulder arthroplasty: a prospective study. J Shoulder Elb Surg. 2013;22:206–14. https://doi.org/10.1016/j.jse.2012.04.016.
68. Nourissat G, Corsia S, Harris HW, Bouché P-A. Specific design of a press fit humeral stem provides low stress shielding in reverse shoulder arthroplasty at minimum 5 years FU. J Shoulder Elb Arthroplast. 2022;6:247154922211125. https://doi.org/10.1177/24715492221112543.
69. Mazaleyrat M, Favard L, Garaud P, Boileau P, Berhouet J. Press-fit vs. cemented humeral stem fixation for reverse shoulder arthroplasty: functional outcomes at a mean follow-up of 9.5 years. J Shoulder Elb Surg. 2021;30:72–9. https://doi.org/10.1016/j.jse.2020.04.052.

Classifying Humeral Bone Loss in Revision Shoulder Arthroplasty

19

Chad W. Parkes and Peter N. Chalmers

19.1 Introduction

Primary shoulder arthroplasty may fail due to a single cause, or more often, a combination of factors. Failure is often related to soft tissue [1] or osseous deficiencies [2] and may ultimately result in patients experiencing pain, loss of function, instability, component failure, or infection [3]. Humeral bone loss is commonly encountered in the setting of revision shoulder arthroplasty, especially in the clinical scenarios of previous surgery, infection, nonunion, malunion, or resorption of the tuberosities in arthroplasty performed for proximal humerus fracture [4], and iatrogenic bone loss from humeral component removal [5]. The degree of humeral bone loss may vary greatly and possess different implications for reconstructive options and outcomes due to the extent and location of bone loss [6]. Historically, uniform treatment strategies and algorithms for humeral bone loss in revision shoulder arthroplasty have not existed due to the lack of validated classification systems.

In the field of orthopedic surgery, classification systems exist to improve the understanding, communication, documentation, and decision-making for a group of related pathologies [7]. Specifically, a classification system for proximal humeral bone loss following shoulder arthroplasty allows surgeons to (1) communicate and discuss cases, (2) perform surgical planning with choice of implant and need for allograft, (3) anticipate the complexity of humeral reconstruction and likelihood of intraoperative humeral-related complications (i.e. greater tuberosity fracture), and (4) conduct future research to further guide treatment decision-making [8]. To date, no classification system has achieved widespread use for proximal humeral bone loss in revision shoulder arthroplasty. In this chapter, we will discuss the various methods and systems currently utilized to classify humeral bone loss in the setting of revision shoulder arthroplasty.

19.2 Classification Systems

Several different methods and systems of classifying humeral bone loss in the setting of revision shoulder arthroplasty have been previously utilized. Chacon et al. [9] evaluated proximal humeral bone loss in the setting of revision shoulder arthroplasty with proximal humeral allografts by measuring a line parallel to the humeral shaft of the distance from the tip of the allograft greater tuberosity (laterally) to the most proximal level of native humerus (medially) in anteroposterior (A-P) radiographs. However, these measurements were performed on the immediate postop-

C. W. Parkes · P. N. Chalmers (✉)
Department of Orthopaedic Surgery, University of Utah Orthopedic Center, Salt Lake City, UT, USA
e-mail: chad.parkes@hsc.utah.edu; peter.chalmers@hsc.utah.edu

F. Franceschi et al. (eds.), *Revision Shoulder Arthroplasty*,
https://doi.org/10.1007/978-3-031-45944-3_19

erative radiographs after the revision procedure had been performed, and there were no measurements performed on preoperative radiographs utilized to plan for the reconstructive procedure. Rather, intraoperative assessment of proximal humeral bone loss and soft tissue tension following removal of the humeral component was utilized to guide the decision to use proximal humeral allograft [9].

Similarly, Budge et al. [10] describe a method of calculating humeral bone loss by utilizing postoperative plain radiographs (A-P, Y-lateral, and axillary views) to measure the distance from the most proximal-lateral aspect of the humeral component to the most proximal aspect of remaining humeral bone, following the revision procedure. Although not included in their calculations, they note the magnitude of bone loss is likely 10–15 millimeters (mm) beyond their obtained measurement, as this is the estimated distance the native proximal humerus may extend above the humeral component. Similar to Chacon et al., these measurements were not performed preoperatively and thus were not utilized to aid in planning for the revision procedure [10].

Mclendon and colleagues [11] have proposed dividing humeral bone loss into two main categories of less than 5 cm of bone loss and greater than 5 cm of bone loss. They performed measurements intraoperatively during the reconstruction procedure after the glenosphere and trial humeral implant were placed with appropriate length and soft tissue tension. The amount of humeral bone loss was then measured from the superior aspect of the humeral tray medially to the medial humeral shaft. In their study, humeral bone loss via this intraoperative measurement was used as a determinant for the use of proximal humeral allograft [11].

Boileau [12] suggested subdividing humeral bone loss into a three-part system. Type A refers to humeral bone loss of less than 2 cm, limited to the epiphysis. Type B refers to humeral bone loss extending into the metaphyseal region or greater than 2 cm and less than 4 cm. Type C refers to humeral bone with extension to the diaphysis or greater than 4 cm. Boileau recommended utilizing these cutoffs to guide operative plan. The recommended treatment for Type A is "cementoplasty reconstruction," or creating a cement collar around the humeral implant, whereas, recommended treatment for types B and C is proximal humeral allograft [12].

Despite these multiple methods described to measure proximal humeral bone loss in the setting of revision shoulder arthroplasty, none of these methods have been evaluated for reliability or been associated with treatment outcomes or complications. In 2019, Chalmers and colleagues [8] proposed a novel classification system—the Proximal Humeral Arthroplasty Revision Osseous in Sufficiency Classification System—or PHAROS classification system. In Chalmers et al. study, the PHAROS system was evaluated for interrater and intrarater reliability and additionally was reviewed for operative characteristics for each type and subtype. As the PHAROS classification system is currently the only validated classification system to evaluate proximal humeral bone loss preoperatively prior to pursuing revision shoulder arthroplasty, it is our recommendation to use this system for operative planning purposes. We will discuss the PHAROS classification system in more detail in the next section.

19.3 Proximal Humeral Arthroplasty Revision Osseous in Sufficiency (PHAROS) Classification

The PHAROS classification [8] for humeral bone loss, inspired by the ancient Greek word "Pharos," a lighthouse that guides sailors in a storm, was published by Chalmers et al. in 2019. The system was created by the evaluation of pre-revision radiographs (AP, Grashey, and lateral views) and operative reports from revision surgery in 106 patients and 108 shoulders. There is no require-

Table 19.1 Summary table for the PHAROS classification system for proximal humeral bone loss in revision shoulder arthroplasty

PHAROS classification system			
Type	Location	Subtype	Description
1	Epiphyseal bone loss	C	Loss of calcar
		G	Loss of greater tuberosity
2	Metadiaphyseal bone loss	A	Metadiaphyseal cortical thinning of >50% of expected cortical thickness, with epiphyseal bone loss or thinning
	Above deltoid attachment	B	Bone loss above deltoid attachment including the epiphysis and part of metadiaphysis
3	Diaphyseal bone loss	A	Diaphyseal cortical thinning of >50% of the expected cortical thickness with epiphyseal or epiphyseal/metadiaphyseal bone loss or thinning
	Below deltoid attachment	B	Compromise of the majority of the diaphysis with loss of the epiphysis, metadiaphysis, and part of the diaphysis below the deltoid insertion

ment for advanced shoulder imaging (computed tomography (CT) or magnetic resonance imaging (MRI)) in order to assign classification in this system. In their study, Chalmers et al. found the PHAROS classification to have acceptable inter-rater agreement on 65% of shoulders evaluated ($\kappa = 0.545$). Within the same evaluator over a 4-month period, intraobserver agreement was obtained on 71% of shoulders ($\kappa = 0.615$). Additionally, PHAROS classification grades were found to be helpful in the prediction of reconstructive complexity during the revision procedure.

The PHAROS classification is a three-part system, consisting of three main numeric subtypes with further subdivision into alphanumeric subtypes (Table 19.1).

19.3.1 Type 1

Type 1 refers to epiphyseal bone loss, including the articular surface, tuberosities, and calcar. Type 1 is subdivided into subtype C (calcar loss as seen on the Grashey and axillary radiographs) (Fig. 19.1a) and subtype G (compromise (loss or malunion) of the greater tuberosity) (Fig. 19.1b).

19.3.2 Type 2

Type 2 refers to metadiaphyseal bone loss above the deltoid attachment. Type 2 classification consists of two subtypes, type 2A and type 2B. Type 2A refers to >50% cortical thinning of the metadiaphysis with epiphyseal bone loss or thinning, in comparison with expected cortical thickness based on the noninstrumented portion of the humerus (Fig. 19.1c). Type 2B refers to bone loss above the deltoid attachment including the epiphysis and part of the metaphysis (Fig. 19.1d).

19.3.3 Type 3

Type 3 refers to diaphyseal bone loss extending below the deltoid attachment. Type 3 classification consists of two subtypes, type 3A and 3B. Type A refers to >50% cortical thinning of the diaphysis below the deltoid attachment, in comparison with the expected cortical thickness based on the noninstrumented portion of the humerus (Fig. 19.1e). Type 3B refers to compromise of the majority of the diaphysis, with loss of the epiphysis, metadiaphysis, and part of the diaphysis below the deltoid insertion (Fig. 19.1f).

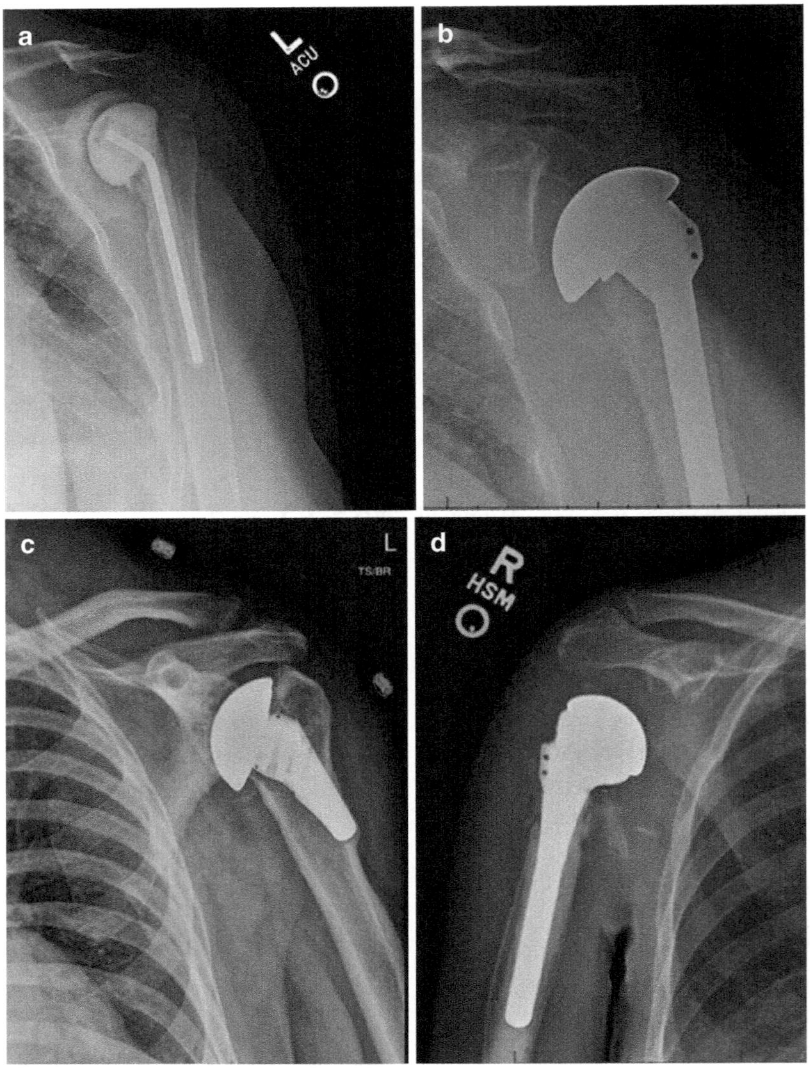

Fig. 19.1 Representative radiographs for each type/subtype of the PHAROS system for humeral bone loss in revision shoulder arthroplasty. (**a**) **PHAROS grade 1C:** epiphyseal bone loss with loss of the calcar. (**b**) **PHAROS grade 1G**: epiphyseal bone loss with loss of the greater tuberosity. (**c**) **PHAROS grade 2A**: metadiaphyseal bone loss above the deltoid tuberosity, >50% cortical thinning of the metadiaphysis with epiphyseal bone loss or thinning. (**d**) **PHAROS grade 2B:**metadiaphyseal bone loss above the deltoid tuberosity, including the epiphysis and part of the metaphysis. (**e**) **PHAROS grade 3A:** diaphyseal bone loss below the deltoid tuberosity with >50% cortical thinning. (**f**) **PHAROS grade 3B:** compromise of the majority of the diaphysis extending below the deltoid insertion, with the loss of the epiphysis and metadiaphysis

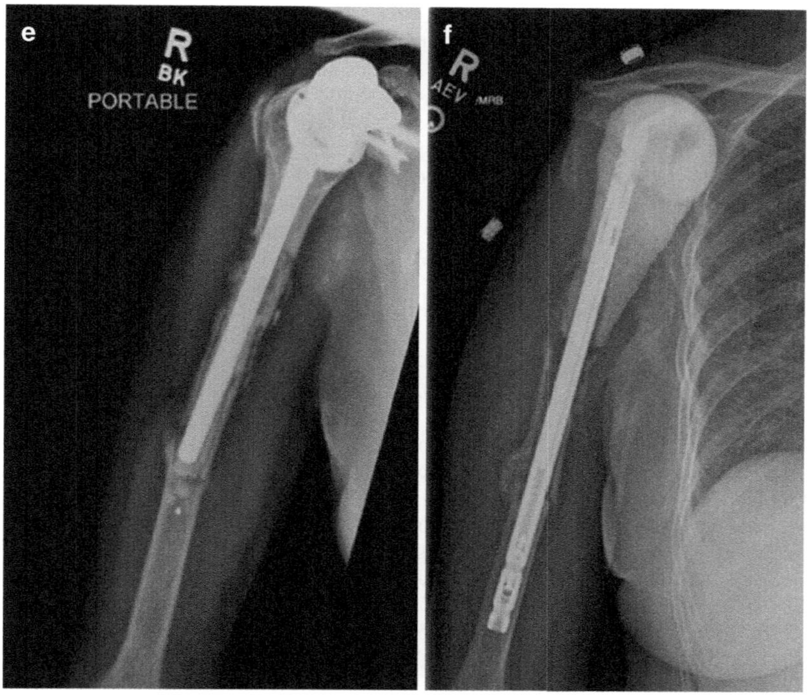

Fig. 19.1 (continued)

19.4 PHAROS Classification Overview

In their study, Chalmers et al. [8] found that the PHAROS classification system was beneficial in directing operative treatment. Types 1 and 2 bone losses were associated with the use of greater tuberosity fixation for intraoperative fractures. Types 2 and 3 were associated with the use of structural humeral bone graft. Type 3 was associated with the use of proximal humeral replacement or total humeral replacement. Additionally, the length of the humeral stem used in the revision procedure increased sequentially with numeric type: 130 mm for type 1, 150 mm for type 2, and 190 mm for type 3.

19.5 Conclusion

To date, there has been no widespread adoption of a classification system for humeral bone loss in the setting of revision shoulder arthroplasty. The PHAROS system by Chalmers et al. [8] is currently the only validated classification system that has been proposed. The PHAROS system allows the shoulder arthroplasty surgeon to evaluate humeral bone loss on plain radiographs of the shoulder and aids in the prediction for the complexity of the revision procedure. Further work to correlate advanced imaging (CT and MRI) and achieving external validity with multiple evaluators/institutions is necessary to achieve further generalizability for the PHAROS classification system.

References

1. Kany J, Jose J, Katz D, Werthel JD, Sekaran P, Amaravathi RS, Valenti P. The main cause of instability after unconstrained shoulder prosthesis is soft tissue deficiency. J Shoulder Elb Surg. 2017;26(8):e243–51. https://doi.org/10.1016/j.jse.2017.01.019. Epub 2017 Feb 27
2. Cox JL, McLendon PB, Christmas KN, Simon P, Mighell MA, Frankle MA. Clinical outcomes following reverse shoulder arthroplasty-allograft com-

posite for revision of failed arthroplasty associated with proximal humeral bone deficiency: 2- to 15-year follow-up. J Shoulder Elb Surg. 2019;28(5):900–7. https://doi.org/10.1016/j.jse.2018.10.023. Epub 2019 Jan 25
3. Gauci MO, Cavalier M, Gonzalez JF, Holzer N, Baring T, Walch G, Boileau P. Revision of failed shoulder arthroplasty: epidemiology, etiology, and surgical options. J Shoulder Elb Surg. 2020;29(3):541–9. https://doi.org/10.1016/j.jse.2019.07.034. Epub 2019 Oct 6
4. Levy J, Frankle M, Mighell M, Pupello D. The use of the reverse shoulder prosthesis for the treatment of failed hemiarthroplasty for proximal humeral fracture. J Bone Joint Surg Am. 2007;89(2):292–300. https://doi.org/10.2106/JBJS.E.01310.
5. Chalmers PN, Boileau P, Romeo AA, et al. Revision reverse shoulder arthroplasty. J Am Acad Orthop Surg. 2019;27:426–36.
6. Stephens SP, Paisley KC, Giveans MR, Wirth MA. The effect of proximal humeral bone loss on revision reverse total shoulder arthroplasty. J Shoulder Elb Surg. 2015;24(10):1519–26. https://doi.org/10.1016/j.jse.2015.02.020. Epub 2015 Apr 7
7. Audigé L, Bhandari M, Hanson B, Kellam J. A concept for the validation of fracture classifications. J Orthop Trauma. 2005;19(6):401–6. https://doi.org/10.1097/01.bot.0000155310.04886.37.
8. Chalmers PN, Romeo AA, Nicholson GP, Boileau P, Keener JD, Gregory JM, Salazar DH, Tashjian RZ. Humeral bone loss in revision total shoulder arthroplasty: the proximal humeral arthroplasty revision osseous insufficiency (PHAROS) classification system. Clin OrthopRelat Res. 2019;477(2):432–41. https://doi.org/10.1097/CORR.0000000000000590.
9. Chacon A, Virani N, Shannon R, Levy JC, Pupello D, Frankle M. Revision arthroplasty with use of a reverse shoulder prosthesis-allograft composite. J Bone Joint Surg Am. 2009;91(1):119–27. https://doi.org/10.2106/JBJS.H.00094.
10. Budge MD, Moravek JE, Zimel MN, Nolan EM, Wiater JM. Reverse total shoulder arthroplasty for the management of failed shoulder arthroplasty with proximal humeral bone loss: is allograft augmentation necessary? J Shoulder Elb Surg. 2013;22(6):739–44. https://doi.org/10.1016/j.jse.2012.08.008.
11. McLendon PB, Cox JL, Frankle MA. Humeral bone loss in revision shoulder arthroplasty. Am J Orthop (Belle Mead NJ). 2018;47(2) https://doi.org/10.12788/ajo.2018.0012.
12. Boileau P. Complications and revision of reverse total shoulder arthroplasty. Orthop Traumatol Surg Res. 2016;102:S33–43.

20 Convertible Humeral Component in Revision Shoulder Arthroplasty

Su Cheol Kim and Jae Chul Yoo

20.1 Introduction

With the increase of shoulder arthroplasty for several decades, the number of revision surgeries is also rising. The incidence of revision shoulder arthroplasty is increasing annually, with 10,290 revision procedures performed in 2017 [1].

Anatomical total shoulder arthroplasty (aTSA) or hemiarthroplasty (HA) can be performed for arthroplasty-indicated patients with preserved rotator cuff function. The survival rate of aTSA or HA is known to be 80% after 15 years of surgery, so 20% of patients require revision surgery [2–4]. One of the most common reasons for the delayed failure of aTSA/HA is rotator cuff dysfunction with aging [5, 6]. For aTSA, aseptic glenoid loosening would be another reason for delayed failure [5]. Also, healing failure of the subscapularis can cause anterior instability after aTSA/HA, which can be observed less than 1 year after the surgery [5].

Failed aTSA/HA can be revised in several ways: revision aTSA/HA, resection arthroplasty, and glenohumeral fusion [5]. Nowadays, conversion to RTSA could be one of the best options because of the predictable outcome [5]. Conversion of aTSA/HA to RTSA requires procedures for the glenoid and humeral parts. During the humeral procedures, the humeral stem should either be removed entirely or retained [5].

Exchanging a complete humeral prosthesis with a new one is challenging [5, 7, 8]. In some cases, the humeral stem can be easily mobilized by hitting it upward [8], but it is impossible for the firmly fixed humeral stem. Vertical humeral osteotomy or a pectoralis-major-pedicled bone window technique is used for mobilizing a well-fixed humeral stem [8–10]. Although various techniques have been introduced, it needs significant efforts to stem extraction, which can cause various complications, including intraoperative humeral fracture, bone loss, and extensive soft tissue dissection, which can lead to long operation times [11]. In addition, the stability of the new humeral stem can be threatened by insufficient humeral bone and osteotomy sites after stem removal [12]. Therefore, attempts to maintain the humeral stem are essential to prevent many complications of stem exchange.

A convertible humeral component is a good option for patients with a well-fixed humeral stem. It is composed of modules, so the humeral head of aTSA/HA can be changed to an RTSA tray and polyethylene without exchanging the humeral stem. This allows surgeons to perform revision RTSA more easily and quickly than stem exchange [7].

Even with these advantages, humeral stem retention is not always possible [13, 14]. There are some preconditions for humeral stem reten-

S. C. Kim · J. C. Yoo (✉)
Department of Orthopedic Surgery, Samsung Medical Center, Sungkyunkwan University School of Medicine, Seoul, South Korea

F. Franceschi et al. (eds.), *Revision Shoulder Arthroplasty*,
https://doi.org/10.1007/978-3-031-45944-3_20

tion. Also, even if the preconditions are met, about 70% of cases achieve humeral stem retention. It comes from the difference in biomechanics between aTSA/HA and RTSA, resulting in soft tissue tension mismatch [13, 14].

20.1.1 Preconditions for Humeral Stem Retention

If the surgeon decides to undergo revision RTSA from aTSA/HA, it is essential to determine whether stem retention can be attempted. Recent implants are mostly designed to be convertible stems; however, much older design needs to be removed due to their design. The history of modular humeral prosthesis goes back over 30 years, and Gartsman et al. reported modular shoulder arthroplasty in 1997, even though it was about aTSA [15]. Also, humeral stem retention can be considered in patients who do not have stem loosening or infection [5].

Aseptic loosening of the humeral stem can be detected from plain radiographs or computed tomography before the surgery [16, 17]. Radio-opaque lines observed around the stem, stem shift, localized cortical hypertrophy, and proximal bony overgrowth are the clues for stem loosening [18, 19]. During the surgery, stem loosening also can be detected by shaking the stem to see if there is any motion [16].

Periprosthetic infection is also a contraindication for stem retention [5]. In chronic infection, moderate to advanced osteolysis and radiolucent line around the humeral stem can be observed in preoperative imaging. Also, other laboratory markers should be considered together to diagnose infection. Usually, the stem is generally loose and easily removed with chronic infection. In acute or low-grade infection, the humeral stem can be firmly fixed without humeral osteolysis and stem loosening. Although controversial, it is generally accepted to perform two-stage revision surgery for periprosthetic infection [20].

If there is no stem loosening or infection, humeral stem retention with humeral head module change can be tried. Conversion to RTSA could be early or delayed after the primary aTSA/HA. There are various reasons for the early failure of primary aTSA/HA. One is the healing failure of tenotomized subscapularis resulting in anterior instability [21]. Tuberosity migration or malunion could be another reason for failed aTSA or HA after proximal humerus fracture [5]. Also, soft tissue tension mismatch can cause overstuff of the glenohumeral joint resulting in early failure [22]. Overstuff can be observed in the high cutting of the humeral head, using a large humeral head, or high position of humeral implant during proximal humerus fracture surgery [22]. Also, it can be observed lateralized glenoid components, especially using metal back glenoid implants [23]. These problems compromise the force couple balance of the shoulder joint, resulting in persistent shoulder pain and loss of motion [21, 22].

Although the survival rate of aTSA/HA is known to be 80–99% after 5 years after surgery [2–4], delayed failure can be observed. The most common reason for the delayed failure of aTSA/HA is rotator cuff deterioration [24]. Even with good function after primary shoulder arthroplasty, the rotator cuff deteriorates with aging, and it could be accelerated in overstuff [24, 25]. Then the humeral head may migrate superiorly, inducing superior polyethylene wear or loosening from glenoid bone stock [23]. In addition, poor implantation of the glenoid implant can be loosened by the rocking horse phenomenon resulting in delayed failure of aTSA/HA [24].

Unlike glenoid prosthesis, humeral prosthesis loosening is much less observed in aTSA/HA [26, 27]. If there is no periprosthetic infection, no evidence of humeral stem loosening from preoperative radiologic examination and intraoperative findings, humeral stem retention can be tried.

20.1.2 Preparing Humeral Stem Retention

Once decided on humeral stem retention, implant manufacturer, type, and version should be checked. It is essential to check whether the currently inserted humeral prosthesis is a modular humeral component. In many cases of conversion

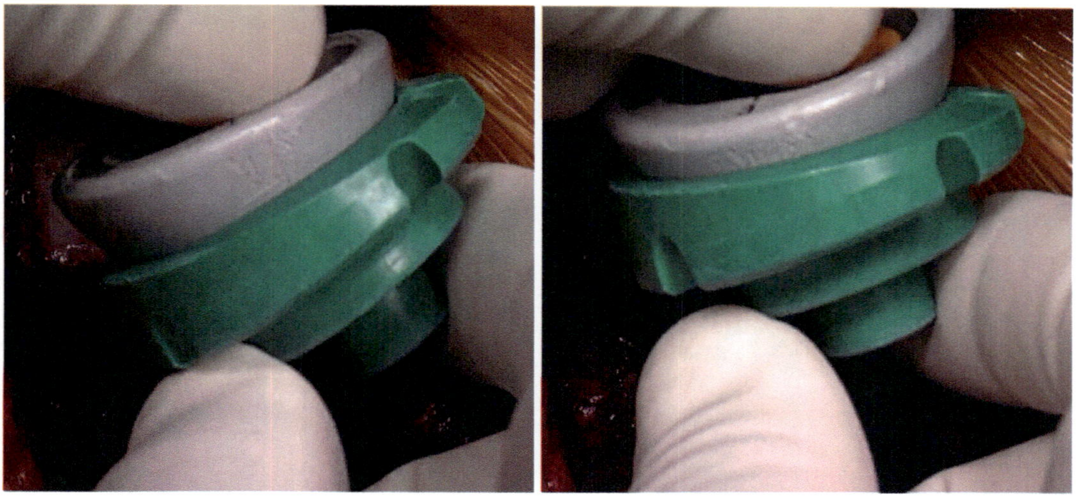

Fig. 20.1 Matching the curvature of humeral polyethylene (Zimmer Trabecular Metal) and glenosphere (Biomet Comprehensive) for hybrid usage

RTSA, a primary arthroplasty was performed long ago, but prostheses are usually improved to new versions over time or discontinued to be produced [3]. If the implant design is improved, the proximal RTSA module could not be compatible with the humeral stem, which causes humeral stem retention to be impossible. When converting old primary arthroplasty to RTSA, surgeons should prepare for unexpected stem exchange.

If humeral and glenoid side implants cannot be matched in some cases, hybrid usage can be another option. If the curvature of humeral polyethylene and glenosphere are matched, these two implants can be used together (Fig. 20.1).

20.1.3 Surgical Techniques

A standard deltopectoral approach should be used to prepare the incision extension to the distal humeral shaft if humeral implant retention is failed. Also, over five cultures are recommended in every case to diagnose unexpected low-grade periprosthetic infection [14]. The stability of the humeral stem should be checked by shaking the stem using hand [16]. If there are visible motions, it could not indicate humeral stem retention.

To dislocate the humeral head, subscapularis detachment and tagging should be performed. The metaphyseal part of the prosthesis should be freed from the scar tissue, bone, and bone cement. Like any revision surgery, five different tissue samples of frozen biopsy are recommended during surgery. If any samples have more than 5 neutrophil counts, thorough debridement and irrigation or second-stage reconstruction are required. During the subdeltoid scar tissue release, unexpected axillary nerve damage might occur, so one should always be cautious during this procedure. Afterward, aTSA/HA head can be removed using the extraction instrument. If the extraction instrument does not engage, metaphyseal bone or cement around the stem should be removed to make space for the extraction instrument. After humeral head removal, the glenoid procedure is performed to insert the glenosphere.

Next, the RTSA tray module can be assembled onto the retained humeral stem. Sometimes, a flat reamer can be used to allow seating of the RTSA tray module. In most conversion RTSA, tight soft tissue tension makes joint reduction difficult [14], so the smallest thickness of humeral tray and polyethylene is recommended for trial reduction. When the proper soft tissue tension is checked, the real implant is inserted, and the surgery is completed after joint reduction (Fig. 20.2).

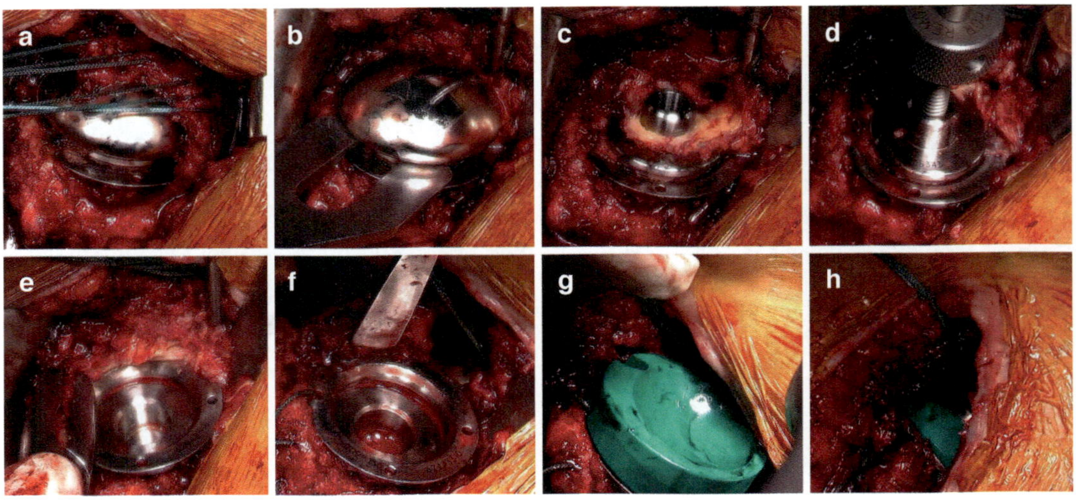

Fig. 20.2 (**a**) Detached subscapularis and tagged with nonabsorbable sutures, (**b**) humeral head distractor engaged (**c**) after removal of the humeral head, (**d**) assembly of humeral head module remover, (**e**) removing scar tissue with a rongeur, (**f**) overgrowth bone at humeral metaphysis with an osteotome, (**g**) humeral polyethylene assembly, and (**h**) glenohumeral reduction was done

20.1.4 Pros and Cons of Humeral Implant Retention Versus Exchange

Various advantages of humeral implant retention have been reported [5, 13, 14, 28]. Lower complication rates during and after surgery, shorter operation times, less blood loss, and fewer re-interventions were reported for humeral implant retention compared to the humeral implant exchange procedure [5, 13, 14, 28].

Well-fixed humeral stem removal needs making humeral shaft longitudinal osteotomy or windows [9–11]. Kang et al. reported router bit extraction technique without making an osteotomy [29]. For the humeral stem with collar, bone–implant interface was grind using router bit, and square-tip impactor is used for upward blows to remove humeral stem. For the humeral stem without a collar, a groove was made along the medial body of the humeral implant, so the impactor can be placed in the groove to remove the stem [29]. However, all of the techniques described earlier can make iatrogenic humeral shaft fracture [7]. If the cemented technique was used for humeral stem fixation during primary surgery, removing bone cement is also required [7]. Humeral stem change would make surgery more difficult and time-consuming. Also, humeral shaft wiring is needed for stable stem fixation and bone healing. Sometimes, nonunion or delayed union can be observed, resulting in humeral stem instability later [10, 13]. In addition, long-term immobilization is necessary for bone healing, which can lead to delayed rehabilitation, which can lead to poor clinical outcomes.

Removing a well-fixed stem could cause iatrogenic humeral bone loss. Making osteotomy and cement removal can damage humeral bone stock [7]. Furthermore, patients who are planned for shoulder revision surgery usually have long-lasting shoulder pain, so they usually have poor proximal humeral bone quality [30]. Also, stress shielding around the humeral stem could occur even one year postoperatively [16, 17]. Recently, to reduce stress shielding, using a small humeral stem with metaphyseal fixation with a lesser filling ratio was recommended rather than a large humeral stem with diaphyseal press-fit [16]. When removing the well-fixed humeral stem, bone stock preservation is crucial, so much care and effort are needed.

Also, extensive soft tissue dissection, more than in primary surgery, is also required during stem removal [31]. To dislocate the humeral head, releasing the adhesion between the humeral metaphysis and deltoid undersurface is required [32]. Extensive soft tissue release near the axillary nerve can cause unexpected axillary nerve injury [32]. In case of severe adhesion, intraoperative neural monitoring can be considered to prevent nerve damage [32, 33].

Humeral stem retention can reduce the complex procedures of removing the well-fixed humeral implant. Weiser et al. reported significantly reduced mean blood loss (48.5 ml vs. 831 ml, $p = 0.001$) and mean surgical time (118 min vs. 176 min, $p < 0.001$) in the stem retention group than the stem exchange group [13]. Crosby et al. reported that patients with humeral stem retention showed significantly shorter operation time ($p < 0.001$) and lower blood loss ($p = 0.034$) than the patients with stem exchange [7]. Furthermore, good effects such as lowering the rate of iatrogenic nerve injury and reducing soft tissue dissection can be obtained [13].

However, not all the convertible humeral stems with proper indication can be successfully retained. Tension mismatch is underlying humeral stem retention. Since aTSA/HA and RTSA usually have different proximal humerus bone cutting levels, soft tissue tension achieved by primary surgery cannot always be appropriate with revision RTSA [5, 7]. Supraspinatus insertion should be preserved during aTSA/HA, which is not essential in revision RTSA. High-level humeral head cutting to preserve supraspinatus insertion during primary surgery may cause tight soft tissue tension during RTSA. Sometimes, reduction cannot be achieved during the revision RTSA. Even if the reduction was possible, tight soft tissue tension could cause neurologic injury, acromion or spine stress fracture, poor deltoid function, limitation of motion, sustained shoulder pain, and causing an unforeseen revision. In contrast, insufficient soft tissue tension can be adjusted by humeral or glenoid side augmentation.

Tight soft tissue tension during revision RTSA largely depends on primary surgery. Despite technically demanding, humeral head cutting should be as low as possible without damaging the supraspinatus and infraspinatus insertion. As mentioned above, insufficient soft tissue tension can be adjusted using a thick humeral tray or polyethylene. However, an initially high position of the humeral implant is difficult to correct during revision. So, if one is using a convertible stem, which nowadays most implants provide, low humeral cutting during primary surgery is mandatory when considering future conversion to RTSA with a convertible humeral prosthesis.

Some convertible humeral implants can adjust the humeral version during the module change. If the proper humeral version was not obtained during the primary operation, it could be corrected during the revision RTSA. The appropriate humeral version during RTSA arthroplasty is still inconclusive. Some recommended that the anatomical humeral version is optimal in RTSA; however, a systematic review reported that only over 20° retroversion showed good outcomes [34].

20.1.5 The Success of Humeral Stem Retention

As mentioned earlier, not all the convertible humeral stems can be retained [13, 14]. Various surgeons reported outcomes of humeral stem retention during revision RTSA; however, the number of cases is still insufficient [13, 14].

Kany et al. reported revision RTSA from aTSA with convertible humeral stem, and 18/25 (72%) patients achieved humeral stem retention [14]. The reason for stem exchange in 7 patients was reduction failure during revision RTSA because of tight soft tissue tension [14]. Wieser et al. reported 13/17 (76.5%) patients of stem retention during conversion RTSA. The reason for failure in 4 patients was tight soft tissue tension in 3 and excessive retroversion in 1 [13]. Other authors reported similar results. Reuther et al. reported that 13/17 (76.5%) patients with fracture HA converted to RTSA without stem removal [5]. The remaining 4/17 patients failed to stem retention and underwent stem removal due to overstuff. They reported 23 mm of mean arm lengthening after conversion RTSA from HA [5].

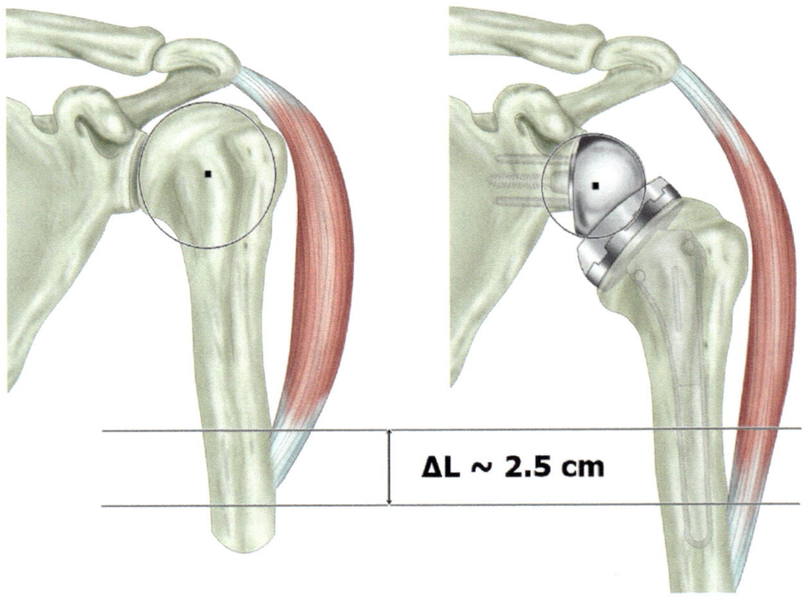

Fig. 20.3 After reverse shoulder arthroplasty, the average humerus distalization is 2.5 cm compared to the original position

Often the failure of stem retention during the surgery is from the high position of the humeral stem [5, 13, 14]. The humeral distalization in RTSA was known to be approximately 11–33 mm from the original position [5, 35]. Werner et al. showed mean 26 mm arm lengthening after conversion aTSA or HA to RTSA using modular humeral stem [36]. Surgeons should be aware that not all revisions in the convertible stem are simple revisions and consider the unexpected humeral stem exchange (Fig. 20.3).

20.1.6 Clinical Outcome of the Convertible Humeral Implant

Good clinical outcomes have been reported for humeral stem retention during the revision RTSA [5, 7, 36]. Ruether et al. reported a case series with stem retention in 17 patients and showed significantly improved PVAS, ASES, Constant score, and ROM even one year after the revision surgery ($p < 0.05$) [5]. Werner et al. showed significantly improved ROM and functional scores in 14 cases of stem retention ($p < 0.05$) [36]. Crosby et al. analyzed the patients with humeral stem retention (convertible humeral implant) versus those with humeral stem change (nonconvertible humeral implant). They reported that ROM was better in the retention group than change group (ER, 26 ± 23 vs. 11 ± 23 [$p = 0.006$]; FF, 112 ± 37 vs. 96 ± 33 [$p = 0.055$]) [7]. However, Weiser et al. compared the patients with stem retention and stem change during revision RTSA and reported similar functional scores between the patient groups [13].

Previous studies showed that stem retention has a lower complication rate than stem exchange [28]. Crosby et al. reported a high prevalence of intraoperative complications in the stem exchange group, including 9/73 greater tuberosity ± humeral shaft fracture, 2/73 nerve injury, and 1/73 revision surgery. However, no intraoperative complication and no humeral stem loosening were observed in the stem retention group [7]. From a recent systematic review, the overall complication rate was 8/123 (6.50%) versus 47/113 (41.6%) in the stem retention and stem exchange group ($p < 0.01$) [28]. In-depth, the fracture was observed in 2/123 (1.63%) and 18/113 (15.9%) patients, and reoperation was performed in 3/123 (2.44%) and 10/113 (8.85%) patients in the stem retention and stem exchange group, respectively [28].

20.1.7 Humeral Implant Retention Case

Eight years ago, a 46-year-old female patient who underwent arthroscopic debridement for infection after arthroscopic subacromial decompression at another hospital came to our clinic. The patient underwent open debridement with an antibiotic-mixed cement spacer insertion. To preserve the subscapularis tendon, rotator interval approach was performed to insert the cement spacer. Four months later, with normalized laboratory results and clinical symptoms, aTSA (Trabecular Metal Reverse Shoulder System, Zimmer Biomet, Warsaw, IN, USA) was performed. Initially, she showed tolerable shoulder ROM and pain but complained of moderate shoulder pain with loss of motion after 3.5 years after the aTSA.

The plain radiograph showed the progressive loosening of the glenoid prosthesis, but humeral stem loosening was not observed. A laboratory study showed no increase of infection markers (ESR and CRP), so it was suspected as the aseptic loosening of the glenoid prosthesis.

Therefore, conversion to RTSA with humeral stem retention was planned. During the surgery, multiple frozen biopsies were performed to evaluate periprosthetic infection, and polymorphonuclear neutrophil was not observed. After removing scar tissue around the humeral prosthesis, the humeral stem was shaken and firm fixation was observed. Then, the humeral head module was changed from aTSA to RTSA without removing the humeral stem. The glenoid implant was easily removed, and the glenosphere was implanted with a hybrid technique (Biomet, Comprehensive). It took 2 h for revision RTSA with humeral stem retention. During and after the surgery, a blood transfusion was not performed.

Two years after the revision RTSA, minimal shoulder pain with functional recovery (ASES 75, Constant-Murray score 62, ROM FF 140, ER 60, IR T12) was observed. There was no neurologic complication and implant loosening after two years of follow-up (Fig. 20.4).

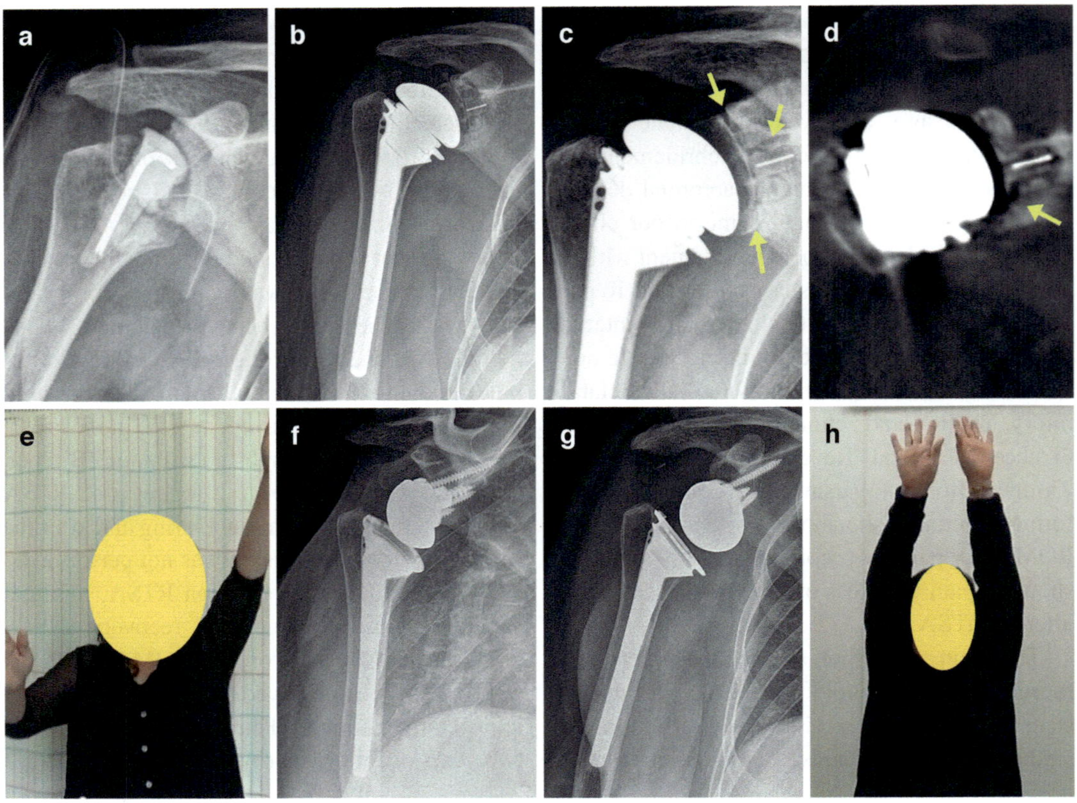

Fig. 20.4 Patient with the conversion from aTSA to revision RTSA. (**a**) Antibiotics mixed cement spacer was inserted through RI to preserve subscapularis for the infectious arthritis, (**b**) conversion to aTSA after infection control, (**c**) glenoid implant loosening (yellow arrows) in X-ray, and (**d**) CT, (**e**) pseudoparalysis of the affected arm, (**f**) conversion to RTSA, the humeral stem was retained, and the glenoid prosthesis was exchanged with hybrid technique, (**g**) 2 years after the RTSA, good X-ray, and (**h**) good function of the affected arm

20.2 Conclusion

A convertible humeral component is a good option for converting failed aTSA/HA to RTSA. Surgeons should carefully consider the preconditions for stem retention before revision RTSA. Stem retention has the advantages of less soft tissue dissection and bleeding, short operation time, fewer intraoperative complications, and neurologic damage than stem exchange. However, not all stem retention can be achieved due to tension mismatch, so always prepare for stem exchange.

References

1. Farley KX, et al. Prevalence of shoulder arthroplasty in the United States and the increasing burden of revision shoulder arthroplasty. JB JS Open Access. 2021;6(3):e20.00156.
2. Sperling JW, Cofield RH, Rowland CM. Minimum fifteen-year follow-up of Neer hemiarthroplasty and total shoulder arthroplasty in patients aged fifty years or younger. J Shoulder Elb Surg. 2004;13(6):604–13.
3. Torchia ME, Cofield RH, Settergren CR. Total shoulder arthroplasty with the Neer prosthesis: long-term results. J Shoulder Elb Surg. 1997;6(6):495–505.
4. Taunton MJ, et al. Total shoulder arthroplasty with a metal-backed, bone-ingrowth glenoid component. Medium to long-term results. J Bone Joint Surg Am. 2008;90(10):2180–8.

5. Reuther F, et al. Conversion of hemiarthroplasty to reverse shoulder arthroplasty with humeral stem retention. J Clin Med. 2022;11(3):834.
6. Hasler A, et al. Joint-line medialization after anatomical total shoulder replacement requires more rotator cuff activity to preserve joint stability. JSES Int. 2021;5(3):406–12.
7. Crosby LA, et al. Conversion to reverse total shoulder arthroplasty with and without humeral stem retention: the role of a convertible-platform stem. J Bone Joint Surg Am. 2017;99(9):736–42.
8. Phipatanakul WP, Bowen JM, Jobe CM. Removal of well-fixed flanged humeral prostheses may require humeral expansion. J Shoulder Elb Surg. 2009;18(5):724–7.
9. Sperling JW, Cofield RH. Humeral windows in revision shoulder arthroplasty. J Shoulder Elb Surg. 2005;14(3):258–63.
10. Sahota S, Sperling JW, Cofield RH. Humeral windows and longitudinal splits for component removal in revision shoulder arthroplasty. J Shoulder Elb Surg. 2014;23(10):1485–91.
11. Gohlke F, Rolf O. Revision of failed fracture hemiarthroplasties to reverse total shoulder prosthesis through the transhumeral approach : method incorporating a pectoralis-major-pedicled bone window. Oper Orthop Traumatol. 2007;19(2):185–208.
12. Dodson CC, et al. Anterior humeral window for revision shoulder arthroplasty. Tech Should Elbow Surg. 2006;7(2):111–5.
13. Wieser K, et al. Conversion of stemmed hemi- or total to reverse total shoulder arthroplasty: advantages of a modular stem design. Clin Orthop Relat Res. 2015;473(2):651–60.
14. Kany J, et al. A convertible shoulder system: is it useful in total shoulder arthroplasty revisions? Int Orthop. 2015;39(2):299–304.
15. Gartsman GM, Russell JA, Gaenslen E. Modular shoulder arthroplasty. J Shoulder Elb Surg. 1997;6(4):333–9.
16. Kim SC, et al. Humeral stem with low filling ratio reduces stress shielding in primary reverse shoulder arthroplasty. Int Orthop. 2022;46(6): 1341–9.
17. Denard PJ, et al. Stress shielding of the humerus in press-fit anatomic shoulder arthroplasty: review and recommendations for evaluation. J Shoulder Elb Surg. 2018;27(6):1139–47.
18. Jakim I, Barlin C, Sweet MB. Radiological signs of loosening of the femoral stem in cementless total hip arthroplasty. S Afr J Surg. 1989;27(3):78–83.
19. Raiss P, et al. Radiographic changes around humeral components in shoulder arthroplasty. J Bone Joint Surg Am. 2014;96(7):e54.
20. Coste JS, et al. The management of infection in arthroplasty of the shoulder. J Bone Joint Surg Br. 2004;86(1):65–9.
21. Shields E, Ho A, Wiater JM. Management of the subscapularis tendon during total shoulder arthroplasty. J Shoulder Elb Surg. 2017;26(4):723–31.
22. Geervliet PC, et al. Overstuffing in resurfacing hemiarthroplasty is a potential risk for failure. J Orthop Surg Res. 2019;14(1):474.
23. Montoya F, et al. Midterm results of a total shoulder prosthesis fixed with a cementless glenoid component. J Shoulder Elb Surg. 2013;22(5):628–35.
24. Young AA, et al. Secondary rotator cuff dysfunction following total shoulder arthroplasty for primary glenohumeral osteoarthritis: results of a multicenter study with more than five years of follow-up. J Bone Joint Surg Am. 2012;94(8):685–93.
25. Dines D. Late-onset rotator cuff dysfunction after total shoulder arthroplasty--the "forgotten" complication. Commentary on an article by Allan A. Young, MD, et al. Secondary rotator cuff dysfunction following total shoulder arthroplasty for primary glenohumeral osteoarthritis: results of a multicenter study with more than five years of follow-up. J Bone Joint Surg Am. 2012;94(8):e53.
26. Denard PJ, et al. Mid- to long-term follow-up of total shoulder arthroplasty using a keeled glenoid in young adults with primary glenohumeral arthritis. J Shoulder Elb Surg. 2013;22(7):894–900.
27. Walch G, et al. Patterns of loosening of polyethylene keeled glenoid components after shoulder arthroplasty for primary osteoarthritis: results of a multicenter study with more than five years of follow-up. J Bone Joint Surg Am. 2012;94(2):145–50.
28. Kirsch JM, et al. Platform shoulder arthroplasty: a systematic review. J Shoulder Elb Surg. 2018;27(4):756–63.
29. Kang JR, et al. The router bit extraction technique for removing a well-fixed humeral stem in revision shoulder arthroplasty. Bone Joint J. 2019;101-B(10):1280–4.
30. Bernatz JT, et al. Prevalence and treatment of osteoporosis prior to elective shoulder arthroplasty. J Am Acad Orthop Surg Glob Res Rev. 2020;4(12):e20 00204.
31. Theelen LMA, et al. Stem retention and survival in revision of anatomical convertible shoulder arthroplasty to reverse arthroplasty: a Dutch registry study. BMC Musculoskelet Disord. 2021;22(1):396.
32. Abboud JA, Anakwenze OA, Hsu JE. Soft-tissue management in revision total shoulder arthroplasty. J Am Acad Orthop Surg. 2013;21(1):23–31.
33. Nagda SH, et al. Neer Award 2005: Peripheral nerve function during shoulder arthroplasty using intraoperative nerve monitoring. J Shoulder Elb Surg. 2007;16(Suppl. 3):S2–8.
34. Jassim SS, Ernstbrunner L, Ek ET. Does humeral component version affect range of motion and clinical outcomes in reverse total shoulder arthroplasty? A systematic review. J Clin Med. 2021;10(24):5745.
35. Teschner H, et al. Conversion of hemi into reverse shoulder arthroplasty: implant design limitations. Arch Orthop Trauma Surg. 2014;134(12):1683–9.
36. Werner BS, Boehm D, Gohlke F. Revision to reverse shoulder arthroplasty with retention of the humeral component. Acta Orthop. 2013;84(5):473–8.

How to Remove a Well Implanted Humeral Component and Complications Associated

21

Amir Abdelmalek, Robert Hurley, Andrew McBride, Phillip Duke, and Mark Ross

21.1 Introduction

The indications and criteria for shoulder arthroplasty have expanded significantly since the inception of the idea by Themistocles Gluck in the 1880s. The first reported successful shoulder arthroplasty was performed by Jules-Emile Péan in 1893 [1].

However, the concept of shoulder arthroplasty did not gain widespread recognition until Charles Neer published his results on replacing the proximal humerus to treat fractures in 1955 [2].

The innovation continued when Paul Grammont laid the foundations of the modern design of reverse shoulder arthroplasty in 1985 [3]. A year later, Stephen Copeland questioned the idea of stemmed implants and developed a humeral head resurfacing implant [4].

Since then, the evolution of techniques and implants have transformed shoulder arthroplasty. Modern designs provide the versatility of platform systems to facilitate revision procedures and different bearing surface materials to increase the longevity of the implants [5, 6].

This has led to improved outcomes and the number of primary procedures has grown exponentially across the years, which inevitably has increased the number of failures and revision procedures [7–10].

Despite modern techniques, revision shoulder arthroplasty remains a complex, challenging problem for the treating surgeon [10, 11]. This is particularly true when involving the removal of a well-fixed humeral component.

The procedure to remove a well-fixed humeral component can have significant complications, including intraoperative fractures, loss of tuberosity integrity or loss of bone stock, which can lead to poor postoperative outcomes [12–14].

In this chapter we discuss our protocol for removing a well-fixed humeral component.

21.2 A Stepwise Approach

21.2.1 Pre-operative Planning

Preoperative planning is of utmost importance when dealing with revision arthroplasty cases. The procedure starts with gathering information regarding the design and features of the implant, i.e. length of the stem, modularity of the stem, method of humeral fixation and operation notes if available. Of paramount importance is the need to identify the implant so that wherever possible implant specific instruments can be ordered to simplify removal. When prior surgical notes are unavailable and the surgeon is unable to identify the implant,

A. Abdelmalek (✉) · R. Hurley · A. McBride
P. Duke · M. Ross
Brisbane Hand and Upper Limb Research Institute, Brisbane, QLD, Australia
e-mail: pdoffice@upperlimb.com; markross@upperlimb.com

F. Franceschi et al. (eds.), *Revision Shoulder Arthroplasty*,
https://doi.org/10.1007/978-3-031-45944-3_21

online services and applications are available to assist. Artificial intelligence (AI) has been increasingly used recently to identify unknown implants or if the operative notes are not available [15–17]. These services currently include mobile phone applications (AIdentyfy, AIdentyfy inc., Mt.Sinai Ortho Center, NYC, USA® and Implant Identifier, Devise Health LLC, Georgia, USA®).

We routinely request bilateral full length humeral x rays to ensure humeral length is restored during the revision operation. Three-dimensional imaging is also essential to assess for bone stock and anticipate the need for strut graft, osseous anatomy, integrity of cement mantle, signs of loosening, soft tissue integrity and signs of infection.

21.2.2 Equipment and Augments

Appropriate internal fixation equipment should be available to deal with unexpected, or planned contingencies including cerclage cables and periprosthetic plating systems. In addition, it is wise to have available strut allografts and milled cancellous allograft. We frequently use options to decrease reliance on reimplanting cemented implants as our preference wherever possible is to perform revision in a fashion that increases bone stock using non cemented implants and bone graft.

21.2.3 Position and Draping in Theatre

The patient is routinely positioned in the beach-chair position. We prefer not to sit the patient at too high an angle as this not only helps the anaesthetist with maintaining cerebral perfusion in patients who may more commonly be medically challenging but also allows easier access to the iliac crest for autograft. In our unit, we prefer not to use a beach chair angle greater than 30° to the horizontal in revision arthroplasty. Care should be taken when draping to allow proximal exposure of the clavicle if clavicular osteotomy or deltoid takedown is needed. A stockinette covering the hand is draped to the level of the elbow-not above – to allow exposure of the entire humerus in case fixation using an anterolateral extension of the delto-pectoral approach is required. Care also should be taken to prepare and drape for iliac crest bone graft if planned.

21.2.4 Approach

A delto-pectoral approach is utilised. This can be extended distally as needed. Adequate exposure of the proximal part of the implant is achieved and scar tissue is excised. Soft tissue releases are performed as necessary. Consideration should be given to maintaining soft tissue attachments to the humerus in the event of requiring humeral osteotomy (these are discussed later in this chapter). If the risk of tuberosity fracture is very high, then early controlled tuberosity osteotomy should be considered over the less ideal uncontrolled fracture. If longitudinal osteotomy as described later in this chapter is thought to be required, then careful consideration of subscapularis and lesser tuberosity management is required. The goal is to maintain soft tissue attachments to any anterior cortical window that may be required and should an extended anterior window be performed it is preferable for this to incorporate the lesser tuberosity (LT) so as to simplify subscapularis management. Should it become apparent that the stem can be removed without an anterior cortical window then our preference, as in primary arthroplasty, is to perform an LT osteotomy for subscapularis mobilisation. The additional access created by the LT osteotomy can simplify the safe removal of a stem, and the removal of 5–8 mm of bone from the anterior aspect of the proximal humerus also improves glenoid exposure.

21.2.5 Removal of a Well-Fixed Stem

21.2.5.1 Head Removal

Usually, the first stage involves removal of the head (unless the rare situation of a monoblock prosthesis). Head removal is usually achieved with a specific u-shaped wedge instrument provided by the implant company. If not available, a standard chisel can usually separate the head from the neck.

The stem is then assessed for stability and whether an attempt to extract the stem can be performed at this stage or not. Unless the stem is clearly loose, we would proceed to the staged interventions below to facilitate atraumatic removal.

The actual removal of the implant, once loosened by some or all of the stages below, can be facilitated either by the specific removal instruments provided by the device manufacturer or by generic techniques. The manufacturer may be able to provide a slap hammer assembly that can be attached to the implant specific coupling instruments. In modular systems, it is important to ensure that specific instruments for breaking morse tapers and uncoupling components are sent. Generic stem extraction systems are available, which combine a slap hammer with some form of locking plier. In circumstances where none of these options are available / feasible, then retrograde impaction with a heavy punch can be utilised. This is simple if the implant has a collar. However, where a collar is not present, a notch to impact into can be created on the neck of the prosthesis using a metal cutting power tool such as the Midas Rex high-speed pneumatic drill system (Medtronic, MN, USA®). We routinely have this system available since we may also use it in removal of a well fixed metallic glenoid base plate.

21.2.5.2 Soft Tissue Clearance

The first stage of removal after the head is removed involves clearance of the soft tissues including scar from around the proximal aspect of the stem/body of the implant. This allows identification of the bone/prosthesis ± cement interface and determination of whether the implant will impact on the greater tuberosity during removal risking fracture. Soft tissue ingrowth in the interface between stem and body in some modular systems can create a potent resistance to extraction.

21.2.5.3 Initial Disruption of Bone/Implant Interface

We use a combination of drilling with long 1.6 mm Kirschner wires down the side of the implant and thin flexible osteotomes circumferentially around the implant to expose and disturb the bone/implant or bone/cement interface. These flexible techniques allow disruption of stem fixation quite distal regardless of implant geometry. Once sufficient disruption between the bone/implant or bone/cement interface has been achieved, stem extraction is attempted using the techniques discussed above. This can be sufficient in some cases.

21.2.5.4 Linear Humeral Osteotomy

If it is established that the previous steps are not adequate, we then progress to linear anterior humeral osteotomy to allow circumferential relaxation around the implant. This is likely to be sufficient in uncemented implants. The line of osteotomy is lateral to the pectoralis major insertion and medial to deltoid insertion, along the lateral border of the bicipital groove (Figs. 21.1 and 21.2, please note that pectoralis major has been removed in the cadaveric specimen in these pictures to facilitate anatomy demonstration, however, this is preserved when creating the linear osteotomy). Once the line of osteotomy is exposed and marked using electrocautery, an oscillating saw is used to create the anterior osteotomy extending down to the level of the implant/cement mantle. This window is then gently spread using a chisel or an osteotome to ease the circumferential fixation. It may be possible to introduce a small dimension flexible osteotome through this gap to assist further in disrupting the interface. Care should be taken not to fracture the humerus during this process. A further attempt can now be made to extract the stem using the above techniques. It is of great importance at this stage to ensure that the proximal part is completely free and the tuberosities are not fixed to the stem/cement.

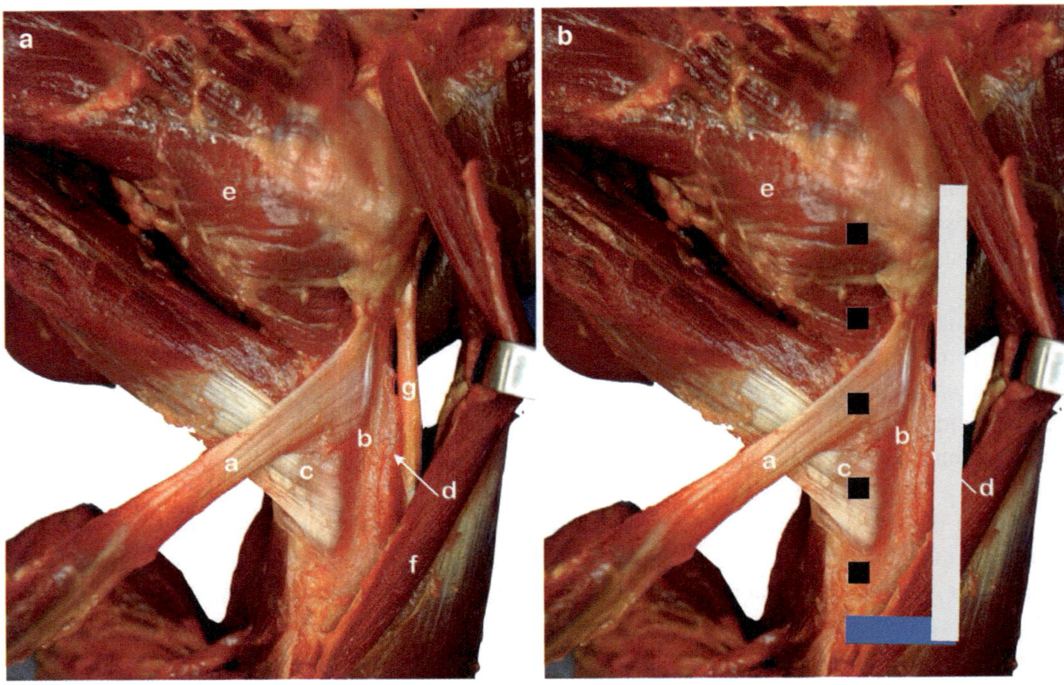

Fig. 21.1 (**a**) Cadaveric dissection showing muscle attachments to proximal humerus, (Anterior view coracobrachialis and short head of biceps retracted laterally). *a*: Latissimus dorsi tendon; *b*: bicipital groove; *c*: teres major tendon; *d*: divided stump of insertion of pectoralis major (insertion was divided to facilitate demonstration of anatomical relationship); *e*: subscapularis; *f*: coracobrachialis; *g*: long head of biceps displaced laterally out of groove. (**b**) Line of Anterior humeral osteotomy. Grey line: anterior humeral osteotomy line; Blue line: L extension; Dotted line: the hinge of the osteotomy when 'opening the book' created using drill holes through the soft tissue attachments and preserving the muscles attachments). Courtesy of The Grasping Hand, Gupta et al., doi: 10.1055/b-0041-180,060, Chap. 12: the Shoulder Joint, M Ross and G Bain, p. 146

21.2.5.5 Extension of Linear Humeral Osteotomy to Anterior Humeral Window

If the linear osteotomy is not sufficient to loosen the interface, the next step would be to create an anterior window with a horizontal limb at the distal end of the osteotomy line and a medial 'postage stamp' osteotomy to create an anterior cortical window. The hinge point for this osteotomy is on the medial side, preserving the muscle attachments (Fig. 21.2). Use of osteotomes to further break any attachment between the implant/cement and this segment of bone is vital to allow mobility in the osteotomy. The dimension of the window is usually approximately 25% of the humeral circumference, and the window is lifted up completely laterally and hinged medially with the preserved soft tissues, which include subscapularis, teres major, latissimus dorsi and pectoralis major. The medial 'tear line' is created by drilling a line of holes through the attached soft tissues using a 2.5 mm drill. Because this cortical window fragment would incorporate the subscapularis attachment to the LT, we do not mobilise the subscapularis until we have decided whether this window osteotomy is required (Fig. 21.3).

21.2.5.6 Canal Debridement

Regardless of whether there is known infection, thorough canal debridement is required. Even in the absence of infection there may be occult infection, and in addition, fixation of uncemented stems and incorporation of graft requires a healthy endosteum devoid of fibrous scar or cement residue. In addition to the usual cement removal instruments which may be sourced from hip revision instrument trays, we have found the

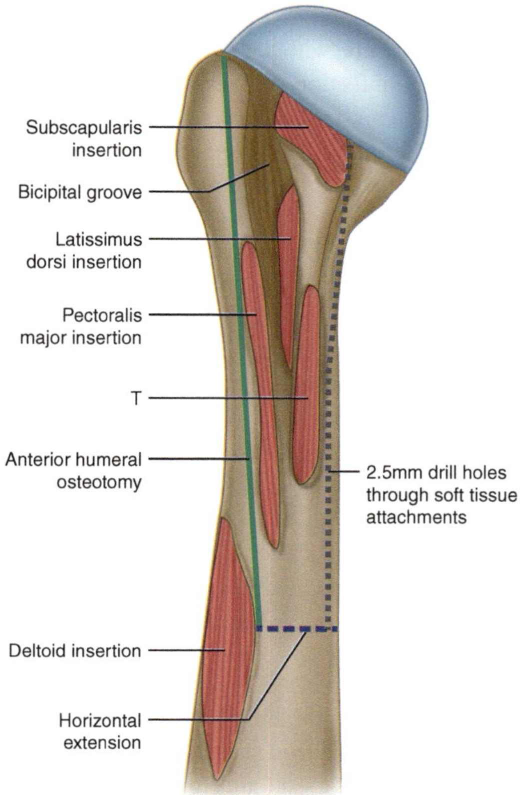

Fig. 21.2 Diagram demonstrating the line of anterior humeral osteotomy in relation to muscle attachments. *S* subscapularis insertion, *BG* bicipital groove, *L* latissimus dorsi insertion, *P* pectoralis major insertion, *D* deltoid insertion; Green line: anterior humeral osteotomy line; blue dotted line: horizontal extension; dotted grey line: 2.5 mm drill holes through soft tissue attachments

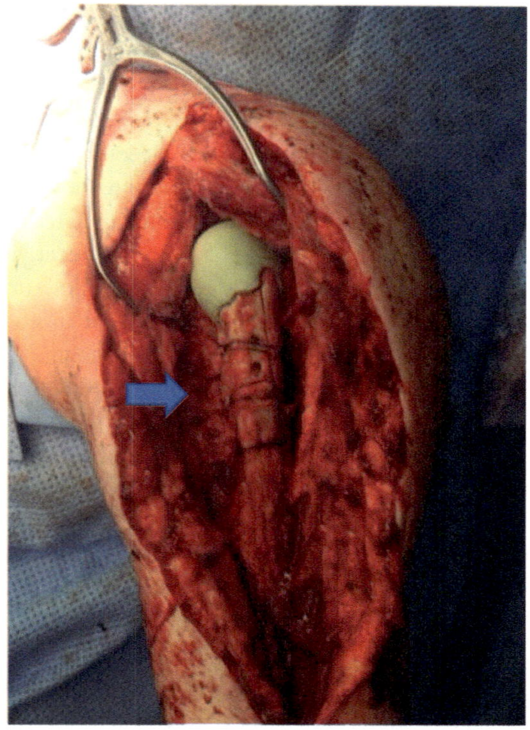

Fig. 21.3 Clinical photograph demonstrating the line of osteotomy and cerclage fixation. Preserved medial soft tissue attachments can be seen (blue arrow)

use of a cannulated reaming system to provide an effective means for internal debridement of the medullary canal. The guide wire position can be checked with fluoroscopy if any doubt and ensures safe debridement without cortical perforation. We have variably used flexible reamers from elbow arthroplasty sets, humeral intramedullary nails, and femoral nails, depending on the dimension required for the individual patient.

21.2.5.7 Osteotomy Fixation

Following canal debridement, the osteotomy is reduced anatomically and fixed with cerclage cables, with care to avoid neurovascular injury during passage. We routinely use impaction bone graft when revising humeral components and/or strut allograft based on bone stock. Strut allograft provides initial additional support and should not be relied upon to heal or unite a fracture. Impaction allografting is performed after solid fixation of the osteotomy.

We find this stepwise technique very reliable in extracting well implanted humeral stems in revision cases. Whether the subsequent part of the revision procedure involves reimplantation of a definitive implant or an antibiotic loaded cement spacer the implant or spacer should extend distal to the osteotomy/ window.

21.3 Discussion

As the number of revision shoulder arthroplasty procedures have grown with time surgeons have developed their surgical techniques to facilitate the removal of humeral components. The challenge is not only present when dealing with chronic cases with poor soft tissue integrity and loss of bone stock but also when dealing with historic implants with no implant-specific extraction equipment.

Van Thiel et al. [18] describe their technique for a single vertical humeral osteotomy and reported 100% success rate in removing the stem with no need to extend to L osteotomy or anterior window. They also reported no intraoperative diaphyseal or metaphyseal fractures. Follow-up radiographs revealed no implant-cement lucencies and no extruded cement. Similar technique and results were also reported by Johnston et al. [19]. In addition, they place a 2.5 mm drill hole at the distal extent of the osteotomy to reduce the risk of longitudinal propagation.

Jouve et al. [20] presented their use of an anterior longitudinal split that starts in the bicipital groove and curves laterally between pectoralis major and deltoid insertions. They reported one patient in whom they failed to extract the prosthesis. Variable amounts of cement extrusion into the surrounding soft tissues were noted, and in each case a cemented component was used.

Sperling and Cofield [13] in their retrospective review reported the use of an anterior and/or medial window(s) in their cohort. The osteotomies were complete, and the cortical piece was removed, then reduced and fixed using heavy sutures, cables, or screws. They needed to supplement the fixation with strut graft in 13 out of 16 patients. They reported a 20% rate of intraoperative fractures.

Sahota et al. [12] reported the use of different techniques in stem revisions including the anterior and medial windows in addition to the longitudinal split. They reported a rate of 23% intraoperative fracture in the humeral windows group, compared to 5% rate of intraoperative fracture in the longitudinal split group (one patient with greater tuberosity fracture). They reported no cases of non-union or malunion in all patients. The anterior humeral window has also been described by Dodson et al. [21] and Phipatanakul et al. [22] with similar techniques.

Other techniques described included vascularised pectoralis major pedicled bone window for converting failed hemiarthroplasty to reverse total shoulder arthroplasty by Gohlke and Rolf [23]. They reported no loosening at final follow-up in 34 patients, with 8 complications including dislocation, infection, and a fracture in the post-operative period. Our technique for postage stamping through the preserved medial soft tissues simplifies creation of a medially hinged vascularised bone flap when required.

More recently, Kang et al. [24] described the use of a handheld high-speed motorised device with a router bit attachment to create a space around the proximal part of the humeral component and use an impactor on the implant to extract, without the need for osteotomy in 98.6% (284/288) of their case series; only 4 patients needed extra humeral window to remove the stem. However, there was no report of the encountered complications.

Recent developments in lower limb arthroplasty have included custom osteotomes for implants. Significant reduction in need for extended trochanteric osteotomy in the removal of uncemented femoral prostheses has resulted in less morbidity, reduced surgical time, and maintained more soft tissue attachments [25]. There may be a role for implant specific osteotomes in the future.

Drawing further from the realm of lower limb arthroplasty, some revision equipment sets have trephines that match the diameter of a cylindrical stem. This often allows a long well-fixed femoral stem to be removed with minimal bone loss and negates the need for extended trochanteric osteotomy. While many modern humeral stems are not cylindrical, some revision stems and some older humeral stems are and would benefit from a trephine.

21.3.1 Summary of Steps

1. Head removal.
2. Soft tissue clearance.
3. Initial disruption of bone / implant interface.
4. Linear humeral osteotomy (optional).
5. Extension of linear humeral osteotomy to anterior humeral window (optional).
6. Canal debridement.
7. Osteotomy fixation.

21.4 Conclusion

In our experience, this stepwise approach is sufficient in removal of a well implanted humeral component during revision shoulder arthroplasty. The adequate proximal exposure of the stem with the help of soft tissue clearance and the use of wires and flexible osteotomes, followed by an anterior osteotomy and 'open book' through medial extension if needed, is usually successful in extracting the stem. This approach allows enough exposure to extract the cement mantle and restore the circumference of the humerus satisfactorily prior the implantation of the new stem or cement spacer, without disrupting the muscular attachments of the humerus.

References

1. Bankes MJ, Emery RJ. Pioneers of shoulder replacement: themistocles Gluck and Jules Emile Péan. J Shoulder Elb Surg. 1995;4(4):259–62.
2. Neer CS. The classic: articular replacement for the humeral head. 1955. Clin Orthop Relat Res. 2011;469(9):2409–21.
3. Baulot E, Sirveaux F, Boileau P. Grammont's idea: the story of Paul Grammont's functional surgery concept and the development of the reverse principle. Clin Orthop Relat Res. 2011;469(9):2425–31.
4. Copeland S. The continuing development of shoulder replacement: "reaching the surface". J Bone Joint Surg Am. 2006;88(4):900–5.
5. McBride AP, Ross M, Hoy G, Duke P, Page R, Peng Y, et al. Mid-term outcomes of pyrolytic carbon humeral resurfacing hemiarthroplasty compared with metal humeral resurfacing and metal stemmed hemiarthroplasty for osteoarthritis in young patients: analysis from the Australian Orthopaedic Association National Joint Replacement Registry. J Shoulder Elb Surg. 2022;31(4):755–62.
6. Bell SN, Christmas MUSI, Coghlan JA. Proximal humeral osteolysis and glenoid radiolucent lines in an anatomic shoulder arthroplasty: a comparison of a ceramic and a metal humeral head component. J Shoulder Elb Surg. 2020;29(5):913–23.
7. Day JS, Lau E, Ong KL, Williams GR, Ramsey ML, Kurtz SM. Prevalence and projections of total shoulder and elbow arthroplasty in the United States to 2015. J Shoulder Elb Surg. 2010;19(8):1115–20.
8. Miura D, Busija L, Page RS, de Steiger R, Lorimer M, Ackerman IN. Lifetime risk of primary shoulder arthroplasty from 2008 to 2017: a population-level analysis using National Registry Data. Arthritis Care Res (Hoboken). 2021;73(10):1511–7.
9. Oppermann J, Celik E, Bredow J, Beyer F, Hackl M, Spies CK, et al. Shoulder arthroplasty in Germany: 2005–2012. Arch Orthop Trauma Surg. 2016;136(5):723–9.
10. Dines JS, Fealy S, Strauss EJ, Allen A, Craig EV, Warren RF, et al. Outcomes analysis of revision total shoulder replacement. J Bone Joint Surg Am. 2006;88(7):1494–500.
11. Wall B, Nové-Josserand L, O'Connor DP, Edwards TB, Walch G. Reverse total shoulder arthroplasty: a review of results according to etiology. J Bone Joint Surg Am. 2007;89(7):1476–85.
12. Sahota S, Sperling JW, Cofield RH. Humeral windows and longitudinal splits for component removal in revision shoulder arthroplasty. J Shoulder Elb Surg. 2014;23(10):1485–91.
13. Sperling JW, Cofield RH. Humeral windows in revision shoulder arthroplasty. J Shoulder Elb Surg. 2005;14(3):258–63.
14. Romeo AACA, Gomoll AH. Revision arthroplasty/revision of loose humeral component. In: Zuckerman JD, Howell S, editors. Advanced reconstruction: shoulder. ISBN-13: 9780892033928. Rosemont, IL: AAOS/ASES; 2007.
15. Karnuta JM, Haeberle HS, Luu BC, Roth AL, Molloy RM, Nystrom LM, et al. Artificial intelligence to identify arthroplasty implants from radiographs of the hip. J Arthroplast. 2021;36(7S):S290–S4.
16. Karnuta JM, Luu BC, Roth AL, Haeberle HS, Chen AF, Iorio R, et al. Artificial intelligence to identify arthroplasty implants from radiographs of the knee. J Arthroplast. 2021;36(3):935–40.
17. Huisman M, Lessmann N. Automatic brand identification of orthopaedic implants from radiographs: ready for the next step? Radiol Artif Intell. 2022;4(2):e220008.
18. Van Thiel GS, Halloran JP, Twigg S, Romeo AA, Nicholson GP. The vertical humeral osteotomy for stem removal in revision shoulder arthroplasty: results and technique. J Shoulder Elb Surg. 2011;20(8):1248–54.
19. Johnston PS, Creighton RA, Romeo AA. Humeral component revision arthroplasty: outcomes of a split osteotomy technique. J Shoulder Elb Surg. 2012;21(4):502–6.
20. Jouve F, Walch G, Wall B, Edwards B. Humeral osteotomy in revision shoulder arthroplasty. Tech Should Elbow Surg. 2006;7(2):106–10.
21. Dodson CC, Nho SJ, Cordasco FA, Craig EV, Dines DM, Warren RF. Anterior humeral window for revision shoulder arthroplasty. Tech Shoulder Elbow Surg. 2006;7(2):111–5.
22. Phipatanakul WP, Bowen JM, Jobe CM. Removal of well-fixed flanged humeral prostheses may require humeral expansion. J Shoulder Elb Surg. 2009;18(5):724–7.
23. Gohlke F, Rolf O. Revision of failed fracture hemiarthroplasties to reverse total shoulder prosthesis through the trans-humeral approach: method

incorporating a pectoralis-major-pedicled bone window. Oper Orthop Traumatol. 2007;19(2):185–208.
24. Kang JR, Logli AL, Tagliero AJ, Sperling JW. The router bit extraction technique for removing a well-fixed humeral stem in revision shoulder arthroplasty. Bone Joint J. 2019;101-B(10):1280–4.
25. Sagers KM, Creech JD, Shields JS, Pollock DC, Langfitt MK, Plate JF. Removing well-fixed, collared and noncollared tapered hip stems without an extended trochanteric osteotomy using a novel stem removal system. Arthroplast Today. 2021;11:146–50.

Revision of a Failed Humeral Stem with Sufficient Bone Stock

22

Edoardo Giovannetti de Sanctis, Alessio Palumbo, Angelo Baldari, Gian Mauro De Angelis D'Ossat, Luca Saccone, Luca La Verde, and Francesco Franceschi

22.1 Introduction

As shoulder arthroplasty is increasingly being implanted, so does the overall number of revisions to be expected in the future.

Revision shoulder arthroplasty is a challenging procedure that has been shown to have inferior outcomes and higher complication rates when compared with primary shoulder arthroplasty.

Reverse total shoulder arthroplasty (rTSA) has been shown to be the only remaining treatment option and an effective treatment in case of failed shoulder arthroplasty with soft tissue (e.g., rotator cuff insufficiency) or bone loss (whether humeral or glenoid) due to its increased constraint and diminished reliance on an intact rotator cuff [1].

Several studies have reported the advantages of retaining the humeral component; however, revision of a failed stem in shoulder arthroplasty is often necessary and presents significant challenges.

Indications for revision of the humeral stem are proximal humeral bone loss (PHBL) (resulting from osteolysis and stress shielding), primary humeral aseptic implant loosening (much less common than with the glenoid component) (Fig. 22.1), periprosthetic fracture, implant malposition and humeral medialization.

The primary goals while revising humeral stems include:

- replication of the physiologic anatomy of the humerus to restore soft tissue tension, providing early implant stability and long-term bony fixation [2];
- creating a stable foundation and secure fixation for the revision stem,
- salvaging as much bone stock as possible.

Both the quantity and quality of remaining humeral bone are important considerations to be assessed before treating these patients.

It influences the risk of stem loosening and deterioration due to mechanical failure [3]. This is particularly true in case of reverse shoulder arthroplasty (rTSA), where due to the specific design, substantial rotational forces are transmitted to the humeral stem.

E. Giovannetti de Sanctis (✉)
Institut Universitaire Locomoteur et du Sport (IULS), Pasteur 2 Hospital, CHU, Nice, France

A. Palumbo · A. Baldari · F. Franceschi
Department of Orthopaedic and Trauma Surgery, San Pietro Fatebenefratelli Hospital, Rome, Italy

UniCamillus-Saint Camillus International University of Health Sciences, Rome, Italy
e-mail: francesco.franceschi@unicamillus.org

G. M. De Angelis D'Ossat · L. Saccone · L. La Verde
Department of Orthopaedic and Trauma Surgery, San Pietro Fatebenefratelli Hospital, Rome, Italy

F. Franceschi et al. (eds.), *Revision Shoulder Arthroplasty*,
https://doi.org/10.1007/978-3-031-45944-3_22

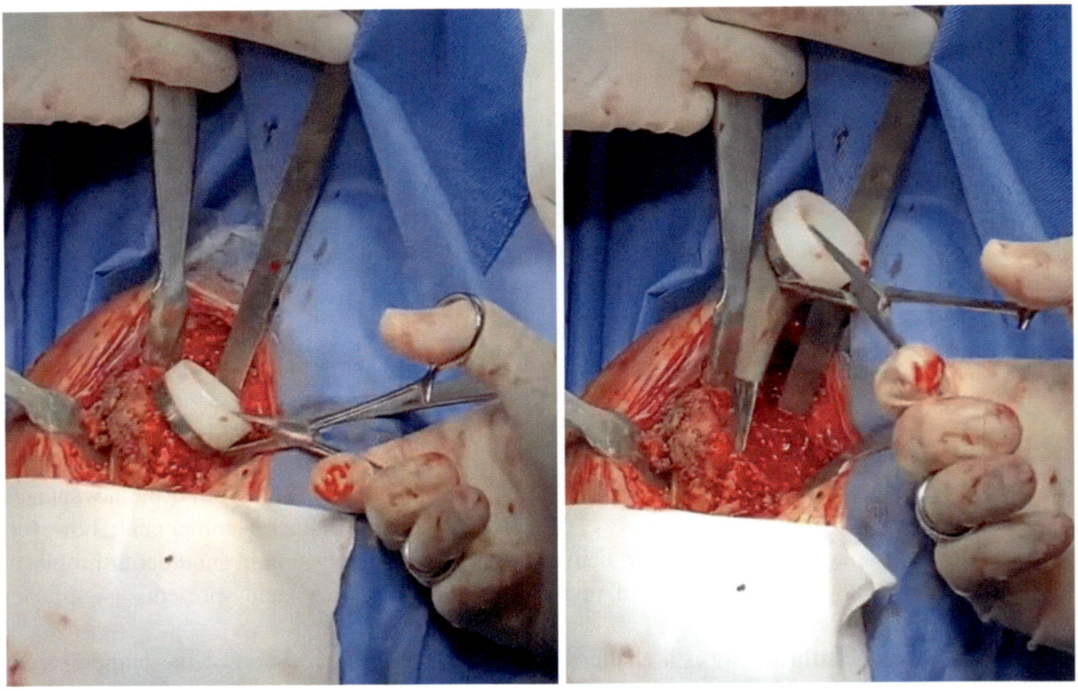

Fig. 22.1 Humeral component mobilization

It also influences the risk of glenohumeral instability and postoperative ROM, affecting the glenohumeral soft tissue envelope. Bone stock lateralizes the pull of the deltoid and improves the contour of the shoulder with enhanced prosthesis stability and allows reattachment of the subscapularis tendon [4]. Furthermore, in case of greater tuberosity absence the ROM is altered, with loss of active external rotation.

PHBL is therefore one of the main challenging obstacles to achieving a well-fixed, stable prosthesis [5]. It occurs in cases of periprosthetic infection, stress shielding, aseptic loosening of previous implant, osteolysis secondary to wear debris, and following humeral resection for tumor. Furthermore, stem extraction and complete removal of the cement may be arduous and can lead to subsequent severe bone loss, cortical perforation, and fracture.

PHBL has driven forward research in newest primary humeral implants with shorter or no stem, relying on fixation at the level of the metaphysis. These innovations have been proposed trying to balance the need for a stable fixation of the humeral component with the potential need for revision surgery.

This implies the advantages of preserved bone stock, less stress shielding, eliminating the diaphyseal stress riser, and easier implant removal at revision.

Boileau et al. and Chalmers et al. have described two systems to classify PHBL [3, 6]. The topic of this chapter is to outline the preoperative planning and revision techniques in case of a failed humeral stem with no or shorter proximal humeral bone defects, classified as A-B according to Boileau et al. [3] or 1 and 2A according to Chalmers et al. [6]. Furthermore, A cut-off value of 5 cm has also been proposed as the threshold to define significant bone loss, with indication to a more aggressive reconstruction [7].

22.2 Preoperative Planning

Anticipating humeral bone deficiency with preoperative appropriate planning is mandatory to success while revising a failed humeral stem and enables the surgeon the achieve adequate fixation and stability.

Both bilateral full-length radiographs of the humeri in neutral rotation and computed tomography (CT) scans are needed preoperatively to evaluate implant migration (whether it occurs in the form of subsidence, tilt, or shift), radiolucency around implant and implant loosening, signs of shoulder displacement, humeral bone resorption and formation, wear of implant articular surfaces, fractures around the implant, and implant breakage and disassembly [8].

Postoperative CT has a greater ability to detect radiolucent lines 36, 37 than do radiographs [8]. Furthermore, 3D planning might help evaluating the cement mantle, the amount of bone that has to be removed, and decide the correct implant sizing and implant position.

Radiographic signs of loosening include component subsidence, cortical scalloping, radiolucent line formation, and pedestal formation around the distal stem.

Component subsidence with proximal bone resorption might appear, without evaluating also the contralateral radiograph, as a normal not loosened stem, resulting in alteration of the humeral length and therefore soft tissue tension.

Attention should be given to measuring the length of the humeral implant in place to provide intraoperative data regarding the possible cortical window length needed to remove a well-fixed stem.

Other important data to be evaluated preoperatively is whether the stem has been cemented and the type/company of the stem previously implanted.

Ladermann et al. outlined a standardised technique to plan preoperatively a reverse shoulder arthroplasty assessing variations in humeral length [9]. This technique might be used to compare the preoperative radiograph to the contralateral or the ipsilateral radiograph taken before implanting the primary shoulder arthroplasty.

Four lines are defined: the epicondylar line (EL) between the most lateral part of the medial and lateral epicondyle; the diaphyseal axis (DI) determined by a line drawn in the centre of the proximal medullary canal; two perpendicular line to DI passing, respectively, through the most lateral and inferior point of the acromion and through the most lateral and superior point of the humerus. Intersection between the EL line and the DI represents the point C; between the DI and top of the humeral head (in preoperative radiograph) is named H, intersection between the two perpendicular lines represent, respectively, point A and P. The distance HC and HP might be used comparing different radiographs to assess humeral bone deficit and humeral length.

In case of humeral component loosening or osteolysis, inflammation-related laboratory data (complete blood count, erythrocyte sedimentation rate, C-reactive protein) are needed preoperatively to exclude any periprosthetic infections.

In case of a high suspicion of infection with normal laboratory values, shoulder aspiration or biopsy should be performed before planning surgery.

22.3 Treatment Strategies

In case of sufficient bone stock, the humeral implant might be well fixed within the native bone and the removal can be challenging.

A number of methods have been described as part of revision shoulder arthroplasty. Initial efforts at removal should be attempted with an osteotome or a carefully used oscillating saw around the stem to mobilize it. However, if no substantial progress is made, consideration might also be given to a vertical humeral window osteotomy made using a saw.

If a vertical osteotomy is performed for stem removal, this should be repaired using a minimum of 3 cerclage wires.

After the humeral component is removed, a final evaluation of the humeral bone stock should be made.

Several treatment strategies have been described to address PHBL, which might be divided essentially in two broad categories based on the amount of proximal bone loss.

The treatment options to restore length and obtain an adequate soft tissue tension in patients with no or shorter proximal humeral bone defects include: the use of thicker polyethylene/metal tray, cementing the stem proportionally proud to re-establish height, implanting an inferior or lateral eccentric glenosphere [10]. Another intraoperative option, which is possible only with few shoulder replacement systems, to alter the soft tissue tension, is to modify the metal tray offset by rotating it.

In case of absence of the greater tuberosity, a proximal cement plasty (a cement collar around the implant) or metaphyseal augments might be used to increase soft tissue wrapping and when possible reattach the rotator cuff still present [11] (Fig. 22.2).

Preoperatively is planned the treatment strategy to be used during surgery. However, the path chosen preoperatively might be modified once the humerus is visible: this might be due to a difference of quality and quantity of the remaining bone compared to preoperative imaging.

Furthermore, intraoperatively the stability and range of motion is assessed to determine whether the humeral component needs to be shortened or lengthened (e.g. increasing the thickness of PE).

Adequate length can be determined through use of a trial component before cementation, by evaluating soft tissue and axillary nerve tension, force required to inferiorly subluxate the humerus, and force required for prosthetic dislocation.

Type of fixation and stem length/size need a special consideration, as knowledge in revision shoulder arthroplasty is improving. Among valuable options, those that should be taken into account when revising a failed humeral stem with sufficient bone stock are cement-on-cement and revising the component with a shorter stem.

Cementing the humeral stem in revision shoulder arthroplasty is a reasonable option and is performed in almost all cases at our institution; using an ingrowth implant might be the alternative. Various intraoperative strategies have been described to provide adequate stability of the stem during revision surgery whether in case of previous cementation or not.

The debate is whether the retained intramedullary cement mantle should be adequately reamed or not and whether efforts should be taken to maximize the added cement volume during reimplantation.

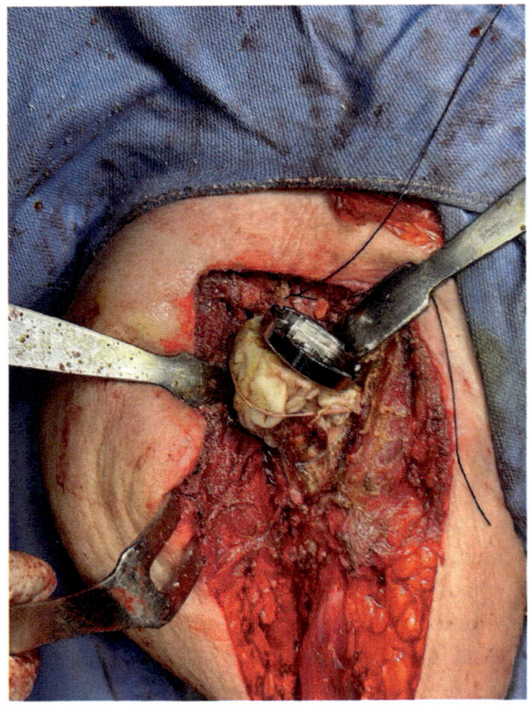

Fig. 22.2 Cement plasty

Implantation of a new cemented revision component into a retained cement mantle is a widely accepted technique in revision hip surgery [12].

In the setting of a revision arthroplasty with previous cementation of the humeral component the options include using the stem with the largest possible diameter in the existing cement mantle thereby minimizing the amount of new cement or implanting the smallest stem possible (smaller than the previous component), allowing for the maximum amount of added cement [12].

Allen Gorman II et al. reported 98 revisions to RSA where a cement-within-cement technique was used at a minimum of 2 years of follow-up [12]. Eight patients developed humeral stem loosening. The authors suggested that efforts to maximise the cement volume during reimplantation may lessen the chance of humeral stem loosening.

Choosing the correct stem is mandatory to achieve good postoperative clinical outcomes and decrease the risk of postoperative complications. It has been shown that modular implants may have a higher risk of mechanical failure in the setting of PHBL. Monoblock implants should be, therefore, preferred for reconstruction constructs in the setting of limited PHBL [5, 13].

Revision shoulder arthroplasty is frequently associated with an increase in stem length chosen by the physician. This practice starts to be debated and might be abandoned in case of primary long stems, where implanting a shorter stem has many advantages, avoiding the need to remove distal cement in patients with cemented primary humeral components and to interfere with any future elbow arthroplasties.

Wagner et al. [14] evaluated 39 patients who underwent revision reverse shoulder arthroplasty using a shorter humeral component. At a follow-up of 3 years, 5 shoulders (13%) were revised due to periprosthetic humerus fracture (1) and glenoid loosening (4). At most recent radiographic follow-up, 1 (5%) patient was shown to have grade 3 humeral lucency.

22.4 Results

Few heterogenous studies describe results of revision of a failed humeral stem with sufficient bone stock. Literature is lacking of trials comparing different treatment options outlined before in patients with short or no PHBL.

Revision of a failed humeral stem is a challenging procedure that has been shown to have inferior outcomes and higher complication rates when compared with primary shoulder arthroplasty [5].

Cil et al. presented 38 revision arthroplasties performed for aseptic loosening of the humeral component [15]. The mean interval from primary arthroplasty to revision was 7.1 years (0.4–16.6) at a mean follow-up of seven years (2–19.3). Humeral components were cemented in 29, with ingrowth implants used in nine cases. There were 19 of standard length and 17 were longer. Intraoperative complications included cement extrusion in eight cases, fracture of the shaft of the humerus in two, and of the tuberosity in four. Revision surgery for aseptic loosening of the humeral component provided reliable pain relief and modest improvement of movement.

Owens et al. evaluated clinically eighty revision shoulder arthroplasties for at least 2 years [16]. The primary indications for use of an intermediate or long stem were proximal bone loss in 40, nonunion in 14, a mispositioned previous stem with bone loss in 10, an acute intraoperative fracture in 7, an acute preoperative periprosthetic fracture in 5, diaphyseal bone loss in 2, and a box-shaped osteotomy to remove a well-fixed stem in 2. Clinical follow-up had an average of 5.9 years, and radiographic follow-up had an average of 4.7 years. Intraoperative complications included fracture removing the previous stem in 5, a cortical perforation in 6, and cement extrusion in 7. Late complications included fracture nonunion in 5, deep infection in 2, and component loosening in 1.

Stephens et al. [13] evaluated 32 revision rTSAs and compared the outcomes of revision rTSA in patients both with and without PHBL. Sixteen patients had PHBL with an average loss of 36.3 mm. Humeral bone deficiency was not associated with significant lower functional or subjective outcomes, except for active motion.

Budge et al. evaluated 15 patients undergoing revision for failed arthroplasty with an average PHBL of 38.4 mm at a minimum 2 years follow up. The satisfaction rate was 87%. CS, ASES, VAS, forward flexion, and external rotation increased significantly. The authors reported a scapular notching rate of, 20%, one humeral stem fracture but no stem loosening, concluding that the use of RTSA for failed shoulder arthroplasty and deficient humeral bone stock provides a significant clinical benefit without the need for allograft augmentation [4].

Holschen et al. reported 60 failed shoulder arthroplasties converted to rTSA, showing that patients with a stemless primary implant achieved a higher constant score than patients with stemmed implants [1]. This study illustrates the benefits of stemless primary implants, which are probably based on a less traumatic revision with a concomitant preservation of humeral bone stock.

Werner et al. evaluated 50 revision reverse shoulder arthroplasty using long-stem cemented humeral components at a mean of 7 years. Progressive humeral radiolucency was present in 24 patients, including 6 patients demonstrating complete loosening or progressive distal migration of the humeral stem. An overall of 12 additional complications in 8 patients, necessitating revision surgery in 16, was noted.

References

1. Holschen M, Franetzki B, Witt KA, Liem D, Steinbeck J. Is reverse total shoulder arthroplasty a feasible treatment option for failed shoulder arthroplasty? A retrospective study of 44 cases with special regards to stemless and stemmed primary implants. Musculoskelet Surg. 2017;101(2):173–80. https://doi.org/10.1007/s12306-017-0467-y.
2. Keener JD, Chalmers PN, Yamaguchi K. The humeral implant in shoulder arthroplasty. J Am Acad Orthop Surg. 2017;25(6):427–38. https://doi.org/10.5435/JAAOS-D-15-00682.
3. Boileau P, Raynier JL, Chelli M, Gonzalez JF, Galvin JW. Reverse shoulder-allograft prosthesis composite, with or without tendon transfer, for the treatment of severe proximal humeral bone loss. J Shoulder Elb Surg. 2020;29(11):e401–15. https://doi.org/10.1016/j.jse.2020.03.016.
4. Budge MD, Moravek JE, Zimel MN, Nolan EM, Wiater JM. Reverse total shoulder arthroplasty for the management of failed shoulder arthroplasty with proximal humeral bone loss: is allograft augmentation necessary? J Shoulder Elb Surg. 2013;22(6):739–44. https://doi.org/10.1016/j.jse.2012.08.008.
5. Kahn T, Chalmers PN. Proximal humeral bone loss in revision shoulder arthroplasty. Orthop Clin North Am. 2020;51(1):87–95. https://doi.org/10.1016/j.ocl.2019.08.003.
6. Chalmers PN, Romeo AA, Nicholson GP, Boileau P, Keener JD, Gregory JM, Salazar DH, Tashjian RZ. Humeral Bone Loss in Revision Total Shoulder Arthroplasty: the Proximal Humeral Arthroplasty Revision Osseous in Sufficiency (PHAROS) classification system. Clin Orthop Relat Res. 2019;477(2):432–41. https://doi.org/10.1097/CORR.0000000000000590.
7. Cuff D, Levy JC, Gutierrez S, Frankle MA. Torsional stability of modular and non-modular reverse shoulder humeral components in a proximal humeral bone loss model. J Shoulder Elb Surg. 2011;20(4):646–51. https://doi.org/10.1016/j.jse.2010.10.026.
8. Durchholz H, Salomonsson B, Moroder P, Lambert S, Page R, Audige L, Sperling J, Schwyzer HK. Core set of radiographic parameters for shoulder arthroplasty monitoring: criteria defined by an International Delphi Consensus Process. JB JS Open Access. 2019;4(4):e0025. https://doi.org/10.2106/JBJS.OA.19.00025.
9. Ladermann A, Williams MD, Melis B, Hoffmeyer P, Walch G. Objective evaluation of lengthening in reverse shoulder arthroplasty. J Shoulder Elb Surg. 2009;18(4):588–95. https://doi.org/10.1016/j.jse.2009.03.012.
10. Sanchez-Sotelo J, Wagner ER, Sim FH, Houdek MT. Allograft-prosthetic composite reconstruction for massive proximal humeral bone loss in reverse shoulder arthroplasty. J Bone Joint Surg Am. 2017;99(24):2069–76. https://doi.org/10.2106/JBJS.16.01495.
11. Boileau P. Complications and revision of reverse total shoulder arthroplasty. Orthop Traumatol Surg Res. 2016;102(Suppl. 1):S33–43. https://doi.org/10.1016/j.otsr.2015.06.031.
12. Gorman RA 2nd, Christmas KN, Simon P, Hess AV 2nd, Brewley EE Jr, Mighell MA, Frankle MA. Optimizing humeral stem fixation in revision reverse shoulder arthroplasty with the cement-within-cement technique. J Shoulder Elb Surg. 2020;29(7S):S9–S16. https://doi.org/10.1016/j.jse.2020.01.094.
13. Stephens SP, Paisley KC, Giveans MR, Wirth MA. The effect of proximal humeral bone loss on revision reverse total shoulder arthroplasty. J Shoulder Elb Surg. 2015;24(10):1519–26. https://doi.org/10.1016/j.jse.2015.02.020.
14. Wagner ER, Statz JM, Houdek MT, Cofield RH, Sanchez-Sotelo J, Sperling JW. Use of a shorter humeral stem in revision reverse shoulder arthroplasty. J Shoulder Elb Surg. 2017;26(8):1454–61. https://doi.org/10.1016/j.jse.2017.01.016.
15. Cil A, Veillette CJ, Sanchez-Sotelo J, Sperling JW, Schleck C, Cofield RH. Revision of the humeral component for aseptic loosening in arthroplasty of the shoulder. J Bone Joint Surg Br. 2009;91(1):75–81. https://doi.org/10.1302/0301-620X.91B1.21094.
16. Owens CJ, Sperling JW, Cofield RH. Utility and complications of long-stem humeral components in revision shoulder arthroplasty. J Shoulder Elb Surg. 2013;22(7):e7–12. https://doi.org/10.1016/j.jse.2012.10.034.

Revision of the Failed Stem Without Sufficient Bone Stock

23

Yousif Atwan, Joseph T. Labrum IV, and Joaquin Sanchez-Sotelo

23.1 Introduction

As the incidence of primary shoulder arthroplasty continues to rise across the world, the number of revision shoulder arthroplasty procedures is expected to increase proportionally [1, 2]. Currently, most revision shoulder arthroplasties are performed with implantation of reverse total shoulder arthroplasty (RSA) components. Dealing with proximal humeral bone loss in the setting of revision arthroplasty continues to be a challenging issue. Humeral bone loss may be encountered at the time of revision shoulder arthroplasty secondary to several reasons, namely stress shielding, osteolysis secondary to wear debris, periprosthetic fracture, and iatrogenic bone loss when removing a well-fixed implant during a revision procedure [3–5]. Occasionally, bone loss was already present at the time of the original primary arthroplasty and was not addressed properly.

In the setting of insufficient proximal humeral bone stock, surgeons are faced with two major issues in the revision procedures: (a) inability to obtain adequate fixation of the new humeral implant and (b) loss of soft-tissue attachments for the rotator cuff, deltoid, and other musculotendinous structures depending on the extent of humeral bone loss [5, 6]. Dislocation of RSA is more common in revision shoulder arthroplasty, especially in the presence of humeral bone loss [3, 7–9]. In the presence of substantial humeral bone loss, RSA dislocation can be facilitated by loss of restoration of humeral length as well as loss of rotator cuff attachment, deltoid insertion, and deltoid wrapping [10, 11]. The extent of bone loss varies depending on the etiology and chronicity of the pathology at the revision setting. As severity and distal extent increase, the management of this problem becomes more challenging.

23.2 Preoperative Planning

Revision RSA procedures with insufficient humeral bone require extensive preoperative planning and decision making. It is important to complete a thorough history and physical examination of patients presenting with this elusive problem. It is imperative to assess patients' expectations and adequately counsel them regarding possible outcomes. The physical examination should include assessment of prior incisions as well as deltoid and axillary nerve function. Care must be taken to evaluate for possible isolated anterior deltoid dysfunction that may have occurred after numerous shoulder procedures.

Y. Atwan · J. T. Labrum IV · J. Sanchez-Sotelo (✉)
Department of Orthopaedic Surgery, Mayo Clinic, Rochester, MN, USA
e-mail: sanchezsotelo.joaquin@mayo.edu

F. Franceschi et al. (eds.), *Revision Shoulder Arthroplasty*,
https://doi.org/10.1007/978-3-031-45944-3_23

The etiology of the humeral bone loss should also be evaluated preoperatively. An infectious cause should be assessed by obtaining C-reactive protein, erythrocyte sedimentation rate, and possibly a joint aspiration and/or biopsy [12]. Our preference is to perform an aspiration for culture and cell count prior to all revision arthroplasty procedures; arthroscopic biopsies are limited to well-fixed implants with unexplained pain and a negative evaluation for infection. Thorough evaluation of plain radiographs should be completed to assess for possible wear debris osteolysis, stress-shielding or evidence of humeral component loosening. Signs of loosening on plain radiographs may include radiolucent line formation, endosteal pedestal at distal aspect of prosthesis, and stem subsidence [4, 13].

It is vital to obtain full length humeral radiographs of the affected and contralateral sides. These radiographs can be useful for determining the true extent and measurement of humeral bone loss that needs to be accounted for in a revision procedure. If the case includes a well-fixed humeral implant, it is important to evaluate the quality of the surrounding bone, since poor bone stock may result in additional iatrogenic bone loss during the implant extraction process. Furthermore, careful landmarking and measurement of the implant in place will allow for efficient planning if a corticotomy or cortical window are required for the extraction of well-fixed humeral implants.

Computed tomography has become an essential image modality for primary shoulder arthroplasty, mostly to assess the glenoid side of the joint and also as the main data input for contemporary preoperative planning software packages. Computed tomography is also extremely useful when planning revision shoulder arthroplasty. Again, most attention is centered on the glenoid side, but careful assessment of the humeral side on computed tomography can be invaluable. In addition, certain preoperative planning software packages (Reflex Complex by Akuna; BluePrint by Stryker Tornier) have revision applications as well.

23.3 Classification of Humeral Bone Loss in Revision Shoulder Arthroplasty

Multiple attempts have been made at classifying proximal humeral bone loss in the setting of revision shoulder arthroplasty. Classifications have been sought to efficiently determine the diagnosis, optimal management, and prognosis for individual cases. Such classification systems aimed to delineate the optimal use of long-stemmed prostheses, allograft, and proximal humeral replacements. Boileau initially proposed a dichotomous classification of proximal humeral bone loss: less or greater than 5 cm of humeral defect. He proposed that bone loss less than 5 cm can be managed by creating a cement collar around a revision humeral implant (cementoplasty), while bone loss in excess of 5 cm was to be managed with an allograft prosthetic composite (APC) [6]. Similarly, McLendon et al. also recommended a 5 cm cut off from medial aspect of the humeral tray as the deciding parameter when considering cementoplasty versus APC reconstruction [14].

More recently, the Proximal Humeral Arthroplasty Revision Osseous inSufficiency (PHAROS) classification system (Table 23.1) was developed to further characterize humeral bone loss in revision shoulder arthroplasty [15]. This alphanumeric system utilized anteroposterior, lateral, and Grashey's radiographic views to classify proximal humeral bone loss. It was found to have an inter-rater reliability of 71% ($\kappa = 0.545$) and intra-rater reliability of 77% ($\kappa = 0.615$) at 4 months [15]. PHAROS type 1 describes epiphyseal bone lose including the articular surface, calcar, and tuberosities. It is further subdivided into type 1C (calcar loss) or type 1G (tuberosity malunion or loss). PHAROS type 2 describes metadiaphyseal bone loss that remains above the deltoid insertion. This was further subdivided into type 2A, which was composed of metadiaphyseal cortical thinning >50% of the expected cortical thickness and type 2B, which was composed of segmental bone loss including part of the metadi-

Table 23.1 The Proximal Humeral Arthroplasty Revision Osseous inSufficiency (PHAROS) classification. Based on work by Chalmers et al. [15]

Type	Description	Subtype	Subtype description
1	Epiphyseal bone loss	C	Loss of the calcar
		G	Loss of the greater tuberosity
2	Metadiaphyseal bone loss above deltoid attachment	A	Metadiaphyseal cortical thinning of >50% of the expected cortical thickness with epiphyseal bone loss or thinning
		B	Bone loss above the deltoid attachment including the epiphysis and part of the metadiaphysis
3	Diaphyseal bone loss extending below deltoid attachment	A	Diaphyseal cortical thinning of >50% of the expected cortical thickness with epiphyseal or epiphyseal/metadiaphyseal bone loss or thinning
		B	Compromise of the majority of the diaphysis with loss of the epiphysis, metadiaphysis, and part of the diaphysis below the deltoid insertion

aphysis. PHAROS type 3 signifies bone loss that extends distal to the deltoid insertion and is subdivided into type 3A, which was composed of diaphyseal cortical thinning >50% of the expected cortical thickness and type 3B, which was composed of bone loss including the majority of the diaphysis (Table 23.1).

23.4 Reconstruction Strategies

The selection of reconstructive strategies in the setting of proximal humeral bone loss largely depends on the distal extent of bone loss as well as the quality of the remaining bone available. The goals of strategies surrounding this problem include restoring humeral length, optimizing implant fixation, and when possible, restoring the function of the posterior rotator cuff and deltoid at a minimum.

Cadaveric studies have determined that the insertion of the upper edge of the pectoralis major tendon is approximately 5.6 cm away from the top of the native humeral head [16, 17]. This landmark can be utilized to estimate the correct height of a humeral stem in the revision setting in shoulders with PHAROS grade 1. However, most surgeons end up selecting length restoration based on soft tissue tension at the time of trial reduction.

Reconstructive options may include use of standard humeral components cemented proud, implantation of modular titanium conical fluted stems, allograft prosthetic composites, and modular segmental (tumor) prostheses. Intraoperatively, humeral length restoration may be based on measurements in preoperative radiographs and CT scans.

23.4.1 Standard Humeral Components

Moderate proximal humerus bone loss can be compensated for by gaining length with the use of standard components. On the glenoid side, length can be gained by placing the baseplate as low as possible and implanting a larger size glenosphere with inferior eccentricity. The humeral component can then be cemented proud so that the overall reconstruction tensions the soft-tissue envelope appropriately. This typically requires used of a standard-length humeral component or even a dedicated cemented revision component, since ultrashort components would be unlikely to gain adequate primary stability when cemented proud.

One concern with the proud implantation of a cemented humeral component is the potential for poor rotational stability of the component; without metaphyseal support, a cylindrical cemented stem is prone to loosening. A second concern with this strategy is loss of restoration of the bulk of the greater tuberosity, which could lead to inadequate deltoid tension (so called loss of deltoid wrapping effect). Some surgeons try to compensate for this phenomenon by "creating" a grater tuberosity shape made of acrylic cement (cementoplasty). Obviously, this strategy does not allow associated soft-tissue reconstructive procedures.

23.4.2 Conical Tapered Fluted Modular Revision Components

In the field of revision hip arthroplasty, titanium conical tapered fluted modular revision components have become the workhorse for most surgeons. Similar implants have been developed for revision shoulder arthroplasty. A metallic cone with flutes provides great primary vertical and rotational stability. The use of titanium minimizes stress shielding when compared to cobalt-chrome alloys. Finally, these components are modular and allow restoration of height independent of where the distal conical portion of the implant achieves primary stability (Fig. 23.1). Currently, these implants do not provide restoration of the shape of the greater tuberosity (deltoid-wrapping), a feature that is likely to be added in the future. There are reports of these modular implants becoming disassembled in vivo; as such, it is imperative to follow the manufacturers' recommendations strictly when the different modules of the final implant are assembled in the back table.

23.4.3 Allograft Prosthetic Composites

In the setting of PHAROS type 2 and 3 bone loss, APC reconstruction has been an increasingly utilized option in order to restore bone, humeral length, and soft tissue tension [18–20]. There are several advantages to this treatment option. Using proximal humeral allograft provides improved bony fixation for a humeral implant as it neutralizes the torsional forces across the implant-bone interface [20, 21]. Furthermore, the presence of a greater tuberosity fills the subdeltoid space and restores deltoid wrapping [20, 21]. Finally, utilizing an allograft with associated allograft tissue (rotator cuff, deltoid, and others) provides an attachment site for soft tissue repair or reconstruction to improve stability of the joint and hopefully improve strength, motion, and function [18, 20, 21] (Fig. 23.2). Nevertheless, the use of APC reconstruction does have inherent risk and possible drawbacks. There are risks of non-union, graft resorption, and infection with the use of allograft bone [21]. The use of APC reconstruc-

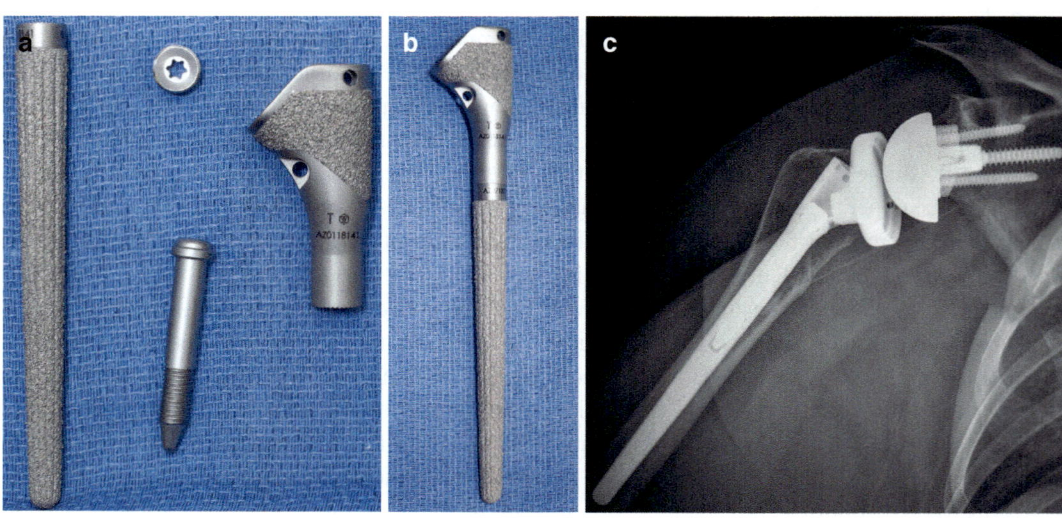

Fig. 23.1 Representation of a modular (**a**) conical tapered fluted revision humeral stem (**b**). Radiographic representation of this implant (**c**)

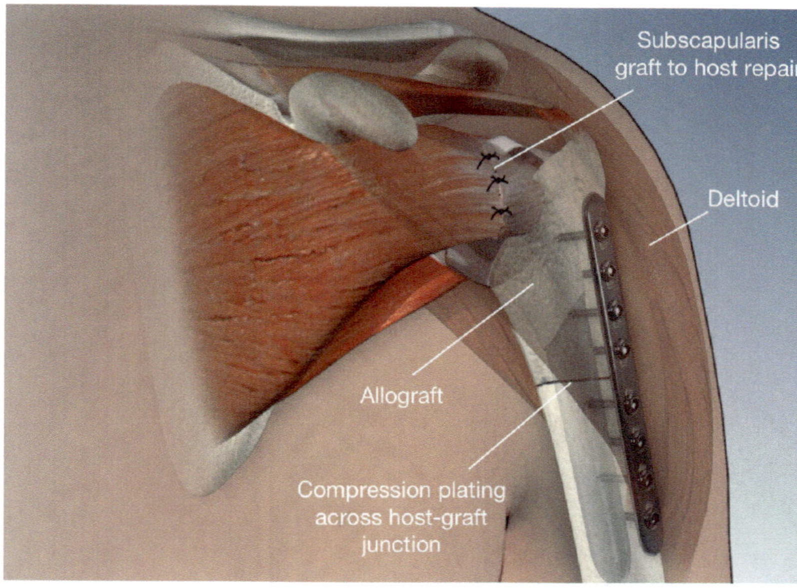

Fig. 23.2 Representation of allograft prosthetic composite reconstruction

tion is not recommended if there is insufficient distal humeral bone stock to allow for optimal graft to host-bone fixation [20].

Generally, a deltopectoral exposure is extended into a distal Henry approach by splitting the brachialis muscle. For shoulders with substantial bone loss, the radial nerve is identified between brachialis and brachioradialis and protected throughout the case. When plate fixation is selected for graft-to-host fixation, sufficient distal humeral exposure is required; less distal exposure may be needed when APC fixation is relied upon just the cemented component across the junction, or when cerclage sutures, wires or cables are used. Once the humeral implant is resected and the glenoid component is implanted, the humeral allograft can be prepared. While the allograft rotator cuff is protected, the allograft proximal humerus is prepared for cemented implantation. The length of allograft is determined either through prior templating or by placing a trial broach and an articulating bearing against the glenoid component. The overlay of the allograft with the native humerus marks the adequate resection level. A step or straight osteotomy may be utilized. If the implant bypasses the allograft osteotomy, a cement restrictor is placed into the distal native humerus, and the allograft and native humerus are subsequently compressed by utilizing a compression plating technique. Next, the trial broach is replaced with a cemented humeral component. Prior to final reduction of the joint, the native posterosuperior cuff is sutured to allograft tendon. The anterior native cuff may be reattached following final reduction [20]. In cuff-deficient shoulders, tendon transfers may be performed at the time of revision shoulder arthroplasty and attached to the allograft tendon present in the proximal humerus allograft.

Clinical outcomes of APC reconstruction have been promising in the setting of proximal humeral bone loss. Cox et al., reported on 73 patients who underwent RSA with APC reconstruction with an average follow up of 67.9 months. Their demonstration significantly improved clinical outcome scores as well as range of motion [22]. Nonetheless, revision procedures were required in 19% of cases for periprosthetic fracture ($n = 6$), instability ($n = 2$), humeral loosening ($n = 2$), and infection ($n = 2$). The reoperation-free survival rate decreased from 88% at 5 years to 67% beyond 10 years [22]. Reif et al., followed 115 similar cases of proximal humeral APC reconstruction with an average follow up of 6.7 years across two different institutions and various osteotomy and fixation methods [18]. Fourteen patients underwent a revision procedure for asep-

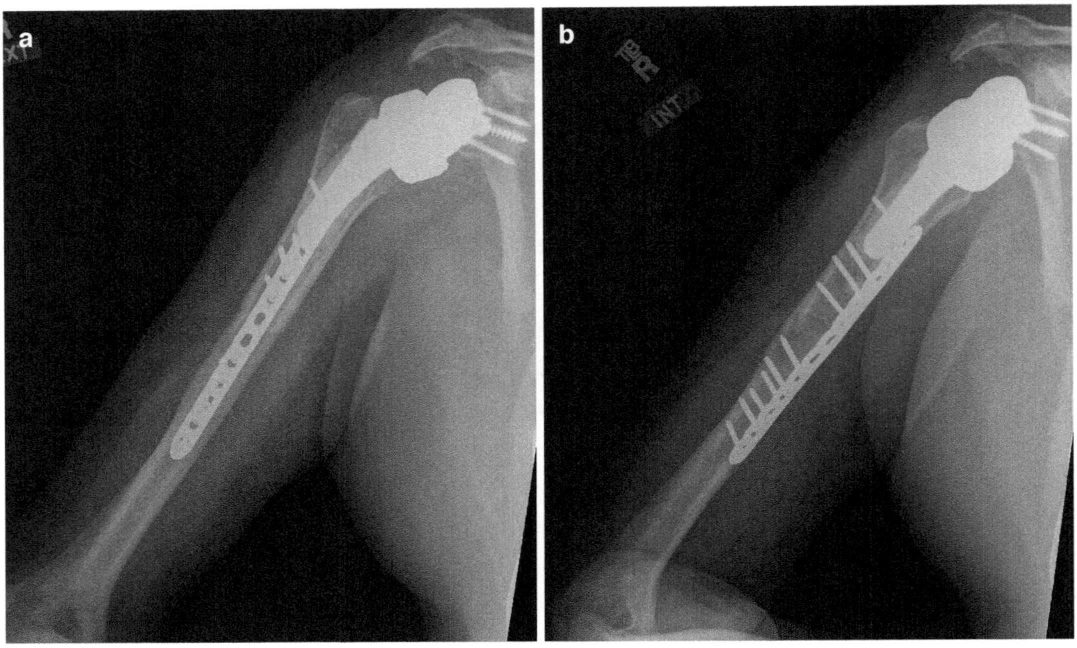

Fig. 23.3 Anteroposterior (**a**) and internally rotated (**b**) views of an allograft prosthetic composite reconstruction

tic causes such as non-union (n = 7), instability (n = 5), and allograft fracture (n = 2) [18]. Sanchez-Sotelo et al., followed 26 patients who underwent APC reconstruction with compression plating techniques. They reported significant improvement in terms of pain relief, external rotation, and elevation. The revision-free survival rate was 96% at 5 years. Interestingly, the mean time to union was reported to be 7 months [20] (Fig. 23.3).

23.4.4 Modular Segmental Metallic (Tumor) Prosthesis

The use of proximal humerus endoprostheses or total humeral replacement in the setting of PHAROS type 3B defects have also been reported as potentially effective treatment options (Fig. 23.4). These modular implants allow for calculated restoration of length and version. Unlike APC reconstructions, the use of endoprosthesis options do not require union between allograft and host bone or the use of plate fixation methods. Nonetheless, disadvantages include the lack of tissue for native rotator cuff deltoid reattachment or for associated tendon transfers. Furthermore, torsional stress at the implant-bone interface can potentially lead to implant loosening, especially when implanted in a non-cemented fashion [21].

Of the limited clinical data available regarding the use of humeral endoprostheses, a large proportion relate to oncological indications. Therefore, it is important to note that this patient population may differ from those undergoing the procedure for a failed arthroplasty with significant bone loss. Guven et al., followed ten patients who underwent a reverse shoulder tumor prosthesis for malignant proximal humeral tumors for a mean of 18.2 months. They reported satisfactory outcome scores and low pain scores [23]. In terms of a comparative study, Potter et al. followed 49 patients who underwent either osteoarticular reconstruction (n = 17), APC (n = 16), or endoprosthesis reconstruction (n = 16) for tumors of the proximal humerus. At a minimum of 24 months, the Musculoskeletal Tumor Society functional scores averaged 71% for osteoarticular reconstruction, 79% for APC, and 69% for endoprosthesis reconstruction [24]. Revision surgery was most common in patients who underwent osteoarticular reconstruction (n = 5), followed by one patient within the APC group

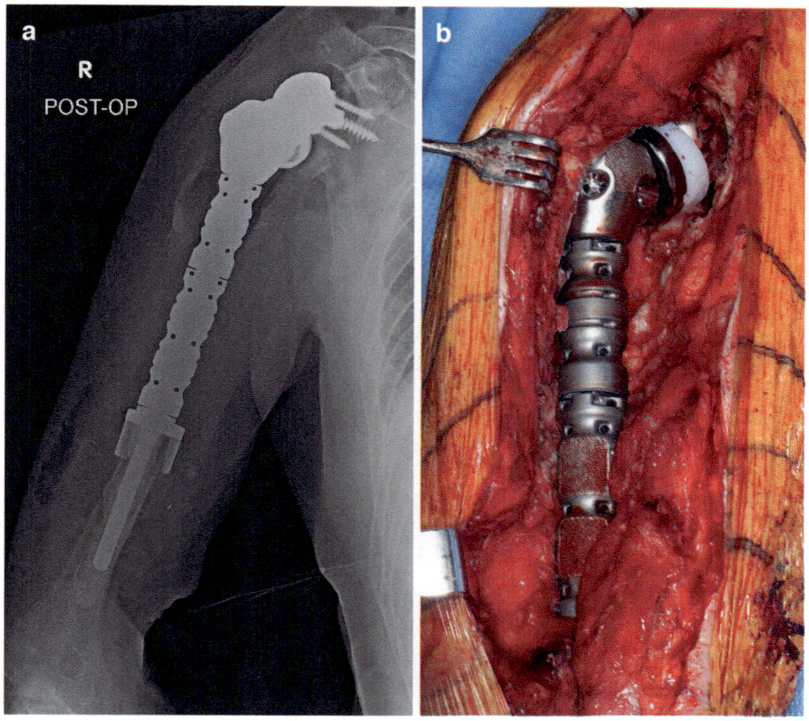

Fig. 23.4 Radiographic (**a**) and intraoperative (**b**) example of proximal humeral endoprosthesis

[24]. We recently reviewed the Mayo Clinic experience using one particular modular segmental prosthesis (Skeletal Reconstruction System, Biomet, Warsaw, In, USA). Seventy-six Skeletal Reconstruction System (SRS) implants were implanted for a variety of indications that mainly included failed arthroplasty (n = 30) and tumor resection (n = 29). Complications occurred in 33% of shoulders and included dislocation (n = 9), humeral loosening (n = 8), infection (n = 4), periprosthetic humeral fracture (n = 3), glenoid loosening (n = 2), and one case of acromial stress fracture. The overall reoperation rate was 20% at 5 years. Based on these studies and other systematic reviews within tumor literature, APC reconstruction appears to result in better functional outcomes while endoprosthesis reconstruction results in decreased revision rates [21].

23.5 Conclusion

Proximal humeral bone loss in the setting of revision RSA is a significant problem. Classification methods have been developed to synthesize the location and significance of the bone loss. Strategies to address this problem include potential APC and endoprosthesis reconstruction. Further studies are required to compare the outcomes of endoprosthesis vs. allograft prosthetic composite reconstruction in the setting of non-oncologic proximal humeral bone loss requiring RSA.

References

1. Best MJ, Aziz KT, Wilckens JH, McFarland EG, Srikumaran U. Increasing incidence of primary reverse and anatomic total shoulder arthroplasty in the United States. J Shoulder Elbow Surg. 2021;30(5):1159–66. https://doi.org/10.1016/j.jse.2020.08.010.
2. Kim SH, Wise BL, Zhang Y, Szabo RM. Increasing incidence of shoulder arthroplasty in the United States. J Bone Joint Surg Am Vol. 2011;93(24):2249–54. https://doi.org/10.2106/JBJS.J.01994.
3. Tashjian RZ, Granger E, Broschinsky K, Kawakami J, Chalmers PN. Effect of complications on outcomes after revision reverse total shoulder arthroplasty. JSES Int. 2020;4(3):662–8. https://doi.org/10.1016/j.jseint.2020.03.016.
4. Kahn T, Chalmers PN. Proximal humeral bone loss in revision shoulder arthroplasty. Orthop Clin N Am. 2020;51(1):87–95. https://doi.org/10.1016/j.ocl.2019.08.003.

5. Cuff D, Levy JC, Gutierrez S, Frankle MA. Torsional stability of modular and non-modular reverse shoulder humeral components in a proximal humeral bone loss model. J Shoulder Elbow Surg. 2011;20(4):646–51. https://doi.org/10.1016/j.jse.2010.10.026.
6. Boileau P. Complications and revision of reverse total shoulder arthroplasty. Orthop Traumatol Surg Res. 2016;102(Suppl. 1):S33–43. https://doi.org/10.1016/j.otsr.2015.06.031.
7. Chalmers PN, Rahman Z, Romeo AA, Nicholson GP. Early dislocation after reverse total shoulder arthroplasty. J Shoulder Elbow Surg. 2014;23(5):737–44. https://doi.org/10.1016/j.jse.2013.08.015.
8. Trappey GJ, O'Connor DP, Edwards TB. What are the instability and infection rates after reverse shoulder arthroplasty? Clin Orthop Rel Res. 2011;469(9):2505–11. https://doi.org/10.1007/s11999-010-1686-9.
9. Gallo RA, Gamradt SC, Mattern CJ, Cordasco FA, Craig EV, Dines DM, et al. Instability after reverse total shoulder replacement. J Shoulder Elbow Surg. 2011;20(4):584–90. https://doi.org/10.1016/j.jse.2010.08.028.
10. Roche CP, Diep P, Hamilton M, Crosby LA, Flurin PH, Wright TW, et al. Impact of inferior glenoid tilt, humeral retroversion, bone grafting, and design parameters on muscle length and deltoid wrapping in reverse shoulder arthroplasty. Bull Hosp Jt Dis. 2013;71(4):284–93.
11. Lemieux PO, Hagemeister N, Tetreault P, Nuno N. Influence of the medial offset of the proximal humerus on the glenohumeral destabilising forces during arm elevation: a numerical sensitivity study. Comput Methods Biomech Biomed Engin. 2013;16(1):103–11. https://doi.org/10.1080/10255842.2011.607813.
12. Garrigues GE, Zmistowski B, Cooper AM, Green A, Group ICMS. Proceedings from the 2018 International Consensus Meeting on Orthopedic Infections: the definition of periprosthetic shoulder infection. J Shoulder Elbow Surg. 2019;28(6S):S8–S12. https://doi.org/10.1016/j.jse.2019.04.034.
13. Nabergoj M, Denard PJ, Collin P, Trebse R, Ladermann A. Radiological changes, infections and neurological complications after reverse shoulder arthroplasty related to different design types and their rates: Part II. EFORT Open Rev. 2021;6(11):1109–21. https://doi.org/10.1302/2058-5241.6.210040.
14. McLendon PB, Cox JL, Frankle MA. Humeral bone loss in revision shoulder arthroplasty. Am J Orthop (Belle Mead NJ). 2018;47(2) https://doi.org/10.12788/ajo.2018.0012.
15. Chalmers PN, Romeo AA, Nicholson GP, Boileau P, Keener JD, Gregory JM, et al. Humeral bone loss in revision total shoulder arthroplasty: the Proximal Humeral Arthroplasty Revision Osseous inSufficiency (PHAROS) classification system. Clin Orthop Rel Res. 2019;477(2):432–41. https://doi.org/10.1097/CORR.0000000000000590.
16. Torrens C, Corrales M, Melendo E, Solano A, Rodríguez-Baeza A, Cáceres E. The pectoralis major tendon as a reference for restoring humeral length and retroversion with hemiarthroplasty for fracture. J Shoulder Elbow Surg. 2008;17(6):947–50. https://doi.org/10.1016/j.jse.2008.05.041.
17. Murachovsky J, Ikemoto RY, Nascimento LG, Fujiki EN, Milani C, Warner JJ. Pectoralis major tendon reference (PMT): a new method for accurate restoration of humeral length with hemiarthroplasty for fracture. J Shoulder Elbow Surg. 2006;15(6):675–8. https://doi.org/10.1016/j.jse.2005.12.011.
18. Reif T, Schoch B, Spiguel A, Elhassan B, Wright T, Sanchez-Sotelo J, et al. A retrospective review of revision proximal humeral allograft-prosthetic composite procedures: an analysis of proximal humeral bone stock restoration. J Shoulder Elbow Surg. 2020;29(7):1353–8. https://doi.org/10.1016/j.jse.2019.10.029.
19. Boileau P, Raynier JL, Chelli M, Gonzalez JF, Galvin JW. Reverse shoulder-allograft prosthesis composite, with or without tendon transfer, for the treatment of severe proximal humeral bone loss. J Shoulder Elbow Surg. 2020;29(11):e401–e15. https://doi.org/10.1016/j.jse.2020.03.016.
20. Sanchez-Sotelo J, Wagner ER, Houdek MT. Allograft-prosthetic composite reconstruction for massive proximal humeral bone loss in reverse shoulder arthroplasty. JBJS Essent Surg Tech. 2018;8(1):e3. https://doi.org/10.2106/JBJS.ST.17.00051.
21. Friedman LGM, Garrigues GE. Management of humeral and glenoid bone defects in reverse shoulder arthroplasty. J Am Acad Orthop Surg. 2021;29(17):e846–e59. https://doi.org/10.5435/JAAOS-D-20-00964.
22. Cox JL, McLendon PB, Christmas KN, Simon P, Mighell MA, Frankle MA. Clinical outcomes following reverse shoulder arthroplasty-allograft composite for revision of failed arthroplasty associated with proximal humeral bone deficiency: 2- to 15-year follow-up. J Shoulder Elbow Surg. 2019;28(5):900–7. https://doi.org/10.1016/j.jse.2018.10.023.
23. Guven MF, Aslan L, Botanlioglu H, Kaynak G, Kesmezacar H, Babacan M. Functional outcome of reverse shoulder tumor prosthesis in the treatment of proximal humerus tumors. J Shoulder Elbow Surg. 2016;25(1):e1–6. https://doi.org/10.1016/j.jse.2015.06.012.
24. Potter BK, Adams SC, Pitcher JD Jr, Malinin TI, Temple HT. Proximal humerus reconstructions for tumors. Clin Orthop Rel Res. 2009;467(4):1035–41. https://doi.org/10.1007/s11999-008-0531-x.

24 Periprosthetic Humeral Fracture: Management and Outcomes

Fabrizio Mocini, Lorenzo Proietti, Dario Candura, Gianluca Ciolli, Katia Corona, and Simone Cerciello

24.1 Background

In the last 30 years, there here has been a progressive increase in the number of total shoulder arthroplasty (TSA) surgeries (369% from 1993 to 2007) due to the expansion of the indications and to aging of population [1]. More recently, in the last decade, the frequency increased 2.5-fold [2, 3]. Current evidence shows that primary, anatomic TSA improves both pain and function in up to 90–95% of patients [4, 5] and reverse total shoulder arthroplasty (rTSA) is effective in treating rotator cuff arthropathy, as well as failure of primary anatomic TSA [6–9]. Although long-term data show the survivorship of these implants at 10 years and 20 years is over 90% and 80%, respectively [10, 11], the direct consequence of the increased volume of implants is the increased number of intraoperative or postoperative complications. Complications rate ranges from 19 to 68% [12] and although earlier studies suggested a higher overall complication rate in rTSA when compared to anatomic TSA, more recent reports show more contradictory results [13]. A recent systematic review showed an overall downward trend in complications over the last decade overall probably because of improved implant designs and surgical technique [12]. Finally, the incidence of complications requiring reoperation is 5–11% and has been shown to be more frequent following revision procedures [14]. The most common complications are infection, instability, neurologic injury, stiffness, tuberosity migration, and periprosthetic fractures. Periprosthetic fractures incidence ranges from 1.6 to 2.8% for anatomic TSA, up to 2.3% for hemiarthroplasty, and up to 3.45% in the rTSA where the fracture represents 20% of whole complications [12, 15, 16]. They can occur intraoperatively or in the early or late postoperative period [17, 18]. Periprosthetic shoulder fractures include fractures of the acromion and spine of the scapula, of the glenoid, and of the humerus (PHF).

The incidence of PHF widely ranges across the literature (1.2–19.4%) [15, 18]. They are particularly relevant as they have a higher non-union rate than native humerus fractures [19], and therefore, they frequently lead to the need for revision surgery [20]. These fractures can occur both intraoperatively or postoperatively

F. Mocini (✉) · L. Proietti
Casa di Cura Villa Betania, Rome, Italy

D. Candura · G. Ciolli
Fondazione Policlinico Universitario Agostino Gemelli, Rome, Italy

K. Corona
Department of Medicine and Health Sciences "Vincenzo Tiberio", University of Molise, Campobasso, Italy
e-mail: katia.corona@unimol.it

S. Cerciello
Casa di Cura Villa Betania, Rome, Italy

Fondazione Policlinico Universitario Agostino Gemelli, Rome, Italy

F. Franceschi et al. (eds.), *Revision Shoulder Arthroplasty*,
https://doi.org/10.1007/978-3-031-45944-3_24

(0.9–3.5% and 1.0–3.0% of the time respectively) [21, 22]. They are more frequent during revision procedures, especially during extraction of a well-fixed humeral stem [23].

24.2 Risk Factors

The risk factors for PHF can be divided into two main categories: patient related and surgery related.

24.2.1 Patient-Related Risk Factors

Patient related risk factors include female sex (more associated with intraoperative fractures), advanced age, poor bone quality (osteoporosis, osteonecrosis, or rheumatoid arthritis), posttraumatic glenohumeral arthritis, higher number of medical comorbidities, and all conditions that increase the risk of falling such as neurological (with dementia increasing the risk by 27% compared to a patient without), cardiovascular diseases or diabetes (due to hypoglycemic episodes) [15, 24]. When analyzing risk factors for intraoperative and postoperative PHF interesting data emerge. Female sex (odds ratio [OR], 4.19) and post-traumatic arthritis (OR, 2.55) have to be considered important risk factors for an intraoperative PHF [15]. Underlying comorbidities, as measured by the Deyo-Charlson index (OR, 1.27), has shown to be a risk factor for postoperative PHF [15]. Osteonecrosis is another risk factor for postoperative PHF: the incidence in patients with corticosteroid-induced osteonecrosis was 6.0%, compared with 1.5% in the control group ($p = 0.002$), 5.0% in alcohol-related osteonecrosis (n.s.), and 5.9% posttraumatic osteonecrosis (n.s.) [25].

24.2.2 Surgery-Related Risk Factors

Factors related to surgery are adjacent implants such as elbow prostheses or prior osteosynthesis and preexisting humeral deformities due to the presence of altered humeral contours, stress riser formation, and local osteopenia [26]. Uncemented stems were thought to be at risk for PHF (proximal metaphysis and greater tuberosity) due to the stress-shielding that occurs proximally. However, several studies revealed no difference between cemented and cementless prostheses [27, 28]. Intraoperative fractures are less common in primary cases than revisions and usually occur during reaming or broaching of the humerus (up to 31%) during trial or implant insertion (up to 18–19%), or because of excessive humeral torque or forceful retractor placement during exposure or reduction (up to 13–15%) [29]. Revision procedures are at greater risk of intra-operative fracture, which is estimated at 3.3% compared to 1.2% for primary procedures (RR, 2.8) [18]. They usually occur during implant removal (up to 81%) and tend to involve the greater tuberosity at the proximal implant-bone interface [29]. The reported PHF rate is 16% when revising RSA or TSA to TSA, with specific risk factors including female sex (OR, 2.41), history of instability (OR, 2.65), and a prior hemiarthroplasty (OR, 2.34) [29]. The increased risk in revision surgery is often the consequence of aggressive soft tissue retraction and torsional solicitations on the humerus to expose the joint in presence of extensive scar tissue in the deltopectoral interval, subacromial space, around the rotator cuff, and capsule. Finally, implant removal often requires extensive use of scalpels, which increases the risk of humeral fracture especially at the level of the tuberosities.

24.3 Diagnosis

Most PHF occur after traumatic events, most of which are falls with the arm extended [17, 30, 31]. In most cases, the diagnosis of a PHF is quite simple and is based primarily on the history of a trauma and clinical examination. In rare cases, PHF can occur even without trauma, due to the continuous stress effect of the implant to the bone, leading to cortical weakening [17, 32].

Clinical manifestations are those of any fracture and include pain, functional impotence, hematoma, and preternatural movement. During the examination, it is very important to evaluate any neurovascular involvement.

Radiographs are useful to show the fracture pattern, the type of implant, any humeral deformities, and signs of osteolysis with the Grashey and axillary views being the most useful. A CT scan with metal suppression is usually performed because it provides more detailed information of the fracture pattern, implant loosening, bone stock and quality, glenoid retroversion, and the state of the rotator cuff [5, 33].

It is essential to evaluate the stability of the stem to plan an adequate treatment. If there are radiolucent lines greater than 2 mm in at least 3 of the 8 humeral areas described by Sperling et al., the risk of stem loosening is very high and it is necessary to plan a revision of the stem as well as fracture fixation [34, 35].

24.4 Classification

Over the years, numerous classifications have been developed for PHF and there is not one that is uniquely used. The oldest is the one by Wright and Cofield, published in 1995 that divides fractures into three categories based on their relationship to the stem: type A includes fractures that start at the tip of the stem and extend proximally for more than a third of the length of the stem, type B includes fractures which extend from the tip of the stem proximally less than one third of the length of the stem, and type c includes fractures distal to the stem [36] (Fig. 24.1). A second classification system was proposed by Campbell et al. in 1998 dividing PHF into 4 types according to the fracture location: tuberosities (type A), metaphysis (type B), proximal shaft (type C), middle and distal shaft (type D) [37] (Fig. 24.2). A similar classification was proposed by Worland et al. in 1999 with type A fractures occurring at the level of the tuberosities, type B at the level of the stem (further subdivided into B1 if spiral, B2 if oblique, and B3 if associated with mobilized implant), and type C distal to the stem [31]. The authors suggested conservative treatment with bracing in case of type B2 fractures and surgery in case of type B3 fractures. Duncan et al. proposed a classification system which is based on the stability of the implant, patient's bone quality, and location of the fracture in relation to soft tissue insertions [38]. Groh et al. in 2008 published a new classification based on the relationship between the fracture and the stem. Type 1 fractures are proximal to the tip of the stem, type 2 are proximal to the tip of the stem but extend distally, and type 3 are distal to the stem [39] (Fig. 24.3). The most recent classification is the one by Kirchhoff et al. in 2018 and it takes into account several aspects such as the fracture pattern, the prosthetic design on the humerus and glenoid, and the integrity of the rotator cuff (Fig. 24.4). The 6 sub-categories: prosthesis type (stemless, anatomic, reversed), fracture location (humeral, glenoidal, or acromial), presence of a glenoid component, rotator cuff condition, relation of the fracture to the stem, and implant stability (stable or loose) allowed for an algorithm of treatment [40] (Fig. 24.5).

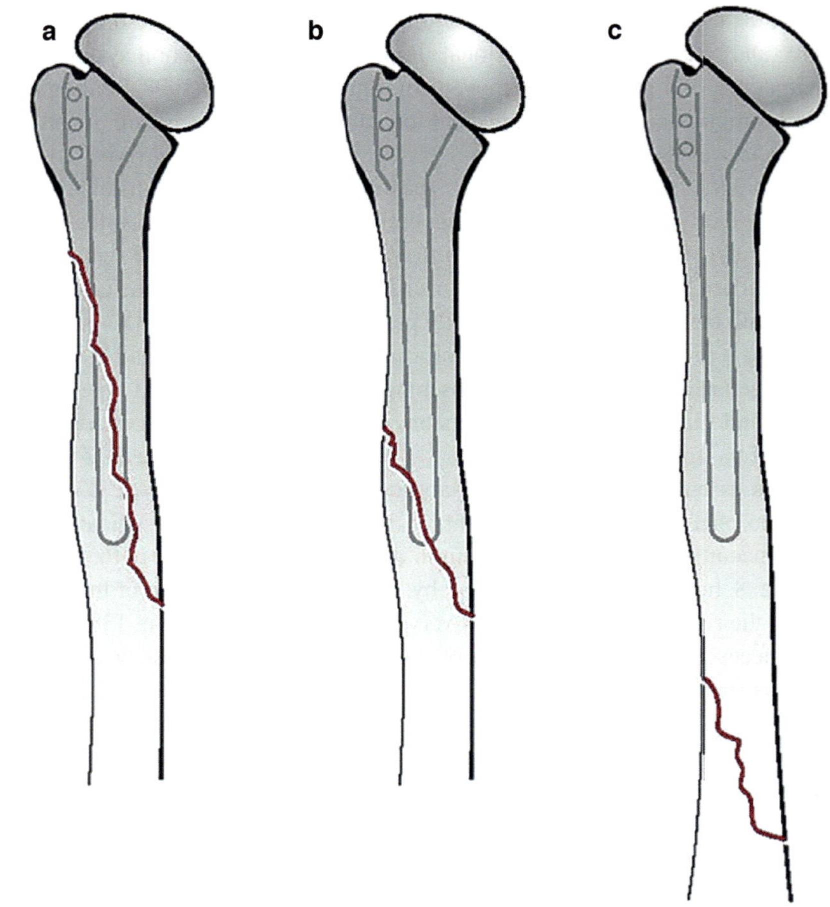

Fig. 24.1 The Wright and Cofield classification of periprosthetic humeral fractures (1995). Type (**a**) fractures begin at the tip of the prosthesis and extend proximally. Type (**b**) fractures begin at the tip of the prosthesis and extend distally. Type (**c**) fractures occur well distal to the stem. (Source: T. W. Wright and R. H. Cofield, “Humeral fractures after shoulder arthroplasty,” J Bone Joint Surg Am, vol. 77, no. 9, pp. 1340–1346, Sep. 1995, doi: 10.2106/00004623-1995 09000-00008)

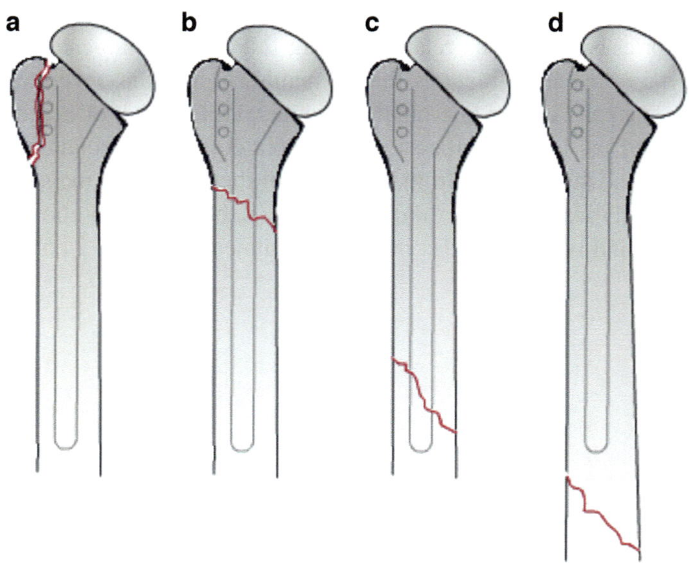

Fig. 24.2 Campbell et al. classification (1998). Type (**a**) Fracture of the greater or lesser tuberosity; Type (**b**) Fracture of the proximal humeral metaphysis. Type (**c**) Fracture of the proximal humeral diaphysis; Type (**d**) Fracture of the mid and distal humeral shaft. (Source: J. T. Campbell, R. S. Moore, J. P. Iannotti, T. R. Norris, and G. R. Williams, “Periprosthetic humeral fractures: mechanisms of fracture and treatment options,” J Shoulder Elbow Surg, vol. 7, no. 4, pp. 406–413, Aug. 1998, doi: 10.1016/s1058-2746(98)90033-7)

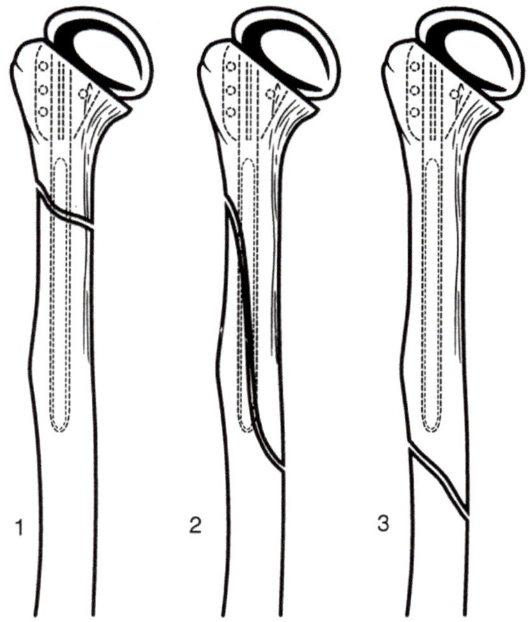

Fig. 24.3 Groh et al. classification (2008). Type I fractures occur proximal to the tip of the prosthesis. Type II fractures occur proximal to the tip of the prosthesis and extend beyond the tip. Type III fractures originate below the tip of the prosthesis. (Source: G. I. Groh, M. M. Heckman, M. A. Wirth, R. J. Curtis, and C. A. Rockwood, "Treatment of fractures adjacent to humeral prostheses," J Shoulder Elbow Surg, vol. 17, no. 1, pp. 85–89, Feb. 2008, doi: 10.1016/j.jse.2007.05.007)

Type	Localisation	Glenoid	Cuff	Height	Prosthesis	Therapy
A Stemless 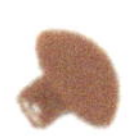	A acromial G glenoidal H humeral	H Hemi T Total	I Intact T Tear	1 Tuberosities 4 Distal 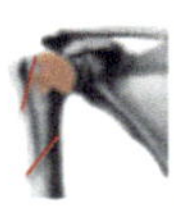	S stable L loose	A-A-X-X-X-X → conservative vs. ORIF A-G-H-I-X-X → conservative vs. ORIF vs. TEP A-G-H-T-X-X → convert to reversed A-G-T-I-X-S → conservative A-G-T-I-X-L → revision glenoid A-G-T-T-X-X → convert to reversed A-H-H-I-1-S → ORIF A-H-H-I-1-L → convert to anatomic stem A-H-H-T-1-L → convert to reversed A-H-H-T-4-L → convert to reversed + ORIF vs. reversed long stem
B Anatomic 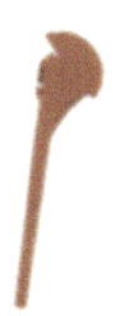	A acromial G glenoidal H humeral	H Hemi T Total	I Intact T Tear	1 Tuberosities 2 Spiral 3 Oblique 4 Distal 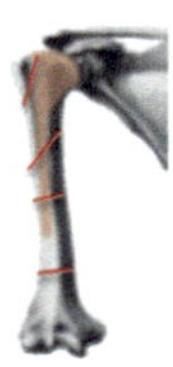	S stable L loose	B-A-X-X-X-X → conservative vs. ORIF B-G-H-I-X-X → conservative vs. ORIF vs. TEP B-G-H-T-X-X → convert to reversed B-G-T-I-X-S → conservative B-G-T-I-X-L → revision glenoid B-G-T-T-X-X → convert to reversed B-H-H-I-X-S → ORIF B-H-H-I-X-L → revise to TEP + new stem B-H-H-T-X-S → convert to reversed B-H-H-T-1-L → convert to reversed B-H-H-T-2-L → convert to reversed + ORIF B-H-H-T-3-L → convert to reversed + long stem B-H-H-T-4-L → convert to reversed long stem + ORIF
C Reversed 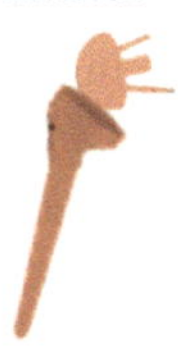	A acromial G glenoidal H humeral			1 Tuberosities 2 Spiral 3 Oblique 4 Distal 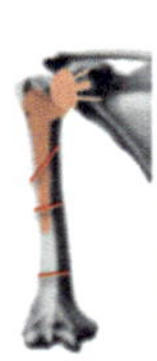	S stable L loose	C-A-X-X → conservative vs. ORIF C-G-X-L → revision glenoid C-H-1-S → conservative vs. ORIF C-H-2-S → ORIF C-H-3-S → ORIF C-H-X-L → convert to reversed long stem vs. convert to reversed long stem + ORIF

Fig. 24.4 Kirchhoff classification system. (Source: C. Kirchhoff, M. Beirer, and U. Brunner, "Periprothetische Humerusfraktur: Strategien und Techniken der Revisionsendoprothetik," Unfallchirurg, vol. 119, no. 4, pp. 281–287, Apr. 2016, doi: 10.1007/s00113-016-0158-4)

Type	Treatment	Type	Treatment	Type	Treatment
A-A-X-X-X-X	Conservative vs ORIF	B-A-X-X-X-X	Conservative vs ORIF	C-A-X-X	Conservative vs ORIF
A-G-H-I-X-X	Conservative vs ORIF vs TEP	B-G-H-I-X-X	Conservative vs ORIF vs TEP	C-G-X-L	Revision glenoid
A-G-H-T-X-X	Convert to reversed	B-G-H-T-X-X	Convert to reversed	C-H-1-S	Conservative vs ORIF
A-G-T-I-X-S	Conservative	B-G-T-I-X-S	Conservative	C-H-2-S	ORIF
A-G-T-I-X-L	Revise glenoid	B-G-T-I-X-L	Revision glenoid	C-H-3-S	ORIF
A-G-T-T-X-X	Convert to reversed	B-G-T-T-X-X	Convert to reversed	C-H-X-L	Convert to reversed long stem +/- ORIF
A-H-H-I-1-S	ORIF	B-H-H-I-X-S	ORIF		
A-H-H-I-1-L	Convert to anatomic stem	B-H-H-I-X-L	Revise to TEP + new stem		
A-H-H-T-1-L	Convert to reversed	B-H-H-T-X-S	Convert to reversed		
A-H-H-T-4-L	Convert to reversed + ORIF vs reversed long stem	B-H-H-T-1-L	Convert to reversed		
		B-H-H-T-2-L	Convert to reversed + ORIF		
		B-H-H-T-3-L	Convert to reversed + long stem		
		B-H-H-T-4-L	Convert to reversed long stem + ORIF		

Fig. 24.5 Treatment algorithm based on Kirchhoff's classification. (Source: Gebrelul A, Green A, Schacherer T, Khazzam M. Periprosthetic humerus fractures: classification, management, and review of the literature. Ann Joint 2018;3:49. doi: 10.21037/aoj.2018.06.02)

24.5 Treatment

The correct management of a PHF must consider many variables. The first major distinction must be made between intraoperative and postoperative fractures. Other characteristics that affect the choice of treatment are: the type of fracture and its location, the age and sex of the patient and his functional requirements, any comorbidities, the quality of the bone, the stability of the humeral stem [41]. The treatment of a PHF ranges from conservative treatment, to ORIF, up to revision arthroplasty.

24.5.1 Intraoperative Fractures

They account for approximately three quarters of all PHF and about 50% of these occurred in the diaphyseal region of the humeral shaft [37]. The reasons for intraoperative fractures are a combination of poor bone quality and poor surgical techniques. The steps at greatest risk of fracture during primary implants are the reaming of the humerus and the external rotation of the arm for exposure of the glenoid [42]. For this reason, there is a greater risk of humeral fracture in total prostheses than in endoprostheses [31]. In revision surgery also, the step at greatest risk of fracture is the removal of the humeral stem due to the rigidity and contracture of the soft tissues (up to 81%) [29]. To try to minimise the risk of fracture, it is important to practice adequate and careful dissection of the soft tissues, use specific implant extraction tools, and when necessary, practice techniques such as corticotomy or humeral shaft windows to reduce the force to remove the stem. The use of modular and convertible implants could reduce the need to remove the stem and the incidence of fractures. The aim of the treatment is to achieve solid internal fixation to prevent any delay in patient's postoperative rehabilitation [27]. Fractures of the greater tuberosity are at risk of displacement due to the rotator cuff pull and must be carefully followed.

Non-displaced fractures that do not extend distally are usually treated with temporary immobilization [18]. Displaced fractures of the tuberosities are generally managed with suture or cerclage wiring [21, 39] or by converting to a reverse arthroplasty, depending on the clinical condition. Sutures or cable cerclages are also indicated in case of tuberosity fractures involving the metaphyseal area. The treatment of humeral shaft fractures depend on their location, when they are proximal to the tip of the stem they usually require longer stem that exceed the fracture location by at least 2–3 cortical diameters with the addition of plates and cerclages and with or without allograft struts [23]. Fractures distal to the stem require internal fixation with hybrid plate/cerclage wire [39].

24.5.2 Postoperative Fractures

In case of fractures with minimal displacement and without stem loosening, conservative treatment with a brace is indicated, although the results reported in literature indicate an unsatisfactory healing rate [32]. Conservative treatment is not recommended in case of obese patients or female patients with large breasts as the body mass tends to abduct the arm and can result in varus displacement. Sometimes, conservative treatment is indicated in case of displaced fractures in those patients who have very low functional requirements or high risks to undergo surgery [40]. Fractures involving the tuberosities in an anatomic arthroplasty are usually managed with transosseous sutures or by conversion to reverse implants. In the event of fractures in the metaphyseal or diaphyseal region of the humerus, the stability of the stem must first be considered. If the stem is stable, an osteosynthesis with plate and screws is carried out leaving the original implant in place; conversely, if the stem is loose, it is necessary to replace it with the longer stem and additional osteosynthesis with plate and screws, and cerclage wires with the possibility of additional strut graft to achieve a biologic support [43, 44]. In case of ORIF, the use of a single 4.5 mm plate is usually sufficient to ensure adequate stability. The use of a double plate has been described in the literature but has never been supported by valid biomechanical data.

When the revision of the stem is needed it is possible to choose whether or not to cement it depending on the quality of the bone and the design of the implant. Up to date, the literature does not report statistically significant clinical results between the two options [45]. When revising the humeral stem, it is important the tip of the implant exceeds at least 2–3 cortical diameters, the most distal part of the fracture, to avoid creating areas of increased stress on the metal bone interface [37]. Different surgical approaches can be used in the setting of fracture reduction and internal fixation, and they depend both on the type and location of the fracture and on the experience of the surgeon. Usually, the deltopectoral and the lateral approaches are used for proximal humerus fractures, and the posterior approach is considered for more distal fractures. Valenti et al. [46] suggested the deltopectoral approach to make stem extraction easier avoiding excessive torsional forces and thus reducing the risk of fracture of the humeral shaft. Identification and exploration of the radial nerve, which can often be involved in bony fragments or in the reduction and osteosynthesis maneuvers, is always recommended, especially before the passage of the cerclage wires, to avoid its entrapment [47].

In complex cases, fracture management can be difficult. In the setting of multiple revisions with poor residual bone stock, restoring the function of the arm can be very challenging. Many surgical techniques have been described in the literature [48]. A cortical strut allograft is the most common option to add structural and biologic support to the osteosynthesis. In case of diaphyseal bone loss, an interesting technique is the one described by Thes et al. [49] in which two hemi cylinders of tibial allografts are placed against each other to create a knock around the fracture called sarcophagus and fixed with cerclage wires. When there is a bone loss of the proximal humerus and the metaphyseal area, which extends distally for more than 5 cm, a viable option is the use of allograft-prosthesis composite [50]. Finally, in cases where a graft is not available, modular implants derived from oncology can be used; in fact, they allow the reconstruction of large bone defects [51]. The postoperative course involves immobilization in a sling for 4–6 weeks depending on the stability of the osteosynthesis, and the clinical characteristics of the patient. Then, initially passive, and subsequently active mobilization is progressively allowed. Radiographic checks are normally performed at 1, 3, and 6 months.

The reported complication rate of these operations ranges from 20 to 40% with the most frequent complication being non-union or malunion (especially in conservatively treated fractures) having a rate up to 13% at 18 weeks [52]. Other complications with a fairly high rate of frequency are radial nerve apraxia, adhesive capsulitis, and wound infection.

24.6 Outcomes

Union rate after surgery is high. Andersen et al. analyzed the outcomes in a series of 36 patients treated either with revision arthroplasty or ORIF. They reported a union rate of 97% and a statistically significant increase in ASES score [53]. However, they reported a 39% complication rate and 19% reoperation rate.

Other studies have shown similar data with notable complication rates and although an increase was observed in all clinical parameters, patients did not recover a shoulder function comparable to what they had after the index procedure [30, 36].

24.7 Conclusions

Although not very frequent, PHF are an emerging problem over the years due to the increased number of shoulder arthroplasty performed and represent a severe complication worsening the clinical outcomes. Correct PHF management is based on the pattern of the fractures and their relation to the implant and on the characteristics of the patient. Several classification systems have been proposed, and they help to choose the most suitable treatment option. Conservative treatment is used only in fractures with non or minimal displacement or in those patients with very low functional demand. In all other cases, surgery is indicated and includes ORIF with plate and screws and wire cerclages if the implant is stable, or revision with a longer stem (cemented or press-fit) and additional osteosynthesis if the implant is mobilized. More complex cases with severe bone loss are treated using strut graft or modular implants. A correct indication and intraoperative and post-operative management normally lead to satisfactory results, although the complication rate is relatively high. Future research will have to establish a unique treatment algorithm and new solutions for more complex cases.

References

1. Day JS, Lau E, Ong KL, Williams GR, Ramsey ML, Kurtz SM. Prevalence and projections of total shoulder and elbow arthroplasty in the United States to 2015. J Shoulder Elb Surg. 2010;19(8):1115–20. https://doi.org/10.1016/j.jse.2010.02.009.
2. Kim SH, Wise BL, Zhang Y, Szabo RM. Increasing incidence of shoulder arthroplasty in the United States. J Bone Jt Surg Am. 2011;93(24):2249–54. https://doi.org/10.2106/JBJS.J.01994.
3. Roberson TA, et al. Outcomes of total shoulder arthroplasty in patients younger than 65 years: a systematic review. J Shoulder Elb Surg. 2017;26(7):1298–306. https://doi.org/10.1016/j.jse.2016.12.069.
4. Norris TR, Iannotti JP. Functional outcome after shoulder arthroplasty for primary osteoarthritis: a multicenter study. J Shoulder Elb Surg. 2002;11(2):130–5. https://doi.org/10.1067/mse.2002.121146.
5. Buck FM, Jost B, Hodler J. Shoulder arthroplasty. Eur Radiol. 2008;18(12):2937–48. https://doi.org/10.1007/s00330-008-1093-8.
6. Gerber C, Pennington SD, Nyffeler RW. Reverse total shoulder arthroplasty. J Am Acad Orthop Surg. 2009;17(5):284–95. https://doi.org/10.5435/00124635-200905000-00003.
7. Boileau P, Gonzalez J-F, Chuinard C, Bicknell R, Walch G. Reverse total shoulder arthroplasty after failed rotator cuff surgery. J Shoulder Elb Surg. 2009;18(4):600–6. https://doi.org/10.1016/j.jse.2009.03.011.
8. Cuff DJ, Pupello DR, Santoni BG, Clark RE, Frankle MA. Reverse shoulder arthroplasty for the treatment of rotator cuff deficiency: a concise follow-up, at a minimum of 10 years, of previous reports. J Bone Jt Surg Am. 2017;99(22):1895–9. https://doi.org/10.2106/JBJS.17.00175.
9. Vanhove B, Beugnies A. Grammont's reverse shoulder prosthesis for rotator cuff arthropathy. A retrospective study of 32 cases. Acta Orthop Belg. 2004;70(3):219–25.
10. Cil A, Veillette CJH, Sanchez-Sotelo J, Sperling JW, Schleck CD, Cofield RH. Survivorship of the humeral

component in shoulder arthroplasty. J Shoulder Elb Surg. 2010;19(1):143–50. https://doi.org/10.1016/j.jse.2009.04.011.
11. Favard L, Levigne C, Nerot C, Gerber C, De Wilde L, Mole D. Reverse prostheses in arthropathies with cuff tear: are survivorship and function maintained over time? Clin Orthop Relat Res. 2011;469(9):2469–75. https://doi.org/10.1007/s11999-011-1833-y.
12. Bohsali KI, Bois AJ, Wirth MA. Complications of shoulder arthroplasty. J Bone Jt Surg Am. 2017;99(3):256–69. https://doi.org/10.2106/JBJS.16.00935.
13. Kiet TK, et al. Outcomes after shoulder replacement: comparison between reverse and anatomic total shoulder arthroplasty. J Shoulder Elb Surg. 2015;24(2):179–85. https://doi.org/10.1016/j.jse.2014.06.039.
14. Gonzalez J-F, Alami GB, Baque F, Walch G, Boileau P. Complications of unconstrained shoulder prostheses. J Shoulder Elb Surg. 2011;20(4):666–82. https://doi.org/10.1016/j.jse.2010.11.017.
15. Singh JA, Sperling J, Schleck C, Harmsen W, Cofield R. Periprosthetic fractures associated with primary total shoulder arthroplasty and primary humeral head replacement: a 33-year study. J Bone Jt Surg Am. 2012;94(19):1777–85. https://doi.org/10.2106/JBJS.J.01945.
16. Zumstein MA, Pinedo M, Old J, Boileau P. Problems, complications, reoperations, and revisions in reverse total shoulder arthroplasty: a systematic review. J Shoulder Elb Surg. 2011;20(1):146–57. https://doi.org/10.1016/j.jse.2010.08.001.
17. Greiner S, Stein V, Scheibel M. Periprosthetic humeral fractures after shoulder and elbow arthroplasty. Acta Chir Orthop Traumatol Cechoslov. 2011;78(6):490–500.
18. Athwal GS, Sperling JW, Rispoli DM, Cofield RH. Periprosthetic humeral fractures during shoulder arthroplasty. J Bone Jt Surg Am. 2009;91(3):594–603. https://doi.org/10.2106/JBJS.H.00439.
19. Choo AMT, Hawkins RH, Kwon BK, Oxland TR. The effect of shoulder arthroplasty on humeral strength: an in vitro biomechanical investigation. Clin Biomech (Bristol, Avon). 2005;20(10):1064–71. https://doi.org/10.1016/j.clinbiomech.2005.06.013.
20. Ingoe HM, Holland P, Cowling P, Kottam L, Baker PN, Rangan A. Intraoperative complications during revision shoulder arthroplasty: a study using the National Joint Registry dataset. Shoulder Elb. 2017;9(2):92–9. https://doi.org/10.1177/1758573216685706.
21. García-Fernández C, Lópiz-Morales Y, Rodríguez A, López-Durán L, Martínez FM. Periprosthetic humeral fractures associated with reverse total shoulder arthroplasty: incidence and management. Int Orthop. 2015;39(10):1965–9. https://doi.org/10.1007/s00264-015-2972-7.
22. Della Rocca GJ, Leung KS, Pape H-C. Periprosthetic fractures: epidemiology and future projections. J Orthop Trauma. 2011;25(Suppl 2):S66–70. https://doi.org/10.1097/BOT.0b013e31821b8c28.
23. Steinmann SP, Cheung EV. Treatment of periprosthetic humerus fractures associated with shoulder arthroplasty. J Am Acad Orthop Surg. 2008;16(4):199–207. https://doi.org/10.5435/00124635-200804000-00003.
24. Ziere G, Dieleman JP, Hofman A, Pols HA, Van Der Cammen TJ, Stricker BC. Polypharmacy and falls in the middle age and elderly population. Br J Clin Pharmacol. 2006;61(2):218–23. https://doi.org/10.1111/j.1365-2125.2005.02543.x.
25. Burrus MT, Cancienne JM, Boatright JD, Yang S, Brockmeier SF, Werner BC. Shoulder arthroplasty for humeral head avascular necrosis is associated with increased postoperative complications. HSS J. 2018;14(1):2–8. https://doi.org/10.1007/s11420-017-9562-8.
26. Carroll EA, Lorich DG, Helfet DL. Surgical management of a periprosthetic fracture between a total elbow and total shoulder prostheses: a case report. J Shoulder Elb Surg. 2009;18(3):e9–12. https://doi.org/10.1016/j.jse.2008.10.003.
27. Williams GR, Iannotti JP. Management of periprosthetic fractures: the shoulder. J Arthroplast. 2002;17(4 Suppl 1):14–6. https://doi.org/10.1054/arth.2002.32683.
28. Werthel J-D, Lonjon G, Jo S, Cofield R, Sperling JW, Elhassan BT. Long-term outcomes of cemented versus cementless humeral components in arthroplasty of the shoulder: a propensity score-matched analysis. Bone Jt J. 2017;99-B(5):666–73. https://doi.org/10.1302/0301-620X.99B5.BJJ-2016-0910.R1.
29. Wagner ER, Houdek MT, Elhassan BT, Sanchez-Sotelo J, Cofield RH, Sperling JW. What are risk factors for intraoperative humerus fractures during revision reverse shoulder arthroplasty and do they influence outcomes? Clin Orthop Relat Res. 2015;473(10):3228–34. https://doi.org/10.1007/s11999-015-4448-x.
30. Boyd AD, Thornhill TS, Barnes CL. Fractures adjacent to humeral prostheses. J Bone Jt Surg Am. 1992;74(10):1498–504.
31. Worland RL, Kim DY, Arredondo J. Periprosthetic humeral fractures: management and classification. J Shoulder Elb Surg. 1999;8(6):590–4. https://doi.org/10.1016/s1058-2746(99)90095-2.
32. Kumar S, Sperling JW, Haidukewych GH, Cofield RH. Periprosthetic humeral fractures after shoulder arthroplasty. J Bone Jt Surg Am. 2004;86(4):680–9. https://doi.org/10.2106/00004623-200404000-00003.
33. Gilot G, et al. The incidence of radiographic aseptic loosening of the humeral component in reverse total shoulder arthroplasty. J Shoulder Elb Surg. 2015;24(10):1555–9. https://doi.org/10.1016/j.jse.2015.02.007.
34. Sperling JW, Cofield RH, O'Driscoll SW, Torchia ME, Rowland CM. Radiographic assessment of ingrowth total shoulder arthroplasty. J Shoulder Elb Surg. 2000;9(6):507–13. https://doi.org/10.1067/mse.2000.109384.
35. Sanchez-Sotelo J, O'Driscoll SW, Torchia ME, Cofield RH, Rowland CM. Radiographic assessment

of cemented humeral components in shoulder arthroplasty. J Shoulder Elb Surg. 2001;10(6):526–31. https://doi.org/10.1067/mse.2001.118482.
36. Wright TW, Cofield RH. Humeral fractures after shoulder arthroplasty. J Bone Jt Surg Am. 1995;77(9):1340–6. https://doi.org/10.2106/00004623-199509000-00008.
37. Campbell JT, Moore RS, Iannotti JP, Norris TR, Williams GR. Periprosthetic humeral fractures: mechanisms of fracture and treatment options. J Shoulder Elb Surg. 1998;7(4):406–13. https://doi.org/10.1016/s1058-2746(98)90033-7.
38. Duncan CP, Haddad FS. The Unified Classification System (UCS): improving our understanding of periprosthetic fractures. Bone Jt J. 2014;96-B(6):713–6. https://doi.org/10.1302/0301-620X.96B6.34040.
39. Groh GI, Heckman MM, Wirth MA, Curtis RJ, Rockwood CA. Treatment of fractures adjacent to humeral prostheses. J Shoulder Elb Surg. 2008;17(1):85–9. https://doi.org/10.1016/j.jse.2007.05.007.
40. Kirchhoff C, Beirer M, Brunner U. Periprothetische Humerusfraktur: Strategien und Techniken der Revisionsendoprothetik. Unfallchirurg. 2016;119(4):281–7. https://doi.org/10.1007/s00113-016-0158-4.
41. Cho C-H, Song K-S, Koo T-W. Clinical outcomes and complications during the learning curve for reverse total shoulder arthroplasty: an analysis of the first 40 cases. Clin Orthop Surg. 2017;9(2):213–7. https://doi.org/10.4055/cios.2017.9.2.213.
42. Brusalis CM, Taylor SA. Periprosthetic fractures in reverse total shoulder arthroplasty: current concepts and advances in management. Curr Rev Musculoskelet Med. 2020;13(4):509–19. https://doi.org/10.1007/s12178-020-09654-8.
43. Kirchhoff C, Brunner U, Biberthaler P. Periprosthetic humeral fractures: strategies and techniques for osteosynthesis. Unfallchirurg. 2016;119(4):273–80. https://doi.org/10.1007/s00113-016-0161-9.
44. Updegrove GF, Mourad W, Abboud JA. Humeral shaft fractures. J Shoulder Elb Surg. 2018;27(4):e87–97. https://doi.org/10.1016/j.jse.2017.10.028.
45. King JJ, Farmer KW, Struk AM, Wright TW. Uncemented versus cemented humeral stem fixation in reverse shoulder arthroplasty. Int Orthop. 2015;39(2):291–8. https://doi.org/10.1007/s00264-014-2593-6.
46. Valenti P, Kilinc AS, Sauzières P, Katz D. Results of 30 reverse shoulder prostheses for revision of failed hemi- or total shoulder arthroplasty. Eur J Orthop Surg Traumatol. 2014;24(8):1375–82. https://doi.org/10.1007/s00590-013-1332-9.
47. Fu MC, Hendel MD, Chen X, Warren RF, Dines DM, Gulotta LV. Surgical anatomy of the radial nerve in the deltopectoral approach for revision shoulder arthroplasty and periprosthetic fracture fixation: a cadaveric study. J Shoulder Elb Surg. 2017;26(12):2173–6. https://doi.org/10.1016/j.jse.2017.07.021.
48. Sewell MD, Kang SN, Al-Hadithy N, Higgs DS, Bayley I, Falworth M, Lambert SM. Management of peri-prosthetic fracture of the humerus with severe bone loss and loosening of the humeral component after total shoulder replacement. J Bone Jt Surg Br. 2012;94:1382–9.
49. Thés A, Klouche S, de Tienda M, Bauer T, Hardy P. Cortical onlay strut allograft with cerclage wiring of periprosthetic fractures of the humerus without stem loosening: technique and preliminary results. Eur J Orthop Surg Traumatol. 2017;27(4):553–7. https://doi.org/10.1007/s00590-017-1961-5.
50. McLendon PB, Cox JL, Frankle MA. Humeral bone loss in revision shoulder arthroplasty. Am J Orthop (Belle Mead NJ). 2018;47(2):12. https://doi.org/10.12788/ajo.2018.0012.
51. Wang ML, Ballard BL, Kulidjian AA, Abrams RA. Upper extremity reconstruction with a humeral tumor endoprosthesis: a novel salvage procedure after multiple revisions of total shoulder and elbow replacements. J Shoulder Elb Surg. 2011;20(1):e1–8. https://doi.org/10.1016/j.jse.2010.07.018.
52. Wierks C, Skolasky RL, Ji JH, McFarland EG. Reverse total shoulder replacement: intraoperative and early postoperative complications. Clin Orthop Relat Res. 2009;467(1):225–34. https://doi.org/10.1007/s11999-008-0406-1.
53. Andersen JR, Williams CD, Cain R, Mighell M, Frankle M. Surgically treated humeral shaft fractures following shoulder arthroplasty. J Bone Jt Surg Am. 2013;95(1):9–18. https://doi.org/10.2106/JBJS.K.00863.

Part V

Infection

25 Diagnosing Shoulder Prosthetic Joint Infections

Corey J. Schiffman and Surena Namdari

25.1 Introduction

Prosthetic joint infection (PJI) of the shoulder is unique because it is most frequently caused by less virulent organisms, with the most common organism being *Cutibacterium acnes* [1–3]. As a result, infection after shoulder arthroplasty often presents without the typical signs of infection such as warmth, erythema, and drainage. Instead, it typically presents with more subtle symptoms of pain and stiffness after a "honeymoon" period and without overt clinical or radiographic signs of infection. This lack of a substantial host response makes diagnosing shoulder PJIs challenging, and surgeons should have a high index of suspicion when patients return with shoulder dysfunction without another clear explanation.

25.2 Imaging

When evaluating a patient for shoulder PJI, standard radiographs should be obtained as early loosening may be a sign of infection (Fig. 25.1). Pottinger et al. found that humeral component loosening and humeral osteolysis on radiographs were associated with threefold and tenfold increases in the risk of positive *Cutibacterium* cultures, respectively [4]. However, humeral osteolysis secondary to stress shielding is also a common finding after use of a press-fit component, so it is not always a clear indicator of infection [5]. Advanced imaging in the form of CT or MRI scan can demonstrate signs of implant loosening or soft tissue collection but is of limited utility in diagnosing infection.

C. J. Schiffman (✉) · S. Namdari
Rothman Orthopaedic Institute,
Philadelphia, PA, USA
e-mail: Corey.Schiffman@rothmanortho.com;
Surena.Namdari@rothmanortho.com

F. Franceschi et al. (eds.), *Revision Shoulder Arthroplasty*,
https://doi.org/10.1007/978-3-031-45944-3_25

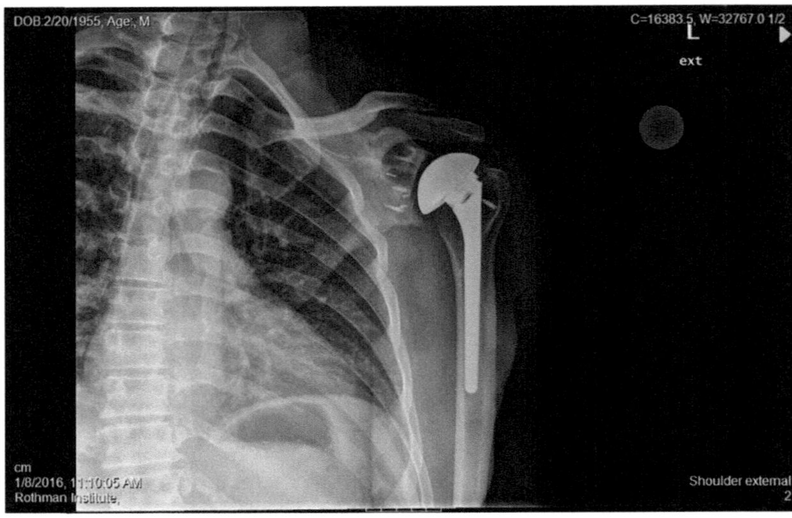

Fig. 25.1 Radiograph of an anatomic total shoulder arthroplasty concerning for infection

25.3 Serology

Basic infectious serologic testing including WBC count, erythrocyte sedimentation rate (ESR), and C-reactive protein (CRP) are standard in the work up for infection. These tests are specific and have a high positive predictive value (PPV) but have low sensitivity and negative predictive value (NPV) because they are often within normal limits in the setting of an indolent infection. In a systematic review performed by Nelson et al. evaluating patients with shoulder PJIs, only 6.8% had an elevated WBC count, 37.6% had elevated ESR, and 62.1% had elevated CRP. Because of the low sensitivity of basic infectious labs, other tests such as serum Interleukin-6 (IL-6) and D-dimer have been evaluated as potential tests with more diagnostic utility. Unfortunately, both IL-6 and D-dimer were also found to have low sensitivity in diagnosing shoulder PJI [6, 7].

25.4 Synovial Fluid Culture and Analysis

While arthrocentesis is a standard test when working up a hip or knee PJI, its utility when evaluating a shoulder PJI is less clear. Shoulder arthrocentesis typically yields only a small amount of synovial fluid, and there is no established cutoff for synovial fluid cell count. When enough fluid is collected, culture results have low sensitivity. In a study of patients being evaluated for chronic shoulder PJIs, fluoroscopic-guided glenohumeral aspiration had a sensitivity of 16.7% but specificity and positive predictive value of 100% [8]. Therefore, while a negative arthrocentesis does not provide much guidance, a positive culture is useful for diagnosing infection.

Multiple studies have also been performed investigating the utility of synovial fluid analysis. While IL-6, IL-2, and leukocyte esterase have been studied, alpha-defensin is the most clinically available test [9, 10]. Frangiamore et al. found that alpha-defensin had a sensitivity of 63% and specificity of 95% [10]. Similarly, Unter Ecker et al. found that alpha-defensin had a sensitivity of 75%, specificity of 93%, negative predictive value of 93%, and positive predictive value of 86% in detecting shoulder PJI [11]. However, the widespread use of alpha-defensin testing has been curtailed due to its limited accessibility.

25.5 Tissue Culture and Histopathology

Because of the low sensitivity of bacterial cultures after arthrocentesis, some surgeons advocate for arthroscopic tissue biopsy (Figs. 25.2 and 25.3). In a study comparing arthroscopic tis-

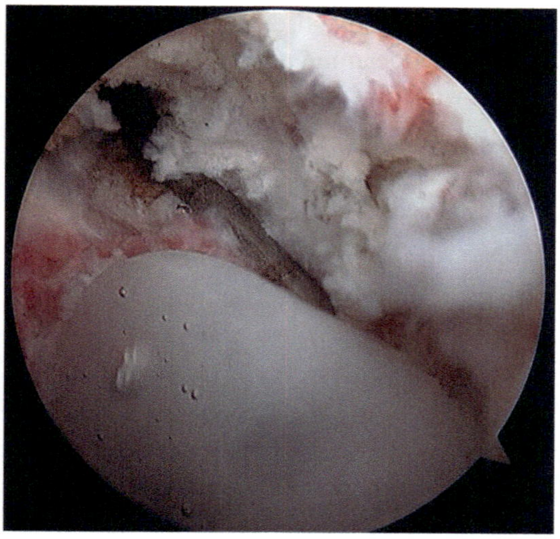

Fig. 25.2 Arthroscopic view of a polyethylene glenoid component during arthroscopic biopsy

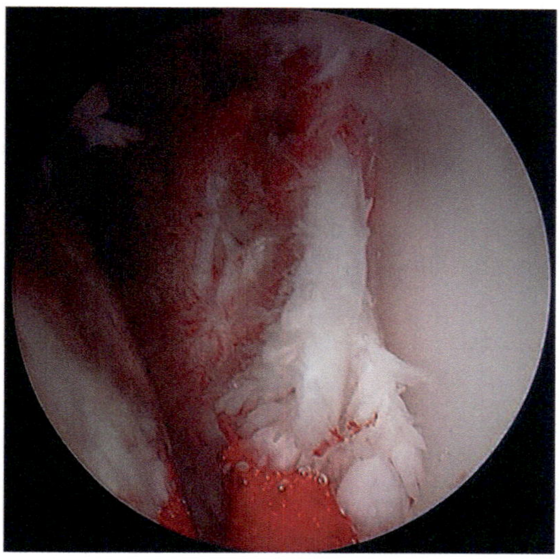

Fig. 25.3 Synovitic peri-glenoid tissue during arthroscopic tissue biopsy

sue biopsy to arthrocentesis prior to revision arthroplasty, Dilisio et al. found that tissue biopsy had a sensitivity and negative predictive value of 100% compared to arthrocentesis having a sensitivity and negative predictive value of only 16.7% and 58.3%, respectively [8]. However, the benefit of performing prerevision arthroscopic tissue biopsy needs to be weighed against the risk, cost, and inconvenience of an additional procedure and general anesthetic. It is best indicated in the setting of persistent shoulder pain without mechanical source for failure and negative infection workup.

During revision surgery, frozen section histopathology samples may provide more timely guidance for the surgeon when the presence of infection may change the operative plan. While the hip and knee literature typically describes a threshold of more than five neutrophils in five or more high-power microscopic fields, Grosso et al. advocated for lowering the threshold to 10 or more total neutrophils in five high-power fields in shoulder PJIs because lower virulent bacteria typically mount a less robust inflammatory response [12]. In this study, they found a sensitivity of 72% and specificity of 100% for infection. However, utilization of frozen section histopathology relies on the presence of a histology lab on site that can analyze and report the results in a timely manner.

Tissue cultures should also be obtained during revision surgery when there is any concern for infection as it can direct post-operative antibiotic therapy. At our institution, we typically obtain five tissue cultures. Cultures should be held in the laboratory for at least 14 days in aerobic, anaerobic, and broth media [13]. In order to quantify the bacterial load, Ahsan et al. developed a semi-quantitative scoring system, known as the Shoulder Propi Score [14].

While tissue cultures are critical to guide antibiotic management in cases of infection, the utility of obtaining cultures when there is a low suspicion for infection is less clear. Some surgeons advocate against obtaining cultures when there is mechanical cause for the symptoms leading to revision because it is unclear if an unexpected positive culture (UPC) is indicative of an infection, a commensal bacterium or a contaminant. Wong et al. evaluated culture positivity in patients undergoing primary total shoulder arthroplasty and found a positive culture rate of 38%, with the most common organism being *Cutibacterium* [15]. Hsu et al. and Padegimas et al. both evaluated culture positivity during revision shoulder arthroplasty for noninfectious reasons and found a positivity rate of 49% and

23.9%, respectively [16, 17]. Subsequent revision surgery rate was similar between patients with and without UPCs in both studies.

25.6 Next-Generation Sequencing

Because of the difficulty with interpreting positive cultures, there has been recent interest in next-generation sequencing (NGS), a technique that sequences the entire microbial DNA and identifies bacteria within a soft tissue or synovial fluid sample. This technique allows the generation of thousands of bacterial DNA sequences, providing a comprehensive analysis of the bacterial environment within a sample. Namdari et al. performed a prospective study comparing culture data and NGS in patients undergoing shoulder arthroscopy for rotator cuff tears or primary arthroplasty for shoulder osteoarthritis and found limited concordance between the two methods, with only 4 of the 18 cases (22.2%) with positive *Cutibacterium* cultures also having *Cutibacterium* identified by NGS (kappa – 0.238) [18]. NGS identified bacteria in 23% of cases, all of which were polymicrobial. In a similar study comparing tissue cultures and NGS in patients undergoing primary arthroplasty without signs of infection, Rao et al. found a substantially higher positivity rate and presence of polymicrobial bacteria with NGS compared to tissue cultures [19]. *E. coli,* a bacterium uncommonly cultured during shoulder surgery, was identified by NGS in 20% (5/25) of skin samples and 16% (4/25) of deep tissue samples. These authors concluded that the increased sensitivity of NGS may lead to an increase in false-positive findings, and more research is needed to better determine proper bacterial thresholds of NGS testing. Another study by Namdari et al. comparing these two methods during revision shoulder arthroplasty found that NGS data was more frequently polymicrobial, while culture data was monomicrobial and more prone to being defined as a "probable contaminant" [20]. While NGS shows promise as a sensitive tool for isolating bacteria, further research is necessary in determining its role in identifying clinically relevant infection.

25.7 International Consensus Meeting (ICM)

Because of the unique characteristics of shoulder PJI, the commonly used Musculoskeletal Infection Society (MSIS) published criteria for hip and knee PJI is not translatable to shoulder PJI. As a result, a definition of shoulder PJI was established at the 2018 International Consensus Meeting (ICM) [21]. Meeting one major criteria, including a sinus tract communicating with the prosthesis, gross intra-articular purulence, or 2 positive cultures with identical virulent organisms, is diagnostic of a definite infection. For less clear situations, a scoring system with minor criteria was developed with weighted values for positive tests performed during work up for infection (Table 25.1). Based on this scoring, likelihood of infection is determined (Table 25.2). Validation studies on the ICM criteria have found it to be an accurate and reliable tool for risk stratifying for infection [20–22].

Table 25.1 Minor criteria with weighted scoring

Minor criteria	Weight
Wound drainage	4
Single virulent positive tissue culture	3
Single low-virulent positive tissue culture	1
2nd identical low-virulent positive tissue culture	3
Humeral loosening	3
Positive frozen section (5 PMNs in ≥5 high-power fields)	3
Positive preoperative aspirate culture	3
Elevated synovial neutrophil percentage (>80%)	2
Elevated synovial WBC (>3000 cells/μL)	2
Elevated ESR (>30 mm/h)	2
Elevated CRP (>10 mg/L)	2
Elevated synovial alpha-defensin	2
Cloudy fluid	2

Table 25.2 Interpretation of minor criteria score

Score	Likelihood of infection
≥6 w/identified organism	Probable PJI
≥6 w/no identified organism	Possible PJI
≤6 w/1 virulent organism	Possible PJI
≤6 w/2 low-virulent organisms	Possible PJI
≤6 w/negative cultures	Unlikely PJI
≤6 w/1 low-virulent organism	Unlikely PJI

25.8 Conclusion

While we continue to make progress in our ability to diagnose shoulder PJIs, the typical indolent presentation and difficulty with interpreting positive cultures from the shoulder continue to make it a challenging problem to identify and treat. Future studies should focus on identifying a tool with improved sensitivity and negative predictive value that can be used to supplement the currently available tests with high specificity and positive predictive value.

References

1. Patel A, Calfee RP, Plante M, Fischer SA, Green A. Propionibacterium acnes colonization of the human shoulder. J Shoulder Elb Surg. 2009;18(6):897–902.
2. Nelson GN, Davis DE, Namdari S. Outcomes in the treatment of periprosthetic joint infection after shoulder arthroplasty: a systematic review. J Shoulder Elb Surg. 2016;25(8):1337–45.
3. Singh JA, Sperling JW, Schleck C, Harmsen WS, Cofield RH. Periprosthetic infections after total shoulder arthroplasty: a 33-year perspective. J Shoulder Elb Surg. 2012;21(11):1534–41.
4. Pottinger P, Butler-Wu S, Neradilek MB, Merritt A, Bertelsen A, Jette JL, et al. Prognostic factors for bacterial cultures positive for Propionibacterium acnes and other organisms in a large series of revision shoulder arthroplasties performed for stiffness, pain, or loosening. J Bone Jt Surg Am. 2012;94(22):2075–83.
5. Cole EW, Moulton SG, Gobezie R, Romeo AA, Walker JB, Lederman E, et al. Five-year radiographic evaluation of stress shielding with a press-fit standard length humeral stem. JSES Int. 2020;4(1):109–13.
6. Villacis D, Merriman JA, Yalamanchili R, Omid R, Itamura J, Rick Hatch GF 3rd. Serum interleukin-6 as a marker of periprosthetic shoulder infection. J Bone Jt Surg Am. 2014;96(1):41–5.
7. Zmistowski B, Chang M, Shahi A, Nicholson T, Abboud J, Lazarus M, et al. Is D-dimer a reliable serum marker for shoulder periprosthetic joint infection? Clin Orthop Relat Res. 2021;479(7):1447–54.
8. Dilisio MF, Miller LR, Warner JJ, Higgins LD. Arthroscopic tissue culture for the evaluation of periprosthetic shoulder infection. J Bone Jt Surg Am. 2014;96(23):1952–8.
9. Frangiamore SJ, Saleh A, Kovac MF, Grosso MJ, Zhang X, Bauer TW, et al. Synovial fluid interleukin-6 as a predictor of periprosthetic shoulder infection. J Bone Jt Surg Am. 2015;97(1):63–70.
10. Frangiamore SJ, Saleh A, Grosso MJ, Kovac MF, Higuera CA, Iannotti JP, et al. Alpha-defensin as a predictor of periprosthetic shoulder infection. J Shoulder Elb Surg. 2015;24(7):1021–7.
11. Unter Ecker N, Koniker A, Gehrke T, Salber J, Zahar A, Hentschke M, et al. What is the diagnostic accuracy of alpha-defensin and leukocyte esterase test in periprosthetic shoulder infection? Clin Orthop Relat Res. 2019;477(7):1712–8.
12. Grosso MJ, Frangiamore SJ, Ricchetti ET, Bauer TW, Iannotti JP. Sensitivity of frozen section histology for identifying Propionibacterium acnes infections in revision shoulder arthroplasty. J Bone Jt Surg Am. 2014;96(6):442–7.
13. Matsen FA 3rd, Butler-Wu S, Carofino BC, Jette JL, Bertelsen A, Bumgarner R. Origin of propionibacterium in surgical wounds and evidence-based approach for culturing propionibacterium from surgical sites. J Bone Jt Surg Am. 2013;95(23):e1811–7.
14. Ahsan ZS, Somerson JS, Matsen FA 3rd. Characterizing the Propionibacterium load in revision shoulder arthroplasty: a study of 137 culture-positive cases. J Bone Jt Surg Am. 2017;99(2):150–4.
15. Wong JC, Schoch BS, Lee BK, Sholder D, Nicholson T, Namdari S, et al. Culture positivity in primary total shoulder arthroplasty. J Shoulder Elb Surg. 2018;27(8):1422–8.
16. Hsu JE, Gorbaty JD, Whitney IJ, Matsen FA 3rd. Single-stage revision is effective for failed shoulder arthroplasty with positive cultures for Propionibacterium. J Bone Jt Surg Am. 2016;98(24):2047–51.
17. Padegimas EM, Lawrence C, Narzikul AC, Zmistowski BM, Abboud JA, Williams GR, et al. Future surgery after revision shoulder arthroplasty: the impact of unexpected positive cultures. J Shoulder Elb Surg. 2017;26(6):975–81.
18. Namdari S, Nicholson T, Abboud J, Lazarus M, Ramsey ML, Williams G, et al. *Cutibacterium acnes* is less commonly identified by next-generation sequencing than culture in primary shoulder surgery. Shoulder Elb. 2020;12(3):170–7.
19. Rao AJ, MacLean IS, Naylor AJ, Garrigues GE, Verma NN, Nicholson GP. Next-generation sequencing for diagnosis of infection: is more sensitive really better? J Shoulder Elb Surg. 2020;29(1):20–6.
20. Namdari S, Nicholson T, Abboud J, Lazarus M, Ramsey ML, Williams G, et al. Comparative study of cultures and next-generation sequencing in the

diagnosis of shoulder prosthetic joint infections. J Shoulder Elb Surg. 2019;28(1):1–8.
21. Garrigues GE, Zmistowski B, Cooper AM, Green A. Proceedings from the 2018 international consensus meeting on orthopedic infections: rationale and methods of the shoulder subgroup. J Shoulder Elb Surg. 2019;28(6S):S4–7.
22. Patel VV, Ernst SMC, Rangarajan R, Blout CK, Lee BK, Itamura JM. Validation of new shoulder periprosthetic joint infection criteria. J Shoulder Elb Surg. 2021;30(7S):S71–S6.

26 Managing the Infected Arthroplasty: Antibiotic Suppression, Debridement, One- Versus Two-Stage Revision

Franziska Eckers, Bettina Hochreiter, Gregory A. Hoy, and Eugene T. Ek

Periprosthetic joint infection (PJI) is a significant complication following joint replacements and is one of the most common indications for revision surgery [1, 2]. While the overall incidence is relatively low [3], a high index of suspicion for shoulder PJI should be considered when treating patients with increased risk factors. These include male gender, younger age, previous surgery, repeated cortisone injections, primary arthroplasty in the context of both trauma and rotator cuff arthropathy compared to osteoarthritis, reverse total shoulder arthroplasty (rTSA) compared to anatomic total shoulder arthroplasty (aTSA), as well as patients on immunocompromising medications and conditions such as rheumatoid arthritis, diabetes mellitus, alcohol overuse, and iron-deficiency anemia [2–4].

Treatment aims to eradicate infection while preserving or restoring satisfactory shoulder function. Historically, in the absence of a reliable and consistent definition of shoulder PJI, treatment approaches have varied and have been based on available evidence from the hip and knee PJI literature [5, 6]. The most common treatment protocols have comprised of aggressive and thorough debridement, antibiotics and implant retention with exchange of the polyethylene liner, which is often referred to as DAIR or alternatively, staged revision arthroplasty in combination with targeted antimicrobial treatment [7, 8]. The first option is typically employed in cases of early postoperative or acute hematogenous infection without signs of implant loosening. Exchange arthroplasty is indicated for delayed or chronic PJI [9], either as single-stage or as staged revision arthroplasty; all important aspects of which will be discussed below. In select cases, antibiotic suppression without surgical intervention, definitive spacer implantation, or resection arthroplasty may be further options [7, 10–12].

Recently, a consensus definition for shoulder PJI [13] was included in the recommendations of the International Conference on Periprosthetic Infections, which was identified through systematic literature review and a Delphi process. With this in place, the development of a uniform treatment algorithm for periprosthetic shoulder infections can be developed. Notably, there are certain factors that set the diagnostic and treatment algorithms of shoulder PJI apart from that of hip and knee PJI. First, the microbial spectrum of shoulder PJI tends to be somewhat different from that of the lower limb.

F. Eckers · B. Hochreiter
Melbourne Orthopaedic Group,
Melbourne, VIC, Australia

G. A. Hoy · E. T. Ek (✉)
Melbourne Orthopaedic Group,
Melbourne, VIC, Australia

Department of Surgery, Monash University,
Melbourne, VIC, Australia

F. Franceschi et al. (eds.), *Revision Shoulder Arthroplasty*,
https://doi.org/10.1007/978-3-031-45944-3_26

Low-virulence pathogens such as *Cutibacterium acnes* (*C. acnes*) and *coagulase-negative Staphylococci* (*CNS*) predominate, both in case of "real infection" and in the context of "unexpected positive cultures" (UPC) [1, 14–18]. UPC are a frequent finding in revision procedures of the shoulder; their significance and implications have not yet been well understood [10]. Symptoms caused by these pathogens may vary considerably, ranging from subtle pain to stiffness and mechanical symptoms due to implant loosening, at the same time typically lacking the typical features such as wound erythema, swelling, fever, or increased inflammatory markers [3, 19]. This variability can make the diagnostic process of shoulder PJI difficult and invariably delay commencement of appropriate treatment [19].

Second, suspected shoulder PJI, as opposed to other joints, may require operative tissue sampling to confirm the diagnosis and to identify the causative microorganism, as fluid aspiration is often difficult to obtain and also it frequently provides unreliable results [20–22]. This may constitute a certain threshold in decision-making and call for some preoperative consideration and planning.

As a result of the relative difficulty in detecting a shoulder PJI, this often leads to a delay in diagnosis, giving biofilm producing pathogens such as *C. acnes* and *CNS* time to become stationary on the prosthetic material and reducing their antibiotic susceptibility [14]. Thus, the "window" to successfully perform DAIR is often already closed by the time treatment is initiated, thus necessitating revision surgery. The main characteristics and indications for the management options will be described in the following.

26.1 Antibiotic Suppression

(Prolonged) suppressive antibiotic therapy ((P) SAT) describes the long-term, usually life-long—administration of antibiotics in the presence of PJI, with the goal to avoid local and systemic spreading of the infection, and to improve symptoms. It is thus a palliative form of treatment with no intention to eradicate infection, as the likelihood to attain elimination of microorganisms in the presence of a mature biofilm is very low.

The indication for SAT may be adequate in two scenarios: (1) As stand-alone treatment in very frail patients with comorbidities that would preclude safe surgical intervention. (2) After failed DAIR or staged revision arthroplasty, when further exchange surgeries are medically or mechanically no longer feasible, e.g., in the presence of severe cardiopulmonary conditions not compatible with anesthesia or in massive bone loss situations.

To date, very little literature is available on the topic of stand-alone SAT in the context of shoulder PJI, with only eight shoulders ever to be included in publications [10]. These were enclosed in articles that comprised very heterogeneous findings mainly from research into hip/knee arthroplasty but also on other overlapping fields of study such as osteomyelitis [12, 23]. Prendki et al. [23] published a study on a group of 21 patients with PJI of different joints, one of which being a shoulder. With a mean follow-up of 9.2 months, it was concluded that SAT protected patients from acute sepsis while being relatively well tolerated. A 2020 publication by Sandiford et al. [12] looked at 26 patients with PJI of the hip and knee, who underwent SAT and were observed for a mean of 3.2 years. Treatment success was defined as no admissions due to sepsis arising from the affected joint, no progression to further surgery or death from related causes. Overall, SAT was found to be a successful form of managing medically frail patients. Side effects of antibiotics such as gastrointestinal problems and drug interactions, e.g., with anticoagulants, may, however, complicate this course of treatment and sometimes lead to its termination, putting patients at risk for relapse of infection [10, 24].

Hence, stand-alone SAT remains a rare choice but retains a role in the treatment of shoulder PJI. Long-term antibiotic suppression in the aftermath of surgical procedures shall be discussed below.

26.2 Debridement, Antibiotics, and Implant ReteNTION (DAIR)

DAIR involves radical surgical debridement of the periprosthetic tissue, synovectomy, irrigation, exchange of the polyethylene liner and glenosphere in the setting of reverse shoulder arthroplasty, or the humeral head in anatomic prostheses. No evidence of prosthetic loosening is a prerequisite [25]. Postoperatively, empiric antibiotic treatment is commenced and transitioned into targeted antibiotic therapy once intraoperative tissue samples have been cultured and sensitivities are determined. In such cases, where the infection is assumed to have been eradicated, antibiotic treatment is discontinued after 6–12 weeks, based on consultation with an infectious diseases department [25].

26.2.1 Indications for DAIR

DAIR for treatment of PJI is indicated during the early postoperative period (<3 months after prosthetic implantation) or in the setting of delayed-onset acute hematogenous onset (<3 weeks after start of symptoms) PJI, no matter if caused by a low-virulence pathogen such a *C. acnes* or *CNS* or by a high-virulence pathogen such as *MSSA, MRSA,* or *E. coli* [10]. Some authors propose shorter time limits, the rationale being the formation of biofilm which largely determines the success of treatment [26]. The earlier treatment is commenced, the higher the chances of successful eradication of the infection [27]. From research on infected hip arthroplasty, it is known that hematogenous infections have a worse prognosis than early postoperative infections when treated with DAIR [28]. Negative prognostic factors are the presence of bacteriaemia or of a sinus tract, failure to exchange convertible components of the prosthesis during surgery, severe immunosuppression, PJI of a revision prosthesis, and certain microbiological factors (e.g., fungal infections or the refrain to use biofilm-penetrating antibiotics) [25].

Whether or not the treatment principles and the expectations that have been translated from the knee and hip arthroplasty literature are applicable in the setting of shoulder PJI has yet to be determined. The particularities of shoulder PJI, as described in the beginning of this chapter, make it particularly challenging to adequately draw a direct comparison when indicating DAIR versus revision arthroplasty in shoulder arthroplasty.

26.2.2 Outcomes of DAIR

Previous publications on the outcome of DAIR in the presence of shoulder PJI are scarce and consist mainly of small, retrospective case series and have reported inconsistent treatment details and heterogeneous outcomes [5, 29, 30], which, in summary, are not encouraging.

A 2016 systematic review by Nelson et al. [31] included a total of 22 studies to evaluate outcome of shoulder PJI treatment. Thirty-five patients were treated with DAIR, two-thirds had successful treatment, whereas one-third was classified as failures. The authors suggested that some of the patients might have been undertreated, given their history and local status. More recently conducted studies have not been able to demonstrate better results. In 2021, Lemmens et al. [32] reported about a total of 36 patients who were treated for chronic shoulder PJI, six of which with DAIR due to their complex comorbidities. Discouragingly, the infection recurrence rate for this subgroup was 80%. In 2016, Dennison et al. published the outcome of ten shoulders treated with DAIR. In three patients, infection control could only by attained by subsequent resection arthroplasty. In all other patients, it was decided to continue long-term SAT in order to avoid recurrence of symptomatic infection [29]. Better, yet still inadequate appearing results were presented by Jacquot et al. [18] in 2015. Thirteen cases of infected rTSA, where seven were acute and six were subacute or chronic infections, were treated with DAIR. Fifty-seven percent of acute infections and 50% for subacute/chronic infections could be treated successfully, and when combined with polyethylene and glenosphere exchange, 75% could achieve successful eradication.

26.2.3 DAIR: Surgical Technique

In principle, DAIR can be performed either arthroscopically or by open arthrotomy. Regarding this question, there is no relevant shoulder-specific literature available, which could guide decision making. Literature on PJI of hip and knee, however, indicates that arthroscopic DAIR is associated with poorer outcomes than open DAIR [18, 33]. This is probably because the mobile parts of the prosthesis are not being exchanged during arthroscopic DAIR, thus not reducing the potential impact of the residual biofilm.

Open DAIR is performed by revision of the previous scar, followed by debridement of all underlying scar tissue. The exchangeable components of the implant are then removed to allow for extensive synovectomy, debridement, and irrigation of all tissue and prosthetic surfaces. At this stage, it is unclear what type of irrigation solution should best be used [34]. New mobile components are then implanted, and wound closure is performed.

26.2.4 Antibiotic Treatment

There are currently no guidelines regarding the recommended agent(s), treatment route, and duration of peri- and postoperative antibiotics [14]. Orthopedic literature tends to recommend collaboration with an infectious disease specialist and decision-making on a case-by-case basis. However, some aspects of antimicrobial treatment will be reviewed here.

First, it is still controversially discussed whether preoperative prophylactic antibiotics should be held until biopsies are retrieved. The benefit of increasing the chance to avoid wound infection is weighed against the possibility of lowering the chances to isolate the microorganism responsible for the suspected PJI, which may be a germ difficult to culture [35]. Several studies have now demonstrated, though, that the administration of preoperative antibiotics does not significantly influence the detectability of microorganisms in tissue samples [36, 37]. This has prompted the *International Consensus Group* on orthopedic infections to now recommend administration of antibiotic prophylaxis in the setting of suspected PJI [19].

Regarding postoperative antibiotic protocols, there are certain "rules" that should be respected. Initial empirical treatment should cover *C. acnes* and gram-positive microorganisms, e.g., by using Vancomycin combined with a ®-lactam antibiotic, such as Cefazolin or Ceftriaxone [24, 38]. Once the infecting organism and its sensitivities are identified, treatment should be modified accordingly. Commonly, Rifampicin, which has the ability to penetrate into bacterial biofilms and to affect stationary-phase bacteria, is also introduced [14, 24, 39], in combination with a second potent drug to avoid Rifampicin resistance [14]. Notably, the use of Rifampicin in hardware-related infections has improved success rates significantly [40]. If no adverse effects such as gastrointestinal problems and drug interactions, arise, the preferred treatment duration is between 6 and 12 weeks [10, 24].

Due to the nature of shoulder PJI and, above all, its unique microbial profile, the role of DAIR in treatment of shoulder PJI seems to be limited. Failure rates have been reported to be high, however to date, and to the best of our knowledge, no large-scale studies with consistent inclusion criteria and treatment algorithms have been performed, which would allow for unequivocal recommendations. Therefore, treatment indications should be made very cautiously, especially in cases of delayed-onset hematogenous PJI and patients that have a high risk of treatment failure. Nevertheless, if successful, DAIR does have its advantages, mainly that it is far less disruptive for patients than exchange revision arthroplasty.

26.3 One- Versus Two-Stage Revision Arthroplasty

As in PJI of the lower limb, two-stage revision arthroplasty has also been proposed as the gold standard for shoulder PJI [5]. Specifically, implant removal, aggressive debridement, placement of an antibiotic spacer, and subsequent delayed reimplantation have been favored over single-stage replacement revision arthroplasty [5, 6, 41]. However, the additional surgical procedure invariably carries a risk of postoperative complications and leads to higher patient morbidity. Therefore, single-stage revision has been proposed to avoid the need for a second surgery. To date, there are conflicting data on one- and two-stage revisions, and there is no consensus as to whether one option is better than the other in terms of infection eradication or postoperative outcome [42]. The British Elbow and Shoulder Society (BESS) has established an evidence-based algorithm for the treatment of PJI in the shoulder. However, the recommendation of whether to perform a one- or two-stage revision is limited because there are few comparative analyses of one- and two-stage revisions in the current literature [43].

The first few systematic reviews on this topic, comprising approximately 30 studies, were published in 2016. George et al. [44] and Nelson et al. [31], found comparable results in infection eradication and functional outcomes for different treatment modalities, including resection arthroplasty or arthrodesis, DAIR, antibiotic spacer, one- or two-stage revision arthroplasty. Since then, the available literature on shoulder PJI has expanded, and this will be summarized in the following section.

26.3.1 Indication

According to the Proceedings from the 2018 International Consensus Meeting on Orthopedic Infections the indications for one- versus two-stage revision are at this time unclear [10]. Two-stage revision is highly recommended when the microorganism responsible for the infection is unknown [45]. Otherwise, there are no clear distinctions. Even the presence of a productive fistula, which has previously been proposed to be a contraindication for one-stage revision, does not appear to be one in the end [46, 47]. Beekman et al. [47] performed one-stage revisions in 11 cases of rTSA, among which eight had a fistula, and achieved infection eradication in 90%.

26.3.2 One-Stage Revision Arthroplasty: Surgical Technique

A standard deltopectoral approach is performed, excising the fistula, if present. The infected tissue is radically debrided, and the implant is removed with the standard extractors. Preparation of the medullary canal requires radical excision of infected tissue, including all cement, if present [47]. In subacute or chronic situations, the glenoid component should also be removed, even when well-fixed, as the reinfection rate is higher with component retention [10, 48]. Special attention should then be paid to the inferior part of the glenoid, where extensive synovitis can usually be found, especially in the presence of severe scapular notching. This pseudocapsule should then be detached from the lateral scapular pillar, which will allow for correct placement of the inferior screw of the new baseplate [47]. The operation site is thoroughly irrigated by (pulsatile) lavage. After removal of all used gloves, gowns and surgical instruments utilized during the initial stage, the surgical team will then implant the new prosthesis using new sterile equipment. Some institutions who advocate one-stage revision would, after explantation and prior to reimplantation, close the wound and re-desinfect the patient's skin and apply new drapes and then re-open the wound for the reimplantation of the new prosthesis.

26.3.3 Two-Stage Revision Arthroplasty: Surgical Technique

The initial steps of the first stage correspond to the technique described above and consist of thorough tissue debridement and complete removal of all prosthetic components including all cement. After collection of a minimum of four tissue samples [49] and thorough irrigation, a

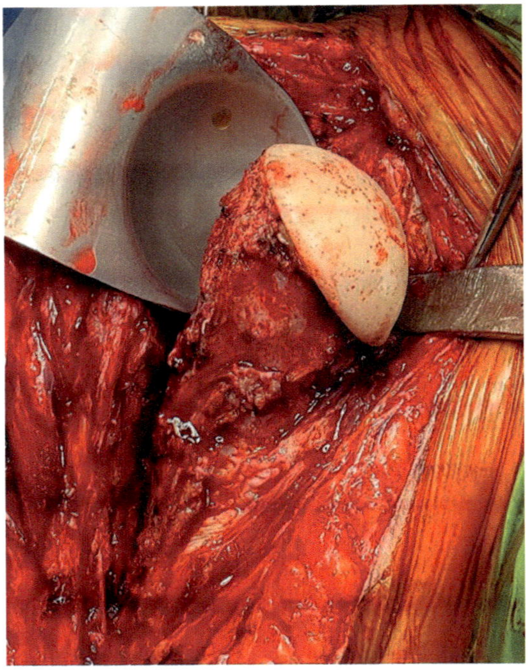

Fig. 26.1 shows an antibiotic cement spacer (StageOne™, Zimmer Biomet, Warsaw, IN, USA) during the second stage of a two-stage revision arthroplasty

cement spacer loaded with antibiotics is implanted. Options are to use either prefabricated spacers (e.g., InterSpace®, Exactech, Gainesville, FL, USA) or molds (StageOne™, Zimmer Biomet, Warsaw, IN, USA; Fig. 26.1), which are available on the market, or to handmake spacers intraoperatively by surrounding a metal core structure, e.g., a 3.5 mm locking compression plate, with antibiotic loaded cement, e.g., Palacos® R + G (Heraeus Medical GmbH, Wehrheim, Germany). This technique has previously been described by Grubhofer et al. [50] and has the advantages of being able to press-fit the stem and to adjust the antibiotic content. There is no consensus on the optimal class of antibiotics to use in the spacer preparation. Heat-stable antibiotics (vancomycin, gentamicin, and tobramycin) have been used alone or in combination [10]. The mean antibiotic concentration peaks on the first day and decreases dramatically over the following 7 days [51].

Cement spacers thus deliver antibiotics to the local tissues, eliminate dead space, and maintain soft tissue tension and (limited) shoulder function [50, 52] during the interval between the first and second stage of the revision. If a patient declines medically and is no longer a good surgical candidate, or if significant bone loss due to the infection and/or explantation procedure impedes a second stage of the revision, the spacer can be considered as a permanent solution [53, 54]. Inflammatory markers such as CRP or IL-6 have been shown to be valuable in predicting infection eradication and thus the timing of reimplantation [55, 56]. In case of persistent infection, another irrigation and debridement should be considered.

For re-implantation, rTSA has become the implant of choice [57]. First, it allows for uncompromised debridement during the first stage, with little concern for soft tissue (rotator cuff) preservation. Second, in most cases, it allows for more reliable treatment the glenoid bone deficiency during the second stage, either with or without bone grafting. Adequate implant positioning and soft tissue management should allow for recovery of acceptable function. In rare instances, however, when the glenoid bone loss is severe, this may require the consideration of alternative implants or techniques, such as large-head hemiarthroplasty [57] or hemi-reverse revision arthroplasty [58] either as a temporizing measure to allow the glenoid bone graft to incorporate or a permanent solution in non-reconstructable cases. This will be described in further detail in a previous chapter of this book.

26.3.4 Antibiotic Treatment

As far as postoperative antibiotic treatment after one-stage revision is concerned, the literature is scarce and primarily based on heterogeneous case series with inconsistent definitions for infection and variable treatment protocols. As a practical approach to management, the 2018 International Consensus Meeting on Orthopedic Infections suggested that a course of oral antibiotics may be initiated that covers the potential organism until intraoperative cultures are finalized. If the cultures are positive and PJI with a nonvirulent organism (*C. acnes* or CNS) is diagnosed, a continued course of antibiotics (up to 6 weeks) should be pursued. There is no evidence to support a preferred route [oral vs. intravenous (IV)], type, and duration of antibiotic treatment. If cultures are positive and PJI with a virulent organism is diagnosed, IV antibiotics and IV antibiotics followed by oral antibiotics are both reasonable options. As there is no consensus on the route or duration, these treatment parameters should be selected in consultation with an infectious disease specialist [10].

Antibiotic treatment in conjunction with two-stage revision commences perioperatively with the first stage revision. As stated above, and analogous to the antibiotic treatment accompanying DAIR procedures, the *International Consensus Group* on orthopedic infections now recommends the start of empiric antibiotics preoperatively and before tissue sampling, even when the causative microorganism is still unknown [19]. Once it is identified, empiric coverage is transitioned into tailored pathogen-specific therapy, in order to decrease the unnecessary coverage of broad-spectrum antibiotics as well as to minimize adverse effects [59]. Treatment duration is typically between 4 weeks and 3 months, with the patient under clinical and laboratory observation. In the absence of ongoing signs and symptoms of infection, re-implantation of a new shoulder prosthesis is then performed.

26.3.5 Outcomes After One- Versus Two-Stage Revision Arthroplasty

26.3.5.1 Infection Eradication

The most recent systematic review on one- versus two-stage revision arthroplasty was published in 2021. Ruditsky et al. [60] were able to include 26 articles with a total of 452 shoulders (one-stage revision: n = 163; two-stage revision: n = 289). Four studies reported results for one-stage revision only, 15 for two-stage revision only, and seven for both one- and two-stage revisions. Interestingly, the overall infection clearance rate was 95.6% for one-stage procedures and only 85.2% for two-stage procedures. Previously, George et al. [44] published a systematic review with six articles reporting on one-stage revision (n = 75), 13 on two-stage revision (n = 142), eight on resection arthroplasty (n = 83) and eight on permanent spacers (n = 68). The average infection eradication rates were 94.7% at a mean follow-up of 47 months after one-stage revision, 90.8% at 38 months after two-stage revision, 86.7% at 40 months after resection arthroplasty and 95.6% at 31 months following a permanent spacer. The differences were not statistically significant. Similarly, Belay et al. [42], including a total of 43 articles with 798 shoulders, found a non-significant trend for higher infection eradication rates in single stage approaches (6.3% versus 10.1%). Notably, the one-stage group had a higher percentage of *C. acnes* (48.7% versus 33.6%) infections and of (sub-) acute infections (63% versus 46.1%), whereas the two-stage group had a higher percentage of virulent (MRSA; 0% versus 2.6%) and chronic infections (53.9% versus 37%). This likely represents a significant selection bias by the treating surgeons and highlights the significant limitation of the interpretation.

Akgün et al. [61], reporting on 49 patients treated with a two-stage revision strategy, looked at the topic from a slightly different angle. While infection eradication could be achieved in 85.7% of re-implanted shoulders—comparing to the numbers above—it was found that the second stage was completed in only 71% of patients. The reasons for which were varied including satisfaction with the current status, but above all, high morbidity and premature death with a mortality rate of 10% within 90 days after implant removal.

Overall, these results suggest that—in a select group of patients—single-stage revision arthroplasty is at least as effective as two-stage procedures, at the same time being associated with the advantage of fewer surgeries, lower costs and reduced risks. However, these findings should be interpreted cautiously due to an inherent selection bias with regard to factors that guide treatment, such as severity and timing of infection, as well as perioperative clinical findings. In older patients with a more severe comorbid profile, surgeons may lean towards a two-stage concept.

Remarkably, a considerable subset of these patients may end up never undergoing the second stage of the intended treatment.

26.3.5.2 Clinical Outcomes

Ruditsky's 2021 review [60] compared the change in outcome scores between one-stage and two-stage revision from preoperatively to postoperatively: the Constant-Murley Score (CMS) improved by 21.0 points versus 22.8 points, respectively, the American Shoulder and Elbow Surgeons (ASES) score by 26.2 points versus 33.6 points, respectively, and the Simple Shoulder Test (SST) score by 3.5 points versus 6.4 points, respectively. However, the included studies varied in terms of reported outcome scores and of the 26 included studies only a fraction of studies reported pre- and postoperative clinical outcome. According to the paper by George et al. [44], patients treated with one-stage revision had statistically significant better postoperative CMS scores (51 ± 13) than patients who had undergone two-stage revision (44 ± 9), resection arthroplasty (32 ± 7) or a permanent spacer (31 ± 9). However, when considering only studies comparing pre- and postoperative CMS, the difference was not statistically significant. Along the same lines, Kunutsor et al. [62] reported no significant differences in clinical outcome. Two-stage revision patients, though, suffered a significantly higher non-infection complication rate (18.9% versus 12.1%), including dislocations, periopera-tive fractures, nerve lesions, non-union, glenoid baseplate failure, glenosphere dissociation, and arthrofibrosis. Klingebiel et al. [57] also reported a significant percentage of non-infection complications, which, in 31%, resulted in revision surgery. Not surprisingly, when rTSA was the implant of choice at reimplantation, rather than megaprosthesis or large-head hemiarthroplasty, patients experienced less disability and fewer long-term complications, with better subjective stability and function.

Several studies have evaluated the outcome of patients with permanent cement spacers. Pellegrini et al. [63] reported no recurrence of infection in a cohort of 19 elderly, low-demand patients. At a mean follow-up of 8 years, all patients reported satisfactory subjective and objective outcomes. Levy et al. [53] retrospectively reviewed nine patients with shoulder PJI who elected not to undergo prosthetic reimplantation. At a mean follow-up of 25 months, patients had acceptable function in the absence of recurring infection. Only one patient (11%) was unsatisfied with the result. As summarized in a 2022 review article on antibiotic spacers for shoulder PJI by Namdari et al. [31], further publications of similar scale offer comparable results.

Definitive spacer retention may therefore well be a viable option in some patients but does not come without the possibility of complications such as fractures, glenoid erosion, or spacer dislocation [64]. Nevertheless, from the various studies, the reported outcomes appear to be relatively favorable.

The indications for one- versus two-stage revision are still unclear at this present time. However, both treatment strategies seem to be effective in treating periprosthetic shoulder infection. Studies showing better results for one-stage revisions should be interpreted cautiously due to a high probability of a relevant treatment bias.

26.4 Summary and Outlook

Shoulder PJI is a relatively uncommon but potentially catastrophic complication of shoulder arthroplasty, which is most commonly caused by biofilm producing low-virulent microorganisms such as *C. acnes* and CNS. Due to its often subtle symptomatology, shoulder PJI may be difficult to diagnose and therefore treatment initiation is often delayed.

Treatment generally comprises surgical intervention, paired with targeted antibiotic therapy. Long-term stand-alone antibiotic suppression therapy or other salvage procedures may be an option in select cases, but DAIR or exchange revision arthroplasty is usually necessary to eradicate infection. According to the *International Consensus Meeting on Orthopedic Infections*, DAIR is indicated in early postoperative or acute hematogenous PJI, while revision arthroplasty is

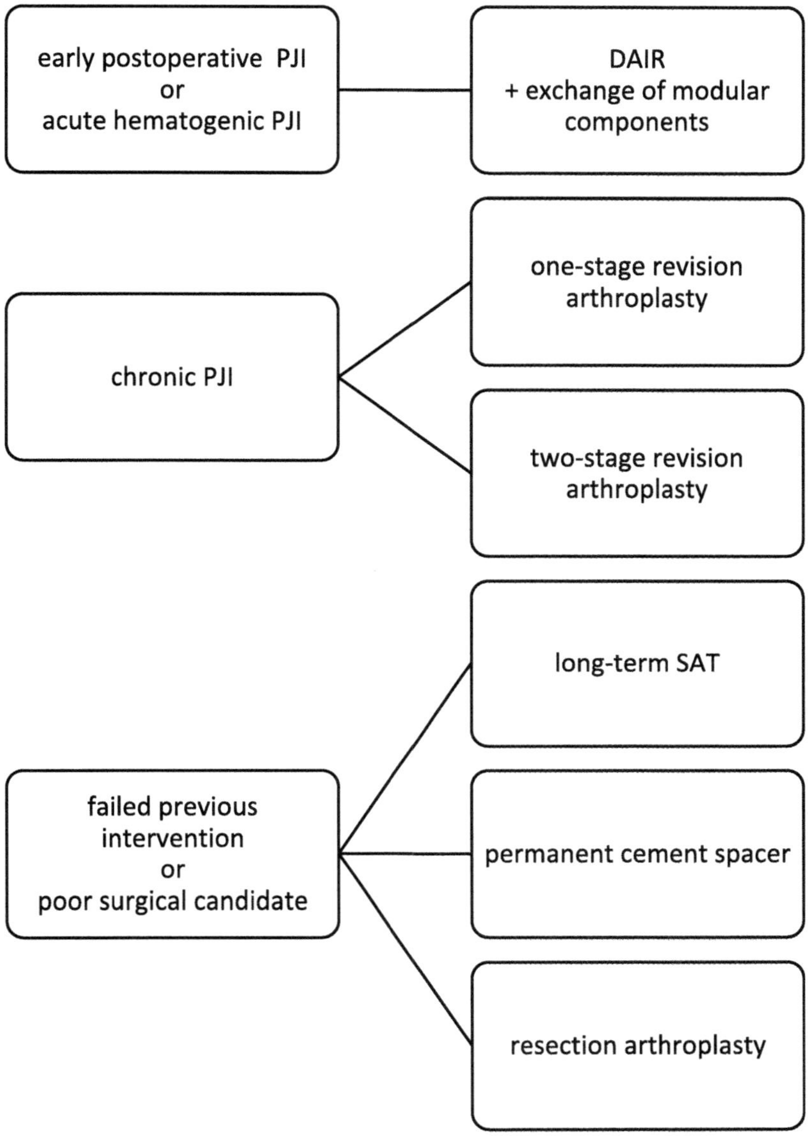

Fig. 26.2 illustrates a treatment algorithm for shoulder PJI. A more refined universal algorithm is yet to be defined. *PJI* periprosthetic joint infection, *DAIR* debridement, antibiotics and implant retention, *SAT* suppressive antibiotic therapy

to be indicated in delayed and chronic cases (Fig. 26.2). When deciding whether to proceed with a one- and two-stage procedure, the following factors need to be considered: the type of pathogen, the timing of the infection, the findings on preoperative clinical examination, the patient's own decision, the surgeon's preference, and the intraoperative appearance of the soft tissues/bone. However, at this stage, there is still no consensus recommending single-stage versus 2-stage revision arthroplasty.

Bibliography

1. Pottinger P, Butler-Wu S, Neradilek MB, Merritt A, Bertelsen A, Jette JL, et al. Prognostic factors for bacterial cultures positive for Propionibacterium acnes and other organisms in a large series of revision shoulder arthroplasties performed for stiffness, pain, or loosening. J Bone Jt Surg Am. 2012;94(22):2075–83.
2. Kunutsor SK, Barrett MC, Whitehouse MR, Craig RS, Lenguerrand E, Beswick AD, et al. Incidence, temporal trends and potential risk factors for prosthetic joint infection after primary total shoulder and elbow replacement: systematic review and meta-analysis. J Infect. 2020;80(4):426–36.

3. Richards J, Inacio MCS, Beckett M, Navarro RA, Singh A, Dillon MT, et al. Patient and procedure-specific risk factors for deep infection after primary shoulder arthroplasty. Clin Orthop Relat Res. 2014;472(9):2809–15.
4. Seok HG, Park JJ, Park SG. Risk factors for periprosthetic joint infection after shoulder arthroplasty: systematic review and meta-analysis. J Clin Med. 2022;11(14):4245.
5. Coste JS, Reig S, Trojani C, Berg M, Walch G, Boileau P. The management of infection in arthroplasty of the shoulder. J Bone Jt Surg Br. 2004;86(1):65–9.
6. Cooper ME, Trivedi NN, Sivasundaram L, Karns MR, Voos JE, Gillespie RJ. Diagnosis and management of periprosthetic joint infection after shoulder arthroplasty. JBJS Rev. 2019;7(7):e3.
7. Fink B, Sevelda F. Periprosthetic joint infection of shoulder arthroplasties: diagnostic and treatment options. Biomed Res Int. 2017;2017:4582756. https://www.ncbi.nlm.nih.gov/pmc/articles/PMC5750516/
8. Choi HR, von Knoch F, Zurakowski D, Nelson SB, Malchau H. Can implant retention be recommended for treatment of infected TKA? Clin Orthop Relat Res. 2011;469(4):961–9.
9. Parvizi J, Gehrke T, Chen AF. Proceedings of the International Consensus on periprosthetic joint infection. Bone Jt J. 2013;95-B(11):1450–2.
10. Garrigues GE, Zmistowski B, Cooper AM, Green A, ICM Shoulder Group. Proceedings from the 2018 International Consensus Meeting on Orthopedic Infections: management of periprosthetic shoulder infection. J Shoulder Elb Surg. 2019;28(6S):S67–99.
11. Toms AD, Davidson D, Masri BA, Duncan CP. The management of peri-prosthetic infection in total joint arthroplasty. J Bone Joint Surg Br. 2006;88(2):149–55.
12. Sandiford NA, Hutt JR, Kendoff DO, Mitchell PA, Citak M, Granger L. Prolonged suppressive antibiotic therapy is successful in the management of prosthetic joint infection. Eur J Orthop Surg Traumatol. 2020;30(2):313–21.
13. Garrigues GE, Zmistowski B, Cooper AM, Green A, ICM Shoulder Group. Proceedings from the 2018 international consensus meeting on orthopedic infections: the definition of periprosthetic shoulder infection. J Shoulder Elb Surg. 2019;28(6S):S8–12.
14. Achermann Y, Sahin F, Schwyzer HK, Kolling C, Wüst J, Vogt M. Characteristics and outcome of 16 periprosthetic shoulder joint infections. Infection. 2013;41(3):613–20.
15. Kim SJ, Kim JH. Unexpected positive cultures including isolation of Propionibacterium acnes in revision shoulder arthroplasty. Chin Med J. 2014;127(22):3975–9.
16. Dodson CC, Craig EV, Cordasco FA, Dines DM, Dines JS, Dicarlo E, et al. Propionibacterium acnes infection after shoulder arthroplasty: a diagnostic challenge. J Shoulder Elb Surg. 2010;19(2):303–7.
17. Kadler BK, Mehta SS, Funk L. Propionibacterium acnes infection after shoulder surgery. Int J Shoulder Surg. 2015;9(4):139–44.
18. Jacquot A, Sirveaux F, Roche O, Favard L, Clavert P, Molé D. Surgical management of the infected reversed shoulder arthroplasty: a French multicenter study of reoperation in 32 patients. J Shoulder Elb Surg. 2015;24(11):1713–22.
19. Garrigues GE, Zmistowski B, Cooper AM, Green A, ICM Shoulder Group. Proceedings from the 2018 international consensus meeting on orthopedic infections: evaluation of periprosthetic shoulder infection. J Shoulder Elb Surg. 2019;28(6S):S32–66.
20. Zanna L, Sangaletti R, Akkaya M, Shen T, Abuljadail S, Gehrke T, et al. What is the concordance rate of preoperative synovial fluid aspiration and intraoperative biopsy in detecting periprosthetic joint infection of the shoulder? J Shoulder Elb Surg. 2022;32(3):492–9.
21. Dilisio MF, Miller LR, Warner JJP, Higgins LD. Arthroscopic tissue culture for the evaluation of periprosthetic shoulder infection. J Bone Joint Surg Am. 2014;96(23):1952–8.
22. Morman M, Fowler RL, Sanofsky B, Sanosky B, Higgins LD. Arthroscopic tissue biopsy for evaluation of infection before revision arthroplasty. J Shoulder Elb Surg. 2011;20(3):e15–22.
23. Prendki V, Sergent P, Barrelet A, Oziol E, Beretti E, Berlioz-Thibal M, et al. Efficacy of indefinite chronic oral antimicrobial suppression for prosthetic joint infection in the elderly: a comparative study. Int J Infect Dis. 2017;60:57–60.
24. Marschall J, Lane MA, Beekmann SE, Polgreen PM, Babcock HM. Current management of prosthetic joint infections in adults: results of an Emerging Infections Network survey. Int J Antimicrob Agents. 2013;41(3):272–7.
25. Boyer B, Cazorla C. Methods and probability of success after early revision of prosthetic joint infections with debridement, antibiotics and implant retention. Orthop Traumatol Surg Res. 2021;107(1S):102774.
26. Zimmerli W, Moser C. Pathogenesis and treatment concepts of orthopaedic biofilm infections. FEMS Immunol Med Microbiol. 2012;65(2):158–68.
27. Fehring TK, Odum SM, Berend KR, Jiranek WA, Parvizi J, Bozic KJ, et al. Failure of irrigation and débridement for early postoperative periprosthetic infection. Clin Orthop Relat Res. 2013;471(1):250–7.
28. Bryan AJ, Abdel MP, Sanders TL, Fitzgerald SF, Hanssen AD, Berry DJ. Irrigation and debridement with component retention for acute infection after hip arthroplasty: improved results with contemporary management. J Bone Jt Surg Am. 2017;99(23):2011–8.
29. Dennison T, Alentorn-Geli E, Assenmacher AT, Sperling JW, Sánchez-Sotelo J, Cofield RH. Management of acute or late hematogenous infection after shoulder arthroplasty with irrigation, débridement, and component retention. J Shoulder Elb Surg. 2017;26(1):73–8.
30. Weber P, Utzschneider S, Sadoghi P, Andress HJ, Jansson V, Müller PE. Management of the infected shoulder prosthesis: a retrospective analysis and review of the literature. Int Orthop. 2011;35(3):365–73.

31. Nelson GN, Davis DE, Namdari S. Outcomes in the treatment of periprosthetic joint infection after shoulder arthroplasty: a systematic review. J Shoulder Elb Surg. 2016;25(8):1337–45.
32. Lemmens L, Geelen H, Depypere M, De Munter P, Verhaegen F, Zimmerli W, et al. Management of periprosthetic infection after reverse shoulder arthroplasty. J Shoulder Elb Surg. 2021;30(11):2514–22.
33. Triantafyllopoulos GK, Poultsides LA, Zhang W, Sculco PK, Ma Y, Sculco TP. Periprosthetic knee infections treated with irrigation and debridement: outcomes and preoperative predictive factors. J Arthroplast. 2015;30(4):649–57.
34. Siddiqi A, Abdo ZE, Rossman SR, Kelly MA, Piuzzi NS, Higuera CA, et al. What is the optimal irrigation solution in the management of periprosthetic hip and knee joint infections? J Arthroplast. 2021;36(10):3570–83.
35. Zappe B, Graf S, Ochsner PE, Zimmerli W, Sendi P. Propionibacterium spp. in prosthetic joint infections: a diagnostic challenge. Arch Orthop Trauma Surg. 2008;128(10):1039–46.
36. AlBuhairan B, Hind D, Hutchinson A. Antibiotic prophylaxis for wound infections in total joint arthroplasty: a systematic review. J Bone Jt Surg Br. 2008;90(7):915–9.
37. Matsen FA, Russ SM, Bertelsen A, Butler-Wu S, Pottinger PS. Propionibacterium can be isolated from deep cultures obtained at primary arthroplasty despite intravenous antimicrobial prophylaxis. J Shoulder Elb Surg. 2015;24(6):844–7.
38. Pinder EM, Ong JC, Bale RS, Trail IA. Ten questions on prosthetic shoulder infection. Shoulder Elb. 2016;8(3):151–7.
39. Coenye T, Spittaels KJ, Achermann Y. The role of biofilm formation in the pathogenesis and antimicrobial susceptibility of *Cutibacterium acnes*. Biofilms. 2022;4:100063.
40. Renz N, Trampuz A, Zimmerli W. Controversy about the role of rifampin in biofilm infections: is it justified? Antibiotics (Basel). 2021;10(2):165.
41. Mook WR, Garrigues GE. Diagnosis and management of periprosthetic shoulder infections. J Bone Jt Surg Am. 2014;96(11):956–65.
42. Belay ES, Danilkowicz R, Bullock G, Wall K, Garrigues GE. Single-stage versus two-stage revision for shoulder periprosthetic joint infection: a systematic review and meta-analysis. J Shoulder Elb Surg. 2020;29(12):2476–86.
43. Rangan A, Falworth M, Watts AC, Scarborough M, Thomas M, Kulkarni R, et al. Investigation and management of periprosthetic joint infection in the shoulder and elbow: evidence and consensus based guidelines of the British Elbow and Shoulder Society. Shoulder Elb. 2018;10(1 Suppl):S5–19.
44. George DA, Volpin A, Scarponi S, Haddad FS, Romanò CL. Does exchange arthroplasty of an infected shoulder prosthesis provide better eradication rate and better functional outcome, compared to a permanent spacer or resection arthroplasty? A systematic review. BMC Musculoskelet Disord. 2016;17:52.
45. Bonnevialle N, Dauzères F, Toulemonde J, Elia F, Laffosse JM, Mansat P. Periprosthetic shoulder infection: an overview. EFORT Open Rev. 2017;2(4):104–9.
46. Klatte TO, Junghans K, Al-Khateeb H, Rueger JM, Gehrke T, Kendoff D, et al. Single-stage revision for peri-prosthetic shoulder infection: outcomes and results. Bone Jt J. 2013;95-B(3):391–5.
47. Beekman PDA, Katusic D, Berghs BM, Karelse A, De Wilde L. One-stage revision for patients with a chronically infected reverse total shoulder replacement. J Bone Jt Surg Br. 2010;92(6):817–22.
48. Ince A, Seemann K, Frommelt L, Katzer A, Loehr JF. One-stage exchange shoulder arthroplasty for peri-prosthetic infection. J Bone Jt Surg Br. 2005;87(6):814–8.
49. Ahsan ZS, Somerson JS, Matsen FA. Characterizing the Propionibacterium load in revision shoulder arthroplasty: a study of 137 culture-positive cases. J Bone Jt Surg Am. 2017;99(2):150–4.
50. Grubhofer F, Imam MA, Wieser K, Achermann Y, Meyer DC, Gerber C. Staged revision with antibiotic spacers for shoulder prosthetic joint infections yields high infection control. Clin Orthop Relat Res. 2018;476(1):146–52.
51. Anagnostakos K, Wilmes P, Schmitt E, Kelm J. Elution of gentamicin and vancomycin from polymethylmethacrylate beads and hip spacers in vivo. Acta Orthop. 2009;80(2):193–7.
52. Jawa A, Shi L, O'Brien T, Wells J, Higgins L, Macy J, et al. Prosthesis of antibiotic-loaded acrylic cement (PROSTALAC) use for the treatment of infection after shoulder arthroplasty. J Bone Jt Surg Am. 2011;93(21):2001–9.
53. Levy JC, Triplet J, Everding N. Use of a functional antibiotic spacer in treating infected shoulder arthroplasty. Orthopedics. 2015;38(6):e512–9.
54. Mahure SA, Mollon B, Yu S, Kwon YW, Zuckerman JD. Definitive treatment of infected shoulder arthroplasty with a cement spacer. Orthopedics. 2016;39(5):e924–30.
55. Villacis D, Merriman JA, Yalamanchili R, Omid R, Itamura J, Rick Hatch GF. Serum interleukin-6 as a marker of periprosthetic shoulder infection. J Bone Jt Surg Am. 2014;96(1):41–5.
56. Coffey MJ, Ely EE, Crosby LA. Treatment of glenohumeral sepsis with a commercially produced antibiotic-impregnated cement spacer. J Shoulder Elb Surg. 2010;19(6):868–73.
57. Klingebiel S, Theil C, Gosheger G, Schneider KN, Ackmann T, Timme M, et al. Clinical outcome of two-stage revision after periprosthetic shoulder infection. J Clin Med. 2021;10(2):E218.
58. Walch A, Edwards TB, Kilian CM, Boileau P, Walch G, Athwal GS. Hemi-reverse revision arthroplasty in the setting of severe glenoid bone loss. J Shoulder Elb Surg. 2022;31(9):1859–73.

59. Miller R, Higuera CA, Wu J, Klika A, Babic M, Piuzzi NS. Periprosthetic joint infection: a review of antibiotic treatment. JBJS Rev. 2020;8(7):e1900224.
60. Ruditsky A, McBeth Z, Curry EJ, Cusano A, Galvin JW, Li X. One versus 2-stage revision for shoulder arthroplasty infections: a systematic review and analysis of treatment selection bias. JBJS Rev. 2021;9(9):e20.
61. Akgün D, Wiethölter M, Maziak N, Paksoy A, Karczewski D, Scheibel M, et al. Two-stage exchange arthroplasty for periprosthetic shoulder infection is associated with high rate of failure to reimplant and mortality. J Clin Med. 2021; 10(21):5186.
62. Kunutsor SK, Wylde V, Beswick AD, Whitehouse MR, Blom AW. One- and two-stage surgical revision of infected shoulder prostheses following arthroplasty surgery: a systematic review and meta-analysis. Sci Rep. 2019;9(1):232.
63. Pellegrini A, Legnani C, Macchi V, Meani E. Management of periprosthetic shoulder infections with the use of a permanent articulating antibiotic spacer. Arch Orthop Trauma Surg. 2018;138(5):605–9.
64. Namdari S, Sudah SY, Menendez ME, Denard PJ. Antibiotic spacers for shoulder periprosthetic joint infection: a review. J Am Acad Orthop Surg. 2022;30(19):917–24.

27 Preventing Infection in Revision Shoulder Arthroplasty

Adam Z. Khan, Mohamad Y. Fares, and Joseph A. Abboud

27.1 Introduction

Total shoulder arthroplasty (TSA), both anatomic and reverse, utilization has significantly increased in the last few decades [1]. A total of 39,000 shoulder replacements are estimated to be performed per year, and growth rates are approximated at 5–9% annually [2]. This progression looks to continue with increasing life expectancies and a trend of exponentially increasing shoulder replacement rates [1]. While outcomes of reverse total shoulder arthroplasty (rTSA) have proven to be generally favorable, the procedure is still limited by a burden of complications that can significantly impair recovery and change patient prognosis for the worse [3]. These complications include infection, nerve injury, periprosthetic fractures, component loosening, instability, and dislocation [3].

Adam Z. Khan and Mohamad Y. Fares have contributed equally and should be designated as co-first authors.

A. Z. Khan
Southern California Permanente Medical Group, Panorama City, CA, USA

M. Y. Fares
Division of Shoulder and Elbow Surgery, Rothman Orthopaedic Institute, Philadelphia, PA, USA

J. A. Abboud (✉)
Division of Shoulder and Elbow Surgery, Rothman Orthopaedic Institute, Philadelphia, PA, USA

The Sidney Kimmel Medical College, Thomas Jefferson University, Philadelphia, PA, USA

With this surge in primary shoulder arthroplasty, there is a subsequent increased potential for revision arthroplasty, which conceivably magnifies prosthetic joint infection (PJI) prevalence and the consequential medical resource as well as economic burden [4]. The current incidence of PJI in the setting of revision shoulder arthroplasty is estimated between 4 and 15.4% compared to a significantly lower incidence in the primary setting (0.7–1.8%) [5–10]. This relative increased burden of PJI in the setting of revision shoulder arthroplasty brings strategies for infection identification, but more importantly prevention to center stage for shoulder arthroplasty surgeons. Failure to effectively prevent PJI in the setting of revision shoulder arthroplasty can result in devastating complications and significant patient morbidity, including systemic infection and sepsis, need for multiple revision surgeries, or lifelong antibiotic suppression.

In the setting of prosthetic shoulder infection, commonly isolated causative microorganisms include *Cutibacterium acnes* (38.9%), followed by *Staphylococcus aureus* (14.8%), and *Staphylococcus epidermidis* (14.0%), and *coagulase-negative Staphylococcus* not otherwise unspecified (CNS) (14.0%) [11]. This microbiological profile, with a higher incidence of indolent, non-suppurative bacteria, is unique to the shoulder compared with other periprosthetic joint infections. It creates a significant diagnostic challenge, as patients do not present with typical

F. Franceschi et al. (eds.), *Revision Shoulder Arthroplasty*,
https://doi.org/10.1007/978-3-031-45944-3_27

clinical signs of infection (erythema, swelling, warmth, or drainage) and abnormal laboratory findings and often have relatively low intraoperative culture yield [12, 13]. Moreover, this creates an even more significant challenge in developing strategies for infection prevention as large patient numbers become necessary to create studies that are powered to create effective treatment modalities [13, 14].

The goal of this chapter is to provide a comprehensive review of risk factors of infection following revision shoulder arthroplasty, identify potential perioperative strategies for infection prevention, and provide recommendations for evidence-based best practices to minimize infection risk in the setting of revision surgery.

27.2 Risk Factors of Periprosthetic Joint Infections

Many factors contribute to the development of infection in arthroplasty procedures, and these can be categorized into non-modifiable risk factors and modifiable risk factors [15]. Several studies explored the different non-modifiable risk factors and were able to identify younger age, male sex, having an rTSA, undergoing arthroplasties for traumatic indications, depression, and revision surgery to be some of the prominent contributors to infection in shoulder arthroplasty procedures [15–18]. A multicenter retrospective study by Richards et al. evaluated a cohort of 4528 shoulder arthroplasty patients in an attempt to extract patient-specific risk factors of deep postoperative infection [16]. The authors reported a 5% lower risk of infection with every 1-year increase in patient age [16]. They also reported that male patients were 2.59 times more likely to develop an infection than female patients; patients undergoing a rTSA were 6.11 times more likely to develop an infection than those undergoing an anatomic total shoulder arthroplasty (aTSA) [16]. In addition, the authors noted that arthroplasties indicated for traumatic events were 2.98 times more likely to acquire a deep infection than those indicated for elective purposes [16]. Another study by Morris et al. identified 301 primary rTSAs from a prospectively collected shoulder arthroplasty registry and conducted bivariate and multivariable regression analyses in order to extract possible risk factors of infection following rTSA [17]. The authors reported that patients undergoing revision arthroplasty and those who are younger than 65 were 5.75 times and 4 times more likely to develop postoperative infections [17]. In addition, a systematic review and meta-analysis conducted by Seok et al. aimed to assess the evidence describing risk factors of periprosthetic joint infections (PJIs) and identify those factors that contribute to infection development [15]. The authors reported that male sex, undergoing a revision arthroplasty, surgical history, acute trauma, and preoperative diagnoses other than osteoarthritis were all risk factors that were highly associated with PJI [15]. Finally, psychiatric disorders such as depression have also been implicated in the development of infection following shoulder arthroplasty [18]. Mollon et al. reviewed the United States Nationwide Inpatient Sample and identified 224,060 patients who had undergone elective total shoulder arthroplasty [18]. Of the entire cohort of included patients, 12.4% had a history of diagnosed depression, which was an independent risk factor for postoperative infection at a significant odds ratio of 2.09 ($p = 0.045$) [18]. As such, it has been established in the literature that non-modifiable risk factors play a prominent role in the development of infection following shoulder arthroplasties and that a meticulous review of patient history is warranted in order to implement any prophylactic measures prior to undergoing any replacement procedures [15–18].

Several studies similarly explored the involvement of modifiable risk factors in the development of PJIs following shoulder arthroplasty [19–22]. Some of the implicated modifiable risk factors include diabetes mellitus (DM), obesity, and interventions prior to surgery [19–22]. Cancienne et al. explored a national database of DM patients who underwent shoulder arthroplasty procedures and assessed the association between perioperative hemoglobin A1c (HbA1c) and the rate of wound infections and complications [19]. Using a receiver operating characteristic (ROC) curve analysis, the authors reported that DM patients with HbA1c greater than 8.0 had significantly higher rates of wound complications and deep infections when compared to control patients [19]. Stryker et al. retrospectively reviewed all patients undergoing primary total joint arthroplasty at their institution for 7 years and explored the association between glycemic blood control and the development of wound complications within 30 days of surgery [20]. The development of wound complications was nine times more likely when preoperative HbA1c was higher than 6.7, 3.75 times more likely when mean postoperative blood glucose was higher than 200 mg/dL, and 3 times more likely when maximum postoperative blood glucose was higher than 260 mg/dL [20]. On the other hand, McElvany et al. conducted a retrospective cohort study with 8819 shoulder arthroplasty patients to explore whether an association between diabetes status and postoperative complications such as deep wound infections exists [21]. In their study, the authors defined poor glycemic control as HbA1c greater than 7.0 and used the Adapted Diabetes Complications Severity Index (aDCSI) to measure diabetes severity [21]. The authors reported that diabetic patients with poor glycemic control had a higher likelihood of 90-day readmission due to complications when undergoing elective shoulder arthroplasty [21]. They also reported that patients with severe diabetes according to aDCSI had a higher likelihood of 90-day readmission for complications in both elective and trauma-related shoulder arthroplasties [21]. Nevertheless, the authors concluded that, using ROC curve analysis, both preoperative HbA1c and aDCSI acted as poor classifiers for differentiating adverse events [21].

With regard to obesity and body mass index (BMI), no specific cutoff has been defined by the literature to determine association with PJI following shoulder arthroplasty [22]. Studies in the literature report conflicting results and views regarding this topic [22]. Nevertheless, some studies examining total joint arthroplasty reported obesity and BMI to be prominent factors that can lead to higher infection rates following procedures [23, 24]. Ward et al. stratified the complication risk of 22,808 patients undergoing total joint arthroplasty based on BMI [23]. Upon conducting multivariable regression, the authors reported that BMI greater than 40 can be considered an independent risk factor for several complications, including superficial infection [23]. Another registry-based study by Qvistgaard et al. explored 460 cases of hip arthroplasty reoperations due to PJIs and reported that obese patients (BMI greater than 30) had a higher risk of infection when compared to underweight, normal, or overweight individuals ($p < 0.001$) [24]. As such, obese patients should be counseled prior to intervention in order to help attenuate the rate of possible infection-related complications.

Other modifiable risk factors implicated in the literature include procedures done on the joint shortly prior to surgery as well as duration of surgery [25, 26]. Werner et al. queried a national database of Medicare patients in order to explore the association between timing of injection prior to index shoulder procedure and rate of postoperative infection [26]. The authors categorized the shoulder arthroplasty patients into three groups: injection within 3 months prior to arthroplasty, injection between 3 and 12 months prior to arthroplasty, and a control group that did not receive any injection [26]. The authors reported that infection rates at 3 months and 6 months postoperatively were significantly higher in patients who had an injection within 3 months before the shoulder arthroplasty procedures [26]. In addition, several studies have reported that shoulder arthroscopy procedures shortly prior to an index shoulder arthroplasty procedures can increase the risk of PJI following the arthroplasty [25]. A study by Nezwek et al. explored patient risk factors that contribute to the development of infection after rTSA and showed that postoperative infection was three times higher in patients with a history of shoulder surgery (6%) than in patients with no prior history of shoulder surgeries (2%) ($p = 0.003$) [25, 27, 28]. Similar results were reported by other studies in the literature such as Wright-Chisem et al. and Malik et al. [27, 28]. These studies highlight important considerations that need to be taken prior to counseling patients who are undergoing a revision arthroplasty procedure.

27.3 Preoperative Measures and Skin Preparations

Several measures taken during surgical site preparation have been explored in the literature to determine whether they induce a significantly protective impact against postoperative infection [29–31]. For example, Kapadia et al. conducted a study to delineate whether chlorhexidine skin preparation can reduce surgical site infection rates in patients undergoing total knee arthroplasty (TKA) [29]. The authors identified 3717 patients who underwent TKA at a single institution and stratified them into a treatment group—i.e., patients who used chlorhexidine skin preparation before surgery—and a control group—i.e., patients who did not use chlorhexidine skin preparation [29]. The authors reported that the use of preoperative chlorhexidine was associated with a reduced periprosthetic infection rate, with a relative risk of 6.4 and a p value of 0.002 favoring the treatment group [29]. Another study by Murray et al. evaluated 100 randomized prospectively recruited patients who underwent shoulder surgery and were assigned either to use 2% chlorhexidine-gluconate cloths (treatment group) or to shower with soap and water prior to surgery (control group) [30]. The authors took cutaneous cultures from the patient's shoulder prior to the surgery and reported that the overall positive culture rate was 94% in the control group, significantly higher than that of the treatment group at 66% ($p = 0.0008$) [30]. The authors noted that the treatment group was more capable of decreasing *coagulase-negative Staphylococcus*, in particular, an agent known to cause postoperative shoulder infections. As such, they concluded that 2% chlorhexidine preps can prove useful in reducing the risk of surgical site infections following shoulder surgery [30]. Similar results were reported by Saltzman et al. who conducted a prospective study to evaluate 150 consecutive patients who were undergoing shoulder surgery at a single institution [31]. Shoulders were randomized into two groups: one group receiving Chloraprep (Duraprep—which consists of 0.7% iodophor and 74% isopropyl alcohol), and another receiving povidone-iodine scrub and paint [31]. Cultures were taken following skin preparation, and overall positive culture rate was reported to be 7% in the Chloraprep group, significantly lower than that of the Duraprep group at 19% ($p = 0.01$), and that of the povidone-iodine group at 31% ($p < 0.0001$) [31]. With regard to *coagulase-negative Staphylococcus*, Chloraprep and Duraprep were significantly more capable of decreasing bacterial load than povidone-iodine ($p < 0.001$); as for the ability to eliminate *Propionibacterium acnes* in specific, there was no difference observed between the three solutions [31].

However, there is some controversy in the literature on this topic. Some studies contend the efficacy of surgical preparation solutions and how prominent an effect they have in eliminating infection risk. Lee et al. wanted to explore whether the use of Chloraprep (2% chlorhexidine gluconate and 70% isopropyl alcohol) could reduce the quantity of dermal Propionibacterium species in the upper back [32]. To do so, the authors recruited ten healthy male volunteers and applied Chloraprep to their backs before culturing two dermal punch biopsies, obtained from each volunteer, for *C. acnes* [32]. The authors reported persistence of the bacteria in seven of ten volunteers, indicating that Chloraprep does not significantly reduce the quantity of dermal *C. acnes* species in the back prior to surgery [32]. This carries heavy implications regarding infection in shoulder surgery patients, as this area falls in proximity to the usual surgical sites.

Hydrogen peroxide has been presented as a potential player in helping decrease intraoperative culture positivity in shoulder arthroplasty, specifically *C. acnes* species [33, 34]. Several studies explored the potential protective efficiency of hydrogen peroxide and reported promising results. Chalmers et al. conducted a prospective trial with a consecutive series of shoulder arthroplasty patients and categorized patients into two groups: the control group had a standard skin preparation, while the treatment group had hydrogen peroxide added to the standard skin preparation protocol [33]. The treatment group recorded no triple-positive cultures (i.e., skin, dermis, and joint) while that of the control group had a triple-positive rate of 19% ($p = 0.024$) [33]. In addition, the treatment group had lower rates of positive joint cultures at 10% compared to that of the control group at 35% ($p = 0.031$) [33]. The authors then conducted a post hoc gender stratified subgroup analysis and reported that the differences in culture-positive rates were only significant in male patients [33]. Regardless, they stated that hydrogen peroxide may offer a low-cost, low-risk method to help reduce PJI following shoulder arthroplasty procedures, particularly in males [33]. Similar findings were reported by Stull et al. who conducted a prospective trial that randomized shoulder arthroscopy male patients into a control group that underwent standard skin preparation and a treatment group that had an additional preparation with 3% hydrogen peroxide [34]. The culture-positive rate for *C. acnes* was found in 34.2% of the control group and 17.1% of the treatment group, indicating a significant reduction in positivity rates ($p = 0.033$) [34]. On the other hand, Grewal et al. reported differing results, and they prospectively randomized 60 patients undergoing shoulder arthroplasty to receive standard skin preparation and antibiotic prophylaxis either with or without dermal hydrogen peroxide after incision [34]. The positive culture rate for *C. acnes* was 20% for the hydrogen peroxide group and 16% for the control group, indicating no significant difference with regard to positivity rates [34].

Benzoyl peroxide solutions are another skin preparation that has been supported by the literature to help combat postoperative infections in the surgical setting [35, 36]. Dizay et al. prospectively enrolled 65 patients undergoing shoulder arthroscopy and had them apply topical benzoyl peroxide and clindamycin one night prior to their surgery [35]. *C. acnes* cultures were obtained in the operating room prior to the administration of chlorhexidine gluconate [35]. The authors reported that the treatment was able to effectively eliminate superficial and deep colonization of the bacterium species and that its use should be considered in shoulder procedures [35]. The effect of benzoyl peroxide has also been explored by Kolakowski et al. who prospectively enrolled 80 patients undergoing shoulder surgery in a double-blind trial and randomized them to receive either benzoyl peroxide or chlorhexidine gluconate for three consecutive days [36]. The authors then obtained *C. acnes* culture from skin surrounding the surgical incision site of the patients and compared the positivity rates between the two groups [36]. Their results showed that benzoyl peroxide was more effective in reducing *C. acnes* species in the shoulder when compared to chlorhexidine preparation and noted that its utility should be highly considered in the setting of shoulder surgery [36].

Another agent that has been explored in the literature as a preoperative measure that can help reduce bacterial load prior to surgery is blue light [37]. In the recent years, light therapies have emerged as a treatment modality for many skin pathologies, and the clinical application of blue light, in particular, has been proposed to be an effective agent to combat microbial proliferation in the skin [37]. Boyd et al. conducted a comparative in vitro study to compare the effects of blue light irradiation in the presence and absence of oxygen on the proliferation of *P. acnes* species, a prominently causative agent of skin infections following different surgical procedures (including shoulder arthroplasty) [37]. The authors reported that blue light was able to effectively kill the bacterial species in planktonic culture, demonstrating the efficiency and potential applicability of this modality as a prophylactic measure for infection [37]. On the other hand, Cotter et al. investigated the antimicrobial effects of blue light therapy in the clinical setting by conducting a trial that randomized 60 male volunteers to three treatment groups: a group receiving benzoyl peroxide alone, a group receiving blue light therapy alone, and a group receiving both benzoyl peroxide and blue light therapy [38]. Swab cultures were then taken from the skin of each treated shoulder, and after applying chlorhexidine to both treated shoulders and controls (contralateral shoulder), comparisons between the reduction in *C. acnes* positivity rates of each group were made [38]. The authors reported that the benzoyl peroxide and combined blue light and benzoyl peroxide groups were able to effectively eliminate *C. acnes* in most cases, whereas the blue light (alone) group was not able to demonstrate effective antibacterial properties against *C. acnes* species [38]. These results challenged clinical potential of blue light in combatting shoulder infections following surgical procedures and implied the need for additional research in order to accurately assess its utility and benefit.

27.4 Intraoperative Measures

Several studies have explored the efficacy and value of different intraoperative measures in the prevention of postoperative infection. These include the administration of antibiotics, tranexamic acid (TXA), laminar air flow and space suits, use of different surgical instrumentation, and betadine irrigation, among others. The use of different prophylactic antibiotics has been widely discussed in the literature. Cefazolin, in specific, is considered a prominent prophylactic antibiotic in different orthopedic procedures. Crane et al. explored the susceptibility of *C. acnes* isolates from the shoulder with the aim to determine the efficacy of different antibiotics on this bacterial species [39]. The authors reported that the antibiotics with the lowest minimal inhibitory concentrations were penicillin, cephalothin, and ceftriaxone [39]. Marigi et al. conducted a retrospective study to examine whether prophylactic cefazolin can help reduce the rate of PJIs in shoulder arthroplasty procedures [40]. In this study, the authors compared the rate of PJIs after shoulder arthroplasty in patients who had received cefazolin to those receiving alternative regimens like vancomycin or clindamycin [40]. The authors reported that patients who received cefazolin had significantly lower rates of PJIs when compared to patients who received non-cefazolin alternatives [40]. A similar study by Yian et al. retrospectively reviewed 7140 patients undergoing shoulder arthroplasty to investigate the efficacy of cefazolin to that of vancomycin and clindamycin [41]. The authors, however, reported no difference in infection rate between cefazolin and vancomycin but a 3.5 times higher infection risk in patients who received clindamycin alone when compared to cefazolin [41]. This had prominent implications for shoulder arthroplasty patients with a penicillin allergy.

Intra-incisional use of topical vancomycin powder has also been adopted by many surgeons during shoulder arthroplasty as a prophylactic measure to combat PJIs. One in vitro study by Miquel et al. explored the prophylactic efficacy of vancomycin in combatting *C. acnes* species on a biomimetic shoulder arthroplasty model [42]. The authors reported effective prevention of *C. acnes* growth in the shoulder joint model and stated that its use may help limit infection following shoulder arthroplasty [42]. Hatch et al. further investigated the utility of vancomycin powder administration by conducting a cost-effectiveness analysis of its use in preventing PJI following shoulder arthroplasty [43]. Using vancomycin costs reported in the literature (between 2.5 USD and 44 USD per 1000 mg), the authors stated the antibiotic powder would be cost-effective if its absolute risk reduction has a range of 0.005% (for 2.5USD/1000 mg) to 0.19% (for 44USD/1000 mg) [43]. As such, vancomycin powder was found to be a highly cost-effective measure, as reported efficacy rates in the literature vary between 2.6% and 25.1% in different medical specialties [44–47]. Other intraoperative measures used during shoulder arthroplasty include intraarticular antibiotic injections and the use of antibiotic cement [48, 49]. Lovallo et al. retrospectively reviewed 507 shoulder arthroplasty cases and compared patients who received prophylactic antibiotics and an intraarticular injection of gentamycin at the end of the surgery to those just receiving prophylactic antibiotics [48]. The authors reported lower infection rates in the gentamicin group and supported this use as an intraoperative prophylactic measure against infection in shoulder arthroplasty [48]. As for the use of antibiotic-loaded bone cement, Nowinski et al. retrospectively reviewed 501 reverse shoulder arthroplasties and compared the deep infection rate between patients who received antibiotic cement for humeral fixation (n = 236) to those that received cement with no antibiotics (n = 265) [49]. After a mean follow-up of 37 months, no deep infection was reported in the antibiotic cement group, whereas 8 deep infections (3%) were reported in the control group [49]. The authors suggested that the antibiotic-loaded bone cement can have prominent prophylactic benefit in combatting deep infections after shoulder arthroplasty [49].

Other intraoperatively administered drugs and measures have also been discussed as potential prophylactic factors against infection in shoulder arthroplasty but have been proven to have equivocal effects in the literature [50–52]. For example, TXA is an antifibrinolytic agent that helps prevent excessive bleeding in the clinical setting, thereby reducing the amount of blood loss and the need for transfusions after a surgical procedure [50]. As such, through a potential decreased risk of postoperative hematoma as well as decreased transfusion need, TXA may play a role in decreasing the rate of postoperative infections [50]. Rojas et al. conducted a meta-analysis to assess the effects of TXA administration in shoulder arthroplasty procedures [53]. The authors examined postoperative infection as a secondary outcome measure and noted no conclusive effect played by TXA in decreasing infection rates [53]. Another measure that has conflicting results in the literature is the use of laminar air flow and space suits during arthroplasty procedures [51]. The use of laminar air flow and space suits has been classically thought to decrease the risk of wound contamination and lower postoperative infection rate. Nevertheless, a registry-based study by Hooper et al. investigated the use of these two measures in total hip and total knee replacement procedures and conveyed unfavorable results [51]. The authors reported a significant increase in early infection when space suits were worn (against when they were not), a laminar-flow setting was used (against a conventional surgical setting), and a laminar-flow with space suits was used (against a conventional surgical setting with no space suit) [51]. Another study by Davis et al. analyzed the cost-effectiveness of the use of laminar flow and stated that for the procedure to be deemed cost-effective, it has to reduce the incidence of PJI by 35.1%, implying that the high cost of implementation of this measure in the setting of shoulder arthroplasty procedures may not be justified [52].

The use of different surgical instrumentation has also been explored as a potential player in postoperative infection [54–56]. In 2006, Schindler et al. studied the contamination of surgical knife blades from 203 elective orthopedic procedures and suggested the use of separate skin and inside knives when operating, as that can reduce the risk of deep infection [54]. Levy et al. analyzed the cost-effectiveness of this routine practice [55]. The authors explored the presence of *C. acnes* on the blades used for initial skin incision, and after noting the high rate of *C. acnes* contamination found on these blades, they concluded that the practice of discarding initial blades is economically founded [55]. As for the use of electrocautery, Callaway et al. compared the *C. acnes* contamination rate between a scalpel blade and an electrocautery blade (heated to 41 °C) and noted no significant difference in bacterial transference between the two instruments [56]. As such, there was no concrete evidence supporting the use of electrocautery for infection prevention, whereas good evidence was found to advocate for the routine practice of discarding the initial skin incision blade in the setting of infection prevention.

Different measures are taken upon the termination of a surgical procedure, often with the intention to reduce wound contamination and eliminate risk infection, and these include betadine irrigation and application of special wound dressings. Published evidence corroborating both of these measures has been found in the literature [57–59]. Brown et al. evaluated the efficacy of dilute betadine lavage in the prevention of early deep infection after total hip and total knee replacements [57]. The authors compared the rate of PJIs between 688 cases where betadine lavage was applied and 1862 cases where it was not (control) [57]. The PJI rate was 0.15% in the betadine group and 0.97% in the control group, indicating a significant difference and justifying the use of this inexpensive preparation solution as a potential preventive tool against postoperative infection [57]. As for special wound dressings, silver-containing dressings have been reported to reduce the risk of surgical site infections. Bowler et al. conducted an in vitro study to investigate the antibacterial efficacy of silver-containing wound dressings on *P. acnes* species [58]. Using a simulated wound model, the authors demonstrated that the dressing exerted bactericidal effects on *P. acnes* over the course of 7 days and that it may play an important role in minimizing the risk of associated surgical site infections [58]. Similar results were reported by Cai et al. who retrospectively compared the PJI rate of 903 arthroplasty patients receiving Aquacel Surgical dressing to 875 arthroplasty patients receiving standard gauze dressing [59]. The incidence of PJI was significantly lower in the Aquacel dressing group after a follow-up of 3 months, indicating a potential protective role in preventing infection following arthroplasty procedures [59]. As such, it would make sense to state that betadine lavage and the application of special wound dressings play a potential role in preventing infection following arthroplasty procedures of the shoulder.

Duration of surgical procedure is one of the major contributors to postoperative infection, with numerous studies showing close associations between length of operative time and infection [24, 60, 61]. Procter et al. explored the American College of Surgeons National Surgical Quality Improvement Program database to investigate whether operative duration is associated with an increased risk of infectious complications [60]. The authors reported that infectious complication risk increased for every 30 min over an hour of operative time, almost doubling at 2.1–2.5 h [60]. In another registry-based study conducted to explore risk factors leading to postoperative infections in hip arthroplasty reoperations, Qvistgaard et al. reported that for every additional 10 min of surgery time, the risk of PJI increases by 6% [24]. Similar findings were reported by Jonsson et al. who investigated the prevalence of intraoperative contamination of joint replacement procedures and its relationship with the development of postoperative PJIs [61]. When assessing for possible risk factors, the authors reported that 13% of samples were contaminated when collected prior to 130 min of surgery, whereas 35% of them were contaminated when collected after 130 min of surgery [61]. This indicated a potential relationship between length of operation and rate of infection.

27.5 Oral Antibiotic Prophylaxis

In addition to perioperative intravenous as well as topical antibiotic prophylaxis, there is some recent literature that has evaluated the efficacy of prophylactic preoperative or postoperative antibiotic utilization. Much of this literature has centered around the ability to decolonize the skin or deeper tissues for *C. acnes*, the predominant isolate seen in PJI around the shoulder. In a study that evaluated *C. acnes* strains isolated from hip, knee, and shoulder implants in the setting of PJI, there was a 98% susceptibility of these strains to doxycycline [62]. Therefore, doxycycline has been the focus of a few research investigations.

Namdari et al. [63] performed a randomized trial of 74 male patients undergoing shoulder arthroscopy comparing those who received an oral doxycycline regimen (100 mg twice a day for 7 days) preoperatively with patients who did not receive any preoperative oral antibiotics. Two skin punch biopsies were performed at that time of surgery. They found 59.5% of patients in the no treatment group compared to 43.2% of patients in the doxycycline treatment group had at least one positive culture for *C. acnes*; however, this was not statistically significant ($p = 0.245$). Unfortunately, this study did not evaluate the susceptibilities of these isolated species to see if they were resistant to doxycycline. Furthermore, with only 74 patients, this study may not have been powered and was susceptible to type II error in not showing a difference between groups. Ultimately, the authors concluded that the risk of resistance was not worth it.

Rao et al. [64] performed a randomized controlled trial of 56 patients that evaluated giving doxycycline in addition to cefazolin compared to just giving cefazolin at the time of primary shoulder arthroplasty. They also found no reduction in culture positivity for samples taken from the skin, dermal tissue, or glenohumeral joint for *C. acnes* (37% in the cefazolin-only group versus 38% in the cefazolin plus doxycycline group in the patients who received doxycycline) when treated with doxycycline. No studies to date have specifically evaluated preoperative antibiotic administration in the setting of revision shoulder arthroplasty. Further investigation into preoperative and perioperative antibiotic regimens is indicated, as there is still significant controversy over the ideal treatment regimen [65].

With regard to postoperative antibiotic suppression, there is limited literature on shoulder arthroplasty to guide surgeons. The literature available evaluating postoperative antibiotic usage for suppressive purposes following treatment of PJI has primarily focused on lower extremity arthroplasty cases. Pradier et al. [66] retrospectively evaluated the use of oral doxycycline as a suppressive agent in 36 patients following the surgical management of PJI in patients with *S. aureus* infections of the hip and knee. They found a total of 74.4% of patients remained infection-free at a mean follow-up of 2.72 years with a low side effect profile from the doxycycline. This same group also retrospectively evaluated the use of oral tetracycline (doxycycline or minocycline) as a suppressive agent in 78 patients following surgical management of PJI for knee (37), hip (35), elbow (4), or shoulder (2) PJI with various bacterial species identified [67]. They found 71.8% of patients to remain infection-free at a mean follow-up of 2.79 years but did identify 3 cases (3.8%) that developed tetracycline-resistant bacterial strains. Both of these studies lacked a comparison control group to truly evaluate the benefit of postoperative oral antibiotic suppression. Larger cohort studies need to be performed with comparison arms to better elucidate if there is value in postoperative antibiotic suppression in patients undergoing aseptic revision arthroplasty, as this has currently not been evaluated in the literature.

27.6 Conclusion

Over the past two decades, there has been exponential growth in primary shoulder arthroplasty cases performed with significant innovation with regard to product design and implant modernization [68]. Along with this growth comes an increased volume of revision arthroplasty cases and a potential burden of shoulder PJI moving into the future. The low virulence of the most commonly isolated organisms in the setting of shoulder PJI, specifically *C. acnes*, creates a significant challenge with regard to evaluating and creating effective prevention strategies for these organisms.

Current strategies for prevention include a comprehensive preoperative evaluation of patient-associated risk factors, specifically ones that are modifiable and can be optimized preoperatively. Intraoperatively, reduction in surgical time has been shown to be effective in reducing infection risk with mixed literature on the best perioperative skin preparation formulation. Furthermore, laminar flow had not been shown to be effective from a preventative or cost standpoint. With limited studies, preoperative oral antibiotics have yet to show a significant reduced bacterial load in the shoulder at the time of surgery, and there are limited studies currently available on the effectiveness of postoperative suppressive antibiotics. Therefore, caution should be taken prior to administration of a prolonged prophylactic antibiotic course, as this could increase the development of antibiotic resistance.

There is significant associated morbidity when a patient develops a shoulder PJI with an increased risk of PJI following revision shoulder arthroplasty compared to primary cases. Investigation and innovation in the field of PJI prevention needs to continue to be a focal point moving forward.

Competing Interests JAA would like to disclose royalties from: DJO GLOBAL, ZIMMER-BIOMET, SMITH AND NEPHEW, STRYKER, GLOBUS MEDICAL, INC.; research support from as a PI from: LIMA CORPORATION - ITALY, ORTHOFIX, ARTHREX, OREF; royalties, financial or material support from:

WOLTERS KLUWER; and board member/committee appointments for: AMERICAN SHOULDER AND ELBOW SOCIETY, PACIRA.

Funding None.

References

1. Farley KX, et al. Prevalence of shoulder arthroplasty in the United States and the increasing burden of revision shoulder arthroplasty. JB JS Open Access. 2021;6(3):156.
2. Steinhaus ME, et al. Outpatient total shoulder arthroplasty: a cost-identification analysis. J Orthop. 2018;15(2):581–5.
3. Reddy AK, et al. Complication and revision rates after reverse total shoulder revision from hemiarthroplasty: a systematic review. Shoulder Elb. 2022;14(5):481–90.
4. Padegimas EM, et al. Periprosthetic shoulder infection in the United States: incidence and economic burden. J Shoulder Elb Surg. 2015;24(5):741–6.
5. Coste JS, et al. The management of infection in arthroplasty of the shoulder. J Bone Jt Surg Br. 2004;86(1):65–9.
6. Dodson CC, et al. Propionibacterium acnes infection after shoulder arthroplasty: a diagnostic challenge. J Shoulder Elb Surg. 2010;19(2):303–7.
7. Ramsey ML, Fenlin JM Jr. Use of an antibiotic-impregnated bone cement block in the revision of an infected shoulder arthroplasty. J Shoulder Elb Surg. 1996;5(6):479–82.
8. Singh JA, et al. Periprosthetic infections after total shoulder arthroplasty: a 33-year perspective. J Shoulder Elb Surg. 2012;21(11):1534–41.
9. Sperling JW, et al. Infection after shoulder arthroplasty. Clin Orthop Relat Res. 2001;382:206–16.
10. Verhelst L, et al. Resection arthroplasty of the shoulder as a salvage procedure for deep shoulder infection: does the use of a cement spacer improve outcome? J Shoulder Elb Surg. 2011;20(8):1224–33.
11. Paxton ES, Green A, Krueger VS. Periprosthetic infections of the shoulder: diagnosis and management. J Am Acad Orthop Surg. 2019;27:e935.
12. Garrigues GE, et al. Proceedings from the 2018 International Consensus Meeting on Orthopedic Infections: evaluation of periprosthetic shoulder infection. J Shoulder Elb Surg. 2019;28(6S):S32–66.
13. Shields MV, Abdullah L, Namdari S. The challenge of Propionibacterium acnes and revision shoulder arthroplasty: a review of current diagnostic options. J Shoulder Elb Surg. 2016;25(6):1034–40.
14. Contreras ES, et al. Periprosthetic infection after reverse shoulder arthroplasty: a review. Curr Rev Musculoskelet Med. 2020;13(6):757–68.
15. Seok H-G, Park J-J, Park SG. Risk factors for periprosthetic joint infection after shoulder arthroplasty: systematic review and meta-analysis. J Clin Med. 2022;11(14):4245.
16. Richards J, et al. Patient and procedure-specific risk factors for deep infection after primary shoulder arthroplasty. Clin Orthop Relat Res. 2014;472(9):2809–15.
17. Morris BJ, et al. Risk factors for periprosthetic infection after reverse shoulder arthroplasty. J Shoulder Elb Surg. 2015;24(2):161–6.
18. Mollon B, et al. The influence of a history of clinical depression on peri-operative outcomes in elective total shoulder arthroplasty: a 10-year national analysis. Bone Jt J. 2016;98(6):818–24.
19. Cancienne JM, et al. Ambulatory total shoulder arthroplasty: a comprehensive analysis of current trends, complications, readmissions, and costs. JBJS. 2017;99(8):629–37.
20. Stryker LS, et al. Elevated postoperative blood glucose and preoperative hemoglobin A1C are associated with increased wound complications following total joint arthroplasty. J Bone Jt Surg Am. 2013;95(9):808–14.
21. McElvany MD, et al. Diabetes disease severity was not associated with risk of deep infection or revision after shoulder arthroplasty. Clin Orthop Relat Res. 2019;477(6):1358–69.
22. De Martino I, Gulotta LV. The effect of obesity in shoulder arthroplasty outcomes and complications. Orthop Clin N Am. 2018;49(3):353–60.
23. Ward DT, et al. Complications of morbid obesity in total joint arthroplasty: risk stratification based on BMI. J Arthroplast. 2015;30(9 Suppl):42–6.
24. Qvistgaard M, et al. Risk factors for reoperation due to periprosthetic joint infection after elective total hip arthroplasty: a study of 35,056 patients using linked data of the Swedish Hip Arthroplasty Registry (SHAR) and Swedish Perioperative Registry (SPOR). BMC Musculoskelet Disord. 2022;23(1):275.
25. Nezwek TA, et al. Prior shoulder surgery and rheumatoid arthritis increase early risk of infection after primary reverse total shoulder arthroplasty. JSES Int. 2021;5(6):1062–6.
26. Werner BC, et al. The timing of elective shoulder surgery after shoulder injection affects postoperative infection risk in Medicare patients. J Shoulder Elb Surg. 2016;25(3):390–7.
27. Wright-Chisem J, et al. The impact of prior ipsilateral arthroscopy on infection rates after shoulder arthroplasty. J Shoulder Elb Surg. 2021;30(7):1596–602.
28. Malik AT, et al. Undergoing an arthroscopic procedure prior to shoulder arthroplasty is associated with greater risk of prosthetic joint infection. Arthrosc J Arthrosc Relat Surg. 2021;37(6):1748–54.
29. Kapadia BH, et al. Does preadmission cutaneous chlorhexidine preparation reduce surgical site infections after total knee arthroplasty? Clin Orthop Relat Res. 2016;474(7):1592–8.
30. Murray MR, et al. Efficacy of preoperative home use of 2% chlorhexidine gluconate cloth before shoulder surgery. J Shoulder Elb Surg. 2011;20(6):928–33.
31. Saltzman MD, et al. Efficacy of surgical preparation solutions in shoulder surgery. J Bone Jt Surg Am. 2009;91(8):1949–53.

32. Lee A, et al. Clinical and functional outcomes by graft type in superior capsular reconstruction: a systematic review and meta-analysis. Am J Sports Med. 2021;50:3635465211040440.
33. Chalmers PN, et al. Hydrogen peroxide skin preparation reduces *Cutibacterium acnes* in shoulder arthroplasty: a prospective, blinded, controlled trial. J Shoulder Elb Surg. 2019;28(8):1554–61.
34. Stull JD, et al. Addition of 3% hydrogen peroxide to standard skin preparation reduces *Cutibacterium acnes*-positive culture rate in shoulder surgery: a prospective randomized controlled trial. J Shoulder Elb Surg. 2020;29(2):212–6.
35. Dizay HH, Lau DG, Nottage WM. Benzoyl peroxide and clindamycin topical skin preparation decreases Propionibacterium acnes colonization in shoulder arthroscopy. J Shoulder Elb Surg. 2017;26(7):1190–5.
36. Kolakowski L, et al. Neer Award 2018: benzoyl peroxide effectively decreases preoperative *Cutibacterium acnes* shoulder burden: a prospective randomized controlled trial. J Shoulder Elb Surg. 2018;27(9):1539–44.
37. Boyd JM, et al. Propionibacterium acnes susceptibility to low-level 449 nm blue light photobiomodulation. Lasers Surg Med. 2019;51(8):727–34.
38. Cotter EJ, et al. Efficacy of combinational therapy using blue light and benzoyl peroxide in reducing *Cutibacterium acnes* bioburden at the deltopectoral interval: a randomized controlled trial. J Shoulder Elb Surg. 2021;30(12):2671–81.
39. Crane JK, et al. Antimicrobial susceptibility of Propionibacterium acnes isolates from shoulder surgery. Antimicrob Agents Chemother. 2013;57(7):3424–6.
40. Marigi EM, et al. Antibiotic prophylaxis with cefazolin is associated with lower shoulder periprosthetic joint infection rates than non-cefazolin alternatives. J Bone Jt Surg Am. 2022;104(10):872–80.
41. Yian EH, et al. Perioperative clindamycin use in penicillin allergic patients is associated with a higher risk of infection after shoulder arthroplasty. J Am Acad Orthop Surg. 2020;28(6):e270–6.
42. Miquel J, et al. Vancomycin is effective in preventing *Cutibacterium acnes* growth in a mimetic shoulder arthroplasty. J Shoulder Elb Surg. 2022;31(1):159–64.
43. Hatch MD, et al. The cost effectiveness of vancomycin for preventing infections after shoulder arthroplasty: a break-even analysis. J Shoulder Elb Surg. 2017;26(3):472–7.
44. Levy PY, et al. Propionibacterium acnes postoperative shoulder arthritis: an emerging clinical entity. Clin Infect Dis. 2008;46(12):1884–6.
45. Noskin GA, et al. National trends in *Staphylococcus aureus* infection rates: impact on economic burden and mortality over a 6-year period (1998–2003). Clin Infect Dis. 2007;45(9):1132–40.
46. Sweet FA, Roh M, Sliva C. Intrawound application of vancomycin for prophylaxis in instrumented thoracolumbar fusions: efficacy, drug levels, and patient outcomes. Spine (Phila Pa 1976). 2011;36(24):2084–8.
47. Yan H, et al. Intrawound application of vancomycin reduces wound infection after open release of post-traumatic stiff elbows: a retrospective comparative study. J Shoulder Elb Surg. 2014;23(5):686–92.
48. Lovallo J, et al. Intraoperative intra-articular injection of gentamicin: will it decrease the risk of infection in total shoulder arthroplasty? J Shoulder Elb Surg. 2014;23(9):1272–6.
49. Nowinski RJ, et al. Antibiotic-loaded bone cement reduces deep infection rates for primary reverse total shoulder arthroplasty: a retrospective, cohort study of 501 shoulders. J Shoulder Elb Surg. 2012;21(3):324–8.
50. Reed MR, Woolley LT. Uses of tranexamic acid. Contin Educ Anaesth Crit Care Pain. 2015;15(1):32–7.
51. Hooper GJ, et al. Does the use of laminar flow and space suits reduce early deep infection after total hip and knee replacement?: the 10-year results of the New Zealand Joint Registry. J Bone Jt Surg Br. 2011;93(1):85–90.
52. Davis DE, et al. Cost effectiveness of laminar flow systems for total shoulder arthroplasty: filtering money from the OR? Arch Bone Jt Surg. 2020;8(1):38–43.
53. Rojas J, Srikumaran U, McFarland EG. Inconclusive evidence for the efficacy of tranexamic acid in reducing transfusions, postoperative infection or hematoma formation after primary shoulder arthroplasty: a meta-analysis with trial sequential analysis. Shoulder Elb. 2021;13(1):38–50.
54. Schindler OS, Spencer RF, Smith MD. Should we use a separate knife for the skin? J Bone Jt Surg Br. 2006;88(3):382–5.
55. Levy BJ, et al. Is there value in the routine practice of discarding the incision scalpel from the surgical field to prevent deep wound contamination with *Cutibacterium acnes*? J Shoulder Elb Surg. 2021;30(4):806–10.
56. Callaway LF, et al. Use of electrocautery does not diminish the transmission rate of *Cutibacterium acnes* compared to a scalpel blade. J Orthop. 2020;19:162–5.
57. Brown NM, et al. Dilute betadine lavage before closure for the prevention of acute postoperative deep periprosthetic joint infection. J Arthroplast. 2012;27(1):27–30.
58. Bowler PG, et al. Topical antimicrobial protection of postoperative surgical sites at risk of infection with Propionibacterium acnes: an in-vitro study. J Hosp Infect. 2013;83(3):232–7.
59. Cai J, et al. Aquacel surgical dressing reduces the rate of acute PJI following total joint arthroplasty: a case-control study. J Arthroplast. 2014;29(6):1098–100.
60. Procter LD, et al. General surgical operative duration is associated with increased risk-adjusted infectious complication rates and length of hospital stay. J Am Coll Surg. 2010;210(1):60–5.e1.
61. Jonsson E, et al. Bacterial contamination of the wound during primary total hip and knee replacement. Median 13 years of follow-up of 90 replacements. Acta Orthop. 2014;85(2):159–64.
62. Khassebaf J, et al. Antibiotic susceptibility of Propionibacterium acnes isolated from ortho-

paedic implant-associated infections. Anaerobe. 2015;32:57–62.
63. Namdari S, et al. Preoperative doxycycline does not decolonize Propionibacterium acnes from the skin of the shoulder: a randomized controlled trial. J Shoulder Elb Surg. 2017;26(9):1495–9.
64. Rao AJ, et al. Preoperative doxycycline does not reduce Propionibacterium acnes in shoulder arthroplasty. J Bone Jt Surg Am. 2018;100(11):958–64.
65. Longo UG, et al. Antibiotic prophylaxis in primary and revision shoulder replacement: a systematic review. BMC Musculoskelet Disord. 2020;21(1):292.
66. Pradier M, et al. Suppressive antibiotic therapy with oral doxycycline for *Staphylococcus aureus* prosthetic joint infection: a retrospective study of 39 patients. Int J Antimicrob Agents. 2017;50(3):447–52.
67. Pradier M, et al. Suppressive antibiotic therapy with oral tetracyclines for prosthetic joint infections: a retrospective study of 78 patients. Infection. 2018;46(1):39–47.
68. Leafblad N, Asghar E, Tashjian RZ. Innovations in shoulder arthroplasty. J Clin Med. 2022;11(10):2799.

Part VI

Instability and Soft Tissue Management

Defining Risk Factors for TSA and RSA Instability

28

Emma Lewis, James Conville, Andrew McBride, Phil Duke, and Mark Ross

28.1 Introduction

Primary total shoulder arthroplasty (TSA) and reverse shoulder arthroplasty (RSA) carry a high success rate achieving 95% good and excellent results. Currently, TSA survivorship has been reported at 5, 10, 15 and 20 years as 98%, 93%, 88% and 85%, respectively, with a reported complication rate of approximately 6–10% [1–4]. RSA survivorship is approximately 95% at 10 years with a reported complication rate of approximately 2–15% [1, 3, 5].

Instability has been reported as the most common complication after RSA and the third most common complication after anatomic TSA [3]. The AOANJRR has shown that instability is the primary cause of early revision in both RSA and TSA [6].

The causes for instability are multi-factorial and can be classed as patient related, soft tissue or bone and implant related. Some are common to both anatomic and reverse arthroplasty, and others are specific to one group. Recognition of these risk factors and consideration of them in the preoperative planning phase is imperative for a satisfactory surgical outcome.

28.2 Patient Factors for Instability in TSA and RSA

There are several patient factors that influence stability following shoulder arthroplasty. Joint registry and clinical studies demonstrate a higher rate of instability in younger patients with osteoarthritis. This was noted in patients under the age of 65 undergoing TSA and for RSA in the 55–64-year-old age bracket with a 4% revision rate at 3 years [6, 7]. In the fracture RSA population, an association with instability was noted in patients <75. Instability has also been associated with a high BMI (>30 kg/m^2) [8]. The Australian 2021 Joint registry revealed that for RSA for fracture, obesity correlated with early revision due to instability. This may be as a result of implant malposition given difficult access, or soft tissue abutment leading to at risk postures. Male gender has been identified as a risk factor for instability with these patients having a higher incidence of instability in the first 9 months following RSA [6, 8]. Finally, subscapularis insufficiency and revision arthroplasty were both identified as independent risk factors for prosthetic dislocation [9]. In fact, any multiply operated shoulder is at risk for instability [10–12].

E. Lewis · P. Duke · M. Ross
Brisbane Hand and Upper Limb Clinic, Brisbane, Australia
e-mail: philduke@upperlimb.com; markross@upperlimb.com

J. Conville · A. McBride (✉)
Princess Alexandra Hospital, Brisbane, Australia

F. Franceschi et al. (eds.), *Revision Shoulder Arthroplasty*,
https://doi.org/10.1007/978-3-031-45944-3_28

28.3 Soft Tissue Factors in RSA

The incidence of instability in RSA ranges from 0 to 8%, mean 4.3% [8, 11, 13, 14]. Instability usually occurs in an anterosuperior direction with the arm in the 'at-risk position' of adduction, extension and internal rotation [7].

Balanced the soft tissues are an essential component of a stable joint. Biomechanical studies have demonstrated that the most effective approach to increase stability following RSA is through the joint compressive force. This is generated, for the most part, by the negative pressure in the glenohumeral joint alongside active and passive soft tissue constraints.

Surgical approach is the first consideration. Two approaches have been most commonly described in the literature; the delto-pectoral (DP) approach and antero-superior (AS) approach [15, 16]. Although the subscapular sparing AS approach is a good alternative for RSA, the DP approach remains the 'workhouse' utility approach for arthroplasty. Increased instability has been identified with the AS approach, likely relating to the increased difficulty in achieving adequate clearance of the inferior glenoid margin [17].

Management of the subscapularis is the second soft tissue consideration. RSA converts the subscapularis to a functional adductor and internal rotator. Additionally, its repair can be used to improve stability following RSA. When the deltopectoral approach is used, mobilisation of the subscapularis tendon through excision of both the coracohumeral ligament triangle and anterior capsulectomy is an important step. This provides sufficient excursion for repair under increased tension in the setting of the lateral and distalised center of rotation.

The importance of thorough glenoid exposure and soft tissue clearance cannot be overstated (Fig. 28.1). This is essential in ensuring appropriate visualisation of structures, thereby ensuring appropriate placement of components. Achieving adequate soft tissue and bony clearance of the inferior glenoid rim is paramount to prevent inferior impingement of the humeral tray on the scapula that can lead to notching and subsequent dislocation.

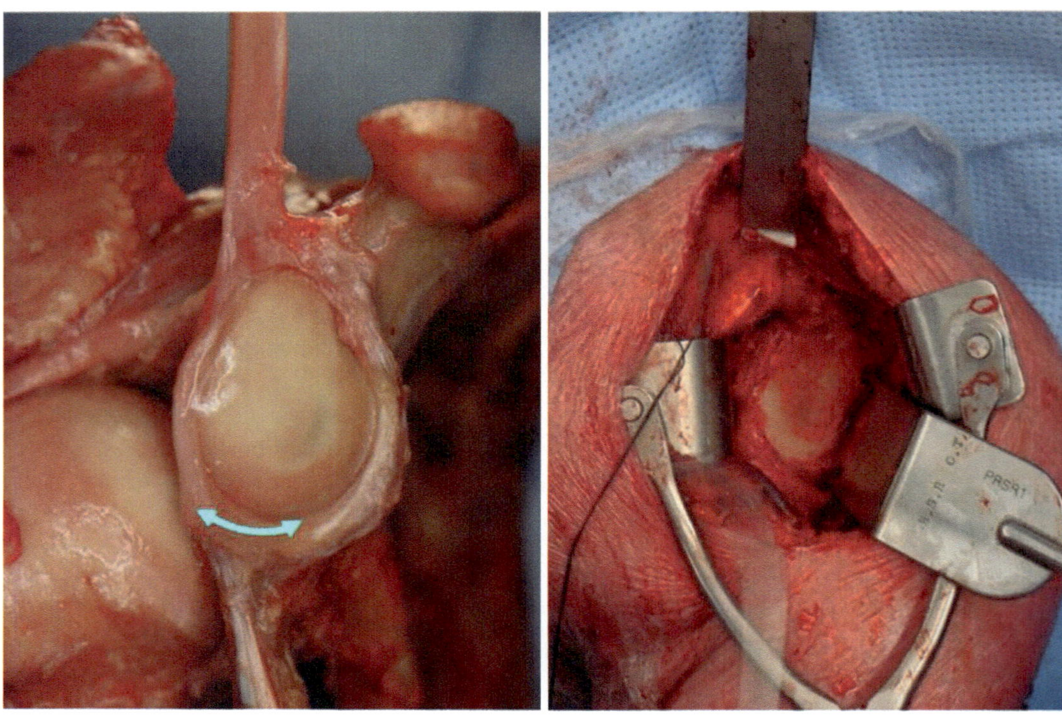

Fig. 28.1 Glenoid exposure

Finally, optional tensioning of the deltoid and conjoint tendon have been extensively referenced as key components to ensure a stable RSA. This can be achieved by way of careful implant positioning, with distalisation and lateralisation of the centre of rotation [10, 11, 18–20].

28.4 Bone/Implant Factors in RSA

28.4.1 The Glenosphere

Joint registry data, which evaluates glenoid morphology, has not shown any association with wear pattern on instability in OA [6]. What has been noted, however, is that glenosphere size greater than 40 mm has been link to lower revision rates as compared to below 40 mm [6]. In CTA, the glenosphere size does not appear to affect the risk of revision [6]. Two studies have evaluated the effect of glenosphere size and design on dislocation rates [21, 22]. In the first study, the rates of instability were 6.3%, 2.8% and 0% for 40 mm, 36 mm and 42 mm, respectively [22]. Cheung et al. found no significant difference in mean glenosphere size in their instability cohort (38.5 mm, 2.8 mm) and stable cohort (37.1 mm, 2.3 mm), $P = 0.06$ [21].

Various studies have demonstrated that glenosphere malposition has a significant association with instability. Higher dislocation rates occur when the glenoid is retroverted greater than 10° or placed in greater than 10° of superior tilt [23]. Placing the glenosphere with >4 mm of overhang relative to the glenoid has also been demonstrated to reduce instability by reducing contact and impingement between the polyethylene and inferior glenoid neck [24].

Glenoid lateralisation may further reduce instability by reducing impingement as well as optimising soft tissue tension, positively influencing the functional role of the subscapularis and deltoid. A cadaveric study by Ferle et al. illustrated that glenosphere lateralization significantly increased anterior stability of the glenohumeral joint without influencing the range of passive external rotation [25] (Fig. 28.2).

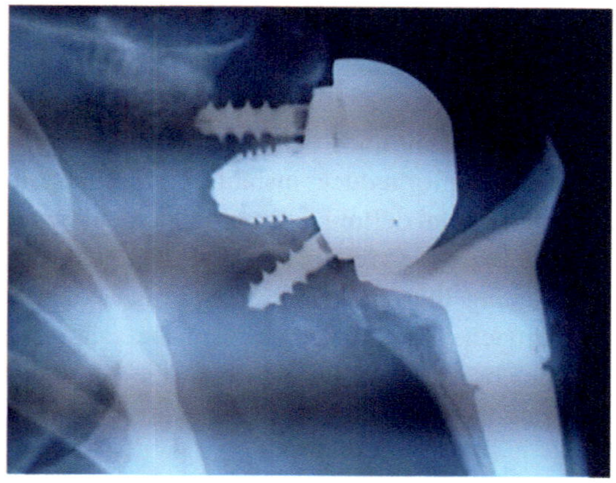

Fig. 28.2 Unstable reverse shoulder arthroplasty due to osteophyte impingement

28.4.2 The Humeral Component

Over the evolution of the RSA, many humeral components have been developed with varying neck shaft angles and options for constraint. Additionally, the surgeon can implant this component in their chosen position, with more retroversion increasing stability at the cost of external rotation.

The ability to restore humeral length and therefore establish appropriate deltoid length and soft tissue tension is critical to avoid instability and has been extensively described in the literature [18, 26]. A fresh cadaver study by Shimada et al. demonstrated that a neck-shaft angle of 155° showed the highest anterior dislocation force among neck-shaft angles, and there was no difference in dislocation force in 60° abduction with any neck-shaft angle [27].

The inlay Grammont style prosthesis (which medialises the centre of rotation with a higher neck-shaft angle) was popularised in the early 2000s with a lower risk of acromial stress fractures and component loosening. However, it has been significantly associated with instability. A systematic review by Shah et al. found that Grammont style prostheses had significantly higher rates of instability (4%) than all others designs combined (1.3%), $P < 0.001$ [28].

With an onlay system, a larger sized glenosphere and a lower neck shaft angle are utilised, thereby increasing the offset and tension of the subscapularis, leading to improved stability and internal rotation [18, 29, 30].

Achieving optimal deltoid tension has also been shown to reduce instability. Methods to achieve optimal deltoid tensioning include lowering the humerus relative to the glenoid [31], lengthening the humerus by inserting a thicker polyethylene humeral component and retaining as much proximal humerus as possible, or by lateralising the humerus [19].

28.5 Soft Tissue Factors in TSA

In anatomic TSA, instability is noted to be the main reason for revision in patients aged <55 years. The reported incidence of instability ranges from 1 to 2% [13]. Instability following TSA is most commonly described in terms of anatomical direction. As with RSA, soft tissue tension and component position are paramount.

Management of the subscapularis tendon both in the approach and in its repair are critical components in the stability of the TSA. The debate between the lesser tuberosity osteotomy and the subscapularis peel has long endured with extensive discussion in the literature. However, studies suggest that lesser tuberosity osteotomy appears to result in improved function and subscapularis integrity relative to tenotomy [32]. Failure of subscapularis repair in TSA is associated with anterior instability, poor range of motion, strength and lower outcome scores [33]. Anterior instability can also occur in the event of axillary nerve injury and deltoid dysfunction [3] (Fig. 28.3).

Tight anterior structures (capsule and subscapularis tendon) and a lax posterior capsule (posterior capsular redundancy) may combine to force the humeral head posteriorly and potentiate instability [34, 35].

Superior instability following TSA is not frequently encountered, however, can become an issue in the longstanding arthroplasty [35]. The underlying cause tends to be related to rotator cuff dysfunction with subsequent superior migration resulting in the 'rocking-horse phenomenon'. An imbalance in the soft tissues, specifically between the rotator cuff muscles and deltoid, can cause eccentric load on the glenoid component resulting in loosening and component failure. Rotator cuff tears and deficiencies in the coracoacromial arch may also lead to humeral component migration superiorly and should be thoroughly evaluated pre and intraoperatively [36–38] (Fig. 28.4).

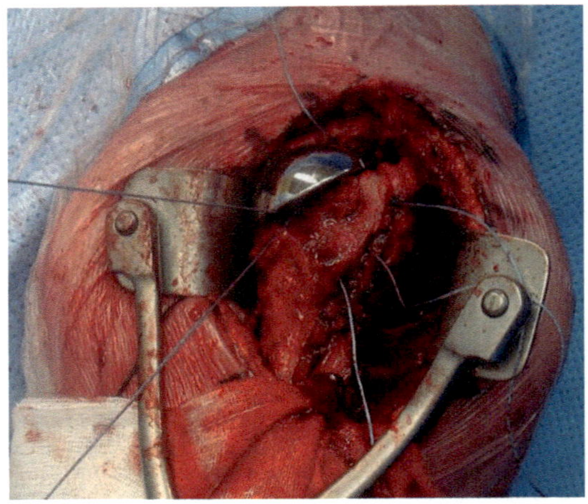

Fig. 28.3 LT osteotomy and sutures placed for repair

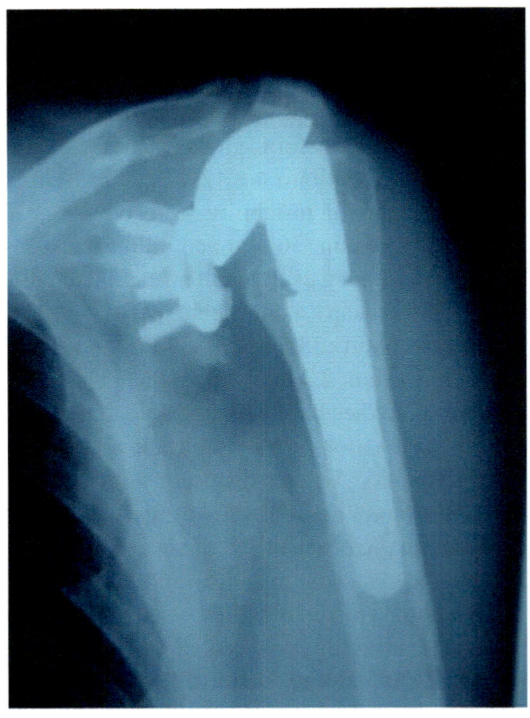

Fig. 28.4 Superior escape of TSA in cuff failure

Pre-existing instability and dislocation arthropathy do not appear to be risk factors for prosthetic dislocation [39].

28.6 Bone/Implant Factors in TSA

In avoiding instability in the TSA, appreciation of the existing bony morphology and natural version of the shoulder as well as careful bony resection and implantation is key. The goal of the anatomic shoulder arthroplasty is to restore anatomical offset and centre of rotation, which can be difficult with severe deformity.

The literature has shown that instability can be associated with component malpositioning. In particular, an aggressive humeral resection with subsequent incorrect humeral height can lead to inferior instability, in the same way a superiorised glenoid component can.

Superior escape of the anatomic shoulder arthroplasty, related to rotator cuff failure, has been linked to a non-anatomic reconstruction [40, 41]. The difficulty in appreciating the original anatomy based on joint wear has been recognised. This led Ianotti et al. to present the concept of the anatomic circle and centre of rotation based on non articular bony landmarks. Their review of the surgeon's ability to assess this has shown that there is a tendency to overstuff the joint, particularly in the hemiarthroplasty but also in the total arthroplasty [41].

Posterior instability following TSA has been attributed to as many as 20% of all complications following TSA [35]. Particularly in the osteoarthritic patient with posterior wear, this has been linked to a patulous posterior capsular in addition to excessive humeral, glenoid or combined retroversion or an undersized glenoid component [38]. Wirth and Rockwood described humeral retroversion of greater than 80° or substantial posterior glenoid erosion as the contributing cause of posterior instability [34].

Other factors to consider include depth or relative constraint of the polyethylene and use of augmentation for glenoid defects. At this stage, these have not been identified in the literature as having a direct effect on instability, but future studies may provide further clarity.

28.7 Conclusion

The cause of instability following RSA and TSA is multifactorial. Avoiding this complication calls for thorough preoperative planning and intraoperative attention to detail. The shoulder surgeon must implement the correct surgical technique, component position and achieve adequate soft tissue balancing, alongside completing a thorough intraoperative stability assessment. Instability postoperatively requires a detailed history and examination supported by plain radiographs, following which appropriate treatment can be performed.

References

1. Ma GC, Bradley KE, Jansson H, Feeley BT, Zhang AL, Ma CB. Surgical complications after reverse total shoulder arthroplasty and total shoulder arthroplasty in the United States. J Am Acad Orthop Surg Glob Res Rev. 2021;5(7):146.
2. Sperling JW, Hawkins RJ, Walch G, Mahoney AP, Zuckerman JD. Complications in total shoulder arthroplasty. Instr Course Lect. 2013;62:135–41.
3. Bohsali KI, Bois AJ, Wirth MA. Complications of shoulder arthroplasty. J Bone Jt Surg Am. 2017;99(3):256–69.
4. Deshmukh A, Koris M, Zurakowski D, Thornhill T. Total shoulder arthroplasty: long-term survivorship, functional outcome, and quality of life. J Shoulder Elb Surg. 2005;14:471–9.
5. Barco R, Savvidou OD, Sperling JW, Sanchez-Sotelo J, Cofield RH. Complications in reverse shoulder arthroplasty. EFORT Open Rev. 2016;1(3):72–80.
6. Australian Orthopaedic Association National Joint Replacement Registry 2021 document. https://aoanjrr.sahmri.com/documents/10180/712282/Hip%2C+Knee+%26+Shoulder+Arthroplasty/bb011aed-ca6c-2c5e-f1e1-39b4150bc693. Accessed 29 Jul 2022.
7. Guarrella V, Chelli M, Domos P, Ascione F, Boileau P, Walch G. Risk factors for instability after reverse shoulder arthroplasty. Shoulder Elb. 2021;13(1):51–7.
8. Chalmers PN, Rahman Z, Romeo AA, Nicholson GP. Early dislocation after reverse total shoulder arthroplasty. J Shoulder Elb Surg. 2014;23(5):737–44.
9. Padegimas EM, Zmistowski BM, Restrepo C, Abboud JA, Lazarus MD, Ramsey ML, et al. Instability after reverse total shoulder arthroplasty: which

patients dislocate? Am J Orthop (Belle Mead NJ). 2016;45(7):E444–50.
10. Affonso J, Nicholson GP, Frankle MA, Walch G, Gerber C, Garzon-Muvdi J, et al. Complications of the reverse prosthesis: prevention and treatment. Instr Course Lect. 2012;61:157–68.
11. Boileau P, Watkinson DJ, Hatzidakis AM, Balg F. Grammont reverse prosthesis: design, rationale, and biomechanics. J Shoulder Elb Surg. 2005;14(1 Suppl S):S147–161S.
12. Dezfuli B, King J, Farmer K, Struk A, Wright T. Outcomes of reverse total shoulder arthroplasty as primary versus revision procedure for proximal humerus fractures. J Shoulder Elb Surg. 2016;25:1133.
13. McBride AP, Ross M, Duke P, Hoy G, Page R, Dyer C, Taylor F. Shoulder joint arthroplasty in young patients: analysis of 8742 patients from the Australian Orthopaedic Association National Joint Replacement Registry. Shoulder Elb. 2021;15:41. https://doi.org/10.1177/17585732211058717.
14. Seebauer L. Total reverse shoulder arthroplasty: European lessons and future trends. Am J Orthop (Belle Mead, NJ). 2007;36(12 Suppl 1):22.
15. Colaço HB, Arnander M, Pearse EO, Tennentf TD. (i) Surgical approaches for shoulder arthroplasty. Orthop Trauma. 2015;29(5):281–6.
16. Chawla H, Gamradt S. Reverse total shoulder arthroplasty: technique, decision-making and exposure tips. Curr Rev Musculoskelet Med. 2020;13(2):180–5.
17. Ross M, Hirpara K. Anterior surgical approaches to the shoulder. In: Bain G, Itol E, editors. Normal and pathological anatomy of the shoulder. New York: Springer; 2015.
18. Gallo RA, Gamradt SC, Mattern CJ, Cordasco FA, Craig EV, Dines DM, et al. Instability after reverse total shoulder replacement. J Shoulder Elb Surg. 2011;20(4):584–90.
19. Gutiérrez S, Keller TS, Levy JC, Lee WE, Luo ZP. Hierarchy of stability factors in reverse shoulder arthroplasty. Clin Orthop Relat Res. 2008;466(3):670.
20. Werner CML, Steinmann PA, Gilbart M, Gerber C. Treatment of painful pseudoparesis due to irreparable rotator cuff dysfunction with the Delta III reverse-ball-and-socket total shoulder prosthesis. J Bone Jt Surg Am. 2005;87(7):1476–86.
21. Cheung EV, Sarkissian EJ, Sox-Harris A, Comer GC, Saleh JR, Diaz R, et al. Instability after reverse total shoulder arthroplasty. J Shoulder Elb Surg. 2018;27(11):1946–52.
22. Sabesan VJ, Lombardo DJ, Shahriar R, Petersen-Fitts GR, Wiater JM. The effect of glenosphere size on functional outcome for reverse shoulder arthroplasty. Musculoskelet Surg. 2016;100(2):115–20.
23. Favre P, Sussmann PS, Gerber C. The effect of component positioning on intrinsic stability of the reverse shoulder arthroplasty. J Shoulder Elb Surg. 2010;19(4):550–6.
24. Karduna AR, Williams GR, Williams JL, Iannotti JP. Joint stability after total shoulder arthroplasty in a cadaver model. J Shoulder Elb Surg. 1997;6:506–11.
25. Ferle M, Pastor MF, Hagenah J, Hurschler C, Smith T. Effect of the humeral neck-shaft angle and glenosphere lateralization on stability of reverse shoulder arthroplasty: a cadaveric study. J Shoulder Elb Surg. 2019;28(5):966–73.
26. Lädermann A, Williams MD, Melis B, Hoffmeyer P, Walch G. Objective evaluation of lengthening in reverse shoulder arthroplasty. J Shoulder Elb Surg. 2009;18(4):588–95.
27. Shimada Y, Ochiai N, et al. Effect of the neck-shaft angle on stability in the onlay type of reverse shoulder arthroplasty: a cadaveric study. Semin Arthroplasty. 2022;32(4):834–41.
28. Shah SS, Roche AM, Sullivan SW, Gaal BT, Dalton S, Sharma A, et al. The modern reverse shoulder arthroplasty and an updated systematic review for each complication: part II. JSES Int. 2021;5(1):121–37.
29. Clark JC, Ritchie J, Song FS, Kissenberth MJ, Tolan SJ, Hart ND, et al. Complication rates, dislocation, pain, and postoperative range of motion after reverse shoulder arthroplasty in patients with and without repair of the subscapularis. J Shoulder Elb Surg. 2012;21(1):36–41.
30. Edwards TB, Williams MD, Labriola JE, Elkousy HA, Gartsman GM, O'Connor DP. Subscapularis insufficiency and the risk of shoulder dislocation after reverse shoulder arthroplasty. J Shoulder Elb Surg. 2009;18(6):892–6.
31. De Wilde L, Mombert M, Van Petegem P, Verdonk R. Revision of shoulder replacement with a reversed shoulder prosthesis (Delta III): report of five cases. Acta Orthop Belg. 2001;67(4):348–53.
32. Bornes T, Rollins M, Lapner P, Bouliane M. Subscapularis management in total shoulder arthroplasty: current evidence comparing peel, osteotomy, and tenotomy. J Shoulder Elb Arthroplasty. 2018;2:247154921880777.
33. Bigdon SF, Bolliger L, Albers CE, Collin P, Zumstein MA. Subscapularis in reverse total shoulder arthroplasty. J Shoulder Elb Arthroplast. 2019;3:2471549219834192.
34. Wirth MA, Rockwood CA. Complications of total shoulder-replacement arthroplasty. J Bone Jt Surg Am. 1996;78(4):603–16.
35. Bohsali KI, Wirth MA, Rockwood CA. Complications of total shoulder arthroplasty. J Bone Jt Surg Am. 2006;88(10):2279–92.
36. Cofield RH, Edgerton BC. Total shoulder arthroplasty: complications and revision surgery. Instr Course Lect. 1990;39:449–62.
37. Jahnke AH, Hawkins RJ. Instability after shoulder arthroplasty: causative factors and treatment options. Semin Arthroplast. 1995;6(4):289–6.

38. Myer D, Bell RH. Instability after total shoulder arthroplasty. Semin Arthroplasty. 2010;21(3):191–4.
39. Lehmann L, Magosch P, Mauermann E, et al. Total shoulder arthroplasty in dislocation arthropathy. Int Orthop (SICOT). 2010;34:1219–25.
40. Franta AK, Lenteres TR, Mounce D, Neradilek B, Matsen FA. The complex characteristics of 282 unsatisfactory shoulder arthroplasties. J Shoulder Elb Surg. 2007;16:555–62.
41. Alobi B, Youderian A, Napolitano L, et al. Radiographic assessment of prosthetic humeral head size after anatomic shoulder arthroplasty. J Shoulder Elb Surg. 2014;23:1740–6.

Management of Shoulder Arthroplasty Instability

29

Jimmy J. Chan, Niraj V. Lawande, and Gregory P. Nicholson

29.1 Introduction

The management of complications after shoulder arthroplasty is critical given the ever-rising incidence of the procedure. Between 2012 and 2017, the incidence of both anatomic and reverse total shoulder arthroplasty (RTSA) increased by 103.7%, with reverse total shoulder arthroplasty (RTSA) increasing by over 2.5-fold [1, 2]. Although shoulder arthroplasty is generally successful, the complication rate is estimated to be around 11% [3, 4]. These complications include instability, component loosening, periprosthetic fracture, infection, and so on.

Instability has consistently been reported to be one of the more common complications following RTSA and anatomic total shoulder arthroplasty (ATSA) [3, 5, 6]. Multiple factors can contribute to the stability of the glenohumeral joint postoperatively, such as glenosphere size, humeral component version, soft tissue and rotator cuff status, and patient factors [7, 8]. In this chapter, we will discuss the epidemiology, evaluation, and treatment of instability after both ATSA and RTSA.

J. J. Chan · N. V. Lawande
Rush University Medical Center, Chicago, IL, USA
e-mail: Niraj.lawande@rushortho.com

G. P. Nicholson (✉)
Department of Orthopedic Surgery, Rush University Medical Center, Chicago, IL, USA
e-mail: Gregory.nicholson@rushortho.com

29.2 Instability in Anatomic Total Shoulder Arthroplasty

29.2.1 Epidemiology

With better understanding of the glenohumeral reconstruction and technique, incidence of instability has continued to decrease in ATSA [3]. In 2006, Bohsali et al. identified the rate of instability as 4.9% following unconstrained ATSA. However, a repeated meta-analysis in 2017 by the same authors focusing on studies published after 2006 saw a decrease in instability to 1% following ATSA. Instability contributed to 10% of overall postoperative complications [3]. Sanchez-Sotelo et al. [8] found 13 out of 777 anatomic total shoulder arthroplasty (TSA) and hemiarthroplasties to have anterior or posterior instability. Furthermore, the authors reported soft tissue imbalance as the leading cause of instability, as 21 of the 33 revisions described in this case series were attributed to soft tissue imbalance intraoperatively [8]. Although the prevalence is decreasing, it is critical for the surgeon to evaluate signs of instability and recommend the appropriate treatment.

29.2.2 Evaluation of Instability in Shoulder Arthroplasty

A thorough history, physical examination, and radiographic evaluation are crucial in diagnosing

F. Franceschi et al. (eds.), *Revision Shoulder Arthroplasty*,
https://doi.org/10.1007/978-3-031-45944-3_29

instability after total shoulder arthroplasty. The glenohumeral joint has dynamic (rotator cuff muscles, periscapular muscles, long head of biceps, and rotator interval) and static (bony architecture, capsule, labrum, and glenohumeral ligaments) restraints to help stabilize the joint. Many of these mechanisms are compromised as part of the shoulder reconstruction procedure, which increases the potential for instability of the prosthetic glenohumeral joint.

A detailed history is important in working up a patient with suspected instability after total shoulder arthroplasty. Soft tissue balance and tensioning are key in maintaining stability as several key anatomic restraints are sacrificed during index arthroplasty [8–10]. Patients with underlying disease processes, such as rheumatoid arthritis or connective tissue disorders, are at higher risk. Twenty to forty percent of rheumatoid patients have been shown to have full-thickness cuff tears [9]. Patients can have instability from subscapularis rupture after a successful arthroplasty [3, 5, 8]. In addition, the timing of instability symptoms can also help determine the cause. Early dislocations are often due to component malposition, soft tissue imbalance, or abnormal bony architecture and patient noncompliance, whereas late dislocation is more likely due to rotator cuff failure [10]. However, one caveat is that most instability symptoms are subluxations and not full dislocations, are unrecognized by patients, and are only diagnosed upon postoperative appointments and careful history and physical examination.

Physical examination can provide clues regarding the direction of instability. Active and passive ranges of motion should be assessed. Manual muscle testing of the rotator cuff, deltoid, and scapular rotators should be documented. Exaggerated external rotation could indicate an insufficient subscapularis, which could be contributing to subtle anterior subluxation. The lift-off test is an exam that can be used to assess the integrity of the subscapularis tendon. Neurologic assessment of the shoulder is crucial to determine the status of the brachial plexus, the axillary nerve and the suprascapular nerve [11].

Radiographic evaluation is necessary for instability after total shoulder arthroplasty. The true anteroposterior (AP) view, or Grashey view, of the glenohumeral joint, lateral, and axillary views should be obtained. Several key radiographic parameters should be assessed. First is the position of the humeral head relative to the tuberosities. The top of the head should be 5–8 mm above the top of the tuberosity. When the prosthetic head height is greater than that value, the humeral component may indeed be proud, or too high. When the distance is smaller or reversed, impingement can occur in overhead position. Size of the humeral head component can also be evaluated. When the humeral head is too big, the joint could be overstuffed. The offset of the glenohumeral joint can be assessed by the distance of tuberosity and lateral edge of acromion. Version of the humeral component can be difficult to assess on plain radiographs. Obtaining an axillary lateral view with the forearm positioned at 30° external rotation (ER) will help confirm the humeral version and the presence of any dislocation or subluxation as the head will oppose the glenoid. The axillary view can be used to determine the position of the humeral head relative to the glenoid. Glenoid version and/or component wear can be evaluated as well. This is also the view used to determine instability or dislocation of the humeral head. Computed Tomography (CT scan) can be used to check the glenoid version and tuberosity healing in cases of proximal humerus fracture. CT arthrogram can be very valuable to check the integrity of the rotator cuff muscles (especially the healing status of the subscapularis) and to evaluate glenoid loosening, and component positioning.

Infection should always be part of the differential diagnosis when treating instability in prosthetic joint replacement. Any history of fever, chills, other areas of infections, or dental procedures should be obtained. Drainage of the wound or erythema and warmth should alarm surgeons about possible infectious etiology. Relevant laboratory values should be obtained, including complete blood count, chemistry, erythrocyte sedimentation rate (ESR), and C-reactive protein (CRP). Should be considered and if fluid obtained, it should be cultured and held for at least two weeks.

29.2.3 Management

29.2.3.1 Anterior Instability

Anterior instability is the most common form of postoperative instability after ATSA [12, 13]. If suspected or diagnosed, early intervention is critical. A frank dislocation is fairly obvious, and a closed reduction should be attempted. If this has occurred in the early postoperative period, early operative intervention to repair the subscapularis is warranted. If it has occurred in a later time period, consideration for a reverse shoulder arthroplasty is appropriate. Most commonly, a dislocation event in ATSA is from either failure of subscapularis anteriorly or malposition of the prosthesis; therefore, tendon repair and component correction are often required in ATSA dislocation [5, 8].

An association between subscapularis insufficiency and anterior instability has been presented throughout the literature [3, 5, 8]. During primary ATSA, tenotomy, lesser tuberosity osteotomy, and tendon peel are the most common ways to take down the subscapularis, and recent evidence suggests no difference in outcomes between the utilization of these techniques [14]. Common causes of postoperative subscapularis rupture include poor tissue quality, aggressive physical therapy, premature or traumatic external rotation or internal rotation, and excessive humeral head size [3, 12]. If subscapularis insufficiency is identified early, within the first month postoperatively, it should be repaired, provided the arthroplasty components are well fixed and in good position (Fig. 29.1). Delayed repair may result in retraction of the subscapularis making results less predictable. Late repairs may require pectoralis major transfer to supplement the repair [9]. While this approach has shown success in a primary setting, caution should be used if utilizing this procedure when there is preoperative anterior subluxation of the humeral head [15, 16]. Achilles tendon allograft can be used as a salvage procedure in those settings. Moeckel et al. [17] presented seven patients who received a revision subscapularis repair after developing anterior instability as a complication after ATSA. Of the seven, three of the revisions failed and instability remained. Those patients received an anterior capsular reconstruction with an Achilles tendon allograft and had successful results.

If repair is delayed, failed, or implant components are the cause of instability, revision to RTSA should be strongly considered. Irreparable subscapularis repairs have a high failure rate [15], which may ultimately require a reverse instead of attempting anterior capsule reconstruction or tendon transfer. The semiconstrained design of components of the RTSA allows for the implant to compensate for the insufficiency of soft tissue, a common cause of anterior instability. However, it is important to consider that RTSA in a revision setting has a higher rate of complications than primary RTSA [6, 18, 19].

29.2.3.2 Posterior Instability

Posterior instability is a rare scenario that is often the result of excessive glenoid or humeral component retroversion or laxed posterior soft tissue [3, 12]. If the instability was due to significant retroversion of the glenoid component, then consideration should be given to revision of the glenoid component. If sufficient bone stock is present, then another glenoid component can be implanted with either corrected glenoid version or utilization of an augmented glenoid component to provide correction. If glenoid bone loss is present, then revision to RTSA should be the next step. There are reports of revision to large-head hemiarthroplasty with selective reaming of glenoid surface, but given significant advancements in RTSA with good reported outcomes recently, this option should be reserved for extreme circumstances. Although quite rare, if the humeral component malposition is the sole culprit of instability after ATSA, then an isolated humeral stem revision can be performed.

There have been attempts of revision ATSA with posterior capsular plication (PCP) to correct posterior instability. However, 7 out of 16 patients

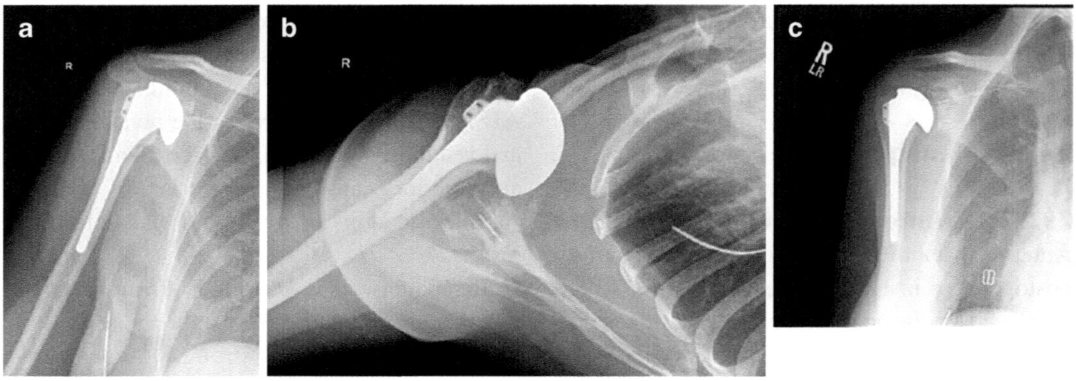

Fig. 29.1 Radiographs demonstrating anterior instability after TSA secondary to subscapularis failure. (**a**) AP radiographs of right shoulder demonstrating dislocation of TSA. (**b**) Lateral XR of right shoulder demonstrating anterior dislocation of TSA. (**c**) Postoperative XR demonstrating open reduction of TSA with subscapularis repair

continued to have posterior subluxations [20]. As a result, the authors recommended revising to RTSA instead of attempting PCP during a revision ATSA.

29.3 Instability in Reverse Total Shoulder Arthroplasty

29.3.1 Epidemiology

Since the contemporary RTSA procedure was first introduced in the 1990s, its indications and design have continued to evolve. As a result, the complication rates and types of complications are shifting [3, 21]. Unlike in ATSA, RTSA can have instability as a complication with higher frequency, and instability is considered one of the more common complications [3, 5, 21, 22]. Instability can make up as much as 38% of complications following RTSA [23]. Tashjian et al. reported that 4% of patients had full dislocations that required reduction. However, when including Grade 2–3 instability (feelings on instability and subluxations), this increases to 13%. Instability is also more prevalent in revision RTSA settings. Boileau reported a 30% reoperation rate due to recurrence after revision RTSA [23]. Abdelfattah [24] reported that 12% of RTSA remained unstable after revision while Kohan et al. [25] reported 32% recurrent instability after revision RTSA.

Increased risk for dislocation following RTSA has been associated with elevated Body Mass Index (BMI), male gender, American Society of Anesthesiologists (ASA) classification, superior glenosphere inclination, and revision surgery [26, 27]. The risk of instability after revision RTSA for failure of anatomic, hemi, or reverse prosthesis or failure of osteosynthesis is three times more than after primary RTSA [28]. Furthermore, a lack of satisfactory subscapularis repair at initial RTSA has been discussed as a contributor to instability [19].

29.3.2 Management

29.3.2.1 Anterior Dislocation

Although a standardized approach to management of RTSA dislocation is lacking, the authors will present an algorithm that has good clinical outcomes in their hands. For first-time dislocation, it is always prudent to attempt a closed reduction with relaxation. This has been shown to be successful in clinical office settings or emergency room or in the operating room setting [19]. This depends on each individual practice and the availability of staff and equipment and support. Ideally, patients should receive relaxation medication to allow easier reduction with more gentle manipulation. The reduction maneuver is a combination of 45° of abduction in neutral rotation, followed by longitudinal traction and a posteriorly and inferiorly directed force applied to the proximal humerus as the limb is elevated in the scapular plane. Chalmers' et al. [19] recommend a trial of closed reduction followed by 6 weeks of sling immobilization. Extension, adduction, and internal rotation are to be avoided, similar to the same precaution in any RTSA postoperative protocol. Teusink et al. [29] reported 21 dislocated RTSA treated with closed reduction and immobilization, and 62% of patients remained stable, 29% required revision procedure, and 9% remained unstable at 28 months; 62% of the dislocation events occurred in the first 90 days, and no difference was seen between early and late dislocations. Therefore, initial closed reduction provides acceptable outcomes and should be attempted as a first-line treatment regardless of the timing of dislocation.

When closed reduction is unsuccessful or if instability persists or there is another dislocation after initial closed reduction, open reduction and component revision are the next appropriate steps. The author's experience has been that when open reduction is required, exchange of the modular component should be performed. Preoperative radiographic workup becomes crucial in this scenario. Barring significant malposition of the glenosphere baseplate or humeral component, the author's recommendation is to keep the well-fixed components. The stability and soft tissue tension can be increased by using a larger glenosphere or a lateralized glenosphere, increasing the thickness of the polyethylene on the humeral component, and in rare cases using a more constrained polyethylene insert [21, 22]. The goal is to either lateralize or distalize the articulation to achieve more myofascial sleeve tension across the joint (Fig. 29.2).

Patients should be placed in abduction sling and immobilized for 4–6 weeks after either open or closed reduction [19]. Subscapularis and capsule repair should always be attempted; however, in the setting of dislocation, the tissues are often irreparable. Thus making strict immobilization of the shoulder a critical step after reduction. The goal is stability over mobility at this point in the clinical course.

When recurrent instability occurred, closed reduction should be attempted again, but a full revision of RTSA should be considered if modular components exchange was already performed. Boileau [23] published his algorithm for revision RTSA based on humeral shortening and medialization. Only in patients with >15 mm of humeral shortening and excessive medialization would a well-fixed component need to be revised. Therefore, good preoperative imaging can be crucial in determining if the revision requires modular components or all components exchange. If humeral shortening >15 mm, then a humeral component revision with and without a proximal humeral allograft should be performed. If humeral medialization >15 mm, then glenoid baseplate revision with augment or lateralizing

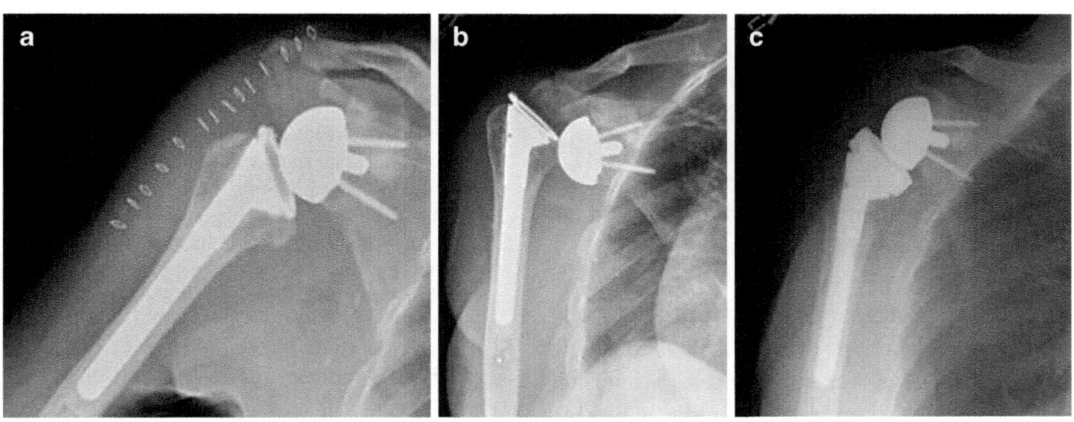

Fig. 29.2 Radiographs demonstrating using metallic spacer to increase myofascial sleeve length. (**a**) Primary RTSA. (**b**) Dislocation of RTSA. (**c**) Postreduction with metallic spacer

structural bone graft would be required [6, 23]. A cerclage suture technique described by Tashjian et al. [30] can be added to the RTSA to provide increased "fixation" to enhance stability and hopefully allow encapsulation of the RTSA at risk.

Besides excessive shortening or medialization, significant malposition of components (version of either humerus or glenoid) is another reason to revise a well-fixed component. If sufficient glenoid bone stock is left, then another glenoid component can be implanted. When there is significant bone deficiency present, bone grafting or a vault reconstruction-type procedure would need to be performed to restore proper glenohumeral relationship.

If instability continues despite well-positioned and well-fixed revision RTSA, then salvage procedure should be considered. Conversion to a large head hemiarthroplasty with reaming of the glenoid socket is a reasonable choice. The cerclage suture technique as described by Tashjian et al. [30] can be added to either RTSA or large head hemiarthroplasty. Typically, a 2-mm drill bit can be passed anterior to posterior, just medial to the glenoid or baseplate. A #5 dyneema unbreakable suture or tape can be passed through and looped around with the posterior limb going around the humeral component in a locking fashion. With the arm in full adduction and neutral position and glenohumeral joint reduced, the anterior and posterior limbs of the cerclage sutures are securely tied down to complete the cerclage procedure. Salazar et al. [31] reported their acromiohumeral cerclage technique in 10 revision RTSA patients. A transosseous tunnel was drilled in acromion, and nonabsorbable, high-tensile suture tape was looped through the tunnels and tied down as an augment to shoulder stability. All patients remained stable with an average follow-up of 23 months.

29.3.2.2 Posterior Dislocation

Posterior dislocation of RTSA is extremely unlikely [32]. However, on rare occasions when it occurs, authors recommend a similar algorithm as anterior dislocation. A closed reduction with relaxation should be attempted first. Open reduction with the exchange of modular components or thicker polyethylene should be performed if closed reduction was unsuccessful. Patients should be immobilized for 4–6 weeks after reduction. In the setting of recurrent instability, component malposition needs to be evaluated, and the possibility of revision of components should be discussed with the patient. Just as for anterior instability, the glenoid inclination and position should be evaluated, and humeral version and length should be adjusted as needed. Cerclage techniques can be added for patients with persistent instability. Large-head hemiarthroplasty is another salvage solution.

29.4 Summary

Reverse TSA is now approximately 65% of all arthroplasty performed, and when instability occurs, it is typically a dislocation and thus more clinically dramatic and impactful than anatomic TSA. Anatomic TSA instability can be more subtle due to the more common subluxation mechanism. With increasing popularity, the instability of ATSA and RTSA requires careful evaluation. Good understanding of the biomechanical principles of implant design will allow surgeons to identify underlying cause and appropriate treatment. When revision surgery is needed, surgeons need to keep in mind the balance of constraint with appropriate freedom of motion.

References

1. Best MJ, Aziz KT, Wilckens JH, McFarland EG, Srikumaran U. Increasing incidence of primary reverse and anatomic total shoulder arthroplasty in the United States. J Shoulder Elb Surg. 2021;30(5):1159–66.
2. Wagner ER, Farley KX, Higgins I, Wilson JM, Daly CA, Gottschalk MB. The incidence of shoulder arthroplasty: rise and future projections compared with hip and knee arthroplasty. J Shoulder Elb Surg. 2020;29(12):2601–9.
3. Bohsali KI, Bois AJ, Wirth MA. Complications of shoulder arthroplasty. J Bone Jt Surg Am. 2017;99(3):256–69.
4. Aldinger PR, Raiss P, Rickert M, Loew M. Complications in shoulder arthroplasty: an analysis of 485 cases. Int Orthop. 2010;34(4):517–24.

5. Parada SA, Flurin PH, Wright TW, Zuckerman JD, Elwell JA, Roche CP, et al. Comparison of complication types and rates associated with anatomic and reverse total shoulder arthroplasty. J Shoulder Elb Surg. 2021;30(4):811–8.
6. Boileau P, Melis B, Duperron D, Moineau G, Rumian AP, Han Y. Revision surgery of reverse shoulder arthroplasty. J Shoulder Elb Surg. 2013;22(10):1359–70.
7. Gutiérrez S, Comiskey CA, Luo ZP, Pupello DR, Frankle MA. Range of impingement-free abduction and adduction deficit after reverse shoulder arthroplasty. Hierarchy of surgical and implant-design-related factors. J Bone Jt Surg Am. 2008;90(12):2606–15.
8. Sanchez-Sotelo J, Sperling JW, Rowland CM, Cofield RH. Instability after shoulder arthroplasty: results of surgical treatment. J Bone Jt Surg Am. 2003;85(4):622–31.
9. Hennigan SP, Iannotti JP. Instability after prosthetic arthroplasty of the shoulder. Orthop Clin N Am. 2001;32(4):649–59.
10. Kany J, Jose J, Katz D, Werthel JD, Sekaran P, Amaravathi RS, et al. The main cause of instability after unconstrained shoulder prosthesis is soft tissue deficiency. J Shoulder Elb Surg. 2017;26(8):e243–51.
11. Lopiz Y, Rodriguez-González A, Martín-Albarrán S, Marcelo H, García-Fernández C, Marco F. Injury to the axillary and suprascapular nerves in rotator cuff arthropathy and after reverse shoulder arthroplasty: a prospective electromyographic analysis. J Shoulder Elb Surg. 2018;27(7):1275–82.
12. Wirth MA, Rockwood CA. Complications of total shoulder-replacement arthroplasty. J Bone Jt Surg Am. 1996;78(4):603–16.
13. Bohsali KI, Wirth MA, Rockwood CA. Complications of total shoulder arthroplasty. J Bone Jt Surg Am. 2006;88(10):2279–92.
14. Buraimoh MA, Okoroha KR, Oravec DJ, Peltz CD, Yeni YN, Muh SJ. A biomechanical comparison of subscapularis repair techniques in total shoulder arthroplasty: lesser tuberosity osteotomy versus subscapularis peel. JSES Open Access. 2018;2(1):8–12.
15. Elhassan B, Ozbaydar M, Massimini D, Diller D, Higgins L, Warner JJP. Transfer of pectoralis major for the treatment of irreparable tears of subscapularis: does it work? J Bone Jt Surg Br. 2008;90(8):1059–65.
16. Updegrove G, Kohler J, Ponnuru P, Armstrong AD. Pectoralis major tendon transfer for management of subscapularis failure after anatomic total shoulder arthroplasty: technique and results. JSES Rev Rep Tech. 2022;2(4):451–7.
17. Moeckel BH, Altchek DW, Warren RF, Wickiewicz TL, Dines DM. Instability of the shoulder after arthroplasty. J Bone Jt Surg Am. 1993;75(4):492–7.
18. Saltzman BM, Chalmers PN, Gupta AK, Romeo AA, Nicholson GP. Complication rates comparing primary with revision reverse total shoulder arthroplasty. J Shoulder Elb Surg. 2014;23(11):1647.
19. Chalmers PN, Rahman Z, Romeo AA, Nicholson GP. Early dislocation after reverse total shoulder arthroplasty. J Shoulder Elb Surg. 2014;23(5):737–44.
20. Alentorn-Geli E, Assenmacher AT, Sperling JW, Cofield RH, Sánchez-Sotelo J. Plication of the posterior capsule for intraoperative posterior instability during anatomic total shoulder arthroplasty. J Shoulder Elb Surg. 2017;26(6):982–9.
21. Chae J, Siljander M, Wiater JM. Instability in reverse total shoulder arthroplasty. J Am Acad Orthop Surg. 2018;26(17):587–96.
22. Garcia-Fernandez C, Lopiz Y, Arvinius C, Ponz V, Alcobía-Diaz B, Checa P, et al. Dislocation after reverse total shoulder arthroplasty using contemporary medialized modular systems. Can we still consider it such a frequent complication? Eur J Orthop Surg Traumatol Orthop Traumatol. 2022;32(8): 1525–34.
23. Boileau P. Complications and revision of reverse total shoulder arthroplasty. Orthop Traumatol Surg Res. 2016;102(1, Supplement):S33–43.
24. Abdelfattah A, Otto RJ, Simon P, Christmas KN, Tanner G, LaMartina J, et al. Classification of instability after reverse shoulder arthroplasty guides surgical management and outcomes. J Shoulder Elb Surg. 2018;27(4):e107–18.
25. Kohan EM, Chalmers PN, Salazar D, Keener JD, Yamaguchi K, Chamberlain AM. Dislocation following reverse total shoulder arthroplasty. J Shoulder Elb Surg. 2017;26(7):1238–45.
26. Padegimas EM, Zmistowski BM, Restrepo C, Abboud JA, Lazarus MD, Ramsey ML, et al. Instability after reverse total shoulder arthroplasty: which patients dislocate? Am J Orthop. 2016;45(7):E444–50.
27. Sinkler MA, Dolan JD, Henderson D, Steflik MJ, Lewis FD, Parada SA, et al. Risk factors of instability following reverse total shoulder arthroplasty in patients with no history of shoulder surgery. J Orthop. 2022;34:339–43.
28. Wall BT, Mottier F, Walch G. 9: Complications and revision of the reverse prosthesis: a multicenter study of 457 cases. J Shoulder Elb Surg. 2007;16(2):e55.
29. Teusink MJ, Pappou IP, Schwartz DG, Cottrell BJ, Frankle MA. Results of closed management of acute dislocation after reverse shoulder arthroplasty. J Shoulder Elb Surg. 2015;24(4):621–7.
30. Tashjian RZ, Broschinsky K, Chalmers PN. Glenohumeral cerclage for salvage of recalcitrant instability after reverse total shoulder arthroplasty. J Shoulder Elb Surg. 2018;27(8):e259–63.
31. Salazar DH, Bialek SE, Garbis NG. Acromiohumeral cerclage in reverse total shoulder arthroplasty for recurrent instability. J Shoulder Elb Surg. 2022;31(8):e376–85.
32. Charalambous CP, Saidapur SK, Alvi F, Birch A, Tsiouri C, Ravenscroft MJ, et al. Fixed posterior dislocation following total shoulder arthroplasty. Shoulder Elb. 2010;2(3):147–50.

Pectoralis Transfer for Deltoid Deficiency After Reverse Shoulder Arthroplasty

30

Ryan Lohre, Abdulaziz F. Ahmed, Karan Dua, and Bassem Elhassan

30.1 Deltoid Deficiency Etiologies

Range of motion (ROM) deficiencies require clear definitions prior to treatment. Loss of active forward elevation or rotation at the glenohumeral joint can occur secondary to traumatic or compressive neuropathies, or dystrophies such as neuralgic amyotrophy (Parsonage-Turner syndrome). A C5 compressive radiculopathy may significantly reduce the strength of the deltoid and can be associated with traumatic or degenerative RC disorders. Patients with C5 nerve palsies will present with extremely reduced ROM of the shoulder secondary to weakness of the deltoid muscle from proximal neuropathy. Axillary nerve palsies will similarly present with extremely limited glenohumeral joint ROM in forward elevation and external rotation and true paralysis of the shoulder. Axillary nerve palsies may also occur secondary to blunt or penetrating trauma, or through iatrogenic injury, either from arthroscopic or open procedures. The axillary nerve is the most injured terminal nerve of the brachial plexus following an anterior shoulder dislocation. The axillary nerve is particularly at risk secondary to its anatomical course, progressing through the quadrilateral space and wrapping around the humerus with multiple branches tethering the nerve to adjacent muscle and fascia. Frequently, the main nerve injury following dislocation is a continuity lesion or avulsion at its branch from the posterior cord near its thoracodorsal origin, though it may also occur at the level of the quadrilateral space, or from the compressive effects of an unreduced humeral shaft.

30.2 Relevant Surgical Anatomy

30.2.1 The Deltoid Muscle

The deltoid muscle is considered the largest muscle of the shoulder joint, and it consists of three parts: anterior, middle, and posterior. The anterior deltoid originates from approximately the lateral half of the clavicle, extending to the anterolateral corner of the acromion. The middle deltoid originates from the anterolateral to posterolateral corners of the acromion. The posterior deltoid originates from the posterolateral corner of the acromion and most of the scapular spine. All three deltoid muscle parts merge to form an arch-like broad tendinous insertion on the deltoid tuberosity on the humeral midshaft [1]. The blood supply of the deltoid is mainly from the posterior humeral circumflex artery, a branch of the third segment of the axillary artery, which supplies the posterior and middle parts of the del-

R. Lohre · A. F. Ahmed · K. Dua · B. Elhassan (✉)
Department of Orthopedic Surgery, Massachusetts General Hospital, Harvard Medical School, Boston, MA, USA
e-mail: afahmed@mgh.harvard.edu; KDUA@mgh.harvard.edu; belhassan@mgh.harvard.edu

F. Franceschi et al. (eds.), *Revision Shoulder Arthroplasty*,
https://doi.org/10.1007/978-3-031-45944-3_30

toid [2], whereas the anterior deltoid is nourished by the deltoid and the acromial branches of the thoracoacromial artery, which originates from the third segment of the axillary artery. The deltoid is innervated by the axillary nerve. In terms of function, forward flexion of the shoulder is mainly produced by the anterior and middle parts of the deltoid in conjunction with the clavicular head of the pectoralis major, whereas forward elevation is a product of anterior and middle deltoid contraction only. Shoulder abduction in the coronal plane is mainly due to the contraction of the middle deltoid, whereas the anterior and posterior parts of the deltoid stabilize the shoulder joint during abduction. The posterior deltoid assists the latissimus dorsi in producing arm extension. Thus, the deltoid muscle is of utmost importance for normal shoulder function [3], and a well-functioning deltoid is an essential prerequisite for a reverse shoulder arthroplasty (RSA).

30.2.2 The Pectoralis Major Muscle

The pectoralis major muscle has two distinct heads: the clavicular head and the sternocostal head. The clavicular head originates from the medial half or two-third of the clavicle, whereas the sternocostal head is the larger of the two heads and broadly originates from the sternum and from the 2-sixth ribs [4]. The clavicular head of the pectoralis major runs in a straight fashion, with all of its fibers being parallel and inserts just lateral to the bicipital groove on the proximal humerus [5]. The sternocostal head shares the same insertion; however, its fibers exhibit two distinct orientations. The upper part of the sternocostal head fibers is parallel and inserts just posterior to the clavicular head fibers. However, the fibers of the lower part of the sternocostal head rotate 180° from their origin to the insertion; as such, the lower fibers insert superiorly on the humerus compared to the upper fibers [6]. The main function of the clavicular head is forward flexion and adduction concurrently with the anterior part of the deltoid. The sternoclavicular head is mainly involved with adduction and internal rotation.

30.2.3 Brachial Plexus Anatomy

When considering pedicled pectoralis major transfers in complex shoulder reconstruction, it is pertinent to review in brief the relevant anatomy of the brachial plexus. The brachial plexus typically consists of five segments: nerve roots, trucks, divisions, cords, and branches. The nerve roots that typically make up the brachial plexus are five: C5, C6, C7, C8, and T1. It is not uncommon for the plexus to receive additional contributions from the C4 or T2 nerve roots. The term "prefixed plexus" indicates that a brachial plexus receives nerve supply from the C4 root, whereas the term "postfixed plexus" denotes that a brachial plexus is also supplied by the T2 nerve root [7]. The nerve roots are a combination of the ventral motor and the dorsal sensory rootlets as they exit the spinal foramen. The dorsal rootlet contains dorsal ganglion, which is an important reference to whether an injury to a specific root is pre- or post-ganglionic. This distinction has important implications for predicting the prognosis of nerve injury recovery, with preganglionic injury having an abysmal prognosis. Nerve trucks are formed as different nerve roots coalesce, except for the middle trunk. The upper trunk forms as the C5 and C6 nerve roots converge, whereas the lower trunk forms as the C8 and T1 nerve roots combine. The middle trunk is merely a continuation of the C7 nerve root. The trucks of the brachial plexus emerge between the anterior and middle scalene muscle bellies. Subsequently, each trunk branches further into an anterior and a posterior division just behind the clavicle. Divisions combine to form the three cords of the brachial plexus, just distal to the clavicle. The cords are intimately related to the axillary artery; as such, each cord is named after its anatomical position in the artery. The posterior divisions combine to form the posterior cord. The lateral cord forms as the anterior divisions of the upper and middle trunks combine, whereas the medial cord forms as the anterior divisions of the lower trunk combine. The branches of the brachial plexus can emerge from nerve roots, trunks, and cords; however, no branches emerge from the divisions. The long thoracic nerve, which supplies the serratus anterior muscle, branches from the C5, C6, and C7 nerve roots. The suprascapular nerve emerges after the C5 and C6 roots meet to form the upper trunk. The lateral pectoral nerve emerges from the lateral cord. Several branches emerge from the posterior cord: the upper subscapular nerve, the thoracodorsal nerve, the lower subscapular nerve, and finally ending with the radial and axillary nerves. The medial cord provides three branches: the medial pectoral nerve, the medial brachial cutaneous nerve, and the medial antebrachial cutaneous nerve.

30.2.4 The Axillary Nerve

The axillary nerve is a terminal branch of the posterior cord of the brachial plexus and carries nerve fibers from carries fibers from the C5 and C6 nerve roots. The axillary nerve lies posteriorly to the axillary artery, given that it branches from the posterior cord. As the axillary descends, it courses anterior to the subscapularis muscle and then passes underneath the inferior edge of the subscapularis muscle at approximately 3–4 cm from the anteromedial aspect of the coracoid tip [8]. Whereas, the axillary nerve crosses underneath the subscapularis at a 3–7 mm distance medial to the subscapular musculotendinous junction [8]. It should be noted that these distances can vary depending on the arm position. After crossing the inferior border of the subscapularis, the axillary nerve courses underneath the glenohumeral capsule, and it then exits the axilla posteriorly through the quadrilateral space. The quadrilateral space borders are the teres minor superiorly, the teres major inferiorly, the humerus laterally, and the long head of the triceps medially. The axillary nerve usually divides into an anterior and posterior branch in the quadrilateral space in 65%–87% of specimens, whereas others have reported that it branches within the deltoid muscle in 35% [9, 10]. The anterior division curves laterally around the humeral surgical neck, accompanied by the posterior humeral circumflex vessels, both of which are within the deep deltoid fascia [10]. The anterior division of the axillary nerve provides motor innervation to the anterior and middle parts of the deltoid. The posterior division of the axillary nerve courses in a posterior direction and does not curve around the humerus in contrast to the anterior branch [11]. The posterior division divides into two branches: the superior lateral brachial cutaneous nerve that provides sensation over the lateral shoulder and a motor nerve to the teres minor muscle.

30.2.5 The Lateral and Medial Pectoral Nerves

The lateral pectoral nerve emerges from the lateral cord distal to the clavicle. Thereafter, it pierces the clavipectoral fascia together with the thoracoacromial artery and courses on the deep surface of the pectoralis major muscle [12]. The lateral pectoral nerve provides motor innervation to the clavicular and upper sternocostal heads of the pectoralis major. The medial pectoral nerve emerges from the medial cord just deep the pectoralis minor. At this level, the medial pectoral nerve receives a branch from the lateral pectoral nerve, which is called the ansa pectoralis. The medial pectoral nerve pierces the pectoralis minor muscle, and it provides motor innervation to the pectoralis minor and courses on the deeper surface of the lower sternocostal head of the pectoralis major [12]. The medial pectoral nerve provides motor innervation to the lower sternocostal head of the pectoralis major and the pectoralis minor muscles. The lateral pectoral nerve is found approximately 9.5–15.5 (mean 12.5 cm) from the pectoralis major humeral insertion and consistently passes medial to the pectoralis minor before inserting into the pectoralis major. The medial pectoral nerve inserts into the pectoralis major 8.6–15.3 (mean 11.9 cm) from the pectoralis major humeral insertion and is consistently inferior to the lateral pectoral nerve [13]. The medial pectoral nerve may pass through the pectoralis minor (75%) or lateral to it (25%) and is consistently at 2 cm from the inferior edge of the lower pectoral head.

30.2.6 Pectoralis Major Blood Supply and Pedicle Anatomy

In terms of blood supply, the pectoralis major is supplied by 3 vessels [14]. The superior thoracic artery, a branch of the upper segment of the axillary artery, is more variable and supplies the clavicular head. Whereas the pectoral branch of the thoracoacromial artery of the second segment of the axillary artery supplies the clavicular head and the upper part of the sternocostal head. The lower part of the sternocostal head is supplied by the lateral thoracic artery, which is a branch of the middle segment of the axillary artery. The pectoralis major pedicle is mainly based on the thoracoacromial artery that branches from the axillary artery at the middle point of the clavicle. The course of the pectoral branch of the thoracoacromial artery can be illustrated by drawing a line from the lateral acromion to the xiphoid process and a line perpendicular to the midpoint between the lateral and middle thirds of the clavicle. The course of the thoracoacromial artery corresponds to the clavicular perpendicular line and the medial part of the acromial-xiphoid line. The pectoral branch of the thoracoacromial artery pedicle can be identified as it is encased by fat on the deeper surface of the pectoralis major muscle once elevated, and it can be clearly dissected from the superficial surface of the pectoralis minor.

30.3 Evaluation of Deltoid-deficient Shoulders

The history of duration and known mechanisms of axillary nerve palsy should be delineated. In traumatic circumstances, penetrating trauma would indicate a high risk of complete nerve injury, and transection and nerve exploration, repair, and grafting should be considered expediently, with improved outcomes shown to occur less than 4–6 months from injury [15]. In settings of dislocation, identifiable independent risk factors for axillary nerve injuries include concomitant fracture (humerus or scapula), vascular injury, delay in reduction >2 h, neurologic deficit identified immediately after in the distribution of the axillary nerve or other distal brachial plexus branches, and immediate or early neuropathic pain. Advanced age should be considered by the surgeon as the risk of any nerve injury increases at an odd of 1.3× for every decade of life [16]. Kosiyatrakul et al. [17] identified a cumulative incidence of nerve injury documented through electromyography for shoulder dislocations as 65%, with 42% remaining symptomatic at 38-month follow-up. Complete, neurotmetic injury to the axillary nerve following dislocation has been described at 2.4–2.7%, increasing to 22.7% when associated with a greater tuberosity (GT) fracture or rotator cuff (RC) injury (terrible triad injury of the shoulder). Robinson et al. [18] analyzed a prospective trauma database of 3633 patients with traumatic anterior shoulder dislocation, identifying 7.8% of patients having a neurologic injury plus a GT fracture and RC tear. Injury mechanism and arm position indicates potential brachial plexus injury, with younger and higher energy mechanisms producing a greater likelihood of single nerve injury versus older (age >50) lower energy falls producing multiple neurologic deficits. Non-traumatic axillary nerve palsies should alert the surgeon to investigate for neuralgic amyotrophy, C5 nerve palsies, or brachial neuritis.

30.4 Physical Examination

Surgeons should evaluate the entire upper extremity along with the axillary nerve to indicate patients for potential reconstructive efforts by brachial plexus specialists or peripheral nerve surgeons. A common misconception is that in an axillary nerve injury, both sensory and motor nerve functions will be affected. The axillary nerve trifurcates at the level of the humeral neck, and the classic "regiment patch" areas' sensation to light touch can be preserved in 15%–50% of patients with a clear motor deficit [16]. Longitudinal, clinical monitoring of nerve recovery is best performed starting 1 week from injury with direct palpation of contraction of deltoid fibers in the anterior, middle, and posterior muscle groups. Clinical assessment of deltoid function by these means has a demonstrable concurrence of 100% with electrophysiologic studies, and clinicians should become attuned to these functions.

Additional deltoid-specific physical examinations include simple range of motion and forward elevation, which will be severely limited to less than 30 degrees. Extension lag tests are performed with the patient seated, leaning forward, and both arms extended at the glenohumeral joint. The patient is asked to hold the arm in this position, and any lag is indicative of posterior deltoid deficiency correlating with a more proximal axillary nerve lesion. This corresponds to a Medical Research Council Manual Muscle Testing scale of less than grade 3. The "swallow-tail sign" tests deltoid abduction with the arm internally rotated to reduce contribution from periscapular muscles [19]. In advanced cases, deltoid atrophy will be apparent on the contralateral side, with visible deep anatomy of the acromion and humeral head and subacromial space (sulcus sign).

Patients will also exhibit weakness in external rotation secondary to associated RC tear, suprascapular neuropathy if not recovered, or teres minor axillary nerve branch injury. Elhassan et al. [14] demonstrated in their series of 21 patients receiving pedicled pectoralis transfer and RSA that 100% ($n = 21/21$) had a positive Jobe test, 38% ($n = 8/21$) had a complete lack of ER although all ($n = 21/21$) had ER <20 degrees, and 57% ($n = 12/21$) had a positive belly-press test. Without a functioning deltoid, the RC will eventually fail secondary to receiving all forces to position the arm in space. Patients may also exhibit anterosuperior escape, when associated with variable patterns of RC deficiency, or cuff tear arthropathy (CTA) and painful, limited arcs of motion.

Periscapular muscles should be assessed for function, including the upper, middle, and lower trapezius, rhomboids, and serratus anterior for scapular stability. The pectoralis major should be assessed by palpation for contractility of the sternal and clavicular heads and through resisted adduction and internal rotation. The pectoralis major is supplied by C5-T1 nerve roots terminating in the medial and lateral pectoral nerves, and complete brachial plexopathies or root injuries will likely affect the function of the pectoralis major and preclude transfer. In patients with deltoid atrophy, the tendinous insertion of the pectoralis major is readily visible in the axillary crease.

30.5 Imaging and Neurophysiologic Evaluation

Initial shoulder evaluation should consist of standard shoulder radiographic series, including a true anteroposterior and axillary radiograph of the glenohumeral joint. In the native glenohumeral joint, deltoid deficiency can manifest as inferior humeral head subluxation. Further radiographic findings that would aid in surgical planning are the degree of arthritic changes, the pattern of wear, and bone loss. In acute injuries, radiographs are valuable to look for dislocations and/or fractures. In the setting of a prior RSA, deltoid deficiency would lead to signs of instability such as subluxation or periprosthetic dislocation. Moreover, radiographs should be scrutinized for humeral shortening, which would lead to deltoid laxity and dysfunction. Arm lengthening can be evaluated by comparing most recent radiographs with those in the immediate post-operative and preoperative periods. Additionally, obtaining radiographs of the contralateral shoulder can be helpful as a benchmark for arm length assessment. Further advanced imaging is warranted in the setting of deltoid deficiency. Computed tomography (CT) scan is helpful in accurately delineating the accompanying bony pathologies, such as glenoid wear pattern and bone loss, which are useful for surgical planning. Magnetic resonance imaging (MRI) is another advanced modality to evaluate soft-tissue pathologies such as deltoid muscle atrophy and compressive lesions along the course of the axillary nerve. Isolated fatty atrophy of the teres minor can also ascertain damage to the axillary nerve. In patients with a prior failed RSA, MRI or CT scans with metal-artifact reduction protocols are useful to rule out other diagnoses associated with failed RSA, such as periprosthetic infection or aseptic loosening. A final radiological evaluation should include the cervical spine to rule out more proximal compressive neuropathies, especially to the C5 and C6 nerve roots.

Neurophysiologic modalities, such as electromyography (EMG) and nerve conduction studies (NCS), are valuable in ascertaining deltoid deficiency due to axillary nerve pathology. These modalities can determine the degree of nerve injury, which has direct implications for prognosis and treatment. Axillary nerve injuries are often low-grade with an expected recovery with non-operative measures at 3–4 months [15, 20]. High-grade axillary nerve injury can be amenable to surgical exploration and repair if detected early. Low-Once an axillary nerve injury has occurred, EMG and NCS can detect early electrophysiologic changes within the axillary nerve. Baseline evaluation with EMG/NCS can be performed between 2–4 weeks post-injury [16]. Recovery of the axillary nerve can be monitored with repeat neurophysiologic studies at 3 and 6 months post-injury [15]. Nerve recovery is signaled by increasing amplitude of compound muscle action potentials and recruitment of motor end plate units [21].

30.6 Deltoid Deficiency

Indications for a pedicled pectoralis major transfer and RSA include true paralysis with atrophic deltoid musculature (particularly anterior and middle deltoid) and associated RC deficiency or CTA. Patients failing prior nerve transfer surgery or not indicated for nerve transfer surgery, as well as those with deltoid deficiency and failing conservative management, should also be considered. Patients with in-situ hardware, including failed open reduction internal fixation (ORIF), hemiarthroplasty, total shoulder arthroplasty (TSA) or RSA, and iatrogenic axillary nerve injury with deltoid atrophy, are also indicated. Select patients with resection of the deltoid and axillary nerves for tumors may be candidates for pedicled pectoralis transfer and RSA if soft tissue coverage is adequate, although other myocutaneous flaps such as latissimus dorsi may be used in these circumstances. Contraindications include active infection, tumor, or axillary neuropraxia with expected recovery. Additional nerve transfer options should be considered prior to reconstructive efforts.

The pedicled pectoralis major transfer attempts to reconstruct the deficient anterior deltoid musculature to improve forward elevation of the arm. The pectoralis major sternal and clavicular heads are detached from their origins and insertion, allowing for the muscle to be rotated on its neurovascular pedicle and reattached to the lateral clavicle and anterior acromion. Reorienting the pectoralis major muscle fibers allows for a vertical line of pull similar to the deltoid. The remaining posterior and middle deltoid that is contractile and non-atrophic can additionally be detached and mobilized anteriorly to assist in forward elevation strength. Performing the pedicled pectoralis major transfer around an RSA allows for improved biomechanics through medializing the COR.

Another MTT option for deltoid deficiency includes a pedicled latissimus dorsi transfer. The broad nature of this muscle may cover greater deltoid defects [22]. A pedicled latissimus dorsi transfer does not provide as much strength or improvements in range of motion (ROM) as reliably as a pedicle pectoralis major transfer, although it provides excellent soft tissue coverage, including skin flaps if necessary. A glenohumeral fusion may also be a treatment option for this patient population. A glenohumeral fusion is also an option following a failed pedicled pectoralis major transfer and RSA, although requires additional bone grafting.

30.7 Pectoralis Major Transfer Technique

The goal of the pectoralis major transfer is to reconstruct the function of the anterior deltoid. To accomplish this, the pectoralis major must change from producing an adductor and internal rotation moment to a flexor moment. This requires a bipolar transfer to be most effective, as seen by detaching both origin and insertion with rotation around the neurovascular pedicle.

The patient is positioned in a recumbent beach chair with draping sufficient to allow access to the sternum and manubrium. The sternal notch and xiphoid process are relevant landmarks to approximate the extent of the surgical field (Fig. 30.1). Posteriorly, the medial border of the scapula may also be accessed if considering a lower trapezius tendon transfer concurrently for external rotation deficiencies secondary to irreparable posterosuperior RC tears or functional deficiencies. If requiring a lower trapezius tendon transfer concurrently, a lateral position has also been described, although implantation of an RSA in a lateral position may be foreign to surgeons.

A large curvilinear incision extending 2 cm proximal to the xiphoid process and medial to the sternocostal junction is produced, traversing over the sternoclavicular joint and extending just distal to the clavicle. The incision continues to extend laterally across the AC joint and then proceeds to the anterolateral acromion before extending distally. A "T" incision can be performed with one limb traversing distally along a standard deltopectoral incision while the other limb proceeds to the posterolateral acromion. The decision to perform either of these is based on prior incisions in the area as well as if transfer of the middle or posterior heads of the deltoid is to be additionally performed. Deep dissection occurs along the incision, and large skin flaps are produced to visualize the entirety of the pectoralis major (Fig. 30.2). Three distinct heads are encountered including the clavicular origin, upper sternal origin, and lower sternal origin.

The insertion of the pectoralis major upper sternal and clavicular heads is released to allow for proper orientation of the muscle (Fig. 30.3).

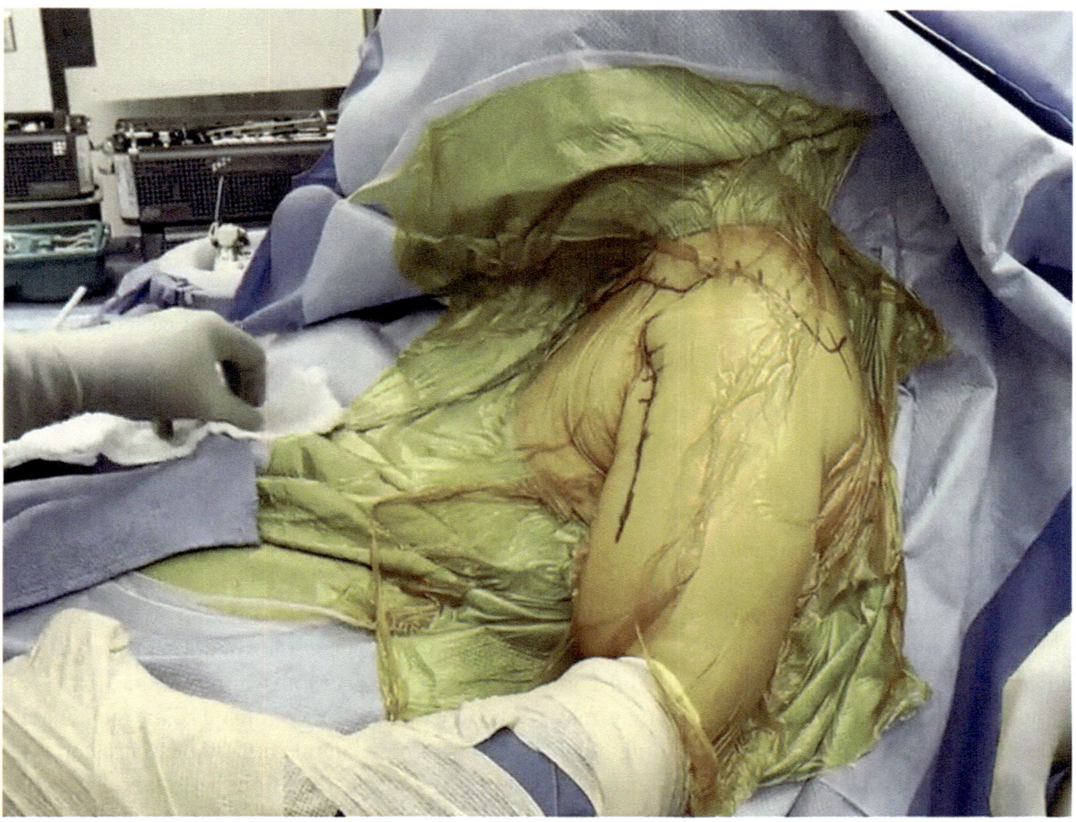

Fig. 30.1 Patient positioned and draped in a beach chair position. The draping is performed to allow unrestricted access to the sternum, clavicle, and scapula

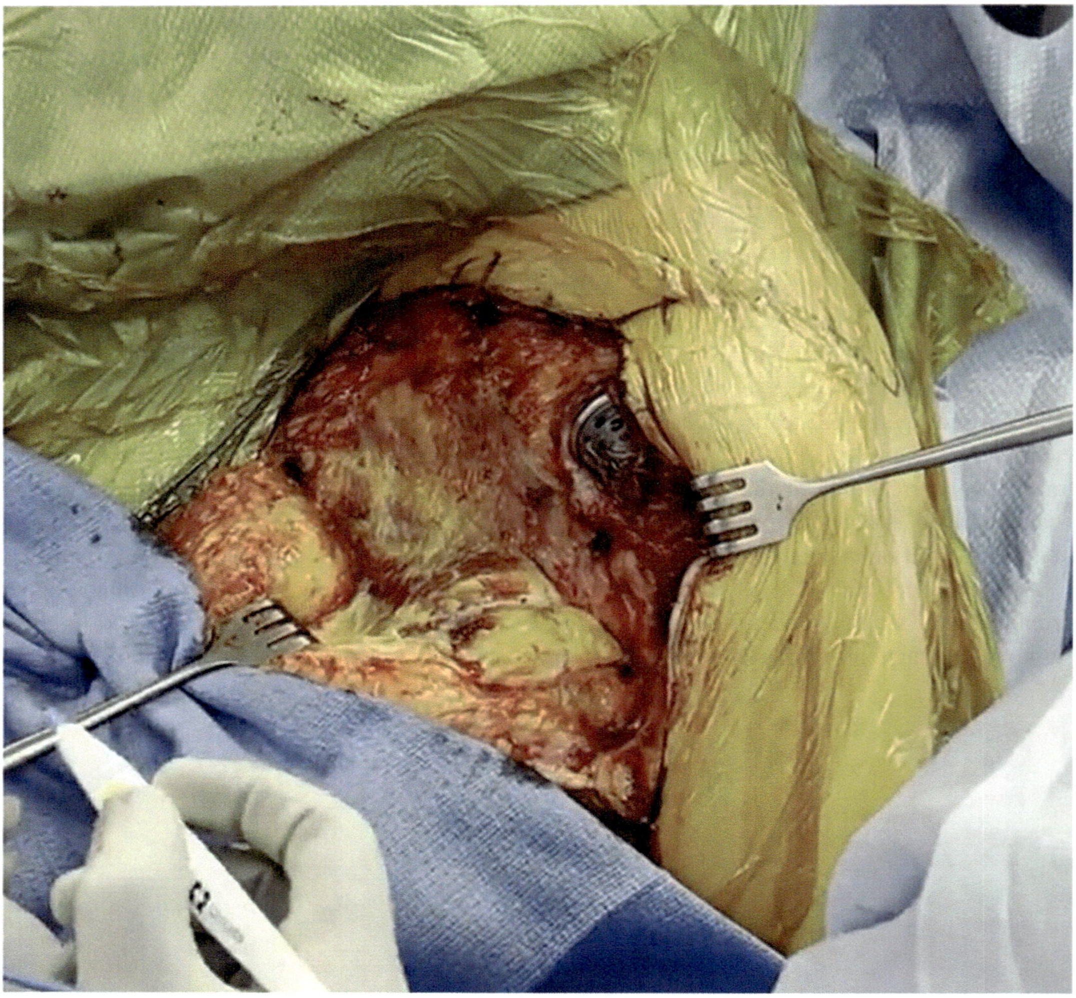

Fig. 30.2 Extensile incision exposing the pectoralis major muscle at its both sternocostal and clavicular origins

The lower pectoral muscle remains attached at its origin and insertion, providing some remaining adduction strength. The upper sternal and clavicular origins are detached using electrocautery from both the sternum and clavicle. These are chosen as the main pectoral muscle groups for transfer based on their innervation and location of neurovascular pedicle. During dissection, costal arterial branches are encountered, and care should be taken to cauterize these as they may retract. The pectoralis minor originating from ribs 3–5 is encountered deep to the pectoralis major during elevation and is a landmark to the neurovascular pedicle in relation to the mid-clavicle. As dissection is continued lateral, the neurovascular pedicle of the pectoralis major is encountered near the middle of the clavicle, distal to the subclavius muscle near the subclavian artery, and vein and brachial plexus. The lateral and medial pectoral nerves are found at an average distance of 8.5 cm medial to the humeral insertion of the pectoralis major and consistently medial to the pectoralis minor (Fig. 30.4) [13]. The free muscle is then rotated so the most medial portion is now lateral (Fig. 30.5). In this orientation, the muscle fibers are all traversing in the long axis of the arm and the neurovascular pedicle remains tension-free (Fig. 30.5). The trans-

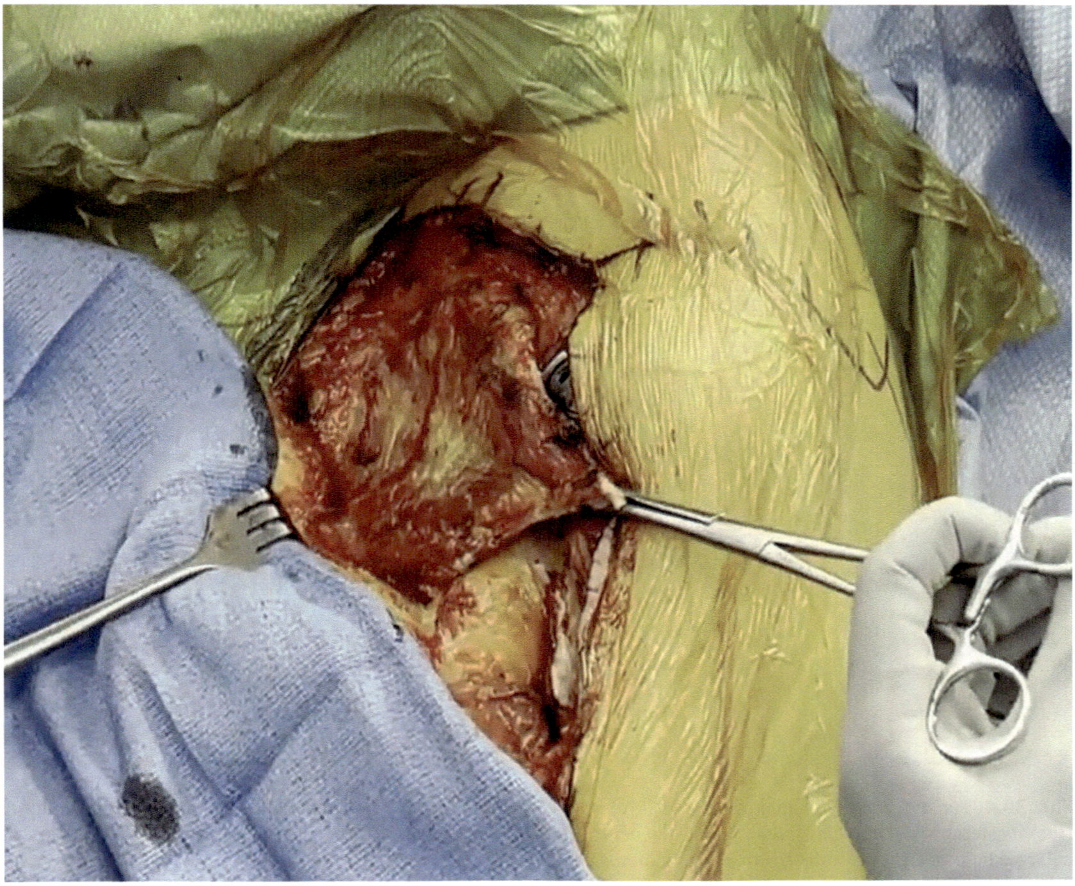

Fig. 30.3 The insertion of the pectoralis major upper sternocostal and clavicular heads are released from their humeral insertion. The lower sternocostal head was not released to retain adduction strength

ferred muscle may then be protected with a moist gauze, checked periodically to assure there is no congestion and RSA is performed through a standard deltopectoral approach.

Atrophic anterior deltoid muscle is excised, and the anterolateral acromion and lateral 1/3 of the clavicle prepared for muscle transfer with a burr. If the subscapularis is detached, this should be reapproximated to aid in soft-tissue coverage and prevent dislocation. At this time, additional muscle transfers may be performed to reconstruct ER strength, including latissimus dorsi or lower trapezius tendon transfers. Latissimus dorsi transfer is performed by releasing the insertion along the bicipital groove, transferred posteriorly under the teres major, and inserted at the infraspinatus or teres minor footprint. In cases of revision surgeries, the latissimus dorsi may have been released and not present, necessitating the use of the lower trapezius transfer. In these circumstances, the lower trapezius is harvested from the acromial spine, and an Achilles allograft is tunneled under the posterior deltoid in the subdeltoid space. The tendon is attached to the infraspinatus footprint and woven through and attached to the lower trapezius tendon with the shoulder in external rotation. Care should be taken when passing the allograft in the subdeltoid space to avoid further iatrogenic injury to the axillary nerve in this region.

The critical fixation point is the medial/lateral extent of the new pectoral origin. This should occur at the medial/lateral distance of the neurovascular pedicle along the clavicle, so it does not

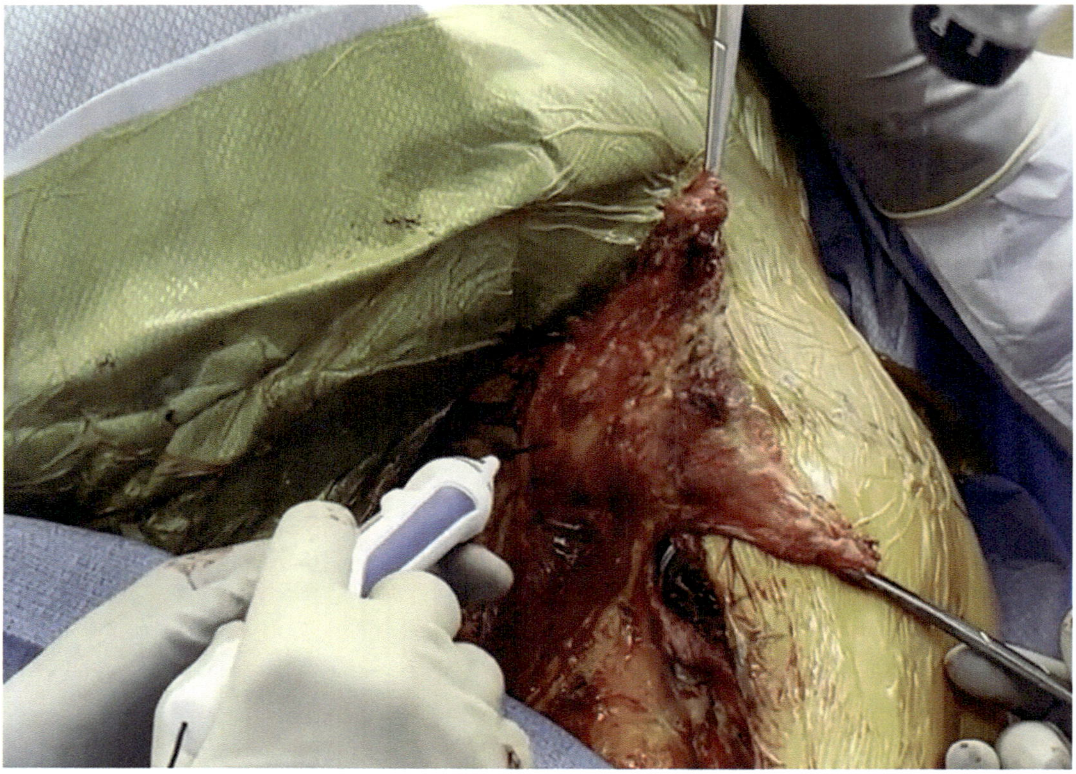

Fig. 30.4 As the pectoralis major muscle is elevated from its sternocostal and clavicular origins, the neurovascular pedicle of the pectoralis major is encountered near the middle of the clavicle, distal to the subclavius muscle near the subclavian artery, and vein and brachial plexus. A nerve stimulator can be used to ascertain the location of the pedicle

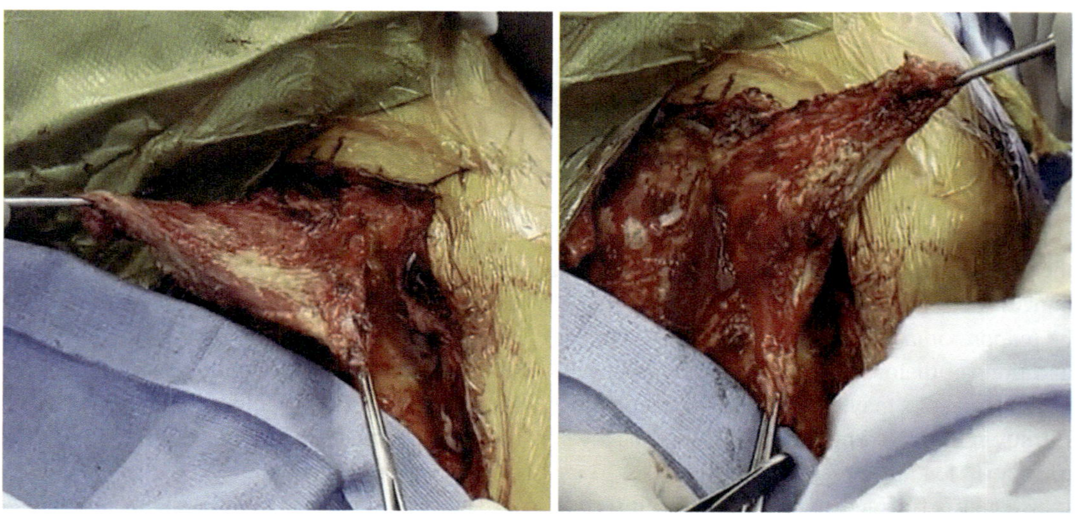

Fig. 30.5 The upper sternal and clavicular origins are detached using electrocautery from both the sternum and clavicle. The image on the left illustrates the anatomical orientation of the pectoralis major muscle, the distal clamp is holding the humeral insertion, and the medial clamp is holding the upper edge of the sternal origin. The image on the right demonstrates the new orientation of the free pectoralis major muscle which is rotated, so the most medial portion is now lateral

tether this structure. Non-absorbable sutures can be placed through bone tunnels in the clavicle and acromion and sequentially fixed from medial to lateral. We typically supplement fixation by using 7–8 buttons with double-loaded sutures tied in a cow-hitch over muscle and tendon. After the new origin has been established, the arm is placed in approximately 60 degrees of flexion, and the insertion is attached again using buttons bicortically to the humeral shaft at the level of the prior deltoid insertion. Any additional deltoid mobilization can now occur if necessary, such as moving the middle deltoid more anteriorly. The interval between the pectoralis major and remaining deltoid is further sutured with non-absorbable suture for added strength. At this time, the surgeon can check the functioning of the pectoral nerve as a shoulder flexor by using a nerve and muscle stimulator. If the arm flexes against gravity, then appropriate tension has been produced. We place two drains into the operative field secondary to the potential space created from the pectoral muscle transfer.

The patient is placed in either a pre-fit brace or a shoulder spica cast for a period of 8 weeks postoperatively. The arm remains in a flexed position of 45–60 degrees with slight internal rotation, or 45–60 degrees of flexion with the addition of 40 degrees of external rotation, akin to singing into a microphone.

Antibiotics are prescribed while the drain is in situ and the drain is removed when less than 30 mL occurs in a 24-hour period. Antibiotics are cessated at this point. The brace or cast is maintained for a period of 8 weeks and subsequently removed with progressive physical therapy. After the brace is removed, the initial period consists of active-assisted range of motion and aquatherapy for 8 weeks, followed by progressive active range of motion as tolerated until 4 months. At 4 months postoperatively, gentle strengthening occurs. At 6 months, activity as tolerated with weight restrictions to 15 lbs. maximum in any direction is recommended. Gradual, progressive stretching, as tolerated, can occur at this point and is prohibited prior to this point to prevent any muscle stretch injuries.

References

1. Rispoli DM, Athwal GS, Sperling JW, Cofield RH. The anatomy of the deltoid insertion. J Shoulder Elb Surg. 2009;18(3):386–90.
2. Hue E, Gagey O, Mestdagh H, Fontaine C, Drizenko A, Maynou C. The blood supply of the deltoid muscle. Application to the deltoid flap technique. Surg Radiol Anat. 1998;20(3):161–5.
3. Groh GI, Simoni M, Rolla P, Rockwood CA. Loss of the deltoid after shoulder operations: an operative disaster. J Shoulder Elb Surg. 1994;3(4):243–53.
4. Fung L, Wong B, Ravichandiran K, Agur A, Rindlisbacher T, Elmaraghy A. Three-dimensional study of pectoralis major muscle and tendon architecture. Clin Anat. 2009;22(4):500–8.
5. Bois AJ, Lo IKY. Surgical anatomy of the pectoralis major tendon insertion revisited: relationship to nearby structures and the pectoral eminence for defining the anatomic footprint. JSES Int. 2020;4(2):324–32.
6. Kakwani RG, Matthews JJ, Kumar KM, Pimpalnerkar A, Mohtadi N. Rupture of the pectoralis major muscle: surgical treatment in athletes. Int Orthop. 2007;31(2):159–63.
7. Noland SS, Bishop AT, Spinner RJ, Shin AY. Adult Traumatic Brachial Plexus Injuries. J Am Acad Orthop Surg. 2019;27(19):705–16.
8. Apaydin N, Tubbs RS, Loukas M, Duparc F. Review of the surgical anatomy of the axillary nerve and the anatomic basis of its iatrogenic and traumatic injury. Surg Radiol Anat. 2010;32(3):193–201.
9. Loukas M, Grabska J, Tubbs RS, Apaydin N, Jordan R. Mapping the axillary nerve within the deltoid muscle. Surg Radiol Anat. 2009;31(1):43–7.
10. Uz A, Apaydin N, Bozkurt M, Elhan A. The anatomic branch pattern of the axillary nerve. J Shoulder Elb Surg. 2007;16(2):240–4.
11. Ball CM, Steger T, Galatz LM, Yamaguchi K. The posterior branch of the axillary nerve: an anatomic study. J Bone Joint Surg Am. 2003;85(8):1497–501.
12. Aszmann OC, Rab M, Kamolz L, Frey M. The anatomy of the pectoral nerves and their significance in brachial plexus reconstruction. J Hand Surg Am. 2000;25(5):942–7.
13. Klepps SJ, Goldfarb C, Flatow E, Galatz LM, Yamaguchi K. Anatomic evaluation of the subcoracoid pectoralis major transfer in human cadavers. J Shoulder Elb Surg. 2001;10(5):453–9.
14. Elhassan BT, Wagner ER, Werthel JD, Lehanneur M, Lee J. Outcome of reverse shoulder arthroplasty with pedicled pectoralis transfer in patients with deltoid paralysis. J Shoulder Elb Surg. 2018;27(1):96–103.
15. Steinmann SP, Moran EA. Axillary nerve injury: diagnosis and treatment. J Am Acad Orthop Surg. 2001;9(5):328–35.
16. Visser CP, Coene LN, Brand R, Tavy DL. The incidence of nerve injury in anterior dislocation of the shoulder and its influence on functional recovery.

A prospective clinical and EMG study. J Bone Joint Surg Br. 1999;81(4):679–85.
17. Kosiyatrakul A, Jitprapaikulsarn S, Durand S, Oberlin C. Recovery of brachial plexus injury after shoulder dislocation. Injury. 2009;40(12):1327–9.
18. Robinson CM, Shur N, Sharpe T, Ray A, Murray IR. Injuries associated with traumatic anterior glenohumeral dislocations. J Bone Joint Surg Am. 2012;94(1):18–26.
19. Nishijma N, Yamamuro T, Fujio K, Ohba M. The swallow-tail sign: a test of deltoid function. J Bone Joint Surg Br. 1995;77(1):152–3.
20. de Laat EA, Visser CP, Coene LN, Pahlplatz PV, Tavy DL. Nerve lesions in primary shoulder dislocations and humeral neck fractures. A prospective clinical and EMG study. J Bone Joint Surg Br. 1994;76(3):381–3.
21. Avis D, Power D. Axillary nerve injury associated with glenohumeral dislocation: a review and algorithm for management. EFORT Open Rev. 2018;3(3):70–7.
22. Le Hanneur M, Lee J, Wagner ER, Elhassan BT. Options of bipolar muscle transfers to restore deltoid function: an anatomical study. Surg Radiol Anat. 2019;41(8):911–9.

31 Tendon Transfers in Shoulder Arthroplasty

Arno A. Macken, Eric R. Wagner, Wouter J. van der Poel, Geert Alexander Buijze, and Thibault Lafosse

31.1 Introduction

Tendon transfers are used to compensate for an irreparable tendon defect responsible for a lack of movement or chronic pain, combined with a loss of strength. It can be used in the setting of primary or revision shoulder arthroplasty with an anatomic or reversed implant. As anatomic total shoulder arthroplasty (ATSA) is indicated primarily in shoulder pathology with an intact rotator cuff, tendon transfers are used most commonly in the setting of reverse shoulder arthroplasty (RSA). However, some specific indications still exist in the setting of ATSA, particularly in young and active patients with irreparable tendon tears.

RSA is effective in improving forward elevation and abduction by altering the center of rotation, specifically in patients with rotator cuff arthropathy. Increased elevation and abduction lead to an improved ability to perform daily tasks and a marked increase in quality of life. However, rotation after RSA is less predictable. RSA may even result in a loss of external rotation or decrease over time [1–3]. External rotation is crucial for control of the arm held in abduction, which plays an essential role in daily activities. A deficient internal rotation is equally limiting in daily activities due to its importance for personal hygiene and dressing. In patients with poor elevation, external rotation, or internal rotation after RSA, a tendon transfer can be considered. Several options are available; the latissimus dorsi, teres major, pectoralis major, or lower trapezius can be transferred. Furthermore, the pectoralis major can be used in the form of a pedicled graft to reconstruct the deltoid. Overall, these procedures provide satisfying results in terms of range of motion and strength. However, the evidence is sparse, and few comparative studies are available.

Although less common, tendon transfers may also be used after ATSA. For example, it may be used in the case of a symptomatic subscapularis tear or subscapularis insufficiency. Loss of subscapularis function in ATSA may result in the loss of balances between the horizontal and vertical forces, leading to variable outcomes ranging from a complete loss of active forward elevation (pseudoparalytic shoulder) in the case of anterior superior escape to decreased strength and range of motion in internal rotation and instability. In these cases, a transfer of the latissimus dorsi or pectoralis major can be used. The literature on

A. A. Macken · W. J. van der Poel
Alps Surgery Institute, Clinique Générale d'Annecy, Annecy, France

Erasmus Medical Centre, Rotterdam, The Netherlands

E. R. Wagner
Emory Musculoskeletal Institute, Atlanta, GA, USA
e-mail: eric.wagner@emory.edu

G. A. Buijze · T. Lafosse (✉)
Alps Surgery Institute, Clinique Générale d'Annecy, Annecy, France

F. Franceschi et al. (eds.), *Revision Shoulder Arthroplasty*,
https://doi.org/10.1007/978-3-031-45944-3_31

tendon transfers in the setting of ATSA is sparse, but positive results in terms of strength and range of motion are reported. However, despite replacing the subscapularis muscle, instability often remains an issue.

Very little literature is available on transfers after RSA or in the setting of revision shoulder arthroplasty. However, techniques and principles are the same for tendon transfers around shoulder arthroplasty whether it is in the setting of a revision or primary arthroplasty. This chapter provides an overview of the indications, techniques, and results of tendon transfers around (revision) shoulder arthroplasty.

31.2 Tendon Transfers in Reverse Shoulder Arthroplasty

31.2.1 Indications and Decision-Making

Careful patient selection is crucial for the success of tendon transfers in the setting of RSA. Anamnestic information and a thorough physical examination play a central role in decision-making and are supported secondarily by imaging. In general, tendon transfers should be reserved for patients with markedly symptomatic lack of movement that limits their daily functioning.

31.2.1.1 Anamnesis

Tendon transfers may be used in cases of symptomatic deficits in active range of motion. A thorough history is important to determine the etiology of the movement deficit. When considering a primary shoulder arthroplasty or in case an anatomic shoulder arthroplasty is in place, a gain in elevation may be expected of a reversed prosthesis. However, rotation after RSA is less predictable. In some cases, RSA may even result in a loss of active external rotation, and the ability to externally rotate the shoulder also deteriorates over time after RSA [3]. The status of the entire cuff should be taken into account. For example, active external rotation is highly dependent on the state of the teres minor and infraspinatus muscles [1, 2]. With a deficient cuff, a significantly worse external rotation can be expected after RSA (40.9° versus 51.7°, $p = 0.006$) [4].

Tendon transfers should be reserved for patients with marked limitations in daily life due to a movement deficit. Elevation and abduction are important for tasks requiring lifting of the arm, such as grabbing objects from shelves. External rotation is crucial for control of the arm held in abduction, which is important for a wide variety of daily tasks requiring working above chest level, including reaching the face, hair, or back of the head. As a result, extensive abduction is required to perform many activities of daily life. Adequate internal rotation is equally important. For example, internal rotation is essential for personal hygiene and personal care, such as dressing and undressing. A limitation in these movements leads to decreased ability to perform daily activities, which has a significant impact on the patient's autonomy and quality of life. It is important to consider the patient's expectations and (desired) type and level of activity. These considerations should form the basis of decision-making for tendon transfers. In our practice, we commonly use the scores of activity of daily living in internal rotation and external rotation to perform an objective preoperative and postoperative evaluation of our patients (ADLIR and ADLER scores, respectively) [5, 6].

31.2.1.2 Physical Examination

Similar to the anamnesis, the physical examination should be centered on identifying and measuring movement deficits. First, passive range of motion should be assessed. Tendon transfers are indicated only in non-stiff shoulders, where the lack of muscle function is responsible for the active range of motion deficit and not the stiffness. Having confirmed the flexibility of the shoulder, active elevation, abduction, external rotation, and internal rotation should be measured in a standardized fashion, assessing both range of motion, strength, and pain. The external rotation lag sign and Hornblower sign may aid in identifying a loss of active external rotation. The shoulder shrug sign, Jobe test, empty can test, or dropping sign may aid in identifying a loss of elevation or abduction. The lift-off test or lag sign may provide information on internal rotation.

Grading each test on pain and strength provides more accurate information than considering only a positive or negative result. We prefer grading each cuff test with 5 points for strength according to the Medical Research Council, to which is added a pain grading system increasing from 0 (severe pain), 5 (moderate pain), 10 (mild pain), to 15 (no pain), resulting in a scale ranging from 0 to 20. For example, a very painful and weak Jobe test would be graded as 5 + 3 = 8/20.

It is important to keep in mind that an arthritic shoulder may not provide a reliable cuff examination as the pain is related to arthritis and that the examiner may underestimate a weakness because of stiffness. We therefore value a true lack of mobility in external rotation (lag sign) with the arm either adducted or abducted. In the case of a weak external rotation without a lag sign, we anticipate the potential need of a tendon transfer to restore external rotation when draping the patient for surgery and decide intraoperatively to perform a tendon transfer according to the status and quality of the remaining posterior cuff attached to the greater tuberosity.

31.2.1.3 Imaging

The findings of conventional radiographs may indirectly suggest rotator cuff pathology. For instance, cortical irregularity of the greater tuberosity at the attachment site of the supraspinatus indirectly indicates the presence of a rotator cuff tear with a sensitivity of 90% and a negative predictive value of 96% [7]. A large rotator cuff tear may lead to superior migration of the humerus, which can be identified on conventional radiographs. Humeral migration is a sign of a chronic tear, for which a direct repair is often not effective, and a tendon transfer may be considered [8, 9].

Computed tomography (CT) has limited value in identifying muscle or tendon pathologies around the shoulder. It can be used to evaluate muscle atrophy and fatty degeneration, but with low reliability [10, 11]. On the contrary, CT arthrography provides reliable information on rotator cuff tears that are in contact with the articular surface, as well as information on the bone, and the quality of cartilage. The authors consider bone assessment on CT imaging to be more reliable than on magnetic resonance imaging (MRI). Similar to conventional CT imaging, CT arthrography also allows for assessment and grading of the trophicity and fatty infiltration of the muscles, which plays an important role in the decision-making for tendon transfers [10–12]. Due to these properties, and the fact that CT arthrography is more cost-effective and more readily available in most clinics compared to MR arthrography, CT arthrography is the authors' preferred method to assess the rotator cuff.

Magnetic resonance (MR) arthrography is the most sensitive and specific technique for diagnosing both full- and partial-thickness rotator cuff tears and is most effective for intra-articular pathology [13]. Ultrasound (US) and MR imaging (MRI) are comparable in both sensitivity and specificity concerning the diagnosis of rotator cuff tears, and both techniques allow for the assessment of fat infiltration and atrophy [14]. However, US is limited in its ability to assess other structures, such as the capsule, labrum, cartilage, and osseous structures, and is highly dependent on the operator [15]. With proper training, a full-thickness rotator cuff tear can be diagnosed with 92.3% sensitivity and 94.4% specificity by using ultrasound, whereas a partial-thickness tear can be diagnosed with 66.7% sensitivity and 93.5% specificity [13, 14]. Advantages of ultrasound include low cost, accessibility, and lack of contraindications. On conventional MRI, the diagnosis of a full-thickness rotator cuff tear can be made with 92.1% sensitivity and 92.9% specificity, whereas a partial-thickness tear can be diagnosed with 63.6% sensitivity and 91.7% specificity [13, 14]. Furthermore, MRI provides the possibility to globally assess all shoulder structures, including muscle fatty degeneration and atrophy [13]. However, the presence of metal may cause substantial artifacts on MRI, making it a less favorable option after arthroplasty. MRI is also less economical and less accessible compared to US or CT imaging.

31.2.1.4 Surgical Options

To treat a functionally limiting lack in range of motion, several options for tendon transfers can be considered in combination with or after shoulder arthroplasty (Table 31.1). In patients with a lack of active external rotation or a combined loss

Table 31.1 Options for tendon transfers in shoulder arthroplasty

Donor	Technique	Origin	Insertion	Function
Reverse shoulder arthroplasty				
Latissimus dorsi	Transfer	Original	Posterodistal aspect of the greater tuberosity	External rotation
Combined latissimus dorsi & teres minor	Transfer	Original	Posterolateral aspect of proximal humerus	Elevation, external rotation
	Transfer	Original	Proximal anterolateral aspect of the humeral metaphysis	Elevation, external rotation
	Transfer	Original	Lateral aspect of the greater tuberosity	Elevation, internal rotation
Lower trapezius	Transfer (+ Achilles tendon graft)	Original	Site of infraspinatus insertion	External rotation
Pectoralis major	Pedicled graft	Lateral clavicle, acromion	Humerus site of deltoid insertion	Elevation, external rotation, abduction
Anatomic total shoulder arthroplasty				
Latissimus dorsi	Transfer	Original	Greater tuberosity	Internal rotation, stability
Pectoralis major	Transfer	Original	Greater tuberosity	Internal rotation

of active elevation and external rotation (CLEER), a transfer of the latissimus dorsi can be considered. The latissimus dorsi transfer can be combined with a teres major transfer (modified l'Episcopo procedure). Insertion sites for these transfers include the anterior aspect of the greater tuberosity and posterodistal aspect of the greater tuberosity, [16] or the posterolateral aspect of the greater tuberosity, the posterolateral aspect of the proximal humerus, and the proximal anterolateral aspect of the humeral metaphysis [17–19]. The main caution when using these transfers is if the patient also has an irreparable subscapularis tear because using this technique removes an additional internal rotator and anterior stabilizer. Alternatively, the lower trapezius can be transferred to the insertion site of the infraspinatus to restore external rotation [20, 21]. In cases of combined loss of active elevation and internal rotation (CLEIR), an anterior latissimus dorsi and teres major transfer to the lateral aspect of the greater are described in a previous study [22]. However, a lack in internal rotation is compensated after the biomechanical changes provided by RSA implantation. The importance of the subscapularis as an internal rotator in the setting of an RSA is debated. Biomechanical studies have shown that the function in internal rotation after a RSA relies mainly on the action of the pectoralis major [23, 24]. Therefore, the authors prefer not to compensate an irreparable subscapularis, and even tend not to reattach a reparable subscapularis to avoid a potential limitation in external rotation. This approach results in satisfactory ADLIR scores [5]. However, further studies are required to determine the exact role of the subscapularis in RSA. Last, to restore elevation and abduction in cases of deltoid paralysis, RSA can be combined with a pedicled pectoralis major transfer, grafted proximally to the lateral clavicle and acromion, and distally to the humerus at the site of the deltoid insertion [21].

31.2.2 Techniques

31.2.2.1 Latissimus Dorsi Transfer to Restore Active External Rotation

The latissimus dorsi originates on the spinous processes of the thoracic, lumbar, and sacral vertebrae, multiple ribs, and pelvis. The insertion site of the latissimus dorsi tendon is located medial to the bicipital groove and distal to the perimeter of the lesser tuberosity, directly adjacent to the teres major [25]. In its original position, the latissimus dorsi provides adduction, internal rotation, and extension of the humerus [25]. Transfer of the latissimus dorsi in combination with RSA to restore active external rotation is performed through a standard deltopectoral incision, including release of the upper part of the pectoralis major tendon. Based on the insertion site, it can be opted to perform the transfer using a second posterolateral incision. After release of the subscapularis tendon, the latissimus dorsi is harvested from its insertion site, either at the tendon interface or with a bone chip [26]. During mobilization of the muscle belly, care is taken to preserve the neurovascular bundle. The glenoid and humerus are prepared for implantation (or revision) of RSA. With the arm in internal rotation, drill holes are made at the intended site of insertion. Most commonly, the tendon is inserted on the humeral head, at the supraspinatus footprint on the greater tuberosity. However, different locations for attachment have been proposed: previous cadaveric and biomechanical studies found greater external rotation torque with a transfer to the proximal lateral aspect of the greater tuberosity and the insertion site of the teres minor compared to a transfer to the lateral humeral shaft [27, 28]. Similar results were found in a randomized trial of 18 patients [29]. However, this location is further from the original insertion site and therefore puts more strain on the transferred tendon and the RSA, and may even limit the range of motion and function in internal rotation. After creating the drill holes at the chosen site of insertion, the humeral component of RSA is implanted. A lateralized humeral component may be considered; a cadaveric study showed substantially increased torque generated by the tendon transfer combined with a humeral component with a greater offset [28]. The tendon is then transferred to the insertion site. When completing the transfer, care is taken to preserve the branches of the axillary nerve. The latissimus dorsi transfer procedure extends the surgical time of RSA by 26 minutes on average [30].

31.2.2.2 Combination of Latissimus Dorsi and Teres Major Transfers to Restore Active External Rotation

The teres major originates from the dorsal surface of the inferior angle of the scapula. The insertion site on the humerus is adjacent to the latissimus dorsi, and cross-links between the two tendons are common [25]. In its original orientation, the teres major provides adduction and internal rotation. The combined latissimus dorsi and teres major transfer was first described by l'Episcopo in 1934 for obstetrical paralyses [31]. The procedure was later adapted to restore active external rotation in cases with an irreparable rotator cuff tear [32]. Currently, the modified l'Episcopo procedure is used for a variety of indications, including restoring active external rotation in the setting of shoulder arthroplasty. The surgical technique is similar to the above-described technique for the transfer of the latissimus dorsi tendon alone. It is performed through a single-incision deltopectoral approach, and both tendons are transferred together (Fig. 31.1a, b). The same insertion sites as described for the latissimus dorsi transfer can be used. It is important to consider that the combination of two muscles makes the transfer bulkier, resulting in difficulty in bringing the tendon to the targeted insertion site. This pitfall should be taken into consideration in muscular men with bulky muscle bellies; in these cases, a single muscle transfer may be sufficient to restore strength. On the contrary, in less muscular or female patients, transferring two muscles may be required to provide sufficient power.

31.2.2.3 Combination of Latissimus Dorsi and Teres Major Transfers to Restore Active Internal Rotation

Although less common, the latissimus dorsi and teres major can also be transferred anteriorly to restore internal rotation, as described by Hee Baek et al. [22] A standard deltopectoral approach is used, and the long head of the biceps is tenotomized. To allow adequate exposure of the tendi-

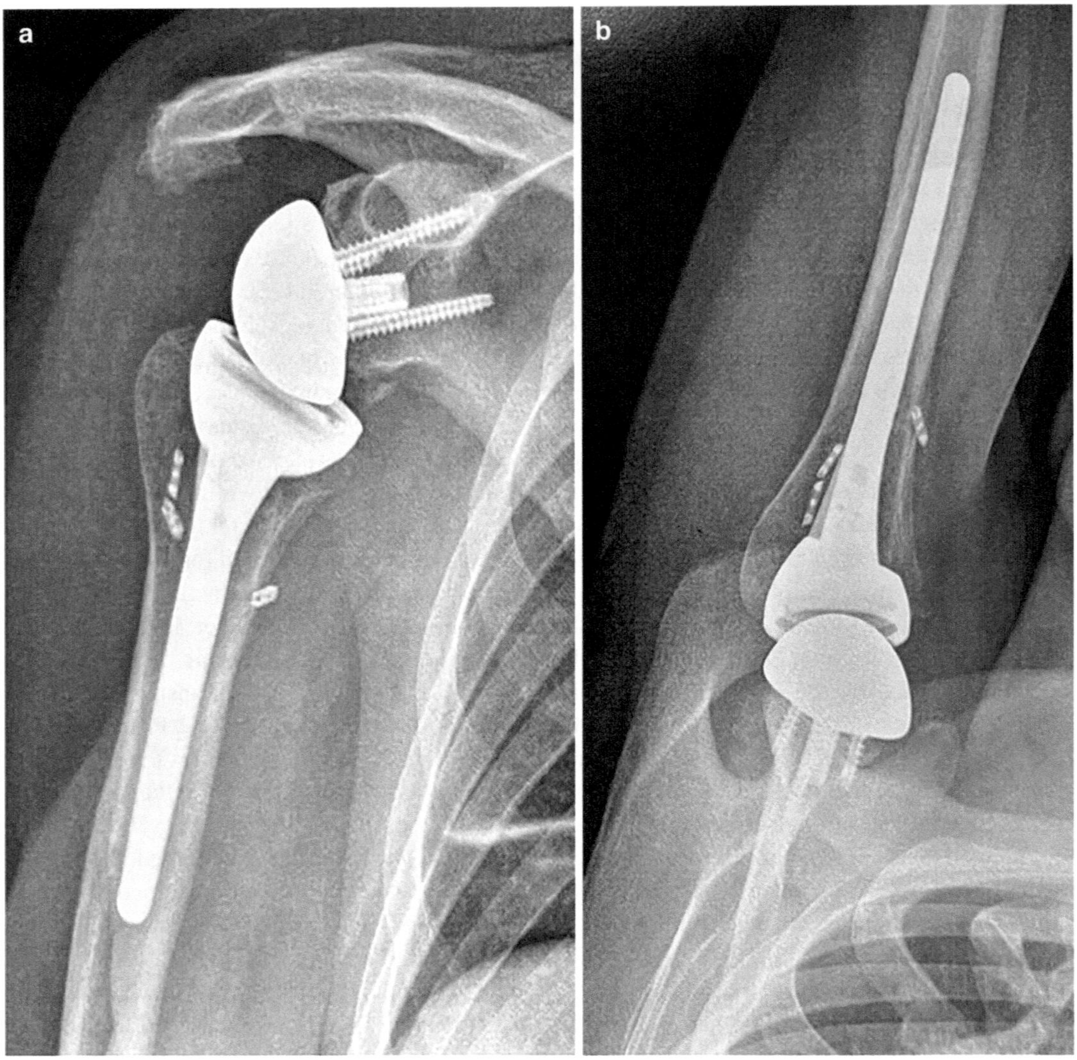

Fig. 31.1 (**a**, **b**) Examples of RSA with latissimus dorsi and teres major transfer fixated with endobuttons

nous portions of the latissimus dorsi and teres major, the proximal third of the pectoralis major is released. The latissimus dorsi and teres major are detached from the humerus and mobilized. After mobilization of the tendons, the humerus and glenoid are prepared for (revision) RSA, and the glenoid component is implanted. Before implantation of the humeral stem, six to eight drill holes are made distally to the lateral edge of the greater tuberosity and laterally to the biceps groove. Three or four sutures are passed through these holes, forming loops. Subsequently, the humeral stem is implanted, and the shoulder is reduced. With the patient's arm positioned in full internal rotation and approximately 45° of abduction, the harvested tendons are tied to previously prepared suture loops [22].

31.2.2.4 Lower Trapezius Transfer to Restore Active External Rotation

For the lower trapezius transfer, as initially described by Elhassan et al., [21] a reverse L-shape vertical incision is performed just medial to the spine of the scapula and extended distally approximately 5 cm. Harvesting the tendon can

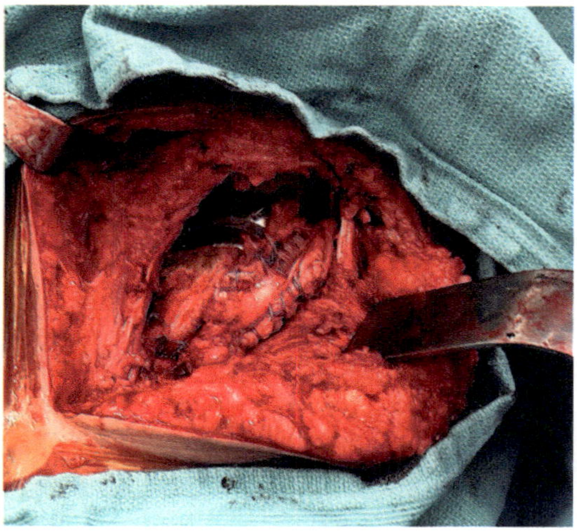

Fig. 31.2 Intraoperative image of a lower trapezius transfer, augmented with a graft, and fixated using endobuttons

also be performed through a smaller horizontal incision, but this is technically more challenging. The lateral and inferior borders of the lower trapezius are identified and detached at the insertion site on the medial scapula. After further dissection of the trapezius muscle, an Achilles tendon allograft is attached to the lower trapezius. A tunnel is created, along the infraspinatus fossa, and the tendon is passed anteriorly toward the deltopectoral window through which the arthroplasty is performed. The tendon is then attached to the lateral aspect of the footprint of the infraspinatus (Fig. 31.2). One cadaveric study showed the lower trapezius generated significantly more torque compared to the latissimus dorsi, although both were effective in restoring active external rotation [20].

31.2.2.5 Pectoralis Major Transfer to Reconstruct the Deltoid Muscle

A pedicled graft of the pectoralis major, as described by Elhassan et al., [21] is performed using an incision starting 2 cm distal to the sternoclavicular joint, extending laterally along the lower border of the clavicle in the direction of the acromioclavicular joint (Fig. 31.3). The incision is continued distally along the deltopectoral groove. The pectoralis major muscle is exposed,

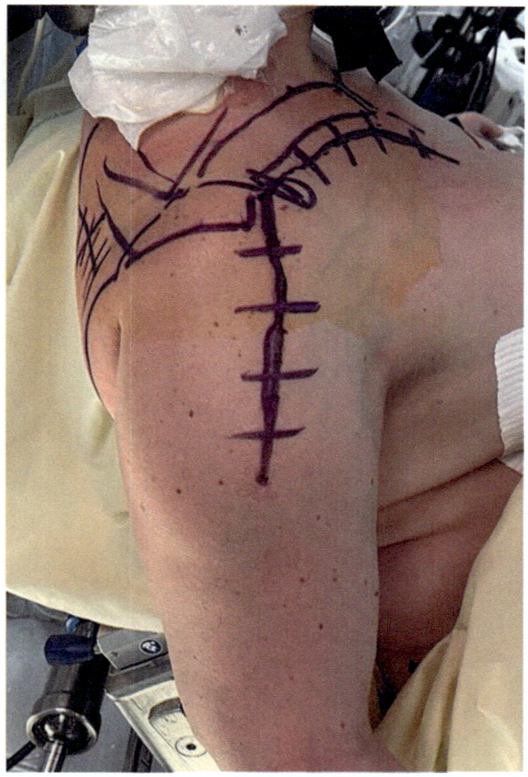

Fig. 31.3 Drawings of the incisions to perform an allograft-prosthetic composite (APC) reconstruction with pedicled pectoralis major and lower trapezius transfer in a right shoulder

creating a large skin flap. Based on the three neurovascular bundles supplying the pectoralis major, the superior third of the muscle is harvested. The upper part of the sternal origin and the complete clavicular origin is detached. It can also be opted to harvest only the clavicular origin, making the dissection easier. However, the power provided by this part of the muscle alone may be insufficient. Caution is taken around the pedicle, which is located distally to the middle of the clavicle. The distal insertion is detached, and the pedicle is mobilized. After mobilization and preparation of the muscle graft, (revision) RSA is performed in a standard fashion. At this stage, additional tendon transfers can be performed if required. Before inserting the muscle graft, the anterior atrophic deltoid is excised and the lateral third of the clavicle and the anterior aspect of the acromion are debrided to create a healthy bleed-

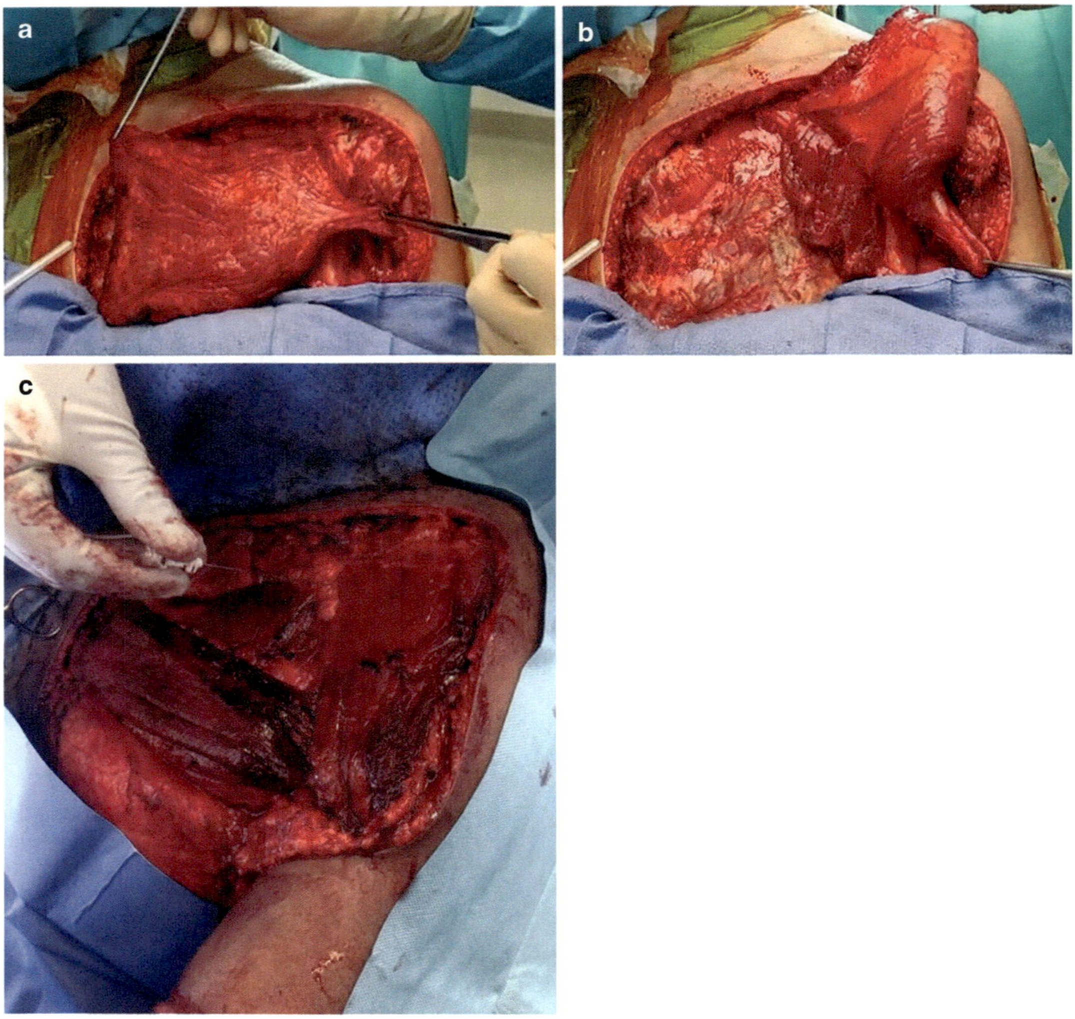

Fig. 31.4 (**a**) Example of a fully harvested pedicled pectoralis major. (**b**) The pectoralis major is flipped around its pedicle. (**c**) Photograph displaying the clavicular belly of the pectoralis major transferred to the anterior deltoid while his muscular activity is being confirmed using a neurostimulator

ing bed. Tunnels are drilled in the clavicle and acromion, and sutures are passed through. A trough is created in the humerus anterior to the deltoid insertion. The pectoralis muscle graft is flipped laterally (Fig. 31.4a–c), and the proximal aspect is attached to the clavicle and acromion holding the shoulder in approximately 60° of flexion. The distal tendon is fixated using buttons and is further reinforced with soft-tissue sutures [21]. Postoperatively, the arm must be immobilized in approximately 60° of anterior flexion for a total of 6–8 weeks.

31.2.3 Outcome

Limited reports are available in the literature on the outcomes of tendon transfers after shoulder arthroplasty or in combination with revision shoulder arthroplasty. In a retrospective study, 10 patients who had poor external rotation after RSA, which impaired their daily functioning, underwent a latissimus dorsi transfer. After latissimus dorsi transfer, they reported a significant increase in mean flexion (86° versus 109°), abduction (80° versus 92°), and external rotation

(−18° versus 2°). The subjective shoulder value (SSV) and Constant score also increased, but this difference was not significant. Regardless of these improvements, most patients rated the final result as poor (2) or fair (6) [18]. Furthermore, Wheelwright et al. reported one case of anterior deltoid weakness from Parsonage-Turner neuropathy and a failed total shoulder arthroplasty with pseudoparalysis for which a revision to RSA with concomitant pectoralis major transfer was performed to substitute for the anterior deltoid [33]. They reported a satisfactory outcome with 130° of active forward elevation, 60° of external rotation, internal rotation to the lumbosacral junction, and a full return to previous activities [33].

With regard to tendon transfers in the setting of primary shoulder arthroplasty, satisfactory outcomes are reported in terms of range of motion, strength, and patient-reported outcome scores. The results after primary tendon transfers in the setting of an arthroplasty are often superior to those in the setting of a revision.

31.2.3.1 Latissimus Dorsi to Restore Active External Rotation

To achieve active external rotation in the setting of the RSA, latissimus dorsi (with or without teres major) has been shown to achieve reliable and reproducible results in achieving external rotation (Fig. 31.5) [17, 34–38]. Latissimus dorsi transfer in the setting of RSA can also significantly modify patient-reported outcome scores. RSA with latissimus dorsi alone can achieve a reported approximate mean increase in anterior elevation of 73° and external rotation ranging between 21° and 23° [36, 38–40]. Studies on RSA with latissimus dorsi alone reported a mean increase in Constant scores ranging from 24 to 42, and approximate increases in American Shoulder and Elbow Surgeons shoulder score (ASES) and SSV of 25 and 42, respectively [26, 36, 38–40]. At least 50% of strength can be restored compared to the contralateral shoulder [41]. Improvements in range of motion may even exceed the baseline expectations of patients undergoing RSA without the need for a tendon transfer; one study compared patients with an external rotation deficit undergoing RSA with latissimus dorsi transfer to patients without external rotation deficit undergoing only RSA. Patients receiving the tendon transfer had up to 22° better postoperative active external rotation than control patients ($P < 0.001$) [30].

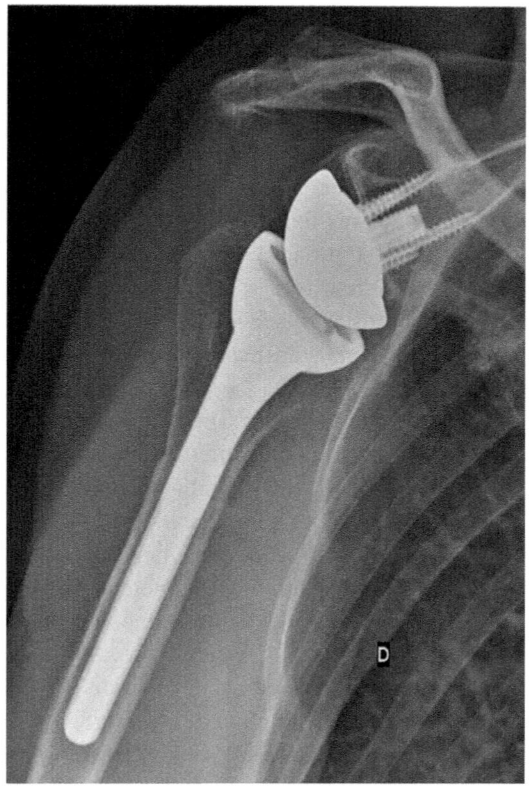

Fig. 31.5 Radiographic image of an RSA with latissimus dorsi transfer at 1-year follow-up

However, few comparative studies are available. In one trial, 28 patients with CLEER undergoing RSA were randomized to tendon transfer or only RSA; no significant difference in the ADLER, Disabilities of the Arm, Shoulder, and Hand (DASH), ASES, Simple Shoulder Test (SST) scores or active range of motion was found between the two groups at the final follow-up [42]. Similar results were found in a comparative retrospective study [43]. These results challenge the added value of the latissimus dorsi transfer to the functional improvements in range of motion that can be expected of RSA. Similarly, a study on 25 patients with a cuff tear arthropathy, pseudoparalysis, and a positive dropping sign found no difference in active external rotation between RSA with a modified l'Episcopo procedure compared to RSA with a lateralized humeral component [44]. Internal rotation was significantly greater in the group with a lateralized humeral component ($p = 0.004$), and a positive dropping sign was found in none of the patients in the lateralized group compared to five patients in the tendon transfer group ($p < 0.001$) [44]. However, it must be taken into account that these studies may lack statistical power due to the small cohorts.

Complications after latissimus dorsi transfers are rare. The rates of infection, dislocation, and aseptic loosening in RSA combined with latissimus dorsi transfer are comparable to RSA alone [45]. Osteolysis may occur at the latissimus dorsi transfer site on the proximal humerus [46, 47]. This is usually without consequence, but one case of a humeral shaft fracture through the site of osteolysis is reported in the literature [46]. Fig. 31.6 shows a radiograph at 1-year follow-up after RSA with a latissimus dorsi transfer with signs of bone loss at the insertion site. In this case, the humeral bone loss did not lead to a complication or clinical consequences. Loss of internal rotation and instability may be a concern in tendon transfers aimed at enhancing external rotation by transferring an internal rotator. Bilateral loss of internal rotation is a severe problem with regard to personal hygiene. One study found that 77% of patients who underwent RSA with latissimus dorsi transfer for an external rotation deficit could not reach the lumbosacral region due to an internal rotation deficit compared to 46% of control patients ($p = 0.010$) [30].

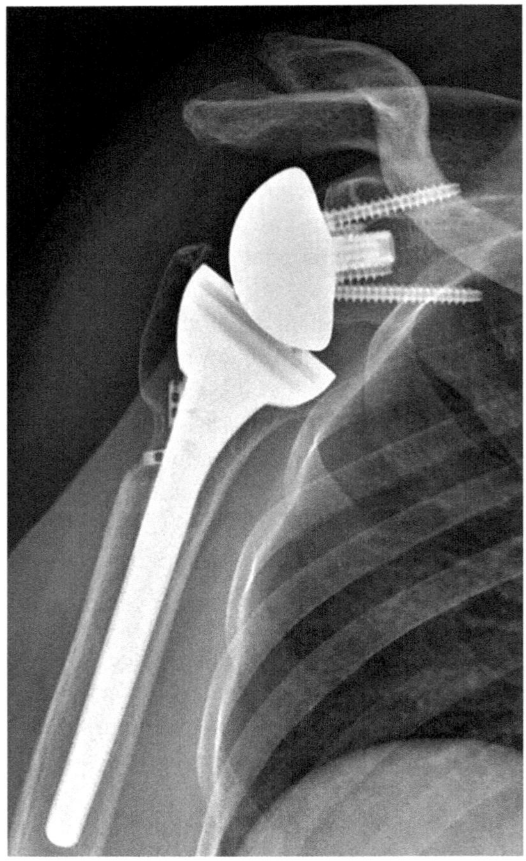

Fig. 31.6 Radiographic image of an RSA with latissimus dorsi transfer at 1-year follow-up showing humeral bone loss

31.2.3.2 Combination Teres Major and Latissimus Dorsi to Restore Active External Rotation

Compared to latissimus dorsi alone, combined latissimus dorsi and teres major transfers in the setting of RSA provide satisfactory improvements in range of motion and patient-reported outcome scores (Fig. 31.7). Latissimus dorsi and teres major transfers can achieve a mean increase in anterior elevation ranging from 58° to 78° and an increase in external rotation ranging from 30° to 36° according to the literature [17, 19, 48–50]. RSA combined with latissimus dorsi and teres major transfers reportedly led to an approximate mean increase of 37 on SSV and an increase in mean Constant scores ranging from 34 to 37 [17, 19].

However, the added value of the teres major is disputed. Theoretically, adding the teres major to the tendon transfer can lead to an increase in strength compared to transferring the latissimus dorsi alone. However, considering the relative size of the teres major compared to the latissimus dorsi, this added value can be expected to be minimal. The effect on functional improvements in practice remains questionable. In one retrospective study of 36 RSAs, there was no difference in external rotation between the patients who received latissimus dorsi combined with teres

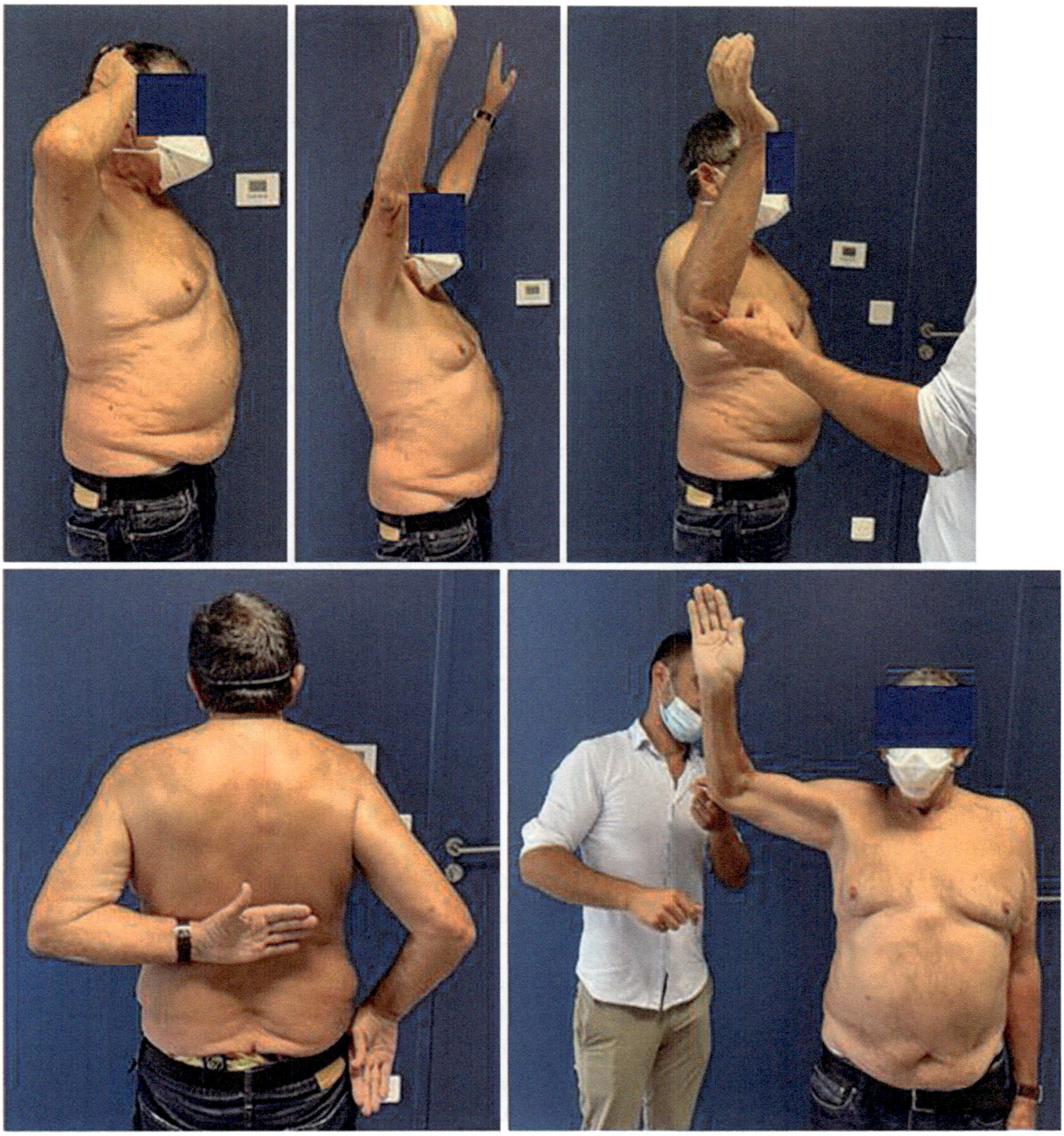

Fig. 31.7 Clinical images demonstrating active range of motion after RSA combined with a latissimus dorsi and teres major transfer in a patient with a preoperative external rotation lag sign

major transfer or latissimus dorsi transfer alone, suggesting that both techniques are equally effective [43].

31.2.3.3 Combination Teres Major and Latissimus Dorsi to Restore Active Internal Rotation

Only one study has been published reporting outcomes after RSA combined with anterior latissimus dorsi and teres major transfer. Baek et al. published a retrospective study including patients with CLEIR receiving either an RSA with the tendon transfer or RSA alone with a minimum follow-up of 2 years [22]. They reported significant improvements in range of motion and patient-reported outcomes in both groups, but the postoperative Constant score, ADLIR score, and internal rotation were greater in the tendon transfer group ($p < 0.008$) [22].

31.2.3.4 Pectoralis Major Transfer to Reconstruct the Deltoid Muscle

A pedicled graft of the pectoralis major is effective in restoring elevation, abduction, and external rotation. However, the available evidence is limited, and there is a large variance in the reported results. One study of RSA in combination with a pedicled pectoralis major graft in patients diagnosed with deltoid paralysis found an improvement in mean elevation from 15° to 83°, in abduction from 12° to 20°, and an overall mean external rotation of 16°. Active external rotation was completely deficient in 8 patients preoperatively and a mean of 20° in the remaining patients [21]. The study reports a mean improvement in SSV from 7 preoperatively to 53 postoperatively ($P < 0.01$) and in the DASH score from 54 preoperatively to 33 postoperatively ($P < 0.01$). However, it must be noted that the pectoralis major graft was combined with a latissimus dorsi transfer in five cases and a lower trapezius transfer in 3 cases, which were not reported separately [21].

Reported complications include acromial fractures at the junction of the acromion and scapular spine. This occurred in two out of 31 patients in a previous study. Regardless of operative or conservative treatment, this complication resulted in persistent pain and limitations in flexion and external rotation [21].

31.3 Tendon Transfers in Anatomic Total Shoulder Arthroplasty

Tendon transfers may be used in ATSA; however, cases are rare and limited literature is available on this subject. Specifically, subscapularis insufficiency is an important consideration in ATSA. If the subscapularis is compromised, the ATSA will be at risk for anterior instability in the form of subluxations or limited function due to a loss of the anterior aspect of the force couple. RSA has emerged as a very reliable and reproducible treatment option for patients with either failed subscapularis repairs after ATSA or in the revision setting with a compromised subscapularis tendon [51]. However, given the difficulty in revising a failed shoulder arthroplasty, [52] tendon transfers can be considered to either reconstruct a failed subscapularis tendon or augment the subscapularis repair.

31.3.1 Latissimus Dorsi

Historically, patients were either treated with a graft augmentation of the retracted tendon or a pectoralis major transfer [53–59]. However, two novel techniques have also emerged in recent years: transfer of the latissimus dorsi transfer alone [60–62] or in combination with an anterior capsular reconstruction [63, 64]. The latissimus dorsi transfer for subscapularis was initially described in an anatomic feasibility study, [60] and subsequently, clinical studies have shown it to be a very reasonable tendon transfer option for subscapularis insufficiency [61, 62]. Given its origin on the posterior chest wall, the force vector of the transferred latissimus dorsi is very similar to the original subscapularis muscle, while both differ almost 90° from the transferred pectoralis major. When performing this transfer in the setting of an ATSA, the latissimus dorsi can be used to either reconstruct or augment the subscapularis. If the subscapularis is completely irreparable, an anterior capsular reconstruction can be considered to augment the latissimus dorsi transfer. The latissimus dorsi transfer in the setting of ATSA is performed with a technique similar to the previously described transfer in the setting of RSA.

31.3.2 Pectoralis Major

An alternative option to address subscapularis insufficiency is a transfer of the pectoralis major tendon. Miller et al. reported 4 cases of pectoralis major transfer for a symptomatic irreparable rupture of the subscapularis muscle after ATSA. Patient-reported outcomes varied greatly, and 2 cases required additional surgery for continued instability [65]. Transfer of the pectoralis major tendon resulted in ASES scores of 82 and 37, satisfaction scores of 9 and 4, and pain scores of 0 and 5, respectively [65].

31.4 Tendon Transfers in the Case of Proximal Humerus Bone Deficiency Using Allograft Prosthetic Composites

Proximal humerus bone loss, whether from tumor, trauma, or failed prior arthroplasty, creates a challenging problem for reconstruction. Historically, shoulder function after reconstruction for proximal humerus bone loss was poor due to the limited options to provide tension to the deltoid, fill the bone defect, and provide soft tissue stability by reattaching the rotator cuff or other tendons [66–68]. One recently developed technique involves using allograft prosthetic composites to allow direct repair of the rotator cuff between the host tendon and cadaver tendon (Fig. 31.8) [66, 69]. Although initial results were published only on allograft prosthetic composites in hemiarthroplasties, [66, 68, 69] in more recent years, allograft prosthetic composites have been used in RSA as well [68, 70]. The semiconstrained nature of this construction provides inherent stability [68] while using the allograft rotator cuff attachments to either repair the rotator cuff or transfer tendons to improve stability and functional outcomes [68, 70].

In the post-traumatic or revision arthroplasty setting, direct repair of the rotator cuff is often not feasible. In these settings, tendon transfers can play a critical role in re-establishing coronal and sagittal plane stability, as well as improving shoulder function. Either the pectoralis major or the latissimus dorsi can be used and transferred to the remnant subscapularis tendon on the allograft to provide added anterior stability and internal rotation function of the shoulder. Although both tendon transfers contribute to anterior stability, due to the force vector of the latissimus dorsi being closer to the subscapularis, [60] it is our preferred transfer if internal rotation is a priority. One disadvantage of the latissimus dorsi tendon is that when the bone loss extends distally beyond its insertion, the tendon harvest could require a posterior axillary fold incision. For the remnant posterosuperior rotator cuff, either the latissimus dorsi tendon or the lower trapezius can be used for the transfer. The advantages of the lower trapezius include its favorable line of pull with respect to the infraspinatus. Furthermore, unlike the "out of phase" latissimus dorsi, [71] the lower

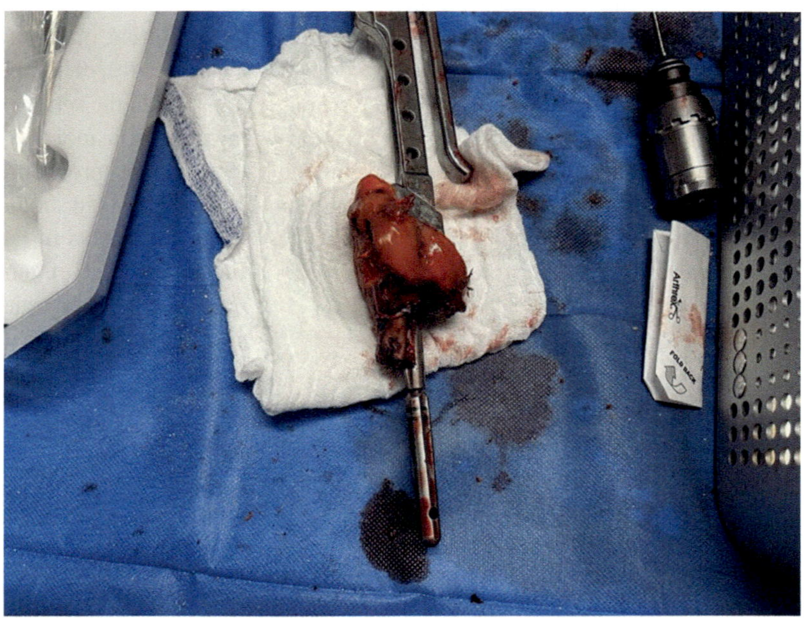

Fig. 31.8 Prepared humeral allograft before implantation

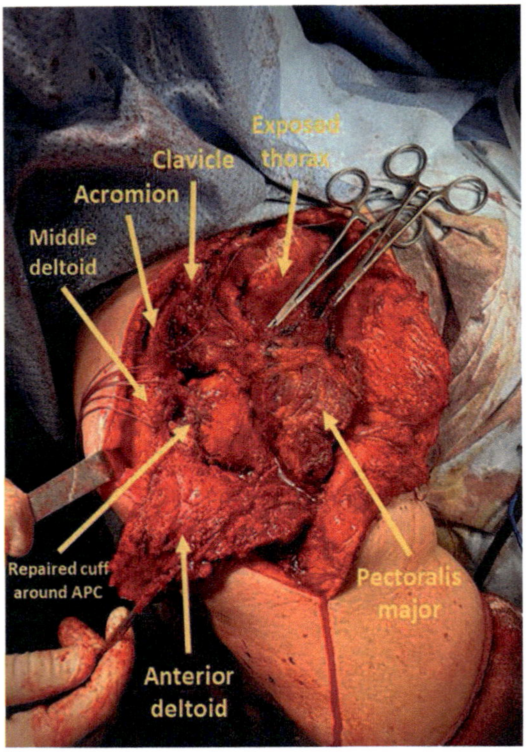

Fig. 31.9 Intraoperative image of the harvested pectoralis major, lower trapezius, and prepared clavicle and acromion after implantation of the APC and arthroplasty

trapezius is considered "in-phase" with shoulder external rotation and elevation [72]. However, the latter does require a separate posterior incision for the harvest and often requires an allograft for augmentation. Furthermore, if the proximal humerus bone loss extends beyond the insertions of the deltoid and pectoralis, these can be mobilized and reattached to their insertions on the allograft. Finally, if the axillary nerve is compromised, a pedicled pectoralis rotational muscle transfer can be used to restore stability and forward flexion (Fig. 31.9) [21].

31.5 Conclusion

Limited evidence is available on tendon transfers after shoulder arthroplasty or in combination with revision shoulder arthroplasty. However, the same principles and similar techniques apply to tendon transfers in primary arthroplasty and revision arthroplasty.

Tendon transfers may be used in the case of a symptomatic deficit in range of motion, resulting in functional limitations. Various options are available, with a transfer of the latissimus dorsi tendon to restore external rotation being the most common, performed alone or in combination with the teres major tendon. In general, positive results are achieved, with marked increases in active range of motion and patient-reported outcome scores. However, few comparative studies are available, and the added value of a tendon transfer is challenged in certain cases. Adequate patient selection is crucial when considering tendon transfers in the setting of shoulder arthroplasty [73].

The advancement toward personalized and evidence-based decision-making for tendon transfers in the setting of (revision) shoulder arthroplasty is yet to be made. Increased awareness of surgical options will result in more personalized treatment based on specific patient characteristics and expectations. Future research could focus on conducting (randomized) comparative studies, which may aid in determining in which cases a tendon transfer is of added value and in which cases it is not, thereby promoting evidence-based decision-making in complex cases. Further reports on less common transfers in the setting of shoulder arthroplasties, such as the lower trapezius, pectoralis major, or tendon transfers in the setting of ATSA, may aid in moving toward a more evidence-based approach to these rare procedures. Furthermore, future advancements in shoulder arthroplasty may result in improvements in range of motion equaling or surpassing that of tendon transfers, potentially rendering tendon transfers unnecessary in specific cases.

References

1. Ackland DC, Richardson M, Pandy MG. Axial rotation moment arms of the shoulder musculature after reverse total shoulder arthroplasty. J Bone Jt Surg. 2012;94:1886–95.

2. Simovitch RW, Helmy N, Zumstein MA, Gerber C. Impact of fatty infiltration of the teres minor muscle on the outcome of reverse total shoulder arthroplasty. J Bone Jt Surg. 2007;89:934–9.
3. Favard L, Levigne C, Nerot C, Gerber C, De Wilde L, Mole D. Reverse prostheses in arthropathies with cuff tear are survivorship and function maintained over time? Clin Orthop Relat Res. 2011;469:2469–75.
4. Waterman BR, Dean RS, Naylor AJ, Otte RS, Sumner-Parilla SA, Romeo AA, Nicholson GP. Comparative clinical outcomes of reverse total shoulder arthroplasty for primary cuff tear arthropathy versus severe Glenohumeral osteoarthritis with intact rotator cuff: a matched-cohort analysis. J Am Acad Orthop Surg. 2020;28:e1042–8.
5. Beckers JJ, Lafosse L, Caruso G, Kopel L, Commeil P, Mariaux S, Lafosse T. A pilot-study focusing on internal rotation after reverse total shoulder arthroplasty using the activities of daily living which require internal rotation (ADLIR) score. Shoulder Elb. 2021;14(6):657–62.
6. Werthel JD, Wagner ER, Elhassan BT. Long-term results of latissimus dorsi transfer for internal rotation contracture of the shoulder in patients with obstetric brachial plexus injury. JSES Open Access. 2018;2:159.
7. Wohlwend JR, Van Holsbeeck M, Craig J, Shirazi K, Habra G, Jacobsen G, Bouffard JA. The association between irregular greater tuberosities and rotator cuff tears: a sonographic study. AJR Am J Roentgenol. 1998;171:229–33.
8. Goutallier D, Le Guilloux P, Postel JM, Radier C, Bernageau J, Zilber S. Acromio humeral distance less than six millimeter: its meaning in full-thickness rotator cuff tear. Orthop Traumatol Surg Res. 2011;97:246–51.
9. Gerber C, Wirth SH, Farshad M. Treatment options for massive rotator cuff tears. J Shoulder Elb Surg. 2011;20:S20–9.
10. Williams MD, Lädermann A, Melis B, Barthelemy R, Walch G. Fatty infiltration of the supraspinatus: a reliability study. J Shoulder Elb Surg. 2009;18:581–7.
11. Oh JH, Kim SH, Choi JA, Kim Y, Oh CH. Reliability of the grading system for fatty degeneration of rotator cuff muscles. Clin Orthop Relat Res. 2010;468:1558–64.
12. Goutallier D, Postel JM, Bernageau J, Lavau L, Voisin MC. Fatty muscle degeneration in cuff ruptures: pre- and postoperative evaluation by CT scan. Clin Orthop Relat Res. 1994;304:78–83.
13. Nazarian LN, Jacobson JA, Benson CB, et al. Imaging algorithms for evaluating suspected rotator cuff disease: Society of Radiologists in ultrasound consensus conference statement. Radiology. 2013;267:589.
14. De Jesus JO, Parker L, Frangos AJ, Nazarian LN. Accuracy of MRI, MR arthrography, and ultrasound in the diagnosis of rotator cuff tears: a meta-analysis. AJR Am J Roentgenol. 2009;192:1701–7.
15. Le Corroller T, Cohen M, Aswad R, Pauly V, Champsaur P. Sonography of the painful shoulder: role of the operator's experience. Skelet Radiol. 2008;37:979–86.
16. Nicholson AD, Apostolakos JM, Mathew JI, et al. Biomechanical comparison of 3 latissimus dorsi transfer sites for reverse total shoulder arthroplasty in the absence of teres minor. J Shoulder Elb Surg. 2022;31:1300–7.
17. Boughebri O, Kilinc A, Valenti P. Reverse shoulder arthroplasty combined with a latissimus dorsi and teres major transfer for a deficit of both active elevation and external rotation. Results of 15 cases with a minimum of 2-year follow-up. Orthop Traumatol Surg Res. 2013;99:131–7.
18. Puskas GJ, Germann M, Catanzaro S, Gerber C. Secondary latissimus dorsi transfer after failed reverse total shoulder arthroplasty. J Shoulder Elb Surg. 2015;24:e337–44.
19. Valenti P, Zanjani LO, Schoch BS, Kazum E, Werthel JD. Mid- to long-term outcomes after reverse shoulder arthroplasty with latissimus dorsi and teres major transfer for irreparable posterosuperior rotator cuff tears. Int Orthop. 2021;45:1263–71.
20. Chan K, Langohr GDG, Athwal GS, Johnson JA. The biomechanical effectiveness of tendon transfers to restore rotation after reverse shoulder arthroplasty: latissimus versus lower trapezius. Shoulder Elb. 2022;14:48–54.
21. Elhassan BT, Wagner ER, Werthel JD, Lehanneur M, Lee J. Outcome of reverse shoulder arthroplasty with pedicled pectoralis transfer in patients with deltoid paralysis. J Shoulder Elb Surg. 2018;27:96–103.
22. Baek CH, Kim JG, Baek GR. Restoration of active internal rotation following reverse shoulder arthroplasty: anterior latissimus dorsi and teres major combined transfer. J Shoulder Elb Surg. 2022;31: 1154–65.
23. Werthel JD, Schoch BS, Hooke A, Sperling JW, An KN, Valenti P, Elhassan B. Biomechanical effectiveness of tendon transfers to restore active internal rotation in shoulder with deficient subscapularis with and without reverse shoulder arthroplasty. J Shoulder Elb Surg. 2021;30:1196–206.
24. Rol M, Favard L, Berhouet J. Factors associated with internal rotation outcomes after reverse shoulder arthroplasty. Orthop Traumatol Surg Res. 2019;105:1515–9.
25. Scholten DJ, Trasolini NA, Waterman BR. Reverse Total shoulder arthroplasty with concurrent latissimus dorsi tendon transfer. Curr Rev Musculoskelet Med. 2021;14:297–303.
26. Ortmaier R, Resch H, Hitzl W, Mayer M, Blocher M, Vasvary I, Mattiassich G, Stundner O, Tauber M. Reverse shoulder arthroplasty combined with latissimus dorsi transfer using the bone-chip technique. Int Orthop. 2014;38:553–9.
27. Favre P, Loeb MD, Helmy N, Gerber C. Latissimus dorsi transfer to restore external rotation with reverse shoulder arthroplasty: a biomechanical study. J Shoulder Elb Surg. 2008;17:650–8.

28. Zafra M, Uceda P, Muñoz F, Ruiz-Bonilla C, Font P. Lack of elevation and external rotation in the shoulder: reverse total shoulder arthroplasty combined with latissimus dorsi transfer to the humerus versus the greater tuberosity. Shoulder Elb. 2021;13:260.
29. Zafra M, Carpintero P, Carrasco C. Latissimus dorsi transfer for the treatment of massive tears of the rotator cuff. Int Orthop. 2009;33:457–62.
30. Flury M, Kwisda S, Kolling C, Audigé L. Latissimus dorsi muscle transfer reduces external rotation deficit at the cost of internal rotation in reverse shoulder arthroplasty patients: a cohort study. J Shoulder Elb Surg. 2019;28:56–64.
31. L'Episcopo JB. Tendon transplantation in obstetrical paralysis. Am J Surg. 1934;25:122–5.
32. Gerber C, Vinh TS, Hertel R, Hess CW. Latissimus dorsi transfer for the treatment of massive tears of the rotator cuff a preliminary report. Clin Orthop Relat Res. 1988;232:51–61.
33. Wheelwright JC, Featherall J, Kazmers NH, Tashjian RZ, Chalmers PN. Revision reverse total shoulder arthroplasty with pectoralis major transfer for anterior deltoid deficiency. JBJS Case Connect. 2022;12(2)
34. Boileau P, Chuinard C, Roussanne Y, Neyton L, Trojani C. Modified latissimus dorsi and teres major transfer through a single delto-pectoral approach for external rotation deficit of the shoulder: as an isolated procedure or with a reverse arthroplasty. J Shoulder Elb Surg. 2007;16:671–82.
35. Boileau P, Walter B, McClelland J, Rumian AP. Massive irreparable rotator cuff tears: how to rebalance the cuff-deficient shoulder. Instr Course Lect. 2014;63:71–84.
36. Gerber C, Pennington SD, Lingenfelter EJ, Sukthankar A. Reverse Delta-III total shoulder replacement combined with latissimus dorsi transfer. a preliminary report. J Bone Joint Surg Am. 2007;89:940–7.
37. Gerhardt C, Lehmann L, Lichtenberg S, Magosch P, Habermeyer P. Modified L'Episcopo tendon transfers for irreparable rotator cuff tears: 5-year follow-up. Clin Orthop Relat Res. 2010;468:1572–7.
38. Puskas GJ, Catanzaro S, Gerber C. Clinical outcome of reverse total shoulder arthroplasty combined with latissimus dorsi transfer for the treatment of chronic combined pseudoparesis of elevation and external rotation of the shoulder. J Shoulder Elb Surg. 2014;23:49–57.
39. Popescu IA, Bihel T, Henderson D, Martin Becerra J, Agneskirchner J, Lafosse L. Functional improvements in active elevation, external rotation, and internal rotation after reverse total shoulder arthroplasty with isolated latissimus dorsi transfer: surgical technique and midterm follow-up. J Shoulder Elb Surg. 2019;28:2356–63.
40. Patel AV, Matijakovich DJ, Brochin RL, Zastrow RK, Parsons BO, Flatow EL, Hausman MR, Cagle PJ. Mid-term outcomes after reverse total shoulder arthroplasty with latissimus dorsi transfer. Shoulder Elb. 2022;14:286–94.
41. Alonso-Rodriguez Piedra J, Souza Virgolino B, Gamez Baños F, Miranda Elstein Q, Ventura Parellada C, Mora Guix JM. Reverse total shoulder arthroplasty with latissimus dorsi and teres major transfer: biomechanical and electromyographical outcomes. Eur J Orthop Surg Traumatol. 2022;33:1003. https://doi.org/10.1007/S00590-022-03238-7.
42. Young BL, Connor PM, Schiffern SC, Roberts KM, Hamid N. Reverse shoulder arthroplasty with and without latissimus and teres major transfer for patients with combined loss of elevation and external rotation: a prospective, randomized investigation. J Shoulder Elb Surg. 2020;29:874–81.
43. Kazum E, Martinez-Catalan N, Caruso G, Schofield BA, Nidtahar I, Zampeli F, Valenti P. Reverse shoulder arthroplasty with isolated latissimus dorsi or combined with teres major transfer for lack of external rotation: a comparative study. Int Orthop. 2022;46(10):2273–81.
44. Merolla G, Cuoghi F, Athwal GS, et al. A kinematic and electromyographic comparison of a Grammont-style reverse arthroplasty combined with a l'Episcopo transfer compared to a lateralized humeral component reverse for restoration of active external rotation. Int Orthop. 2021;45:2061–9.
45. Wey A, Dunn JC, Kusnezov N, Waterman BR, Kilcoyne KG. Improved external rotation with concomitant reverse total shoulder arthroplasty and latissimus dorsi tendon transfer: a systematic review. J Orthop Surg (Hong Kong). 2017;25(2):2309499017718398.
46. Klein JS, Johnston PS, Sears BW, Patel MS, Hatzidakis AM, Lazarus MD. Osseous changes following reverse total shoulder arthroplasty combined with latissimus dorsi transfer: a case series. JSES Int. 2020;4:964–8.
47. Bonnevialle N, Elia F, Thomas J, Martinel V, Mansat P. Osteolysis at the insertion of L'Episcopo tendon transfer: incidence and clinical impact. Orthop Traumatol Surg Res. 2021;107(4):102917.
48. Boileau P, Chuinard C, Roussanne Y, Bicknell RT, Rochet N, Trojani C. Reverse shoulder arthroplasty combined with a modified latissimus dorsi and teres major tendon transfer for shoulder pseudoparalysis associated with dropping arm. Clin Orthop Relat Res. 2008;466:584–93.
49. Boileau P, Rumian AP, Zumstein MA. Reversed shoulder arthroplasty with modified L'Episcopo for combined loss of active elevation and external rotation. J Shoulder Elb Surg. 2010;19:20–30.
50. Shi LL, Cahill KE, Ek ET, Tompson JD, Higgins LD, Warner JJP. Latissimus dorsi and teres major transfer with reverse shoulder arthroplasty restores active motion and reduces pain for posterosuperior cuff dysfunction. Clin Orthop Relat Res. 2015;473:3212–7.
51. Wagner ER, Chang MJ, Welp KM, Solberg MJ, Hunt TJ, Woodmass JM, Higgins LD, Warner JJP. The impact of the reverse prosthesis on revision shoulder

arthroplasty: analysis of a high-volume shoulder practice. J Shoulder Elb Surg. 2019;28:e49–56.
52. Hevesi M, Houdek MT, Cofield RH, Sperling JW, Sanchez-Sotelo J, Wagner ER. Can a reverse shoulder arthroplasty be used to revise a failed primary reverse shoulder arthroplasty?: revision reverse shoulder arthroplasty for failed reverse prosthesis. Bone Jt J. 2018;100B:1493–8.
53. Aldridge JM, Atkinson TS, Mallon WJ. Combined pectoralis major and latissimus dorsi tendon transfer for massive rotator cuff deficiency. J Shoulder Elb Surg. 2004;13:621–9.
54. Elhassan B, Ozbaydar M, Massimini D, Diller D, Higgins L, Warner JJP. Transfer of pectoralis major for the treatment of irreparable tears of subscapularis: does it work? J Bone Joint Surg Br. 2008;90:1059–65.
55. Galatz LM, Connor PM, Calfee RP, Hsu JC, Yamaguchi K. Pectoralis major transfer for anterior-superior subluxation in massive rotator cuff insufficiency. J Shoulder Elb Surg. 2003;12:1–5.
56. Gavriilidis I, Kircher J, Magosch P, Lichtenberg S, Habermeyer P. Pectoralis major transfer for the treatment of irreparable anterosuperior rotator cuff tears. Int Orthop. 2010;34:689.
57. Jost B, Puskas GJ, Lustenberger A, Gerber C. Outcome of pectoralis major transfer for the treatment of irreparable subscapularis tears. J Bone Joint Surg Am. 2003;85:1944–51.
58. Resch H, Povacz P, Ritter E, Matschi W. Transfer of the pectoralis major muscle for the treatment of irreparable rupture of the subscapularis tendon. J Bone Joint Surg Am. 2000;82:372–82.
59. Wirth MA, Rockwood CA. Operative treatment of irreparable rupture of the subscapularis. J Bone Joint Surg Am. 1997;79:722–31.
60. Elhassan B, Christensen TJ, Wagner ER. Feasibility of latissimus and teres major transfer to reconstruct irreparable subscapularis tendon tear: an anatomic study. J Shoulder Elb Surg. 2014;23:492–9.
61. Kany J, Guinand R, Croutzet P, Valenti P, Werthel JD, Grimberg J. Arthroscopic-assisted latissimus dorsi transfer for subscapularis deficiency. Eur J Orthop Surg Traumatol. 2016;26:329–34.
62. Elhassan BT, Wagner ER, Kany J. Latissimus dorsi transfer for irreparable subscapularis tear. J Shoulder Elb Surg. 2020;29:2128–34.
63. Dewing CB, Horan MP, Millett PJ. Two-year outcomes of open shoulder anterior capsular reconstruction for instability from severe capsular deficiency. Arthroscopy. 2012;28:43–51.
64. Pogorzelski J, Hussain ZB, Lebus GF, Fritz EM, Millett PJ. Anterior capsular reconstruction for irreparable subscapularis tears. Arthrosc Tech. 2017;6:e951–8.
65. Miller BS, Joseph TA, Noonan TJ, Horan MP, Hawkins RJ. Rupture of the subscapularis tendon after shoulder arthroplasty: diagnosis, treatment, and outcome. J Shoulder Elb Surg. 2005;14:492–6.
66. O'Connor MI, Sim FH, Chao EYS. Limb salvage for neoplasms of the shoulder girdle. Intermediate reconstructive and functional results. J Bone Joint Surg Am. 1996;78:1872–88.
67. Teunis T, Nota SPFT, Hornicek FJ, Schwab JH, Lozano-Calderón SA. Outcome after reconstruction of the proximal humerus for tumor resection: a systematic review. Clin Orthop Relat Res. 2014;472:2245.
68. Houdek MT, Bukowski BR, Athey AG, Elhassan BT, Barlow JD, Morrey ME, Rose PS, Wagner ER, Sanchez-Sotelo J. Comparison of reconstructive techniques following oncologic intraarticular resection of proximal humerus. J Surg Oncol. 2021;123:133–40.
69. Abdeen A, Hoang BH, Athanasian EA, Morris CD, Boland PJ, Healey JH. Allograft-prosthesis composite reconstruction of the proximal part of the humerus: functional outcome and survivorship. J Bone Joint Surg Am. 2009;91:2406–15.
70. Sanchez-Sotelo J, Wagner ER, Sim FH, Houdek MT. Allograft-prosthetic composite reconstruction for massive proximal humeral bone loss in reverse shoulder arthroplasty. J Bone Joint Surg Am. 2017;99:2069–76.
71. Iannotti JP, Hennigan S, Herzog R, Kella S, Kelley M, Leggin B, Williams GR. Latissimus dorsi tendon transfer for irreparable posterosuperior rotator cuff tears. Factors affecting outcome. J Bone Joint Surg Am. 2006;88:342–8.
72. Smith J, Padgett DJ, Dahm DL, Kaufman KR, Harrington SP, Morrow DA, Irby SE. Electromyographic activity in the immobilized shoulder girdle musculature during contralateral upper limb movements. J Shoulder Elb Surg. 2004;13:583–8.
73. Wieser K. CORR insights ® : latissimus dorsi and teres major transfer with reverse shoulder arthroplasty restores active motion and reduces pain for posterosuperior cuff dysfunction. Clin Orthop Relat Res. 2015;473:3218–20.

Part VII
Others

32 The Role of Arthroscopy After Shoulder Replacement

Javier Ardebol, Simon Hwang, Theresa Pak, Mariano E. Menendez, and Patrick J. Denard

32.1 Introduction

An expanding list of indications, improvement in techniques, and advancement in implant design have increased the popularity of shoulder arthroplasty in the United States. Between 2012 and 2017, the annual incidence of primary anatomic total shoulder arthroplasty (TSA) procedures increased by 31.6% while that of primary reverse shoulder arthroplasty (RSA) increased by 164% [1]. Despite overall high rates of patient satisfaction and long-term implant survival, problems and complications are not infrequent following TSA or RSA. Frequently, reports of patient dissatisfaction following shoulder arthroplasty are persistent pain and limited range of motion, both of which have varying etiologies [2–4]. The most common complications include aseptic glenoid loosening, infection, adhesions, fractures, impingement, and rotator cuff insufficiency [4, 5]. Whereas revision open procedures carry significant additional risk, arthroscopy provides a minimally invasive tool that can be used in both the diagnosis and management of postoperative problems or complications following shoulder arthroplasty.

32.2 Algorithm for Consideration of Arthroscopy

While minimally invasive, arthroscopy following shoulder arthroplasty should be used in a judicious manner. Diagnostically, arthroscopy can be used to evaluate for infection, implant loosening, and postoperative rotator cuff failure. Therapeutically, arthroscopy can be used to treat postoperative stiffness, remove loose implants (e.g., loose glenoid), address postoperative impingement, and treat rotator cuff tears in select cases.

The evaluation for postoperative pain following shoulder arthroplasty should begin with an examination to evaluate for signs of infection and assess for passive and active range of motion loss as well as impingement. The radiographic evaluation, consisting of plain radiographs, and a computed tomography (CT) scan if needed, is vital in considering the role of arthroscopy. Arthroscopy can be considered in 2 primary scenarios: (1) no radiographic evidence of implant loosening or (2) isolated loosening of a TSA glenoid component. Combined glenoid and humeral loosening or isolated glenoid loosening of an RSA both require open revision. Our algorithm for considering arthroscopy following shoulder arthroplasty is summarized in Fig. 32.1.

J. Ardebol · S. Hwang · T. Pak · M. E. Menendez
P. J. Denard (✉)
Oregon Shoulder Institute, Medford, OR, USA

F. Franceschi et al. (eds.), *Revision Shoulder Arthroplasty*,
https://doi.org/10.1007/978-3-031-45944-3_32

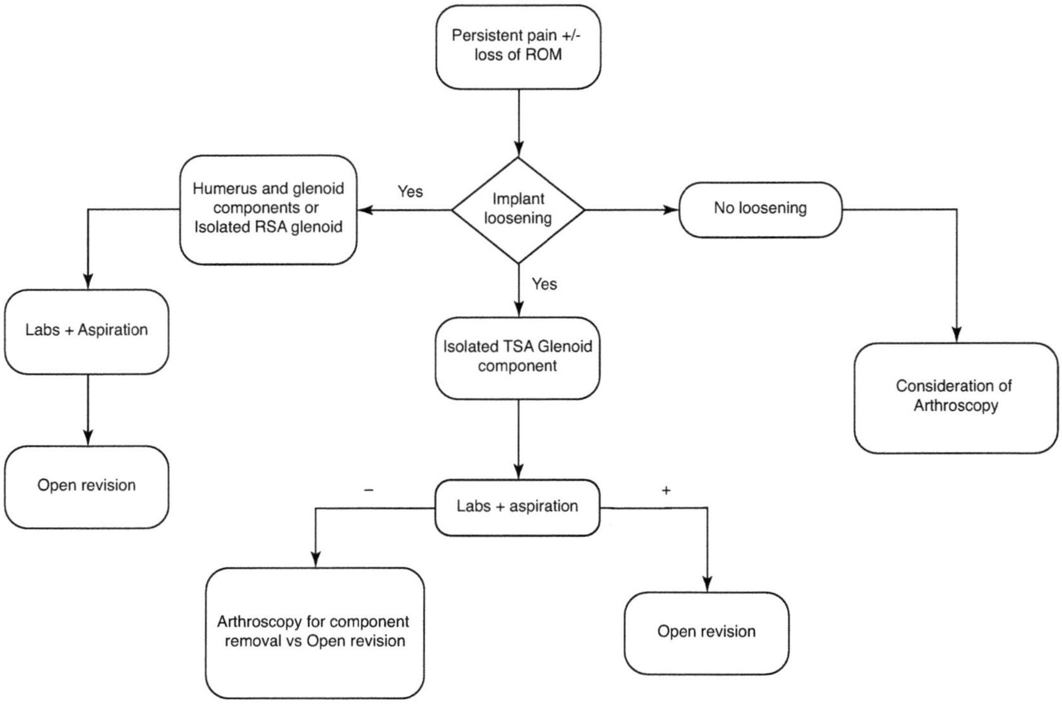

Fig. 32.1 Diagnostic and treatment algorithm for a stiff and painful shoulder after total shoulder arthroplasty

32.3 Evaluation for Infection

The most widely reported use of arthroscopy post-shoulder arthroplasty is for the evaluation of infection [6–8]. Postoperative infection following shoulder arthroplasty is reported in up to 1.8% of primary and 15.4% of revision arthroplasty cases [9]. However, the true incidence may be underreported considering the indolent nature of the most frequently encountered organism, *Cutibacterium acnes* (formerly known as *Propionibacterium*) [8]. This bacteria's lack of classic inflammatory signs typically seen in joint infections often makes the diagnosis difficult [10]. Unfortunately, joint aspirations have a reported sensitivity of only 16.7% [7]. Furthermore, dry taps are common with an estimated 50% of aspirations failing to retrieve fluid [8]. Arthroscopy provides the ability to retrieve multiple tissue samples and is thus useful when the diagnosis of infection is uncertain. This approach is less morbid than open biopsy and has demonstrated high diagnostic value.

Generally, samples are taken from 3 to 5 different sites [6, 8, 11]. Dilisio et al. conducted a retrospective study involving 19 patients who underwent arthroscopic biopsy for evaluation of pain after shoulder arthroplasty [7]. All patients subsequently underwent revision surgery with tissue culture of the periprosthetic sites. They reported perfect consistency (100% sensitivity and specificity) between culture results taken during arthroscopic biopsy and those taken during revision surgery. In a retrospective study, Akgun et al. analyzed arthroscopic biopsies in 23 cases of suspected periprosthetic infection prior to revision surgery [6]. They demonstrated that at least two arthroscopic biopsy samples yielded 80% sensitivity and 94.4% specificity.

32.4 Lysis of Adhesions

Shoulder stiffness after shoulder arthroplasty is a common cause of poor patient satisfaction [2]. Loss of motion may be due to various factors, including overstuffing of the joint, infection, and hypertrophic scar formation [4, 8]. Implant-related factors, such as overstuffing and loosening, are best managed with open surgery. The ideal candidate for lysis of adhesions demonstrates both active and passive range of motion loss refractory to conservative measures and well-positioned components without evidence of loosening. Arthroscopic lysis of adhesions is considered at 6 months postoperatively if conservative measures have failed and the patient is unhappy with their range of motion. Based on our experience, lysis of adhesions is best treated within 1 year of surgery to avoid permanent thixotropy. Muscle thixotropy is a state of muscle stiffness resulting from prolonged inactivity [12]. As opposed to open lysis of adhesions, arthroscopic lysis of adhesions may lead to a lower risk of scar reformation and allow the surgeon to address the capsule post-TSA without violating the subscapularis tendon. If arthroscopy is pursued, there are unique considerations to post-arthroplasty arthroscopy to account for. In contrast to arthroscopy of the native shoulder, post-TSA arthroscopy may result in impaired visualization due to glare from the metal components, while in post-RSA the constrained nature of the prosthesis prevents joint entry. Special attention must also be turned to protecting the integrity of the implanted surfaces.

32.4.1 Surgical Technique Post-TSA

Passive range of motion is assessed under anesthesia. The initial step is to establish a posterior glenohumeral portal. A diagnostic evaluation is first performed, assessing the glenoid component and rotator cuff. Intraarticular biopsies are taken as needed. The release begins by opening the rotator interval, taking care to protect the subscapularis tendon. The coracoid process is dissected with a shaver and electrocautery, beginning at the tip until reaching the coracoid base in order to release the coracohumeral ligament. Then, dissection continues posterior to the subscapularis tendon, releasing the middle glenohumeral ligament and anterior capsule down to the 5 o'clock position of the right shoulder. Range of motion is then reassessed, and a gentle manipulation is performed to propagate the release inferiorly. A posterior release is only performed if internal rotation remains limited. The inferior capsule does not usually require direct release. If required, scissors are preferred over radiofrequency ablators to avoid axillary nerve injury. Additionally, scissors allow for thickness and tissue quality palpation [13]. Upon completion of the intraarticular work, attention is directed to the subacromial space, and additional lysis of adhesions is performed as needed.

Tytherleigh-Strong et al. analyzed patient-reported outcomes in a case series of 29 patients undergoing arthroscopy for persistent pain and loss of motion after arthroplasty [14]. The preoperative Constant score improved from 23 to 62 points at the latest follow-up for all patients, ranging from 5 to 37 months. Similarly, Wagner et al. reported improved range of motion in 19 patients undergoing open or arthroscopic capsular release at a mean follow-up of 2.3 years [15]. Forward flexion, abduction, and internal rotation increased from 77°, 49°, and sacrum to 117°, 98°, and L1, respectively.

32.4.2 Surgical Technique Post-RSA

The surgical technique post-RSA is unique and has been previously described in detail [16]. After RSA, the posterior portal is established slightly higher in order to avoid implant contact. The subacromial space is assessed for interposed adhesions and scar tissue which are cleared with a shaver inserted through the lateral portal. The subcoracoid space is re-established until the anterior glenosphere is visualized.

32.5 Total Shoulder Arthroplasty: Specific Uses

32.5.1 Glenoid Implant Loosening

Classically, one-third of post-TSA complications have been attributed to glenoid component loosening [8, 17]. This complication is often described as the leading cause of failure [17]. In their review of 33 studies with 3360 shoulders, Bohsali et al. found glenoid loosening to be the cause of failure in 37.7% of cases [5]. This is consistent with rates reported by other studies, which range from 18% to 39% [17]. Common causes of glenoid component loosening are infection, aseptic osteolysis, implant wear, and rotator cuff insufficiency [18]. Aseptic loosening seen with rotator cuff insufficiency or component malposition can result in uneven force couples about the glenohumeral joint. The "rocking horse" phenomenon has been used to explain the biomechanical mechanisms involved in glenoid component loosening. Eccentric edge loading of the glenoid component results in lifting of the opposite edge, which, over time, can result in component loosening [19]. Initially, workup includes radiographic imaging. While radiolucent lines and/or implant shift are classically seen, the absence of these radiographic signs does not exclude loosening.

CT arthrography can be utilized if films are equivocal. Mallo et al. evaluated 14 patients with inconclusive films and suspected glenoid loosening with CT arthrography [20]. After comparing results with arthroscopy, CT arthrography demonstrated a sensitivity of 70%, a specificity of 75%, and a negative predictive value of 50%. The authors concluded that the absence of contrast between the glenoid component and bone-cement interface could not reliably predict true stability. Arthroscopy allows for more accurate determination of component loosening through direct visual assessment and probing of the implant. Additionally, concomitant tissue sampling can be performed to evaluate for septic loosening. If glenoid loosening is confirmed either preoperatively or intraoperatively with arthroscopy, arthroscopic removal is a consideration in patients who are either not candidates for open revision or in those who desire an attempt at minimally invasive treatment [21]. The glenoid may be either removed *en bloc* via enlargement of the anterior portal or following segmentation into small pieces with an osteotome.

32.5.2 Rotator Cuff Tears

Rotator cuff tears are a common cause of failure after arthroplasty, representing 9–26% of all complications with a 2–16% incidence overall [8, 22]. Sequelae resulting from these tears include pain, shoulder instability, and glenoid component loosening [23, 24]. Diagnosis of post-operative rotator cuff insufficiency has unique challenges. The physical examination is often difficult as strength may be limited by pain. For instance, Boyd et al. reported low sensitivity and specificity of the belly press test to detect post-TSA subscapularis tears [25]. On plain radiographs, superior or anterior translation of the humeral head can indicate obvious supraspinatus and subscapularis failure, respectively [24, 26, 27]. One report found superior subluxation in 29.9% of patients with supraspinatus tears at 6.6 years post-TSA [24]. However, at other times, the humeral head is well-centered on plain radiographs. Metal artifact interference limits the ability for reliable magnetic resonance imaging (MRI) or CT evaluation of rotator cuff insufficiency post-TSA other than assessment of fatty infiltration. Arthroscopy may thus be an adjunct to diagnosing rotator cuff insufficiency if the diagnosis is unclear. Doherty et al. reported rotator cuff tears in 8 of 12 patients who underwent arthroscopy post-TSA otherwise not identified clinically or radiographically [28]. While primarily used for diagnosis, in select cases, these tears can be repaired arthroscopically.

The incidence of isolated supraspinatus tears after TSA is unknown [29]. Supraspinatus tears are often concomitant with subscapularis tears. It is unclear whether these patterns result from independent supraspinatus tearing or secondary to subscapularis failure. Although repair is a theoretical option, there are limited clinical studies to support this, and the ability to repair the rotator cuff is often decreased from the limited available bone stock following a stemmed prosthesis. Hattrup et al. conducted a case series with 18 patients undergoing open rotator cuff repair for different tear patterns after TSA [30]. Only 4 patients had no pain after long-term restoration of function. They suggested that early interven-

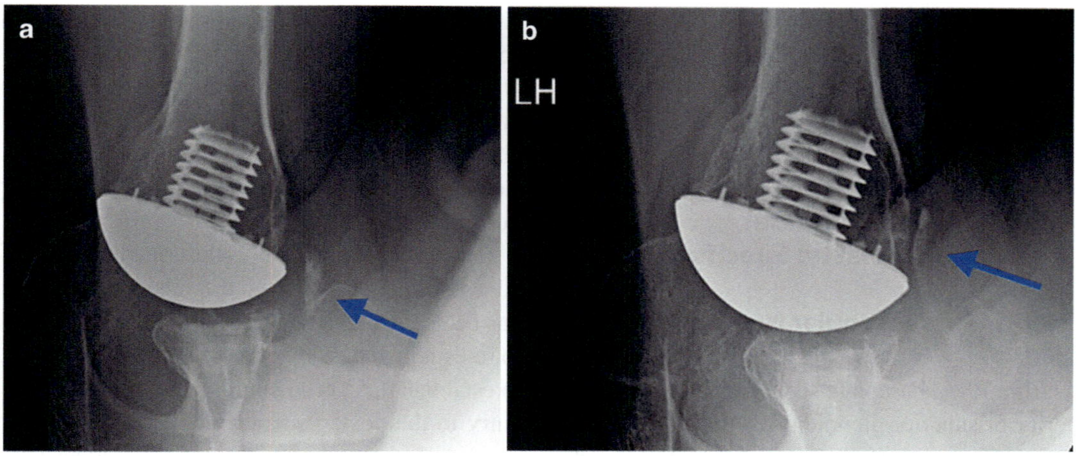

Fig. 32.2 Right shoulder axillary views of a patient with a stemless TSA undergoing rotator cuff repair. (**a**) Preoperative film showing a failed LTO after TSA. (**b**) Postoperative film taken 6 months after repair showing a well-reduced LTO. LTO, lesser tuberosity osteotomy; TSA, total shoulder arthroplasty

tion in traumatic tears could be beneficial, but failures are common.

Subscapularis insufficiency is a common cause of TSA failure [31, 32]. One report showed insufficiency in 78% of failed TSAs [23]. Failure can cause anterior instability, which leads to inferior functional outcomes [31, 32]. When subscapularis tears occur postoperatively, treatment options include soft tissue repair, tendon transfer, and RSA [33]. Revision to RSA is reserved for older patients with chronic attritional tears not amenable to repair. By contrast, repair can be attempted in young patients with acute traumatic tears. Entezzari et al. conducted a retrospective study of 25 patients undergoing subscapularis repair or revision to RSA after failed TSA [33]. Patients in the repair cohort were younger and had a lower injury-to-surgery time than the RSA cohort. Both cohorts had comparable postoperative functional outcomes, but a higher reoperation rate (52.9% vs 0.0%, $p = 0.01$) was seen in the repair group. Similarly, Miller et al. reported a 43% anterior instability rate in a case series of 7 patients undergoing open subscapularis repair after TSA [34]. Revision to RSA generally improves functional outcomes regardless of age; however, there is a higher complication rate in patients <60 years old [35]. As with supraspinatus tears, revision arthroscopic repair of the subscapularis is often limited by the available bone stock. However, with the advent of stemless designs, opportunities may exist to repair post-TSA failures. For instance, biomechanical evaluation has shown that a double-row anchor-based repair showed higher load to failure compared to side-to-side repair [36]. Anchor placement in this study was achieved without contact with a stemless implant. Thus, in young patients with acute tears, soft tissue repair could be considered, especially in the setting of stemless TSA, which allows for anchor placement while avoiding implant contact (Fig. 32.2a, b).

32.5.3 Biceps Tendon Treatment

Most surgeons routinely tenodese or tenotomize the long head biceps tendon during shoulder arthroplasty. If left retained, the biceps tendon can cause increased pain and stiffness postoperatively. A segment can become incarcerated and perched between the humeral component and tuberosities, especially in the case of proximal humeral fractures [37]. Patients undergoing prosthetic replacement for these fractures are vulnerable to segment retention as fracture lines may cross at or near the bicipital groove, and tuberosity repair around the implant can tether a segment of the biceps tendon [8]. Segment removal of the retained portion of the biceps tendon can be achieved arthroscopically. In addition to arthroscopic biceps tenotomy, subpectoral tenodesis may follow using part of the original deltopectoral incision.

32.6 Reverse Shoulder Arthroplasty: Specific Uses

32.6.1 Suprascapular Nerve Injury

During RSA, baseplate screws placed in the posterior or superior glenoid carry the risk of suprascapular nerve (SSN) injury [38]. A cadaveric study analyzing superior and posterior screw placement found nerve contact with a 40-mm screw in 66% and 50% of specimens, respectively [39]. Contact can injure the nerve, leading to postoperative pain and weakness in abduction and external rotation. Although muscle atrophy, if chronic, and ROM suggest SSN injury clinically, electromyography and CT scan are often required. With tomography, prominent screws can be identified and fractures excluded concomitantly. In one report, Wang et al. described a case of SSN entrapment post-RSA treated via open surgery to dissect the nerve and remove the superior screw [40]. Arthroscopically, consideration could be given to the release of the SSN in an effort to avoid open revision.

32.6.2 Subcoracoid Impingement

The constrained nature of the joint with RSA predisposes to mechanical conflict between the humeral component and coracoid, especially with internal rotation [41]. Most commonly, these patients present with lateral coracoid pain to direct palpation as well as an increase in coracoid pain with cross-body adduction [42]. Tashijian et al. proposed an open approach to coracoid pain with conjoined tendon release [43]. In their case series of 11 patients, the authors reported no residual postoperative pain in 55% of patients. Arthroscopy with coracoplasty provides an alternative approach. Additionally, arthroscopy allows the surgeon to address any postoperative adhesions that may also be present in the subcoracoid space [16]. We consider this approach in patients with post-RSA subcoracoid impingement who have persistent pain at a minimum of 6 months postoperatively.

The initial approach is as described for lysis of adhesions post-RSA. After the subacromial space has been cleared, an anterior portal is established to re-establish the subcoracoid space. It is helpful to establish this portal slightly lateral to facilitate entry to the posterior coracoid. Two approaches can be used in cases with extensive adhesions: coracoid tip to anterior glenoid or vice versa. In the first approach, the coracoacromial ligament is identified via the lateral portal and followed to the coracoid tip. Dissection continues towards the base and then laterally to the anterior glenoid (Fig. 32.3a–c). In the second approach, the superior glenoid is identified, and dissection begins between the 12 and 3 o'clock positions on the right shoulder until reaching the anterior glenoid and glenosphere. Then, dissection is turned toward the base of the coracoid and finally to the tip. Care is taken to remain on bone and not to deviate medially toward the coracoid to avoid neurovascular injury. After these structures are visualized, there are anatomical landmarks to clear the subcoracoid space. Anteriorly, dissection is limited to the coracoid tip, medially to the coracoid base, and inferiorly to the lesser tuberosity at the level of the humerus.

32.6.3 Acromial Stress Fractures

Arthroscopy has also been described as a tool for management of select acromial stress fractures following RSA. Acromial stress fractures are reported to occur in approximately 4% of RSA cases [44, 45]. The majority of these fractures occur within the first year postoperatively [46]. Although initially these are treated conservatively, fractures frequently go onto nonunion. Patients often present with pain and tenderness to palpation directly over the acromion. Fracture

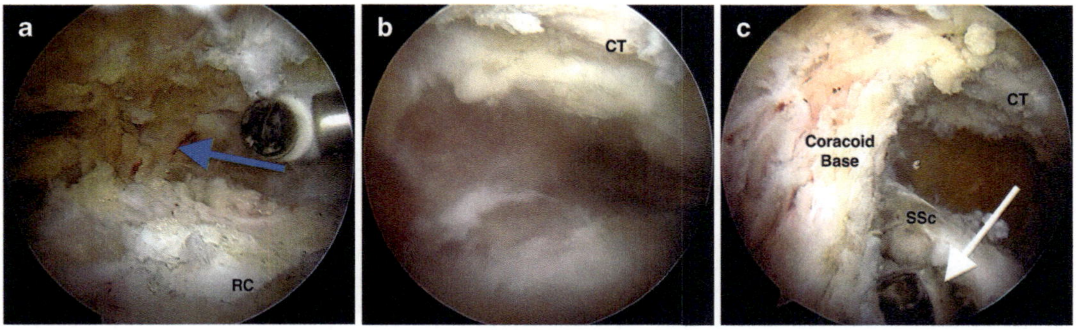

Fig. 32.3 Posterior subacromial view with a 70-degree arthroscope on a right shoulder. (**a**) There are dense adhesions in the subcoracoid space which are cleared by following the rotator cuff (RC) medially until reaching the (**b**) coracoid tip (CT). (**c**) Dissection continues until the base of the coracoid is visualized, and the glenosphere (white arrow) is seen posterior to the subscapularis, if intact

pattern and location determine the extent of deltoid involvement [47]. Those involving the posterior deltoid can be treated with open reduction and internal fixation [46]. By contrast, small fragments involving the anteromedial acromion (Levy type I or Crossby I and II) can be considered for arthroscopic excision without compromising deltoid function [47–49].

32.7 Complications

Complication rates following arthroscopy remain low despite the technical challenges. The reported complication rate of arthroscopy following shoulder arthroplasty is 2.4%, which is comparable to arthroscopy following knee arthroplasty [50]. Additionally, infection rates are significantly lower following shoulder arthroscopy compared to open surgery [51]. In a systematic review, Horner et al. found that although 92% of patients were satisfied with the procedure, 44% had to undergo reoperation after arthroscopy [52]. Subsequently, Heaven et al. analyzed this high revision rate and found that this rate fell to 25% after excluding those treated for prosthetic joint infection [50]. Other aspects to consider are the technical challenges associated with the procedure. Incidental contact between the surgical instruments and the component surfaces is thought to cause abrasion of the components [50, 53]. Avoiding unnecessary contact with the implant components becomes more challenging due to the "mirror" effect. Reflective surfaces of the implant can distort surgical field visualization [54]. However, these consequences have yet to be studied extensively. Surgeon skill and site preparation are important factors in mitigating these adverse effects [8, 50].

32.8 Conclusion

With an ever-increasing number of shoulder arthroplasties performed in the United States, the development of techniques for management of complications is becoming more important. Post-arthroplasty arthroscopy may have a role for patients with equivocal periprosthetic joint infection workup and persistent pain. In addition to its diagnostic role, arthroscopy also has therapeutic potential. Arthroscopy has been described for the treatment of post-operative adhesions, acromial stress fractures, subcoracoid impingement, and rotator cuff repair. While open surgery is well documented for the treatment of these post-arthroplasty complications, arthroscopy is a less invasive alternative with lower morbidity. As the role of arthroscopy after shoulder arthroplasty continues to evolve, more clinical studies are needed to better characterize its diagnostic and therapeutic potential.

References

1. Best MJ, Aziz KT, Wilckens JH, McFarland EG, Srikumaran U. Increasing incidence of primary reverse and anatomic total shoulder arthroplasty in the United States. J Shoulder Elb Surg. 2021;30(5):1159–66.
2. Franta AK, Lenters TR, Mounce D, Neradilek B, Matsen FA. The complex characteristics of 282 unsatisfactory shoulder arthroplasties. J Shoulder Elb Surg. 2007;16(5):555–62.
3. Hasan SS, Leith JM, Campbell B, Kapil R, Smith KL, Matsen FA. Characteristics of unsatisfactory shoulder arthroplasties. J Shoulder Elb Surg. 2002;11(5):431–41.
4. Thorsness RJ, Romeo AA. Stiffness following shoulder arthroplasty: to manipulate or not. Semin Arthroplast. 2016;27(2):104–7.
5. Bohsali KI, Bois AJ, Wirth MA. Complications of shoulder arthroplasty. J Bone Joint Surg. 2017;99(3):256–69.
6. Akgün D, Maziak N, Plachel F, Minkus M, Scheibel M, Perka C, et al. Diagnostic arthroscopy for detection of periprosthetic infection in painful shoulder arthroplasty. Arthroscopy. 2019;35(9):2571–7.
7. Dilisio MF, Miller LR, Warner JJP, Higgins LD. Arthroscopic tissue culture for the evaluation of periprosthetic shoulder infection. J Bone Joint Surg. 2014;96(23):1952–8.
8. Parker DB, Smith AC, Fleckenstein CM, Hasan SS. Arthroscopic evaluation and treatment of complications that Arise following prosthetic shoulder arthroplasty. JBJS Rev. 2020;8(8):e20.00020–8.
9. Padegimas EM, Maltenfort M, Ramsey ML, Williams GR, Parvizi J, Namdari S. Periprosthetic shoulder infection in the United States: incidence and economic burden. J Shoulder Elb Surg. 2015;24(5):741–6.
10. Kapadia BH, Berg RA, Daley JA, Fritz J, Bhave A, Mont MA. Periprosthetic joint infection. Lancet. 2016;387(10016):386–94.
11. Guild T, Kuhn G, Rivers M, Cheski R, Trenhaile S, Izquierdo R. The role of arthroscopy in painful shoulder arthroplasty: is revision always necessary? Arthroscopy. 2020 Jun;36(6):1508–14.
12. Lakie M, Campbell KS. Muscle thixotropy—where are we now? J Appl Physiol. 2019;126(6):1790–9.
13. Barth JRH, Burkhart SS. Arthroscopic capsular release after hemiarthroplasty of the shoulder for fracture: a new treatment paradigm. Arthroscopy. 2005;21(9):1150.e1–5.
14. Tytherleigh-Strong GM, Levy O, Sforza G, Copeland SA. The role of arthroscopy for the problem shoulder arthroplasty. J Shoulder Elb Surg. 2002;11(3):230–4.
15. Wagner ER, Chang MJ, Solberg MJ, Welp KM, Hunt TJ, Woodmass JM, et al. Capsular release following total shoulder arthroplasty: an analysis of early outcomes. Eur J Orthop Surg Traumatol. 2021;31(1):167–73.
16. Ardebol J, Pasqualini I, Hartzler RU, Griffin JW, Lederman E, Denard PJ. Arthroscopic management of stiffness and anterior shoulder pain following reverse shoulder arthroplasty. Arthrosc Tech. 2022;11:1763–e1768.
17. Weatherby PJ, Efejuku TA, Somerson JS. Complications after anatomic shoulder arthroplasty. Orthop Clin N Am. 2021;52(3):269–77.
18. Moore DD, Moravek JE, Baker EA, Salisbury MR, Baker KC, Wiater JM. Exploring failure of Total shoulder arthroplasty systems through implant retrieval, radiographic, and clinical data analyses. J Shoulder Elb Arthroplast. 2017;1:247154921770532.
19. Schrumpf M, Maak T, Hammoud S, Craig E. The glenoid in total shoulder arthroplasty. Curr Rev Musculoskelet Med. 2011;4(4):191–9.
20. Mallo GC, Burton L, Coats-Thomas M, Daniels SD, Sinz NJ, Warner JJP. Assessment of painful total shoulder arthroplasty using computed tomography arthrography. J Shoulder Elb Surg. 2015;24(10):1507–11.
21. Venjakob AJ, Reichwein F, Nebelung W. Arthroscopic removal of a polyethylene glenoid component in Total shoulder arthroplasty. Arthrosc Tech. 2015;4(2):e149–52.
22. Young AA, Walch G, Pape G, Gohlke F, Favard L. Secondary rotator cuff dysfunction following total shoulder arthroplasty for primary glenohumeral osteoarthritis: results of a Multicenter study with more than five years of follow-up. J Bone Joint Surg. 2012;94(8):685–93.
23. Melis B, Bonnevialle N, Neyton L, Lévigne C, Favard L, Walch G, et al. Glenoid loosening and failure in anatomical total shoulder arthroplasty: is revision with a reverse shoulder arthroplasty a reliable option? J Shoulder Elb Surg. 2012;21(3):342–9.
24. Levy D, Abrams G, Harris J, Bach B, Nicholson G, Romeo A. Rotator cuff tears after total shoulder arthroplasty in primary osteoarthritis: a systematic review. Int J Shoulder Surg. 2016;10(2):78.
25. Boyd AD, Aliabadi P, Thornhill TS. Postoperative proximal migration in total shoulder arthroplasty. J Arthroplast. 1991;6(1):31–7.
26. Merolla G, Paladini P, Campi F, Porcellini G. Efficacy of anatomical prostheses in primary glenohumeral osteoarthritis. Chir Organi Mov. 2008;91(2):109–15.
27. Combes D, Lancigu R, Desbordes de Cepoy P, Caporilli-Razza F, Hubert L, Rony L, et al. Imaging of shoulder arthroplasties and their complications: a pictorial review. Insights Imaging. 2019;10(1):90.
28. Doherty C, Furness ND, Batten T, White WJ, Kitson J, Smith CD. Arthroscopy of the symptomatic shoulder arthroplasty. J Shoulder Elb Surg. 2019;28(10):1971–6.
29. Familiari F, Huri G, McFarland EG. Supraspinatus tears after total shoulder arthroplasty: a review of diagnosis and treatment. Semin Arthroplast JSES. 2014;25(1):64–70.
30. Hattrup SJ, Cofield RH, Cha SS. Rotator cuff repair after shoulder replacement. J Shoulder Elb Surg. 2006;15(1):78–83.

31. Buckley T, Miller R, Nicandri G, Lewis R, Voloshin I. Analysis of subscapularis integrity and function after lesser tuberosity osteotomy versus subscapularis tenotomy in total shoulder arthroplasty using ultrasound and validated clinical outcome measures. J Shoulder Elb Surg. 2014;23(9):1309–17.
32. Eichinger JK, Galvin JW. Management of complications after total shoulder arthroplasty. Curr Rev Musculoskelet Med. 2015;8(1):83–91.
33. Entezari V, Henry T, Zmistowski B, Sheth M, Nicholson T, Namdari S. Clinically significant subscapularis failure after anatomic shoulder arthroplasty: is it worth repairing? J Shoulder Elb Surg. 2020;29(9):1831–5.
34. Miller BS, Joseph TA, Noonan TJ, Horan MP, Hawkins RJ. Rupture of the subscapularis tendon after shoulder arthroplasty: diagnosis, treatment, and outcome. J Shoulder Elb Surg. 2005;14(5):492–6.
35. Ernstbrunner L, Suter A, Catanzaro S, Rahm S, Gerber C. Reverse Total shoulder arthroplasty for massive, irreparable rotator cuff tears before the age of 60 years: long-term results. J Bone Joint Surg. 2017;99:1721–9. American Volume Lippincott Williams and Wilkins.
36. Werner BC, McClish SJ, Mealey NC, Wijdicks C, Thompson T, Higgins LD. A biomechanical comparison of subscapularis tenotomy repair techniques for stemless shoulder arthroplasty. J Shoulder Elb Surg. 2022;31(4):711–7.
37. Hersch JC, Dines DM. Arthroscopy for failed shoulder arthroplasty. Arthroscopy. 2000;16(6):606–12.
38. Hart ND, Clark JC, Wade Krause FR, Kissenberth MJ, Bragg WE, Hawkins RJ. Glenoid screw position in the encore reverse shoulder prosthesis: an anatomic dissection study of screw relationship to surrounding structures. J Shoulder Elb Surg. 2013;22(6):814–20.
39. Vance DD, O'Donnell JA, Baldwin EL, Cheah JW, Pereira G, Klifto C, et al. Risk of suprascapular nerve injury during glenoid baseplate fixation for reverse total shoulder arthroplasty: a cadaveric study. J Shoulder Elb Surg. 2021;30(3):532–7.
40. Wang J, Singh A, Higgins L, Warner J. Suprascapular neuropathy secondary to reverse shoulder arthroplasty: a case report. J Shoulder Elb Surg. 2010;19(3):e5.
41. Triplet JJ, Everding NG, Levy JC, Moor MA. Functional internal rotation after shoulder arthroplasty: a comparison of anatomic and reverse shoulder arthroplasty. J Shoulder Elb Surg. 2015;24(6):867–74.
42. Garofalo R, Conti M, Massazza G, Cesari E, Vinci E, Castagna A. Subcoracoid impingement syndrome: a painful shoulder condition related to different pathologic factors. Musculoskelet Surg. 2011;95(S1):25–9.
43. Tashjian RZ, Frandsen JJ, Christensen G, Chalmers PN. Conjoint tendon release for persistent anterior shoulder pain following reverse total shoulder arthroplasty. JSES Int. 2020;4(4):975–8.
44. King JJ, Dalton SS, Gulotta L, v., Wright TW, Schoch BS. How common are acromial and scapular spine fractures after reverse shoulder arthroplasty? Bone Joint J. 2019;101-B(6):627–34.
45. Lau SC, Large R. Acromial fracture after reverse total shoulder arthroplasty: a systematic review. Shoulder Elbow. 2020;12(6):375–89.
46. Joyce CD, Seidl AJ. Managing acromial fractures: prevention and treatment, both nonoperative and operative. Ann Jt. 2019;4:1–1.
47. Levy JC, Anderson C, Samson A. Classification of postoperative acromial fractures following reverse shoulder arthroplasty. J Bone Joint Surg Am Vol. 2013;95(15):e104-1–7.
48. Crosby LA, Hamilton A, Twiss T. Scapula fractures after reverse Total shoulder arthroplasty: classification and treatment. Clin Orthop Relat Res. 2011;469(9):2544–9.
49. Lädermann A, Walch G, Denard PJ, Collin P, Sirveaux F, Favard L, et al. Reverse shoulder arthroplasty in patients with pre-operative impairment of the deltoid muscle. Bone Joint J. 2013;95-B(8):1106–13.
50. Heaven S, de Sa D, Duong A, Simunovic N, Ayeni OR. Safety and efficacy of arthroscopy in the setting of shoulder arthroplasty. Curr Rev Musculoskelet Med. 2016;9(1):54–8.
51. Mayne AIW, AmitS B, Clifford R, Smith MG, Guisasola I, Brownson P. The incidence and causative organisms of infection in elective shoulder surgery. Shoulder Elbow. 2018;10(3):179–85.
52. Horner NS, de Sa D, Heaven S, Simunovic N, Bedi A, Athwal GS, et al. Indications and outcomes of shoulder arthroscopy after shoulder arthroplasty. J Shoulder Elb Surg. 2016;25(3):510–8.
53. Raab GE, Jobe CM, Williams PA, Dai QG. Damage to cobalt-chromium surfaces during arthroscopy of Total knee replacements. J Bone Joint Surg Am Vol. 2001;83(1):46–52.
54. Bonutti PM, Hawkins RJ, Saddemi S. Arthroscopic assessment of glenoid component loosening after total shoulder arthroplasty. Arthroscopy. 1993;9(3):272–6.

33 The Role of Resection and Hemiarthroplasty After RSA

Michael Warnock and Ruth A. Delaney

33.1 Introduction

Reverse shoulder arthroplasty (RSA) can be a challenging procedure with a steep learning curve. There is often variability in a surgeon's choice of implant and philosophy with regard to optimal implant placement. This, coupled with the expanding and variable indications of its use, including fracture surgery, will lead to increased complications and revision surgery despite the ever-improving understanding, implant design, and surgical techniques. Severe complications discussed at length in this book including infection, refractory instability, and poor bone stock may lead to the surgeon being faced with the very difficult reality of impossible retention of a stable reverse prosthesis in any revision surgery. Given also that RSA is increasingly used in the frail and elderly in complex proximal humeral fractures, those patients who develop complications requiring reintervention may not have the comorbid fitness to undergo lengthy revision surgery. Options in both of these scenarios to treat pain and optimize function include excision arthroplasty or hemiarthroplasty.

This chapter will summarize what is known about indications and outcomes in both of these options.

M. Warnock · R. A. Delaney (✉)
Dublin Shoulder Institute, UPMC Sports Surgery Clinic, Dublin, Ireland
e-mail: michael.warnock@doctors.org.uk; ruth@dublinshoulder.com

33.2 Resection Arthroplasty After RSA

The literature reflects that resection arthroplasty (RA), in the majority of cases, is in the setting of infection. This is appealing to the treating surgeon as it allows for removal of all foreign material that could be a harbor for bacteria. A proximal humeral antibiotic spacer, traditionally used as part of a 2-stage treatment for infection, may have superseded RA as a long-term option however, as it adds little to surgical time and has the advantages of (1) local antibiotic delivery, (2) maintenance of joint space and better soft tissue tension, and (3) potentially improved function. A study of 22 patients with an average of 5.6 years follow-up of antibiotic spacer retention for chronic infection showed an average of forward flexion (FF) of 68 degrees and 35 degrees of external rotation (ER) with an average American Shoulder and Elbow (ASES) standardized shoulder score of 54 and visual analog scale (VAS) pain score of 2.8 [1].

RA is a salvage option indicated in frail patients with resistant infection or after failure of other surgical interventions to treat infection according to *Boileau* [2]. Other authors have described indication in extreme weakness of the acromion or glenoid, massive irreparable rotator cuff tear with deltoid dysfunction (due to axillary nerve lesion), or in the setting of deltoid dehiscence problems [3].

F. Franceschi et al. (eds.), *Revision Shoulder Arthroplasty*,
https://doi.org/10.1007/978-3-031-45944-3_33

Muh et al. described 13 patients undergoing resection arthroplasty after RSA and showed an average improvement of 3.3 in VAS from preoperative levels, an average ASES of 38.3, and an average Constant-Murley score (CMS) of 26.8. The average FF was 32.7 degrees with ER of only 6.5 degrees on average [4]. In 12 of these 13 cases, the RA was performed for infection, and in one case, the indication for RA was poor bone quality. It is highlighted that the outcomes of RA may be worse, specifically after RSA due to minimal musculature to maintain any remaining shoulder function. In another study of 17 patients who did not differentiate the type of index arthroplasty procedure, RA for infection yielded significant pain relief (VAS average preoperatively 8.8 versus 4.5 postoperatively) and FF improved on average from 39 degrees preoperatively to 70 degrees postoperatively, but ER decreased slightly on average from 33 to 31 degrees postoperatively. The mean ASES score was 36 [5]. In one study solely looking at infection and describing a treatment algorithm for infected shoulder arthroplasty, the results of eight RA cases are described. Only one of these was for RSA however, with the rest being hemiarthroplasty (HA) revision or total shoulder arthroplasty (TSA). In this chapter, good pain relief is described with a mean VAS of 3.6; however, function was limited with a mean CMS of 27.8 and mean disability of arm, shoulder, and hand (DASH) score of 46.9 [6].

Stevens et al described similar clinical results of RA in the setting of infection in a series of eight shoulders in seven patients. This included four failed RSA in three patients. Beyond demonstrating good pain relief but poor function, they evaluated surveys of the patient's perspective with five of seven patients happy with the decision to undergo RA. Six of seven patients reported that they would undergo the same surgery again if given the option. Three of seven patients felt that the shoulder function was subjectively better than preoperatively with two of seven saying it was the same. Five of seven patients reported being able to perform most activities of daily living [7].

In a study of 32 infected RSA, the logical conclusion of maintenance of an effective joint articulation versus resection arthroplasty yielded statistically significant better functional results but importantly with no higher rates of residual infection. Debridement and implant retention compared to resection showed comparison CMS of 52 vs 25 and revision arthroplasty (one- or two-step) vs resection CMS of 46 vs 25 [8].

The studies available are of low numbers and low quality and are entirely retrospective in nature with many studies including a variety of index procedures (RSA, HA, TSA) before RA. Most studies agree that it is a valid treatment option in highly painful shoulders in low demand patients. A good result in this salvage surgery has been considered good pain relief but minimal function. The limited evidence and experience suggest that outcomes could be variable both in terms of pain relief and function, and therefore, careful discussions with patients in this difficult scenario should reflect this (Fig. 33.1).

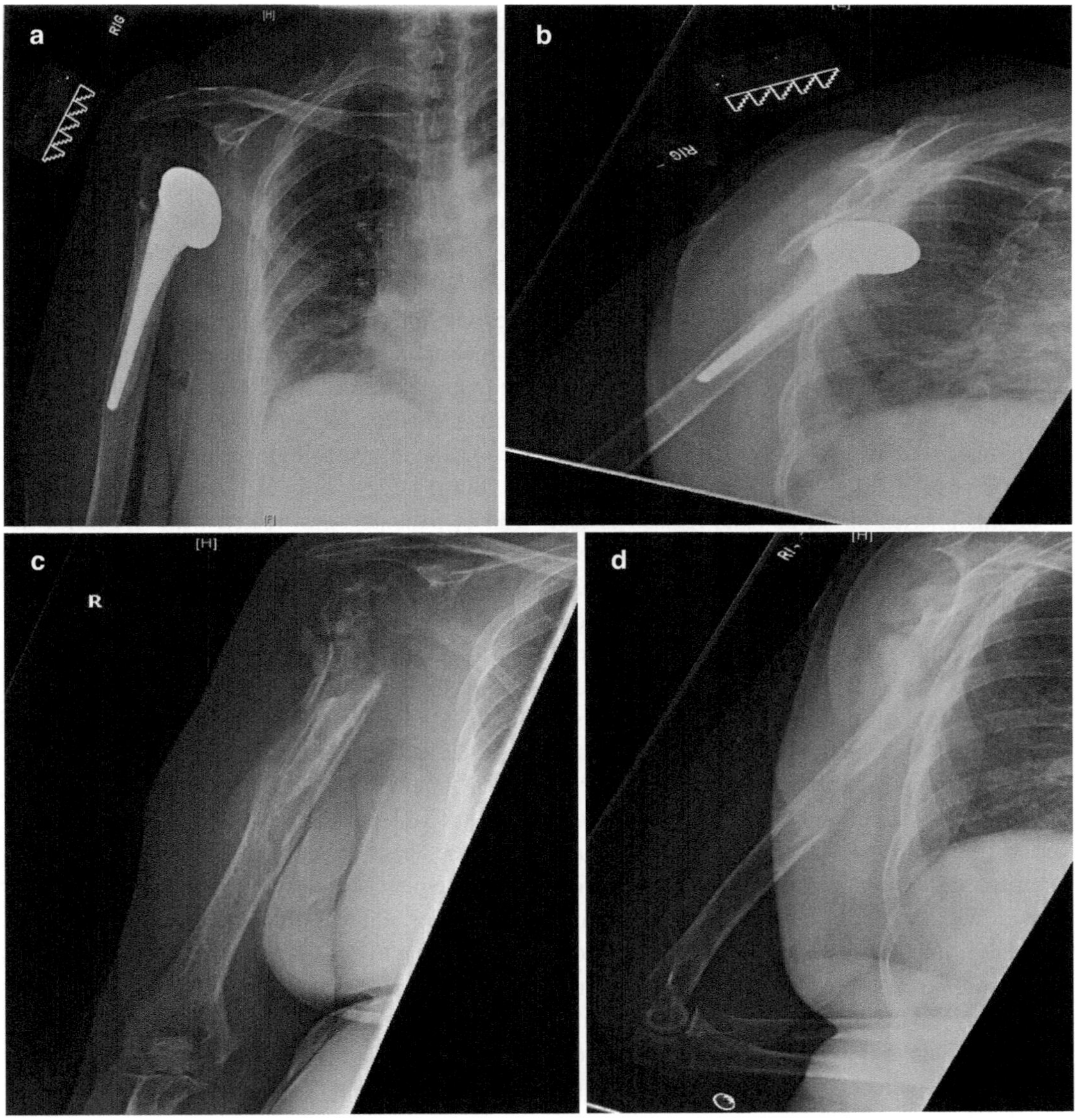

Fig. 33.1 (**a**–**d**) Resection arthroplasty case example. (**a**, **b**) Hemiarthroplasty performed for avascular necrosis following previous fracture fixation. Complicated by aseptic osteolysis and impending periprosthetic fracture causing significant arm pain. The patient presented to the senior author's practice with these X-rays and a chronic axillary nerve palsy. (**c**, **d**) This patient requested RA rather than RSA with tendon transfer

33.3 Hemiarthroplasty After RSA

The management of glenoid component failure and/or glenoid bone loss is discussed at length in Chap. 3. It has been reported that in cases of aseptic glenoid loosening, the need to perform salvage surgery in the form of hemiarthroplasty (HA) can be as high as 33% [9], so it is an important treatment option when there is no chance of stable baseplate fixation. Other less common indications for HA after RSA included unreconstructible scapular spine fractures, instability, and infection sequelae, leading to inadequate glenoid bone stock. Antibiotic-loaded cement hemiarthroplasties used as a medium- and longer-term option for acute and chronic infection and their longer-term outcomes as mentioned above can be considered as a separate part of evidence base for

HA after RSA. Infection is discussed in detail in Chap. 5.

When all other options have been exhausted and no RSA retention revision is possible and/or the patient is too fragile for lengthy revision surgery, HA can be considered [2] to reduce pain, optimize function, and minimize chances of further reintervention. To achieve these aims, newer options include bipolar and/or oversized head sizes to fill dead space and restore soft tissue tension [10]. Modular humeral stems may allow for simple exchange in cases of well-fixed humeral stems, reducing the chances of stem-related complications, and may also reduce surgical time and intraoperative blood loss [11].

A small series of six patients revised to HA following RSA with an average follow-up time of 26.5 months showed an average FF of 42.5 degrees with near 0 degrees ER. Despite poor range of motion, pain levels were low, with a mean VAS score of 2.42. The average ASES score was 52.1. Radiologically, five of the six patients had evidence of anterosuperior escape with the other patient having evidence of anterior dislocation. Of these six patients, three were converted from RSA to HA for glenoid loosening, three for instability, and two were infected and treated with antibiotic-loaded cement hemiarthroplasty. Interestingly, in four patients, glenoid bone graft was used for insufficiency, and later, after follow-up confirmed incorporation and suitability for glenoid component reimplantation, none of the patients chose to have this done despite their significant functional impairment with HA [12].

Glanzmann et al. reported that 16 patients converted to HA as a salvage procedure for failed RSA with a minimum follow-up period of 24 months. The indications were aseptic glenoid loosening in 12 patients (including four patients with an associated scapular spine fracture), infection in three patients, and periprosthetic humeral fracture in another. Postoperative functional outcome was poor with an average FF of 45 degrees and ER of 6 degrees. CMS on average was 25.2, and the QuickDASH score was 63. The median VAS score was 5, and importantly, five of sixteen patients (31%) reported higher levels of pain after HA. Anterosuperior escape was reported in three patients, and medialization beyond the coracoid was reported in six patients with one of these patients requiring RA as a result. Two other patients had periprosthetic fractures postoperatively that were managed conservatively. These three patients were classed as having a significant postoperative complication and were associated with poorer outcomes. The authors highlight, beyond these three patients, the unpredictable nature of outcomes and large differences between individuals that did not correlate, for example, with indication for revision or treatment method (choice of implant/single or staged revision) [13].

In the largest study of HA following RSA, 28 (33%) patients were treated with HA following glenoid loosening and migration. Seventy-nine patients with glenoid loosening in total were included in the study with 29 treated conservatively and 27 undergoing revision RSA. The HA group showed outcomes of mean FF 68.7 degrees and ER 9.2 degrees. Minimal net improvement of FF was gained postoperatively with a reduction in ER noted. CMS was 37.1 with a net improvement of 13.8 points preoperatively. When assessing the pain component of CMS, minimal improvement was shown [9]. The authors highlight poor clinical improvements with HA in comparison to conservative management or revision RSA, but they admit that the treatment choices were obviously not random and that the HA group had poor baseline clinical scores prior to revision.

From a large prospective database (1237 RSAs), a study in Switzerland showed that 1.7% of RSA over a 13-year period starting in 2005 were converted to HA at a mean time of 20 months from index procedure. Of these patients, 12 were available for outcome assessment at a minimum of 2 years after HA. These patients had significant improvements in pain levels but poor function. The average FF was 55, ER was 13, and CMS was 33. The mean follow-up period was 46 months. This study also compared HA to RSA-preserving surgery and highlighted poorer functional outcomes with HA [10].

There is minimal information available in the published literature to inform on different implant choices in HA after RSA. Megahead cuff tear arthropathy prosthesis may have a role in this scenario with the potential advantage of a large lateral extension, allowing for good gliding underneath the acromial arch [3]. This is contraindicated in any compromise to acromial stability, such as significant thinning of acromial bone, fracture, or os acromiale. There is no clear evidence to support megahead prostheses over standard HA.

Drawing any meaningful conclusions from comparisons to other treatment options including revision RSA or indeed RA is very difficult as the evidence is heavily influenced by selection bias. As with patients chosen for RA, patients undergoing HA are likely to have more significant complications and bone loss with poorer baseline function and in many cases worse comorbid fitness than patients in whom revision RSA is considered. The limited level III/IV evidence does suggest that HA after RSA may reduce pain but has significant functional impairment and potentially high rate of radiological complications, such as anterosuperior escape.

While it makes good sense and is widely accepted by many authors that all attempts should be made to preserve shoulder function with a revision RSA in cases of glenoid loosening [2], high-level evidence, such as a randomized controlled trial comparing HA to revision RSA, is now not ethically viable due to the differences in reported outcomes. Preservation of shoulder function following revision RSA has been reported in 90% of cases [2]. However, it should be remembered that revision RSA is a technically demanding procedure with potentially high complication and re-intervention rates. In 2015, *Black* et al reported a major complication rate of 56% and reoperation rate of 38% [14]. With evolving understanding, techniques, experience, and equipment, this will likely fall, but it emphasizes that in patients where further reintervention would be a highly undesirable potential outcome, HA and indeed RA can be an option at the expense of shoulder function. HA, in theory, has the advantage over RA that the implant has some positive effect as a spacer to improve stability and potentially achieve moderate function [13], but there is very little evidence to support any functional difference between RA and HA in this scenario. HA may increase future re-revision options by maintaining an effective joint space but may have a higher risk of future undesirable reintervention compared to RA for pain, infection, or prosthesis migration, for example.

33.4 Summary

Patients in the unfortunate scenario of facing salvage RSA surgery should be counselled at length that outcomes will likely result in FF below 90 degrees with minimal rotational range of motion and that the limited goals are pain relief and reducing chances of further surgery. For the reasons mentioned above, use of HA including cement spacers may give increased options in the future of re-revision to RSA, and in suitable patients, this may be worth discussing and planning for this as opposed to RA.

References

1. Cronin KJ, Hayes CB, Sajadi KR. Antibiotic cement spacer retention for chronic shoulder infection after minimum 2-year follow-up. J Shoulder Elb Surg. 2020;29(9):e325–9. https://doi.org/10.1016/j.jse.2020.01.065.
2. Boileau P. Complications and revision of reverse total shoulder arthroplasty. Orthop Traumatol Surg Res. 2016;102(1 Suppl):S33–43. https://doi.org/10.1016/j.otsr.2015.06.031.
3. Casier S, Middernacht B, Van Tongel A, De Wilde L. Revision of reversed shoulder arthroplasty: is a reoperation possible? Obere Extrem. 2017;12(1):16–24. https://doi.org/10.1007/s11678-017-0400-x.
4. Muh SJ, Streit JJ, Lenarz CJ, McCrum C, Wanner JP, Shishani Y, et al. Resection arthroplasty for failed shoulder arthroplasty. J Shoulder Elb Surg. 2013;22(2):247–52. https://doi.org/10.1016/j.jse.2012.05.025.
5. Rispoli DM, Sperling JW, Athwal GS, Schleck CD, Cofield RH. Pain relief and functional results after resection arthroplasty of the shoulder. J Bone Joint Surg Br. 2007;89(9):1184–7. https://doi.org/10.1302/0301-620X.89B9.19464.
6. Ghijselings S, Stuyck J, Debeer P. Surgical treatment algorithm for infected shoulder arthroplasty: a retrospective analysis of 17 cases. Acta Orthop Belg. 2013;79(6):626–35.

7. Stevens NM, Kim HM, Armstrong AD. Functional outcomes after shoulder resection: the patient's perspective. J Shoulder Elb Surg. 2015;24(9):e247–54. https://doi.org/10.1016/j.jse.2015.03.027.
8. Jacquot A, Sirveaux F, Roche O, Favard L, Clavert P, Molé D. Surgical management of the infected reversed shoulder arthroplasty: a French multicenter study of reoperation in 32 patients. J Shoulder Elb Surg. 2015;24(11):1713–22. https://doi.org/10.1016/j.jse.2015.03.007.
9. Lädermann A, Schwitzguebel AJ, Edwards TB, Godeneche A, Favard L, Walch G, Sirveaux F, Boileau P, Gerber C. Glenoid loosening and migration in reverse shoulder arthroplasty. Bone Joint J. 2019;101-B(4):461–9. https://doi.org/10.1302/0301-620X.101B4.BJJ-2018-1275.R1.
10. Kriechling P, Andronic O, Wieser K. Hemiarthroplasty as a salvage treatment for failed reverse total shoulder arthroplasty. JSES Int. 2021;5(6):1055–61. https://doi.org/10.1016/j.jseint.2021.07.003.
11. Wieser K, Borbas P, Ek ET, Meyer DC, Gerber C. Conversion of stemmed hemi- or total to reverse total shoulder arthroplasty: advantages of a modular stem design. Clin Orthop Relat Res. 2015;473(2):651–60. https://doi.org/10.1007/s11999-014-3985-z.
12. Gamradt SC, Gelber J, Zhang AL. Shoulder function and pain level after revision of failed reverse shoulder replacement to hemiarthroplasty. Int J Shoulder Surg. 2012;6(2):29–35. https://doi.org/10.4103/0973-6042.96991.
13. Glanzmann MC, Kolling C, Schwyzer HK, Audigé L. Conversion to hemiarthroplasty as a salvage procedure for failed reverse shoulder arthroplasty. J Shoulder Elb Surg. 2016;25(11):1795–802. https://doi.org/10.1016/j.jse.2016.03.011.
14. Black EM, Roberts SM, Siegel E, Yannopoulos P, Higgins LD, Warner JJ. Failure after reverse total shoulder arthroplasty: what is the success of component revision? J Shoulder Elb Surg. 2015;24(12):1908–14. https://doi.org/10.1016/j.jse.2015.05.029.

The Role of Hemireverse in Revision Shoulder Arthroplasty

34

Arnaud Walch and Gilles Walch

34.1 Introduction

In the setting of failed shoulder arthroplasty with associated severe glenoid bone loss, revision reconstructive procedures provide several challenges, including bone grafting, questionable remaining glenoid bone stock, implant selection, and intraoperative assessment of acceptable implant stability.

In the setting of extreme glenoid vault deficiency, the major concern is insufficient bone for acceptable stability of the reverse arthroplasty baseplate [1–6], which if present may result in medialization and/or implant migration [7, 8].

34.2 History and Concept

The first hemireverse was performed during a revision total shoulder arthroplasty (TSA) to a planned reverse shoulder arthroplasty (RSA) in a young active male. After implanting the baseplate with an iliac crest bone graft (ICBG) and the glenosphere, the stability of the construct was insufficient to load it with the humeral component. The decision was taken to let the baseplate and glenosphere implanted without any humeral component and to perform another surgery when the bone graft would be healed and the baseplate would be stable enough to implant a humeral component. The patient was totalized to a RSA 6 months after the hemireverse surgery.

Therefore, the concept of the hemireverse is to implant only the glenoid baseplate and glenosphere (Fig. 34.1). This allows reconstructing glenoid bone loss with bone graft, protects the bone graft while it heals, and preserves the joint volume.

A. Walch (✉)
Hôpital Edouard Herriot, Lyon, France

G. Walch
Centre Orthopédique Santy, Lyon, France

F. Franceschi et al. (eds.), *Revision Shoulder Arthroplasty*,
https://doi.org/10.1007/978-3-031-45944-3_34

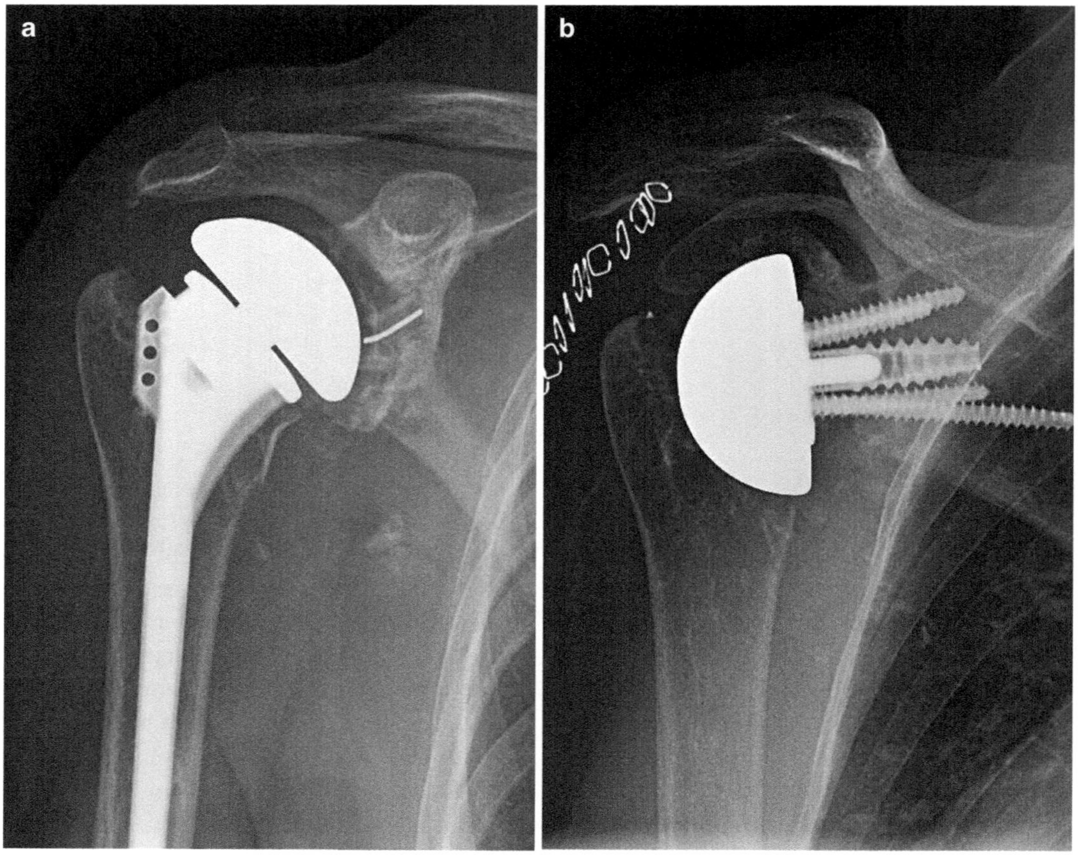

Fig. 34.1 Hemireverse. (**a**) Glenoid loosening after anatomic total shoulder arthroplasty, with subsidence of glenoid component. (**b**) Postoperative radiograph after hemireverse procedure with morseled cancellous iliac crest bone graft. Restoration of a normal joint line with respect to the coracoid process

34.3 Indications

The hemireverse is indicated in revision shoulder arthroplasties when glenoid component stability is deemed insufficient to support a total RSA with the accompanying soft tissue tension. Presently, the literature would recommend a minimum of 10 mm of anchorage in the native bone to predictably provide stability and construct healing [9, 10], but no definitive biomechanical or clinical literature is available regarding the minimal amount of central post depth in host bone. In our experience, it is reasonable to be prepared to perform a hemireverse when the remaining vault thickness is inferior to 5 mm on the preoperative radiographs or computed tomography (CT) scan (Fig. 34.2). The measurements of the remaining vault thickness should be cautious on the CT scan because the CT slices are not always perpendicular to the joint line. Additionally, the maximum bone present is often in the direction of the scapular spine, which is oblique superiorly and posteriorly, and not always in the plane of the CT slices.

The hemireverse has to be used as a salvage procedure: if during the revision surgery the baseplate is stable enough, we recommend to perform a standard RSA.

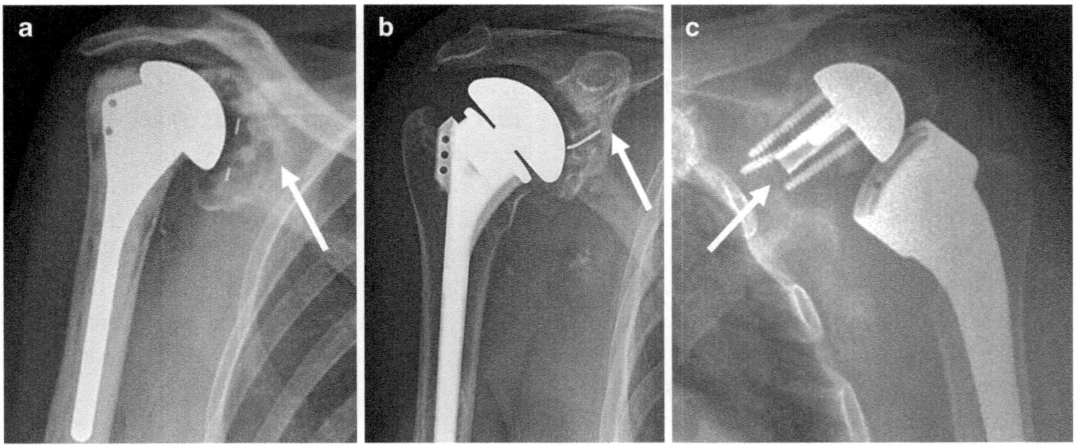

Fig. 34.2 (**a**, **b**) Glenoid loosening after failed anatomic total shoulder arthroplasty with subsidence and migration of glenoid component. (**c**) Glenoid loosening after failed reverse shoulder arthroplasty with a structural iliac crest bone graft. The remaining glenoid bone stock was insufficient to provide a good anchorage of the baseplate. The remaining glenoid vault (white arrows) was inferior to 5 mm in all cases

34.4 Surgical Technique

We describe our current installation, exposure, graft and implant selection, and rehabilitation. These are the steps of a standard revision TSA to RSA.

34.4.1 Installation and Preparation of the Joint

The patient is placed in the beach chair position. We use a deltopectoral approach. The subscapularis, when present, is peeled-off or tenotomized. The humeral component is removed carefully to avoid an iatrogenic greater tuberosity fracture. During revision, intraoperative cultures are taken to rule out infection.

The glenoid is then exposed with the appropriate releases and debridement of fibrotic tissue. The loosen component is carefully removed along with cement. The degree of medialization of the joint line with respect to the base of the coracoid process and the remaining peripheral bone is assessed before advancing a guide pin for central post or screw fixation. In order to find the greatest depth of bone for implant fixation, a 2-mm nonthreaded pin is used to sound the thickness of the remaining vault. Whereas this spot is typically central or inferior for primary RSA, in case of severe glenoid erosion, it is typically more superior and more anteverted within the scapular spine [11]. Glenoid bone grafting is conducted according to each surgeon's preference. When a tricortical ICBG is used, we recommend to perform the Norris technique [12]. During baseplate insertion, screw tightening, and glenosphere implantation, the subjective stability of the glenoid implant is continually assessed by the surgeon. If the construct lacks stability, then a hemireverse is performed. On the other hand, if the construct appears to be stable, then the humeral implant should be inserted.

We recommend not to ream the humerus to accommodate the glenosphere into the humeral metaphysis, so it does not fragilize the humerus and greater tuberosity (GT) and preserve bone stock in case of a further totalization. When a GT fracture occurs, internal fixation is performed with cerclage sutures. To maximize joint stability, whenever possible, the subscapularis is repaired to the lesser tuberosity utilizing transosseous nonabsorbable sutures.

34.4.2 Postoperative Protocol

Rehabilitation is similar to a revision shoulder arthroplasty protocol. This consists of 6 weeks with a sling with early pendulum exercises and active motion of elbow and hand. After 6 weeks, active assisted motion progressing to active motion is started with strengthening at 3 months.

34.4.3 Totalization to RSA

The minimum delay before second-stage revision should be of 6 months to allow for healing and graft incorporation and to ensure sufficient stability to the baseplate. Although we recommend a minimum duration before second stage, there is no maximum delay to proceed to second-stage revision to total RSA. Before totalization, graft healing and glenoid implant stability are carefully assessed on radiographs showing no migration nor loosening of the baseplate and the absence of screw breakage.

The second-stage surgery is performed in a similar fashion through the same deltopectoral incision without any additional procedure on the glenoid side. The stability of the glenoid implant is tested manually during the surgery to assess for any micromotion. The humeral implant is cemented in the previous cement mantle when present without initiative to remove all the cement [13].

34.5 Results

We report the results of a series of 15 hemireverses [14]. Nine patients were women, and 6 dominant sides were involved. The median age at the time of revision to hemireverse was 66 years (interquartile range, 64–74 years). The median number of previous surgeries was 2 (IQR, 1–3).

Reasons for revision included 8 failed anatomic total shoulder arthroplasty (TSA) due to aseptic glenoid loosening, 3 failed RSA due to glenoid component loosening, 3 failed humeral hemiarthroplasties (HHA) (2 due to severe glenoid erosion after previous loose glenoid component removal and 1 primary HHA with secondary rotator cuff tear and severe glenoid erosion), and 1 patient with a cement spacer due to sepsis after a TSA. No patients had any signs of clinical or biological infection at the time of revision to hemireverse.

The glenoid defects were assessed using radiographs, CT scan when available, and intraoperative surgical reports. The types of glenoid bone defects were classified as "combined severe" in all cases. The median remaining thickness of the glenoid vault measured before the revision was 2 mm (IQR, 2–3 mm).

Seven GT fractures occurred during stem extraction and were internally fixed with cerclage sutures. The grafts chosen were 8 tricortical iliac crest bone graft (ICBG), 4 cancellous morcellized ICBG, 2 mixed allograft (structural femoral head and cancellous allograft), and 1 cancellous allograft.

34.5.1 Patients Totalized to RSA

Five patients underwent second-stage revision to total RSA with insertion of a humeral component at a median of 6 months (IQR, 6–8 months). The median follow-up in this group was 73 months (IQR, 45–153 months) after second-stage total RSA (Fig. 34.3). After totalization to RSA, the median anterior forward elevation (AFE) was 135° (IQR, 100°–150°), the median Constant score was 48 points (IQR, 41–56), and the median subjective shoulder value (SSV) was 50% (IQR, 50%–60%). Statistical comparison of the functional results before hemireverse and after totalization to RSA showed a statistically better results for AFE (p = 0.017), Constant score (p = 0.009), pain score (p = 0.002), ADL (p = 0.004), and mobility (p = 0.028).

One patient who underwent total RSA 9 months after hemireverse was further revised 3 years later because of progressive superior migration of the baseplate. The baseplate loosening in this case was attributed to the short post, with absent anchorage in the native glenoid vault. At the time of revision, an extended postbaseplate with anchorage into native glenoid vault was utilized with cancellous morcellized ICBG. At 8-year follow-up after subsequent revision, the baseplate was stable, and the patient had a SSV of 50% and was satisfied.

The sole GT fracture that occurred in this group healed uneventfully. Radiographic examination of the remaining total RSA cases demonstrated no implant failure or migration.

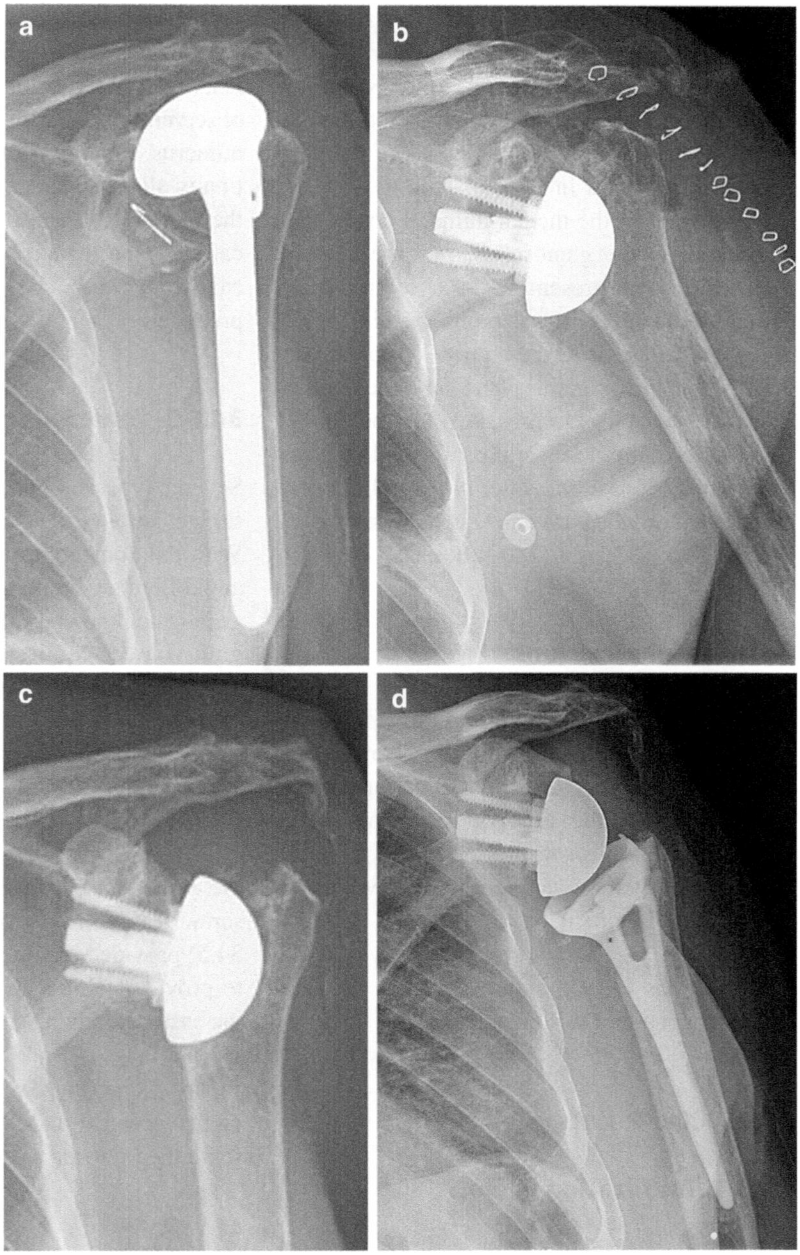

Fig. 34.3 (**a**) Glenoid loosening after anatomic total shoulder arthroplasty, with medialization and superior tilt of loose glenoid. (**b**) Immediate postoperative radiograph showing hemi-reverse implant with morseled cancellous iliac crest bone graft. The graft is 10 mm thick, restoration of a normal joint line. The intraoperative stability of the glenosphere was not strong enough to load the reconstruction with the humeral stem. (**c**) Ten months later, the bone graft healed and there was no instance of graft failure. On the humeral side, there was subsidence of the glenosphere into the humerus with thinning of the greater tuberosity. (**d**) A cemented Aequalis Fracture stem was implanted. A control radiograph at 2 years postoperatively showed no loosening and no notching (Reprinted from Walch A, Edwards BT, Kilian CM, Boileau P, Walch G, Athwal GS. Hemireverse Revision Arthroplasty in the Setting of Severe Glenoid Bone Loss. J Shoulder Elbow Surg. 2022, with permission from Elsevier)

34.5.2 Patients Remained as Hemireverse

Nine patients remained as hemireverse. One patient was unsatisfied with the hemireverse but was too frail for second-stage total RSA. The eight remaining patients were all planned for second-stage total RSA; however, all elected to keep their hemireverse as they were satisfied with the outcome. The median follow-up in this group was 38 months (IQR, 29–60 months), the median AFE was 100° (IQR, 80°–100°), the median Constant score was 41 (IQR, 38–46), and the median SSV was 50% (IQR, 40%–60%). Statistical comparison of the preoperative and postoperative functional results showed a better Constant score ($p = 0.028$), pain score ($p = 0.008$), and ADL ($p = 0.041$). However, with the number available, the comparison of the results between the total RSA group and the hemireverse group did not shown any statistical difference.

Radiographic examinations at the last follow-up demonstrated no glenoid implant failure or migration. Partial inferior osteolysis of the bone graft was observed in 33% of the cases. Slight humeral wear of the medial humeral cortex with subsidence of the glenosphere into the humeral metaphysis was present in 55% of the cases. Thinning of the GT was also observed in 55% of the cases. Sclerosis of the humeral articular contact area with the glenosphere and acetabulization was noted in all cases. Among the six GT fractures present in this group, 5 healed uneventfully while the last one, after structural allograft reconstruction, had complete osteolysis of the GT and superior part of the humerus.

34.5.3 Complications

One patient developed postoperative implant-related infection and had the hemireverse removed 7 months after implantation of the hemireverse. At the time of explantation, the patient had complete resorption of the graft and underwent irrigation and debridement with antibiotic bead placement.

However, we did not observe any specific complications to the hemireverse such as instability or secondary GT fractures.

34.6 Key Points

34.6.1 Totalization or Not?

The decision for totalization or not depends on a case-by-case discussion between the surgeon and the patient. In our experience, the indications for totalization were the incomplete function and pain control or the subjective sensation of instability (Fig. 34.3). Some patients were planned for second-stage total RSA but elected to keep their hemireverse as they were satisfied with the outcome (Figs. 34.4 and 34.5). Although this group is statistically better than their preoperative status regarding Constant score (22 vs 41, $p = 0.028$), pain relief (4 vs 12, $p = 0.008$), and ADL (5 vs 14, $p = 0.041$), their median AFE is not as good as RSA (100° vs 135°, $p = 0.120$). Additionally, we observed cases with secondary wear of the humerus, thinning of the greater tuberosity, and finally slight subsidence of the glenosphere into the humerus. Because of these suboptimal clinical and radiological results, hemireverse should cautiously be considered as a definitive procedure.

34.6.2 Graft Selection

Several types of bone grafts were used in our series: autograft, allograft, or a mix of those. With the numbers available, we did not observe any difference in the rate of healing. As the ideal graft is not known [4, 15–18], the selection of the graft source requires a case-by-case discussion based on the surgeon's experience and graft availability.

34.6.3 Implant Selection

We do not have preferences as the style of central screw (Fig. 34.1) or post (Figs. 34.3, 34.4, and 34.5) provided that the native glenoid is engaged to provide stability to the construct. The size of the baseplate should accommodate to the patient's morphology.

The glenosphere should be the largest and the more eccentric and lateralized possible to preserve the joint space.

34.6.4 Lateralization

Glenoid lateralization is an important parameter in RSA [19, 20]; however, the magnitude of lateralization in the setting of a revision with compromised glenoid bone stock is unknown. Although there is no definitive amount, our series of hemireverse demonstrated that aiming to restore a normal joint line with respect to the coracoid process did not jeopardize stability and healing of the reconstruction (Fig. 34.1). If no glenoid

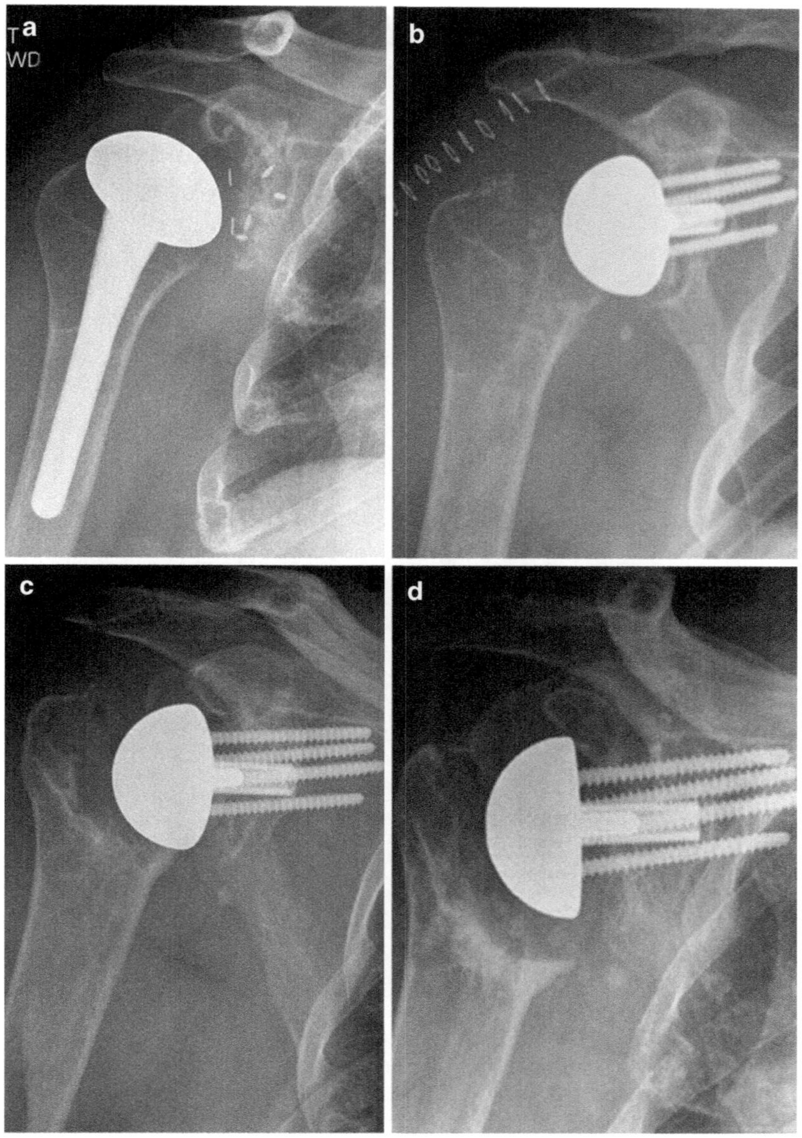

Fig. 34.4 (**a**) Failed anatomic total shoulder arthroplasty for instability arthropathy: glenoid loosening. (**b**) Postoperative radiograph after hemi-reverse procedure with tricortical iliac crest bone graft (Norris technique [12]). (**c**, **d**) The 2- and 5-year postoperative control radiographs showed inferior osteolysis of the graft but no instance of implant loosening. There was progressive thinning of the greater tuberosity, subsidence of the glenosphere into the humerus, and densification and acetabulization of the humerus at the glenosphere contact (Reprinted from Walch A, Edwards BT, Kilian CM, Boileau P, Walch G, Athwal GS. Hemireverse Revision Arthroplasty in the Setting of Severe Glenoid Bone Loss. J Shoulder Elbow Surg. 2022, with permission from Elsevier)

landmarks remain for the determination of the native joint line, we recommend lateralization of the baseplate at least 10 mm and ideally 15 mm with respect to the thin remaining vault (Figs. 34.3 and 34.5).

34.6.5 GT Fracture

Fractures of the humerus are reported to be a frequent intraoperative complication of revision shoulder arthroplasty [13, 21–24], and they greatly influence clinical and radiological results [24]. In our series, we observed a 47% rate of greater tuberosity fractures that occurred during humeral stem extraction. Six out of seven GT fractures healed despite the glenosphere resting in contact with the humeral metaphysis and GT. The hemireverse concept may allow healing of the GT by decreasing the mechanical traction exerted by arm and deltoid lengthening. Therefore, our series suggest that hemireverse could also be an option in case of intraoperative GT fracture in the setting of revision arthroplasty to achieve healing without excessive tension.

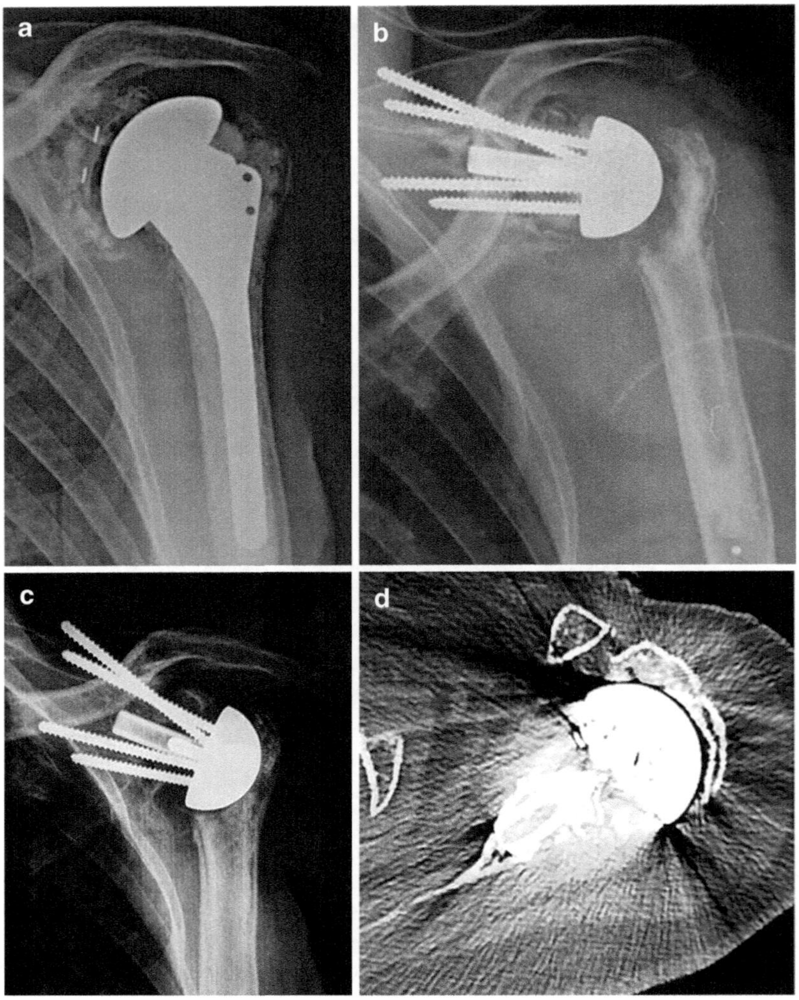

Fig. 34.5 (**a**) Glenoid loosening after anatomic total shoulder arthroplasty with subsidence of glenoid component. (**b**) Postoperative radiograph after hemi-reverse procedure with tricortical iliac crest bone graft (Norris technique [12]). The graft is 12 mm thick, restoration of a normal joint line. (**c**, **d**) The 5-year postoperative control radiograph and computed tomography scan (the patient continued to forego the totalization procedure) showed that the graft was healed with inferior osteolysis. There was thinning of the greater tuberosity and slight subsidence of the glenosphere into the worn humerus (Reprinted from Walch A, Edwards BT, Kilian CM, Boileau P, Walch G, Athwal GS. Hemireverse Revision Arthroplasty in the Setting of Severe Glenoid Bone Loss. J Shoulder Elbow Surg. 2022, with permission from Elsevier)

34.6.6 Humeral Wear

Progressive erosion of the humerus in contact with the metallic glenosphere is similar to glenoid erosion in humeral head replacement and acromial acetabularization in massive rotator cuff tears (Figs. 34.3, 34.4, and 34.5). In cases where the patient elects to maintain the hemireverse as the definitive procedure, we recommend routine radiographic assessment to monitor for bone erosion and subsidence. However, we do not recommend a totalization based only on these radiological features.

34.7 Conclusion

Hemireverse is a relatively safe and effective intermediate salvage procedure to restore glenoid bone stock: it protects the bone graft and preserves the joint space. In revision scenarios with severe glenoid bone deficiency, the rate of bone graft healing was high (86%). Second-stage revision to total reverse arthroplasty leads to satisfactory clinical outcomes. For the patients who elect hemireverse as the definitive procedure, modest improvements in pain and function are observed, however, with adaptative bone changes to the humerus.

References

1. Ho JC, Thakar O, Chan WW, Nicholson T, Williams GR, Namdari S. Early radiographic failure of reverse total shoulder arthroplasty with structural bone graft for glenoid bone loss. J Shoulder Elb Surg. 2020;29(3):550–60. https://doi.org/10.1016/j.jse.2019.07.035.
2. Klein SM, Dunning P, Mulieri P, Pupello D, Downes K, Frankle MA. Effects of acquired glenoid bone defects on surgical technique and clinical outcomes in reverse shoulder arthroplasty. J Bone Joint Surg Am. 2010;92(5):1144–54. https://doi.org/10.2106/jbjs.i.00778.
3. Knowles NK, Columbus MP, Wegmann K, Ferreira LM, Athwal GS. Revision shoulder arthroplasty: a systematic review and comparison of north American vs. European outcomes and complications. J Shoulder Elb Surg. 2020;29(5):1071–82. https://doi.org/10.1016/j.jse.2019.12.015.
4. Mahylis JM, Puzzitiello RN, Ho JC, Amini MH, Iannotti JP, Ricchetti ET. Comparison of radiographic and clinical outcomes of revision reverse total shoulder arthroplasty with structural versus nonstructural bone graft. J Shoulder Elb Surg. 2019;28(1):e1–9. https://doi.org/10.1016/j.jse.2018.06.026.
5. Melis B, Bonnevialle N, Neyton L, Lévigne C, Favard L, Walch G, et al. Glenoid loosening and failure in anatomical total shoulder arthroplasty: is revision with a reverse shoulder arthroplasty a reliable option? J Shoulder Elb Surg. 2012;21(3):342–9. https://doi.org/10.1016/j.jse.2011.05.021.
6. Walker M, Willis MP, Brooks JP, Pupello D, Mulieri PJ, Frankle MA. The use of the reverse shoulder arthroplasty for treatment of failed total shoulder arthroplasty. J Shoulder Elb Surg. 2012;21(4):514–22. https://doi.org/10.1016/j.jse.2011.03.006.
7. Boileau P, Morin-Salvo N, Bessière C, Chelli M, Gauci M-O, Lemmex DB. Bony increased-offset-reverse shoulder arthroplasty: 5 to 10 years' follow-up. J Shoulder Elb Surg. 2020;29(10):2111–22. https://doi.org/10.1016/j.jse.2020.02.008.
8. Favre P, Sussmann PS, Gerber C. The effect of component positioning on intrinsic stability of the reverse shoulder arthroplasty. J Shoulder Elb Surg. 2010;19(4):550–6. https://doi.org/10.1016/j.jse.2009.11.044.
9. Singh J, Odak S, Neelakandan K, Walton MJ, Monga P, Bale S, et al. Survivorship of autologous structural bone graft at a minimum of 2 years when used to address significant glenoid bone loss in primary and revision shoulder arthroplasty: a computed tomographic and clinical review. J Shoulder Elb Surg. 2021;30(3):668–78. https://doi.org/10.1016/j.jse.2020.06.015.
10. Werner BS, Böhm D, Abdelkawi A, Gohlke F. Glenoid bone grafting in reverse shoulder arthroplasty for long-standing anterior shoulder dislocation. J Shoulder Elb Surg. 2014;23(11):1655–61. https://doi.org/10.1016/j.jse.2014.02.017.
11. Frankle MA, Teramoto A, Luo Z-P, Levy JC, Pupello D. Glenoid morphology in reverse shoulder arthroplasty: classification and surgical implications. J Shoulder Elb Surg. 2009;18(6):874–85. https://doi.org/10.1016/j.jse.2009.02.013.
12. Norris TR, Kelly JD, Humphrey CS. Management of Glenoid Bone Defects in revision shoulder arthroplasty. Tech Should Elbow Surg. 2007;8(1):37–46. https://doi.org/10.1097/bte.0b013e318030d3b7.
13. Wagner E, Houdek MT, Hernandez NM, Cofield RH, Sanchez-Sotelo J, Sperling JW. Cement-within-cement technique in revision reverse shoulder arthroplasty. J Shoulder Elb Surg. 2017;26(8):1448–53. https://doi.org/10.1016/j.jse.2017.01.013.
14. Walch A, Edwards BT, Kilian CM, Boileau P, Walch G, Athwal GS. Hemireverse revision arthroplasty in the setting of severe glenoid bone loss. J Shoulder Elb Surg. 2022;31:1859. https://doi.org/10.1016/j.jse.2022.02.018.
15. Jones RB, Wright TW, Zuckerman JD. Reverse total shoulder arthroplasty with structural bone grafting of large glenoid defects. J Shoulder Elb Surg. 2016;25(9):1425–32. https://doi.org/10.1016/j.jse.2016.01.016.
16. Tashjian RZ, Broschinsky K, Stertz I, Chalmers PN. Structural glenoid allograft reconstruction during reverse total shoulder arthroplasty. J Shoulder Elb Surg. 2020;29(3):534–40. https://doi.org/10.1016/j.jse.2019.07.011.
17. Taylor JR, Schrumpf MA, Shea KE, Kelly JD. Distal clavicle autograft augmentation for glenoid bone loss in revision shoulder arthroplasty: results and technique. J Shoulder Elb Surg. 2020;29(10):e386–e93. https://doi.org/10.1016/j.jse.2020.05.009.
18. Wagner E, Houdek MT, Griffith T, Elhassan BT, Sanchez-Sotelo J, Sperling JW, et al. Glenoid bone-grafting in revision to a reverse Total shoulder arthroplasty. J Bone Joint Surg Am. 2015;97(20):1653–60. https://doi.org/10.2106/jbjs.n.00732.

19. Helmkamp JK, Bullock GS, Amilo NR, Guerrero EM, Ledbetter LS, Sell TC, et al. The clinical and radiographic impact of center of rotation lateralization in reverse shoulder arthroplasty: a systematic review. J Shoulder Elb Surg. 2018;27(11):2099–107. https://doi.org/10.1016/j.jse.2018.07.007.
20. Katz D, Valenti P, Kany J, Elkholti K, Werthel JD. Does lateralisation of the Centre of rotation in reverse shoulder arthroplasty avoid scapular notching? Clinical and radiological review of one hundred and forty cases with forty five months of follow-up. Int Orthop (SICOT). 2016;40(1):99–108. https://doi.org/10.1007/s00264-015-2976-3.
21. Dilisio MF, Miller LR, Siegel EJ, Higgins LD. Conversion to reverse shoulder arthroplasty: humeral stem retention versus revision. Orthopedics. 2015;38(9):e773–9. https://doi.org/10.3928/01477447-20150902-54.
22. Favard L. Revision of total shoulder arthroplasty. Orthop Traumatol Surg Res. 2013;99(1 Suppl):S12–21. https://doi.org/10.1016/j.otsr.2012.11.010.
23. Kelly JD, Zhao JX, Hobgood ER, Norris TR. Clinical results of revision shoulder arthroplasty using the reverse prosthesis. J Shoulder Elb Surg. 2012;21(11):1516–25. https://doi.org/10.1016/j.jse.2011.11.021.
24. Zumstein MA, Pinedo M, Old J, Boileau P. Problems, complications, reoperations, and revisions in reverse total shoulder arthroplasty: a systematic review. J Shoulder Elb Surg. 2011;20(1):146–57. https://doi.org/10.1016/j.jse.2010.08.001.

What Is the Value of Revision Shoulder Arthroplasty?

35

Evan K. Stieler, Evan A. O'Donnell, and Jon J. P. Warner

Classically, value is described as a meaningful outcome obtained per unit cost. In other words, Value = Outcome/Cost. Healthcare spending in the United States has grown to an unsustainable level. Part of the problem is failure of critical cost analysis and accounting methods that do not capture true costs. Therefore, value-based cost accounting has been encouraged by some payers [1]. With respect to cost, innovative systems such as capitative methods, diagnosis-related groups, and others are being utilized and studied. Time-driven activity-based costing (TDABC) is a novel approach to quantifying costs in hopes of improving efficiency. While the application of shoulder arthroplasty is growing about 3 times that of hip and knee replacement, so is revision shoulder arthroplasty. While there is a clear value proposition for primary reverse arthroplasty [2, 3], there is little written on this topic for revision shoulder arthroplasty. As such, we propose a triple-tiered approach as a surrogate for the assessment of value:

1. The outcome of the intervention,
2. The recovery arc, and
3. The intervention's durability.

The demand for primary shoulder arthroplasty is increasing and projected to grow [4]. From 2011 to 2017, the incidence of anatomic shoulder arthroplasties (aTSAs) increased by 100% while the incidence of reverse shoulder arthroplasties (rTSAs) increased by 200% [5]. As the incidence of shoulder arthroplasty increases, the number of complications and subsequent revisions will inevitably rise.

Large-registry studies show that revisions for shoulder arthroplasty vary by both indication and procedure. The Australian registry reports an approximate 1% annual revision rate for reverse shoulder arthroplasty (rTSAs), whereas anatomic shoulder arthroplasties (aTSAs) are revised 2% annually (Fig. 35.1) [6].

Kaiser Permanente published a comparative study examining the two-year revision rate between the Australian registry and the Kaiser registry. For all shoulder arthroplasties, the Australian registry and Kaiser registry exhibited two-year revision rates of 5.9% and 1.5%, respectively [7]. Regarding the percentage of TSAs revised after 8 years, the UK registry found a similar rate, 3.9–9.9%, to the Australian registry [8]. The New Zealand Joint Registry study looked at over 8000 primary TSAs from 2000 and 2018 and found its rate of revision to be 4.1% [9]. The

E. K. Stieler
Harvard Orthopaedic Surgery Combined Residency Program, Boston, MA, USA
e-mail: estieler@mgh.harvard.edu

E. A. O'Donnell
Massachusetts General Hospital, Boston, MA, USA
e-mail: eodonnnell4@mgb.org

J. J. P. Warner (✉)
Massachusetts General Hospital Shoulder Service, Boston, MA, USA

F. Franceschi et al. (eds.), *Revision Shoulder Arthroplasty*,
https://doi.org/10.1007/978-3-031-45944-3_35

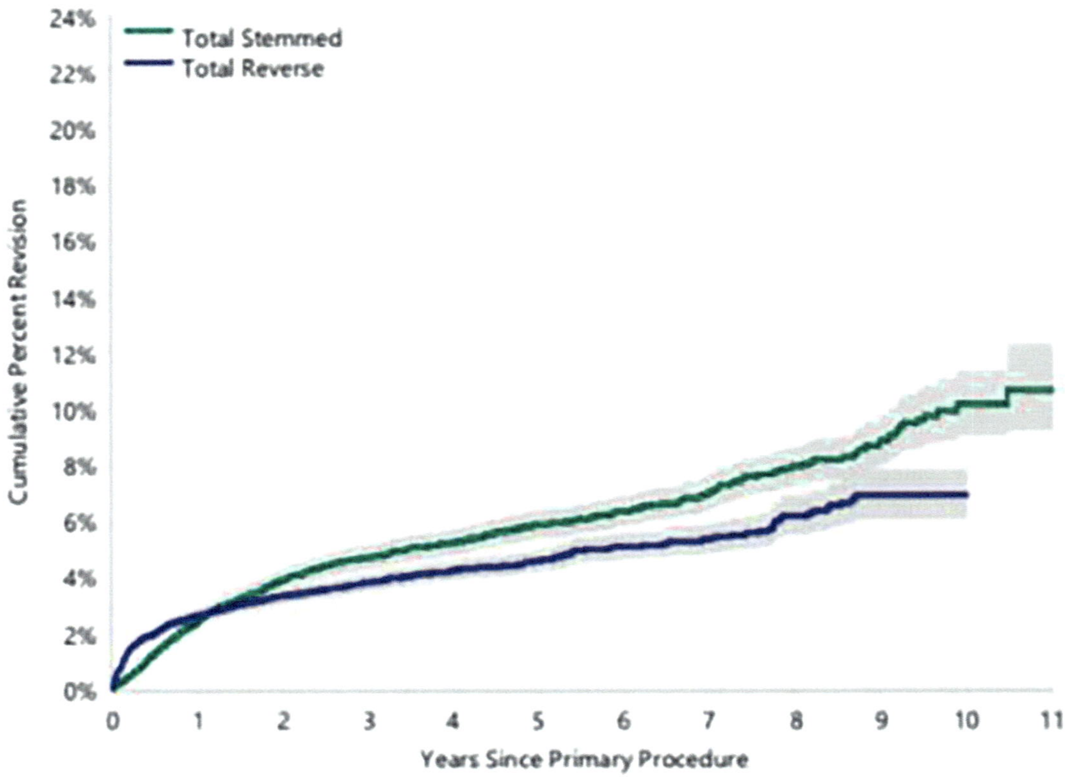

Fig. 35.1 Australian Registry's Cumulative Percent Revision for TSAs [6]

above is significant given that revision shoulder arthroplasty is more expensive, difficult, and associated with poorer patient outcomes [10].

Failure mechanisms differ between aTSA and rTSA. Commonly, aTSAs fail and require revisions for aseptic glenoid loosening, instability, and periprosthetic joint infection (PJI). Aseptic loosening is secondary to inadequate operative fixation, loss of fixation through mechanical wear, soft tissue imbalance, or biological osteolytic loss of fixation. For aTSA, symptomatic aseptic glenoid loosening occurs at rates ranging from 1.2% to 19.3% [11, 12]. Risk factors for PJIs in total shoulder arthroplasties include younger age, male sex, rTSA, and a traumatic indication [13]. The incidence of PJIs after aTSA range from 1% to 3.9% and 1% to 8% after rTSA. There may be a higher incidence of PJIs after rTSA secondary to an increase in dead space and hematoma [14, 15]. There are various forms of instability that can occur postoperatively, and they are caused by glenoid size and version, humeral retroversion and height, humeral head size, soft tissue balancing, and rotator cuff integrity [16]. Infection and instability are the most common causes of rTSA revisions. Scapular notching is commonly associated with rTSA revisions and may negatively impact outcomes, but its clinical significance is debated [17]. Revision TSA consists of great heterogeneity secondary to the aforementioned etiologies and diversity in patients needing the procedure. Operatively, it is challenging because patients have variable scarring, distortion of native tissue planes, reduced bone quality, and various primary implants [10]. Moreover, different prostheses are better suited for revision TSAs depending on the clinical context. Revision TSA procedures involve many variables, and therefore, the cohort who needs them are clinically diverse, and orthopedic surgeons must be flexible in their management.

35.1 Tier 1: Outcome of Revision Shoulder Arthroplasties

Conversion of aTSA to rTSA is one of the more common revision shoulder arthroplasties. A recent meta-analysis of over 5000 revision TSAs showed that rTSAs were used in 67% of cases [10]. rTSA's design addresses prosthetic instability and rotator cuff dysfunction, and therefore, they have become the preferred method in addressing failed anatomic total and hemiarthroplasties. There is a lower risk of further revision surgery in those converted to an rTSA instead of being revised to another aTSA or hemiarthroplasty [18]. Shields and Wiater conducted a matched cohort study that showed the primary and revision rTSA cohorts had similar visual analog score (VAS) and American Shoulder and Elbow Surgeons (ASES) ratings [19]. The revision group, however, had significantly lower subjective shoulder value scores and satisfaction. Moreover, the revision group had a greater rate of complications [19]. Randelli et al. illustrated that revision shoulder arthroplasty can yield a complication rate of 62% and mean revision surgery rate of 27% [20]. Werner et al. reported an 18% revision surgery rate for primary shoulder arthroplasties versus a 38% revision rate in prior revisions [21]. Surgeons discussing conversions to rTSAs should be aware that patients can expect reasonable functional results, although typically inferior to primary rTSAs.

Revision TSA for instability is also common. The incidence of instability after aTSA and rTSA varies, although it has been noted to be 5.2% [22] and 4.7% [23], respectively. Structurally, an rTSA typically fails because of humeral shortening or medialization. The revision options include polyethylene exchange, humeral implant replacement, larger glenosphere implantation, or glenoid implant replacement. The magnitude of shortening and/or medialization influences a surgeon's approach. Revision shoulder arthroplasty for instability has remained a challenging clinical scenario. Outcomes of revision shoulder arthroplasty for instability are inferior to those for primary arthroplasty [7, 10]. Furthermore, studies report as much as 10.1%–22% of revision rTSA procedures will require further revision [23], and unfortunately, half of the revised rTSAs for instability will experience recurrent instability. Although outcomes are inferior to primary rTSA, revision rTSA has been shown to be superior to alternate salvage options [24]. Boileau and colleagues showed that patients retained forward flexion and 89% were satisfied or very satisfied after undergoing a revision rTSA [25]. These data suggest that while revision shoulder arthroplasty for instability has worse outcomes than primary arthroplasty, rTSA remains a reasonable option although with complications and risk of persistent instability.

Periprosthetic joint infections after shoulder arthroplasty are a rare but potentially devastating complication. The incidence of PJIs is 1%–4% in primary shoulder arthroplasty and 4%–15% in revision shoulder arthroplasty [26]. Antibiotic therapy alone is often insufficient with failure rates ranging from 60% to 75% [26], and therefore, these infections often necessitate single or two-staged revision with concurrent antibiosis. The most important risk factors for developing a shoulder PJI are male sex and younger age at initial implantation [27]. Treating a PJI with either single-stage or two-stage revisions has been shown to improve patients' Constant score from 26 preoperatively to 38.3 postoperatively [28]. A recent meta-analysis showed that there was no difference in postoperative flexion and abduction between single-stage and two-stage revision procedures [29]. A 2019 review by Kunutsor et al. demonstrated a recurrent reinfection rate of 16.2% after two-staged revision [30]. Regarding postoperative function after two-staged revisions, Constant scores range improved from 35 to 57, forward elevation ranges from 79 to 118 degrees, and external rotation ranges from 14 to 50 degrees [26]. Failure rates of single-stage revisions, 4%–8.3%, are comparable to those of two-stage revisions, 6%–14% [31]. As described, there is proven benefit in treating PJI, and the choice between single-stage or two-stage revisions depends on various patient and bacterial characteristics.

35.2 Tier 2: Recovery Arc

There has been little effort to chronicle the recovery arc for patients undergoing revision shoulder arthroplasty. Some insight can be gleaned from prior studies—most patients report rapid pain relief, near functional recovery at 6 months after aTSA, and consistent functional improvement 1 year after rTSA [32]. Grubhofer et al. using the pain score showed that 90% and 82% of the total improvement from aTSA and rTSA, respectively, had been accomplished 6 months after the operation [33]. Figure 35.2 illustrates the speed of recovery for aTSA, rTSA, biceps tenodesis, and rotator cuff repair using the SANE score, and Fig. 35.3 illustrates recovery from the same procedures using the ASES [33].

The authors believe that the revision arthroplasty recovery arc is typically slower and with reduced amplitude when compared to the recovery arc of primary shoulder arthroplasty. Older patients should expect to experience greater and longer lasting pain than younger patients [34]. Further research into the recovery arc could create value through more appropriately aligned expectations.

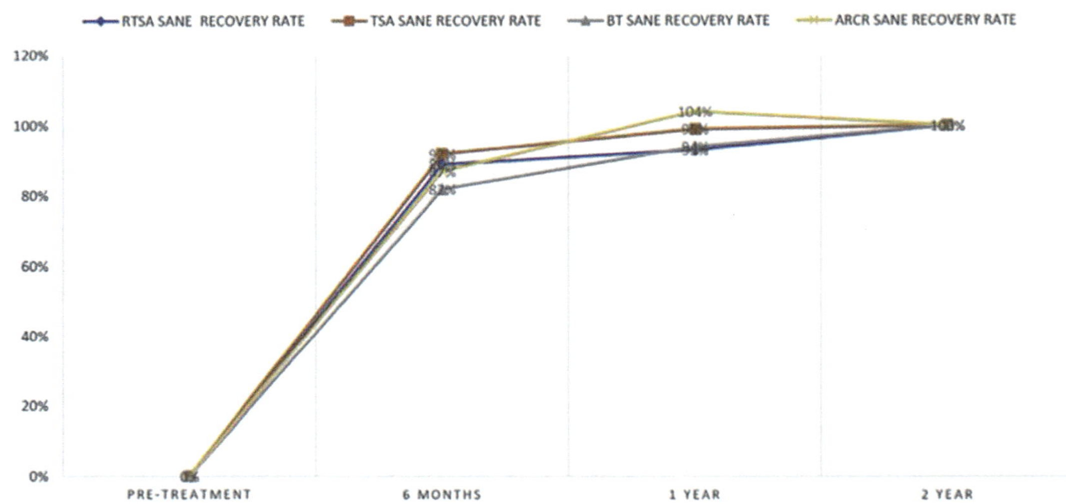

Fig. 35.2 Graphical representation of the speed of SANE recovery for a period of 2 years after shoulder surgery. *SANE* Single Assessment Numeric Evaluation, *rTSA* Reverse total shoulder arthroplasty, *TSA* Total shoulder arthroplasty, *BT* Biceps tenodesis, *ARCR* Arthroscopic rotator cuff repair [33]

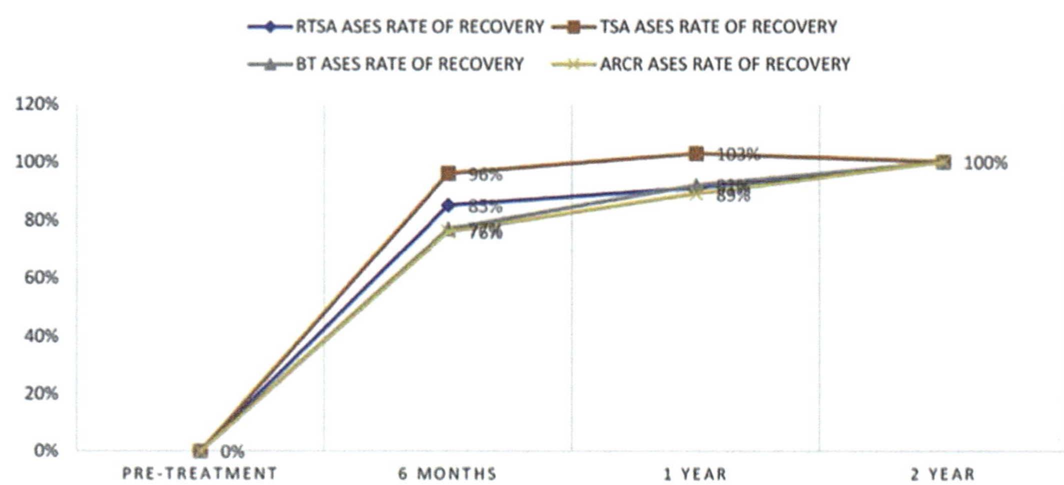

Fig. 35.3 Graphical representation of the speed of ASES recovery for a period of 2 years after shoulder surgery of the four different groups. *ASES* American Shoulder and Elbow Surgeons, *rTSA* Reverse total shoulder arthroplasty, *TSA* Total shoulder arthroplasty, *BT* Biceps tenodesis, *ARCR* Arthroscopic rotator cuff repair [33]

35.3 Tier 3: Durability

The goal of revision arthroplasty is to restore function and provide a lasting solution. Further research needs to be published to further elucidate the survivorship of revision shoulder prostheses. As reported by O'Keefe et al., the rate of re-revision after revision rTSA after 2 years was 13% and increased to 35% at 5 years [18]. Gill et al. found the overall rate of re-revision shoulder arthroplasty to be 13% after 1 year and 24% after 8 years [35]. Complications after revision rTSA remain a significant issue that directly affect durability. Common complications after re-revision surgery include instability, acromion and/or coracoid fracture, infection, and hematoma [36]. The referenced data provide some clarity surrounding revision rTSA survivorship, but larger cohorts and longer follow-up are needed given the high degree of clinical heterogeneity.

35.4 Future Directions

Porter argues that value requires measurement of functional outcomes that patients find truly meaningful. Many studies have used forward elevation, abduction, external rotation, and internal rotation as proxies for functional mobility. These objective measurements are especially useful when compared with preoperative motion. This data alone, however, are insufficient because they do not align with what is most important to patients. Patient-reported outcomes (PROs) are crucial in evaluating the success of a procedure. For revision shoulder arthroplasty, relevant PROs include the previously referenced ASES, Simple Shoulder Test score, and Shoulder Pain and Disability index [5]. Continued improvement is needed in validating and optimizing these measures. Combining functional measures and PROs provides practitioners with the most comprehensive assessment of how patients are progressing toward their goals, aptly describing outcomes in the value equation. Future studies of revision shoulder arthroplasty must include PROs that are meaningful to the patient.

Large-registry data sets are the best way to study the true value of revision arthroplasty. The variation in revision arthroplasty is vast, and studies will only achieve sufficient power if the cohort is large. To date, most PROs measured in revision arthroplasty have featured small cohorts. Large patient sets will allow similar revision indications to be grouped and analyzed further. This would yield a more accurate cost analysis, and subsequently, the true value of revision shoulder arthroplasty could be better known. Moreover, these data sets could exhibit important insights about the recovery process and cost of revision arthroplasty where there is presently a paucity of publications.

35.5 Summary

With healthcare costs continually growing, it is important that orthopedic surgeons can assess the value their interventions are providing. At present, there are few studies that study the value of revision shoulder arthroplasty. Outcomes after revision shoulder arthroplasty show improvement from premorbid states, although the outcomes are guarded. Given the great clinical heterogeneity, few large-cohort studies exist to predict the durability of the outcome or cost. Future large-cohort and registry studies should include the measurement of PROs as well as cost to help delineate the value of revision shoulder arthroplasty.

References

1. Ken Lee KH, Matthew Austin J, Pronovost PJ. Developing a measure of value in health care. Value Heal J Int Soc Pharmacoecon Outcomes Res. 2016;19(4):323–5. https://doi.org/10.1016/j.jval.2014.12.009.
2. Black EM, Roberts SM, Siegel E, Yannopoulos P, Higgins LD, Warner JJP. Reverse shoulder arthroplasty as salvage for failed prior arthroplasty in patients 65 years of age or younger. J Shoulder Elb Surg. 2014;23(7):1036–42. https://doi.org/10.1016/j.jse.2014.02.019.
3. Farley KX, Schwartz AM, Boden SH, Daly CA, Gottschalk MB, Wagner ER. Defining the volume-

outcome relationship in reverse shoulder arthroplasty: a nationwide analysis. J Bone Joint Surg Am. 2020;102(5):388–96. https://doi.org/10.2106/JBJS.19.01012.
4. Schwartz BE, Savin DD, Youderian AR, Mossad D, Goldberg BA. National trends and perioperative outcomes in primary and revision total shoulder arthroplasty: trends in total shoulder arthroplasty. Int Orthop. 2015;39(2):271–6. https://doi.org/10.1007/s00264-014-2614-5.
5. Guy CR, Schoch BS, Frantz R, et al. Revision reverse total shoulder arthroplasty in patients 65 years old and younger: outcome comparison with older patients. JSES Int. 2022;6(2):229–35. https://doi.org/10.1016/j.jseint.2021.11.012.
6. Gill DRJ, Graves SE, Rainbird S, Hatton A. A comparison of revision rates for osteoarthritis of primary reverse total shoulder arthroplasty to primary anatomic shoulder arthroplasty with a cemented all-polyethylene glenoid: analysis from the Australian Orthopaedic Association national joint Repla. Clin Orthop Relat Res. 2021;479(10):2216–24. https://doi.org/10.1097/CORR.0000000000001869.
7. Dillon MT, Page RS, Graves SE, et al. Early revision in anatomic total shoulder arthroplasty in osteoarthritis: a cross-registry comparison. Shoulder Elb. 2020;12(1 Suppl):81–7. https://doi.org/10.1177/1758573219842168.
8. Evans JP, Evans JT, Craig RS, et al. How long does a shoulder replacement last? A systematic review and meta-analysis of case series and national registry reports with more than 10 years of follow-up. Lancet Rheumatol. 2020;2(9):e539–48. https://doi.org/10.1016/S2665-9913(20)30226-5.
9. Mowbray J, Van Niekerk M, Frampton C, Hirner M. The outcomes of shoulder arthroplasty in those aged ≥70 years with glenohumeral arthritis: a New Zealand joint registry study. J Shoulder Elb Surg. 2022;31(4):799–805. https://doi.org/10.1016/j.jse.2021.09.006.
10. Ravi V, Murphy RJ, Moverley R, Derias M, Phadnis J. Outcome and complications following revision shoulder arthroplasty: a systematic review and meta-analysis. Bone Jt open. 2021;2(8):618–30. https://doi.org/10.1302/2633-1462.28.BJO-2021-0092.R1.
11. Papadonikolakis A, Neradilek MB, Matsen FA 3rd. Failure of the glenoid component in anatomic total shoulder arthroplasty: a systematic review of the English-language literature between 2006 and 2012. J Bone Joint Surg Am. 2013;95(24):2205–12. https://doi.org/10.2106/JBJS.L.00552.
12. Neyton L, Kirsch JM, Collotte P, et al. Mid- to long-term follow-up of shoulder arthroplasty for primary glenohumeral osteoarthritis in patients aged 60 or under. J Shoulder Elb Surg. 2019;28(9):1666–73. https://doi.org/10.1016/j.jse.2019.03.006.
13. Richards J, Inacio MCS, Beckett M, et al. Patient and procedure-specific risk factors for deep infection after primary shoulder arthroplasty. Clin Orthop Relat Res. 2014;472(9):2809–15. https://doi.org/10.1007/s11999-014-3696-5.
14. Austin DC, Townsley SH, Rogers TH, et al. Shoulder periprosthetic joint infection and all-cause mortality: a worrisome association. JB JS open access. 2022;7(1) https://doi.org/10.2106/JBJS.OA.21.00118.
15. Namdari S, Sudah SY, Menendez ME, Denard PJ. Antibiotic spacers for shoulder periprosthetic joint infection: a review. J Am Acad Orthop Surg. 2022;30(19):917–24. https://doi.org/10.5435/JAAOS-D-21-00984.
16. Padegimas EM, Zmistowski BM, Restrepo C, et al. Instability after reverse total shoulder arthroplasty: which patients dislocate? Am J Orthop (Belle Mead NJ). 2016;45(7):E444–50.
17. Jang YH, Lee JH, Kim SH. Effect of scapular notching on clinical outcomes after reverse total shoulder arthroplasty. Bone Joint J. 2020;102-B(11):1438–45. https://doi.org/10.1302/0301-620X.102B11.BJJ-2020-0449.R1.
18. O'Keefe DS, Hao KA, Teurlings TL, et al. Survivorship analysis of revision reverse Total shoulder arthroplasty. J Shoulder Elb Surg. 2022;32:e343. https://doi.org/10.1016/j.jse.2022.11.024.
19. Shields E, Wiater JM. Patient outcomes after revision of anatomic Total shoulder arthroplasty to reverse shoulder arthroplasty for rotator cuff failure or component loosening: a matched cohort study. J Am Acad Orthop Surg. 2019;27(4):e193–8. https://doi.org/10.5435/JAAOS-D-17-00350.
20. Randelli P, Randelli F, Compagnoni R, et al. Revision reverse shoulder arthroplasty in failed shoulder arthroplasties for rotator cuff deficiency. Joints. 2015;3(1):31–7.
21. Werner CML, Steinmann PA, Gilbart M, Gerber C. Treatment of painful pseudoparesis due to irreparable rotator cuff dysfunction with the Delta III reverse-ball-and-socket total shoulder prosthesis. J Bone Joint Surg Am. 2005;87(7):1476–86. https://doi.org/10.2106/JBJS.D.02342.
22. Hernandez NM, Chalmers BP, Wagner ER, Sperling JW, Cofield RH, Sanchez-Sotelo J. Revision to reverse Total shoulder arthroplasty restores stability for patients with unstable shoulder prostheses. Clin Orthop Relat Res. 2017;475(11):2716–22. https://doi.org/10.1007/s11999-017-5429-z.
23. Zumstein MA, Pinedo M, Old J, Boileau P. Problems, complications, reoperations, and revisions in reverse total shoulder arthroplasty: a systematic review. J Shoulder Elb Surg. 2011;20(1):146–57. https://doi.org/10.1016/j.jse.2010.08.001.
24. Zhou HS, Chung JS, Yi PH, Li X, Price MD. Management of complications after reverse shoulder arthroplasty. Curr Rev Musculoskelet Med. 2015;8(1):92–7. https://doi.org/10.1007/s12178-014-9252-9.
25. Boileau P. Complications and revision of reverse total shoulder arthroplasty. Orthop Traumatol Surg Res. 2016;102(1 Suppl):S33–43. https://doi.org/10.1016/j.otsr.2015.06.031.
26. Romanò CL, Borens O, Monti L, Meani E, Stuyck J. What treatment for periprosthetic shoulder infection? Results from a multicentre retrospective

series. Int Orthop. 2012;36(5):1011–7. https://doi.org/10.1007/s00264-011-1467-4.
27. Egglestone A, Ingoe H, Rees J, Thomas M, Jeavons R, Rangan A. Scoping review: diagnosis and management of periprosthetic joint infection in shoulder arthroplasty. Shoulder Elb. 2019;11(3):167–81. https://doi.org/10.1177/1758573218779076.
28. Klingebiel S, Theil C, Gosheger G, et al. Clinical outcome of two-stage revision after Periprosthetic shoulder infection. J Clin Med. 2021;10(2) https://doi.org/10.3390/jcm10020218.
29. Mercurio M, Castioni D, Iannò B, Gasparini G, Galasso O. Outcomes of revision surgery after periprosthetic shoulder infection: a systematic review. J Shoulder Elb Surg. 2019;28(6):1193–203. https://doi.org/10.1016/j.jse.2019.02.014.
30. Kunutsor SK, Wylde V, Beswick AD, Whitehouse MR, Blom AW. One- and two-stage surgical revision of infected shoulder prostheses following arthroplasty surgery: A systematic review and meta-analysis. Sci Rep. 2019;9(1):232. https://doi.org/10.1038/s41598-018-36313-3.
31. Paxton ES, Green A, Krueger VS. Periprosthetic infections of the shoulder: diagnosis and management. J Am Acad Orthop Surg. 2019;27(21):e935–44. https://doi.org/10.5435/JAAOS-D-18-00232.
32. Levy JC, Everding NG, Gil CCJ, Stephens S, Giveans MR. Speed of recovery after shoulder arthroplasty: a comparison of reverse and anatomic total shoulder arthroplasty. J Shoulder Elb Surg. 2014;23(12):1872–81. https://doi.org/10.1016/j.jse.2014.04.014.
33. Grubhofer F, Muniz Martinez AR, Ernstbrunner L, et al. Speed of recovery of the most commonly performed shoulder surgeries. JSES Int. 2021;5(4):776–81. https://doi.org/10.1016/j.jseint.2021.03.007.
34. Simon CB, Riley JL 3rd, Coronado RA, et al. Older age as a prognostic factor of attenuated pain recovery after shoulder arthroscopy. PM R. 2016;8(4):297–304. https://doi.org/10.1016/j.pmrj.2015.09.004.
35. Gill DRJ, Page RS, Graves SE, Rainbird S, Hatton A. The rate of 2nd revision for shoulder arthroplasty as analyzed by the Australian Orthopaedic Association National Joint Replacement Registry (AOANJRR). Acta Orthop. 2021;92(3):258–63. https://doi.org/10.1080/17453674.2020.1871559.
36. Tashjian RZ, Granger E, Broschinsky K, Kawakami J, Chalmers PN. Effect of complications on outcomes after revision reverse total shoulder arthroplasty. JSES Int. 2020;4(3):662–8. https://doi.org/10.1016/j.jseint.2020.03.016.

GPSR Compliance

The European Union's (EU) General Product Safety Regulation (GPSR) is a set of rules that requires consumer products to be safe and our obligations to ensure this.

If you have any concerns about our products, you can contact us on ProductSafety@springernature.com

In case Publisher is established outside the EU, the EU authorized representative is:

Springer Nature Customer Service Center GmbH
Europaplatz 3
69115 Heidelberg, Germany

Batch number: 10732799

Printed by Printforce, the Netherlands